T5-CGD-953

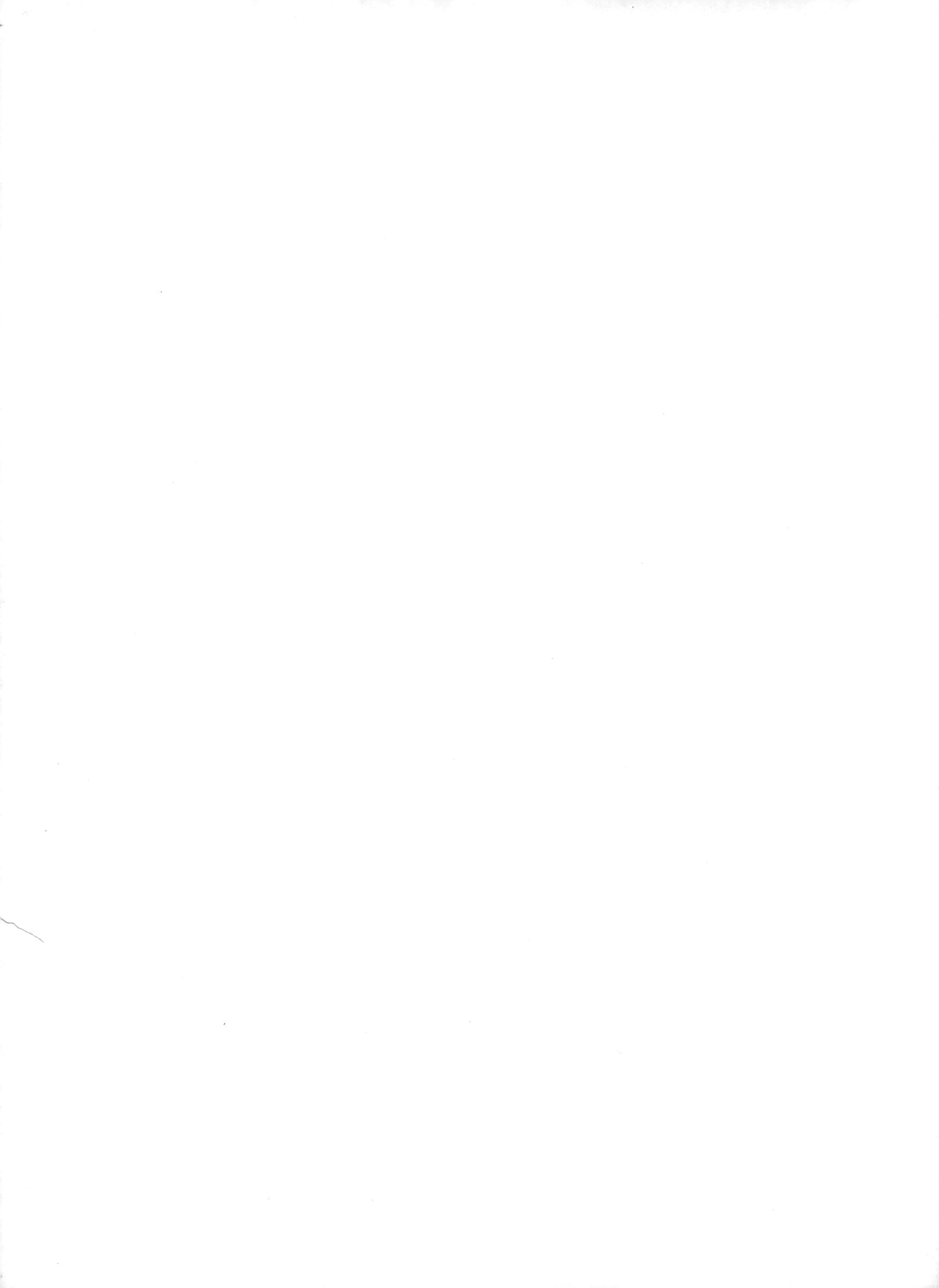

Nutritional Considerations in the Intensive Care Unit

Science, Rationale and Practice

Editors
Scott A. Shikora, M.D., F.A.C.S.
Robert G. Martindale, M.D., Ph.D., F.A.C.S.
Steven D. Schwaitzberg, M.D., F.A.C.S.

American Society for Parenteral
and Enteral Nutrition

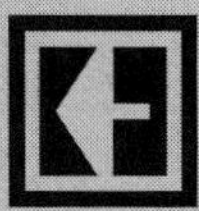

KENDALL/HUNT PUBLISHING COMPANY
4050 Westmark Drive Dubuque, Iowa 52002

Kendall/Hunt Publishing Company Book Team

Chairman and Chief Executive Officer Mark C. Falb
Vice President and Executive Director Emmett Dingley
Professional Education Editor Bridget Hollick
Prepress Editor Charmayne McMurray
Cover Designer Jodi Splinter
Manufacturing Coordinator Tom Mai

A.S.P.E.N. Book Team

Executive Director Robin Kriegel
Director, Marketing and Communications Adrian Nickel
Publications Administrator Carolyn Kohagura

ISBN 0-7872-9072-6

Library of Congress Control Number: 2002100833

Printed in the United States of America
10 9 8 7 6 5 4 3 2 1

Contents

Section 1—Nutritional Derangements and Critical Illness

CHAPTER 1 1
Malnutrition in the Intensive Care Unit
Edward Saltzman, M.D.
Kris M. Mogensen, M.S., R.D.
Paul M. Hassoun, M.D.

CHAPTER 2 11
The Metabolic Response to Stress and Alterations in Nutrient Metabolism
Robert G. Martindale, M.D., Ph.D., F.A.C.S.
Scott A. Shikora, M.D., F.A.C.S.
Reid Nishikawa, Pharm.D., F.C.S.H.P., B.C.N.S.P.
John K. Siepler, Pharm.D., B.C.N.S.P.

CHAPTER 3 21
Nutrition Assessment and Monitoring
Gail A. Cresci, M.S., R.D., L.D., C.N.S.D.

Section 2—Nutritional Support Considerations

CHAPTER 4 31
Estimating Energy Requirements
Carol S. Ireton-Jones, Ph.D., R.D., L.D., C.N.S.D., F.A.C.N.

CHAPTER 5 39
Parenteral Nutrition (Macronutrient Fuels)
David F. Driscoll, Ph.D.
Bruce R. Bistrian, M.D., Ph.D.

CHAPTER 6 51
Micronutrients in Critical Illness
M. Patricia Fuhrman, M.S., R.D., L.D., F.A.D.A., C.N.S.D.
Virginia M. Herrmann, M.D., C.N.S.P.

CHAPTER 7 61
Vitamins and Trace Elements in the Critically Ill Patient
Joel B. Mason, M.D.

CHAPTER 8 79
Assessment and Management of Fluid and Electrolyte Abnormalities
Vincent W. Vanek, M.D., F.A.C.S., C.N.S.P.

CHAPTER 9 101
Assessment and Management of Acid-Base Abnormalities
Vincent W. Vanek, M.D., F.A.C.S., C.N.S.P.

CHAPTER 10 111
Hazards of Overfeeding
Gordon L. Jensen, M.D., Ph.D.
Jeff Binkley, Pharm.D., B.C.N.S.P.

CHAPTER 11 119
Parenteral vs. Enternal Nutrition
Kenneth A. Kudsk, M.D.

CHAPTER 12 131
Intravenous Access for Parenteral Nutrition in the Intensive Care Unit
Dion L. Franga, M.D.

CHAPTER 13 139
Enteral Access—The Foundation of Feeding
William A. Arnold, M.D.
Mark H. DeLegge, M.D., F.A.C.G., C.N.S.P.
Steven D. Schwaitzberg, M.D., F.A.C.S.

CHAPTER 14 153
Drug-Nutrient Interactions
Mary S. McCarthy, R.N., M.N., C.N.S.N.
Janet C. Fabling, R.D., C.N.S.D.
David E. Bell, R.Ph.

Section 3—Designer Nutritional Support for the Critically Ill

CHAPTER 15 175
Nutrition Support in the Critically Ill Diabetic Patient
Polyxeni Koutkia, M.D.
Caroline M. Apovian, M.D.

CHAPTER 16 187
Nutrition Support in Respiratory Failure
Mary S. McCarthy, R.N., M.N., C.N.S.N.
Leonard E. Deal, MAJ., M.C.

CHAPTER 17 199
Nutrition Support in the Patient with Hepatic Failure
James J. Pomposelli, M.D., Ph.D.
David L. Burns, M.D., C.N.S.P.

CHAPTER 18 209
Nutrition Support in Acute Renal Failure
Pamela Charney, M.S., R.D., C.N.S.D.
David Charney, M.D., F.A.C.P.

Chapter 19 219
Nutritional Aspects of Cardiac Disease
Karl V. Hakmiller, M.D.
Mylan C. Cohen, M.D., M.P.H.

Chapter 20 229
Nutritional Support of Trauma Patients
Rosemary A. Kozar, M.D., Ph.D.
Margaret M. McQuiggan, M.S., R.D., C.S.M.
Frederick A. Moore, M.D.

Chapter 21 245
Nutritional Considerations in the Severely Burned Patient
Bruce Friedman, M.D., F.C.C.P., F.C.C.M., C.N.S.P.
Scott A. Deppe, M.D., F.A.C.P., F.C.C.M., F.C.C.P.

Chapter 22 259
Nutritional Considerations in Severe Brain Injury
John R. Vender, M.D.
Gail A. Cresci, M.S., R.D., L.D., C.N.S.D.
Mark R. Lee, M.D., Ph.D.

Chapter 23 269
Nutritional Therapy in Acute Pancreatitis
Stephen A. McClave, M.D.
Gerald W. Dryden, M.D.
James K. Lukan, M.D.

Chapter 24 279
Nutritional Considerations for Dealing with Intestinal Diseases in the Intensive Care Unit
Walter L. Pipkin, M.D.
Thomas R. Gadacz, M.D., F.A.C.S.

Chapter 25 287
Nutrition Support and Pregnancy
Thomas R. Howdieshell, M.D., F.A.C.S., F.C.C.P.
Gail A. Cresci, M.S., R.D., L.D., C.N.S.D.
Robert G. Martindale, M.D., Ph.D., F.A.C.S.

Chapter 26 297
Nutritional Considerations in the Intensive Care Unit: Neonatal Issues
Anjali Parish, M.D.
Jatinder Bhatia, M.D.

Chapter 27 311
Nutritional Support in the Pediatric Intensive Care Unit
Diane L. Olson, R.D., C.N.S.D., C.S.P., L.D.
W. Frederick Schwenk II, M.D., C.N.S.P.

Chapter 28 325
Nutritional Support for the Obese Patient
Scott A. Shikora, M.D., F.A.C.S.
Michael J. Naylor, M.D.

Chapter 29 335
Nutrition in the Immunocompromised Intensive Care Unit Patient
Chris C. Carlson, M.D.

Chapter 30 341
Nutrition in Solid Organ Transplantation
Jeffrey A. Lowell, M.D., F.A.C.S.
Mary Ellen Beindorff, R.D., L.D.

Section 4—Practical Considerations

Chapter 31 347
Anabolic Agents in the Intensive Care Unit
Leah Gramlich, M.D., F.R.C.P.(C)
Demetrios J. Kutsogiannis, M.D., M.H.S., F.R.C.P.(C)

Chapter 32 357
Special Nutrient Formulas (Neutraceuticals)
Hank Schmidt, M.D.
Robert G. Martindale, M.D., Ph.D., F.A.C.S.

Chapter 33 365
Aggressive Perioperative and Intra Operative Enteral Nutrition: Strategy for the Future
Stig Bengmark, M.D., Ph.D.

Chapter 34 381
Probiotics, Prebiotics, and Synbiotics in the Intensive Care Unit
Stig Bengmark, M.D., Ph.D.

Chapter 35 401
Is It Cost Effective to Feed Patients in the Intensive Care Unit?
Stanley A. Nasraway, Jr., M.D., F.C.C.M.
Kris M. Mogensen, M.S., R.D.

Chapter 36 407
The Team Approach to Nutrition Support in the Intensive Care Unit
Nicole M. Daignault, R.D., C.N.S.D.
John R. Galloway, M.D., C.N.S.P.
Glen F. Bergman, M.MSc., R.D., C.N.S.D.
Elaina E. Szeszycki, Pharm.D., B.C.N.S.P.
Therese McNally, R.N., B.S., B.S.N.
Thomas R. Ziegler, M.D., C.N.S.P.

Index 417

Appendix 427

Contributors

Caroline M. Apovian, M.D.
Boston University Medical Center
Boston, Massachusetts

William A. Arnold, M.D.
New England Medical Center
Boston, Massachusetts

Mary Ellen Beindorff, R.D., L.D.
Barnes Hospital
Saint Louis, Missouri

David E. Bell, R.Ph.
Madigan Army Medical Corp
Tacoma, Washington

Stig Bengmark, M.D., Ph.D.
Höganäshamn, Sweden

Glen F. Bergman, M.MSc., R.D., C.N.S.D.
The Emory Clinic
Atlanta, Georgia

Jatinder Bhatia, M.D.
Medical College of Georgia
Augusta, Georgia

Jeff Binkley, Pharm.D., B.C.N.S.P.
Vanderbilt Center for Human Nutrition
Nashville, Tennessee

Bruce R. Bistrian, M.D., Ph.D.
Beth Israel Deaconess Medical Center
Cancer Research Institute
Boston, Massachusetts

David L. Burns, M.D., C.N.S.P.
Lahey Clinic Medical Center
Burlington, Massachusetts

Chris C. Carlson, M.D.
Medical College of Georgia
Augusta, Georgia

David Charney, M.D., F.A.C.P.
Riverside Nephrology Association
Columbus, Ohio

Pamela Charney, M.S., R.D., C.N.S.D.
Consultant, ClinElite Nutrition
Columbus, Ohio

Mylan C. Cohen, M.D., M.P.H.
Maine Medical Center
Portland, Maine

Gail A. Cresci, M.S., R.D., L.D., C.N.S.D.
Medical College of Georgia
Augusta, Georgia

Nicole M. Daignault, R.D., C.N.S.D.
The Emory Clinic
Atlanta, Georgia

Leonard E. Deal, MAJ., M.C.
Madigan Army Medical Corp
Tacoma, Washington

Mark H. DeLegge, M.D., F.A.C.G., C.N.S.P.
Digestive Disease Center
Medical University of South Carolina
Charleston, South Carolina

Scott A. Deppe, M.D., F.A.C.P., F.C.C.M., F.C.C.P.
Doctor's Hospital Burn Center
Augusta, Georgia

Gerald W. Dryden, M.D.
University of Louisville School of Medicine
Louisville, Kentucky

Janet C. Fabling, R.D., C.N.S.D.
Madigan Army Medical Corp
Tacoma, Washington

Dion L. Franga, M.D.
Medical College of Georgia
Augusta, Georgia

Bruce Friedman, M.D., F.C.C.P., F.C.C.M., C.N.S.P.
Doctor's Hospital Burn Center
Augusta, Georgia

M. Patricia Fuhrman, M.S., R.D., L.D., F.A.D.A., C.N.S.D.
Jewish Hospital College of Nursing
Saint Louis, Missouri

Thomas R. Gadacz, M.D., F.A.C.S.
Medical College of Georgia
Augusta, Georgia

John R. Galloway, M.D., C.N.S.P.
The Emory Clinic
Atlanta, Georgia

Leah Gramlich, M.D., F.R.C.P.(C)
Royal Alexandra Hospital
Edmonton, Alberta, Canada

Karl V. Hakmiller, M.D.
Maine Medical Center
Portland, Maine

Paul M. Hassoun, M.D.
USDA Human Nutrition Center on Aging at Tufts University
Pulmonary and Critical Care
Boston, Massachusetts

Virginia M. Herrmann, M.D., C.N.S.P.
Washington University School of Medicine
Saint Louis, Missouri

Thomas R. Howdieshell, M.D., F.A.C.S., F.C.C.P.
Medical College of Georgia
Augusta, Georgia

Carol S. Ireton-Jones, Ph.D., R.D., L.D., C.N.S.D., F.A.C.N.
Coram Healthcare
Carrollton, Texas

Gordon L. Jensen, M.D., Ph.D.
Vanderbilt Center for Human Nutrition
Nashville, Tennessee

Polyxeni Koutkia, M.D.
Boston University Medical Center
Boston, Massachusetts

Rosemary A. Kozar, M.D., Ph.D.
University of Texas Houston Medical School
Houston, Texas

Kenneth A. Kudsk, M.D.
University of Wisconsin
Madison, Wisconsin

Demetrios J. Kutsogiannis, M.D., M.H.S., F.R.C.P.(C)
Royal Alexandra Hospital
Edmonton, Alberta, Canada

Mark R. Lee, M.D., Ph.D.
Medical College of Georgia
Augusta, Georgia

Jeffrey A. Lowell, M.D., F.A.C.S.
Washington University School of Medicine
Saint Louis, Missouri

James K. Lukan, M.D.
University of Louisville School of Medicine
Louisville, Kentucky

Robert G. Martindale, M.D., Ph.D., F.A.C.S.
Medical College of Georgia
Augusta, Georgia

Joel B. Mason, M.D.
Tufts University School of Medicine and New England Medical Center
Boston, Massachusetts

Mary S. McCarthy, R.N., M.N., C.N.S.N.
Madigan Army Medical Corp
Tacoma, Washington

Stephen A. McClave, M.D.
University of Louisville School of Medicine
Louisville, Kentucky

Therese A. McNally, R.N., B.S., B.S.N.
The Emory Clinic
Atlanta, Georgia

Margaret M. McQuiggan, M.S., R.D., C.S.M.
Memorial Herman Hospital Houston Texas
Houston, Texas

Kris M. Mogensen, M.S., R.D.
Frances Stern Nutrition Center
New England Medical Center
Boston, Massachusetts

Frederick A. Moore, M.D.
University of Texas Houston Medical School
Houston, Texas

Stanley A. Nasraway, Jr., M.D., F.C.C.M.
New England Medical Center
Boston, Massachusetts

Michael J. Naylor, M.D.
New England Medical Center
Boston, Massachusetts

Reid Nishikawa, Pharm.D., F.C.S.H.P., B.C.N.S.P.
Nutrishare, Inc.
Fair Oaks, California

Diane L. Olson, R.D., C.N.S.D., C.S.P., L.D.
Mayo Clinic
Rochester, Minnesota

Anjali Parish, M.D.
Medical College of Georgia
Augusta, Georgia

Walter L. Pipkin, M.D.
Medical College of Georgia
Augusta, Georgia

James J. Pomposelli, M.D., Ph.D.
Lahey Clinic Medical Center
Burlington, Massachusetts

Edward Saltzman, M.D.
USDA Human Nutrition Research
and New England Medical Center
Boston, Massachusetts

Hank Schmidt, M.D.
Medical College of Georgia
Augusta, Georgia

Steven D. Schwaitzberg, M.D., F.A.C.S.
New England Medical Center
Boston, Massachusetts

W. Frederick Schwenk II, M.D., C.N.S.P.
Mayo Clinic
Rochester, Minnesota

Scott A. Shikora, M.D., F.A.C.S.
New England Medical Center
Boston, Massachusetts

John K. Siepler, Pharm.D., B.C.N.S.P.
University California Davis Medical Center
Sacramento, California

Elaina E. Szeszycki, Pharm.D., B.C.N.S.P.
The Emory Clinic
Atlanta, Georgia

Vincent W. Vanek, M.D., F.A.C.S., C.N.S.P.
St. Elizabeth's Hospital
Youngstown, Ohio

John R. Vender, M.D.
Medical College of Georgia
Augusta, Georgia

Thomas R. Ziegler, M.D., C.N.S.P.
The Emory Clinic
Atlanta, Georgia

Foreword

Maximally effective, comprehensive and safe management of patients in intensive care units continues to present the greatest challenges to all health care providers committed to this vital responsibility and engaged in the myriad associated therapeutic and supportive activities. Moreover, as health care delivery continues to evolve, and increasing numbers of patients receive required care at home or on an ambulatory out-patient basis, the numbers and percentages of hospitalized patients requiring intensive care, and/or other forms or levels of special care will inevitably expand. This especially applies to the burgeoning geriatric population which will further accentuate the demands for intensive care facilities and services in the near future. Indeed, an increasing number of patients are currently being admitted directly to intensive care or special care units of hospitals, and this is likely to escalate further as the magnitude and sophistication of treatment modalities advance in extended care facilities.

Intensive care units exist primarily to meet the specialized, often critical, and, at times, life-threatening needs of patients with major, complicated, and often multiple diseases, disorders and/or health problems. The special training, expertise and motivation of the physician and nursing personnel are absolutely critical to the success of their valiant endeavors. However, equally important services are provided by other members of this high precision team, which includes dieticians, nursing assistants, respiratory therapists, technicians, pharmacists, clinical pharmacologists, physician assistants, physical therapists, psychologists, sociologists, case managers and other health care delivery specialists.

Clearly, the quality and availability of the facility, together with its access to the most advanced technological adjuncts for the specialized support of its patient population, is a most important **physical** factor in patient outcomes. The provision of timely and optimal dosages of compatible and maximally effective, or even favorably synergistic medications, is a most important **pharmacologic** factor in patient outcomes. Supporting optimal bodily functions including those that are kinetic, somatic, psychological, emotional and personal is a most important **physiological** factor in patient outcomes. However, a most important and fundamental factor in determining patient outcomes in intensive care units is the provision of optimal **nutritional** and **metabolic** support to prevent, minimize or correct malnutrition throughout the continuum of care and concurrently with all of the other integrated intensive care measures. Woefully, nutritional assessment, therapy and monitoring are all too often lowest on the priority scale of critical care teams, possibly because malnutrition only rarely presents as a dire life-threatening emergency demanding their immediate and focused responsiveness. Additionally, the acuity and severity of the patient's primary condition, frequently coupled with multiple collateral health problems, require intense and complex therapeutic regimens which command the attention and efforts of the critical care physicians to the extent that problems related to providing adequate nutrition simultaneously to the seriously compromised patient often frustrate or even overwhelm them.

A primary concern and responsibility of all intensivists, regardless of their specialty, must be the orientation and dedication of their efforts toward maintaining optimal function of the maximum number of cells in the total body cell mass of the patient at all times in order to ensure optimal organ and systems functions. The current strategies for providing nutritional support generally to the whole patient, or more specifically to key organ systems, must proceed and advance to satisfying the substrate needs of all individual cells routinely if the ultimate goal of providing optimal nutrition to all patients under all conditions at all times is to be realized. The important aspects of, and considerations for, achieving this lofty ideal in critically ill patients through a variety of parenteral and enteral feeding techniques and adjuncts are presented and discussed practically and comprehensively by the elite group of authors assembled herein to share their nutritional science, rationale and practices for utilitarian therapeutic application in the intensive care unit.

In its consummate wisdom, and consonant with its vision and mission, the A.S.P.E.N. Board of Directors mandated the production of this monograph to fill the void of data and information available to healthcare providers for the nutritional support of critically ill patients. Accordingly, three of the leaders in this vital field of endeavor, Drs. Scott A. Shikora, Robert G. Martindale and Steven D. Schwaitzberg, were entrusted with the responsibility for determining, organizing and outlining the scope and content of the proposed publication and identifying and recruiting the preeminent experts in the world to make the essential contributions to this comprehensive volume. The resultant book has been designed to provide a state-of-the-art manual for feeding critically ill patients. The authors discuss virtually all of the major types of patients and feeding scenarios encountered in intensive care units in thirty-six outstanding chapters in an orderly, logical, intelligible and useful manner.

All who participated in the conception and production of this extraordinary and unique volume deserve our admiration and gratitude for a job commendably done in fulfilling a crucial need in the optimal management of critically ill patients. On behalf of clinicians of all specialties who expend their energy and talent selflessly caring for nutritionally compromised patients in the intensive care units, I salute the authors and editors for their most impressive accomplishments, and the A.S.P.E.N. Board of Directors for their initiative, direction and stewardship in producing this invaluable tome. I am honored to have been afforded the opportunity to introduce the results of their yeoman collaborative genius to our colleagues throughout the world who strive daily to improve the outcomes of critically ill, nutritionally disadvantaged patients.

Stanley J. Dudrick, M.D.

Preface

Critical care medicine and nutritional support are two distinct fields in medicine that have undergone tremendous advances in the last three decades. Both have benefited from significant advances in scientific research and technology. Both can also be credited with improving the outcome and survival from significant illness or injury. Although these disciplines are quite separate, they are also are closely interwoven and must therefore go hand in hand. Despite the advances in antibiotics, ventilator technology, imaging options, surgical skills, cardiopulmonary assessment, and dialysis, critically ill patients would not survive without the appropriate nutritional intervention. Conversely, despite the use of better nutritional formulations, improvements in access and delivery systems, and the widening use of designer nutrients, patients would also succumb without the appropriate critical care support.

The critically ill represent an extremely diverse group of patients. They vary from the very young to the very old, male and female, severely malnourished to extremely obese, pregnant to organ transplanted. Their reason for admission to a specialized critical care unit may also greatly vary from major trauma to organ failure, to severely septic, and so on. Finally, they may complicate their acute illness with a litany of additional comorbidities. This tremendous degree of diversity prevents a standard nutritional approach from being applicable for the majority of this population. Therefore, it is necessary to individualize the nutritional approach for these patient types. To do so, one needs to understand not only the basics of nutritional medicine but also the impact and/or considerations for determining the most appropriate interventions for a specific patient type. The sophistication and complexity of this subset of hospitalized patients makes it nearly impossible for most practitioners to possess this knowledge and expertise at a level that is up-to-date and sufficiently in depth to meet this challenge. There lies the incentive for this book: to utilize the knowledge of experts in the field to construct a comprehensive, scholarly, and state-of-the-art text to address these issues.

Nutritional Considerations in the Intensive Care Unit: Science, Rationale, and Practice is the result of this endeavor. The book is divided into four sections. The first section, entitled, "Nutritional derangements and critical illness" covers the inter-relationship between critical illness (of any etiology) and nutritional status. The metabolic responses to severe illness or trauma can cause significant nutritional derangements which affects nutritional well-being and nutrient utilization. These issues are covered in detail.

The second section deals with traditional nutritional issues such as determining macronutrient and micronutrient requirements, fluids and electrolytes, acid base disorders, and access issues. Obviously, each of these sections applies these generalized subjects to the critical care environment.

The third section represents the heart of the textbook. Each chapter applies the field of nutritional support to a wide range of critical care conditions as well as to the complex co-morbidities that the critically ill may also suffer from and that require unique nutritional approaches such as diabetes, organ dysfunction, trauma, obesity, immunosuppressive disorders, severe burns, abdominal sepsis, and transplantation. Age-related topics such as pregnancy, neonatal, and pediatric patients are also covered.

The final section ties in other important considerations such as the cost of nutritional support and the use of novel nutritional approaches such as designer formulas, probiotics, and anabolic agents.

Our hope is that this book will help clinicians of all disciplines who work in an intensive care environment to understand the unique interrelationship between nutritional support and critical illness. By understanding these concepts, we hope to improve the provision of nutritional and metabolic support and thus hopefully, decrease complications, and improve outcome.

Scott A. Shikora, M.D., F.A.C.S.
Robert G. Martindale, M.D., Ph.D., F.A.C.S.
Steven D. Schwaitzberg, M.D., F.A.C.S.

CHAPTER

1

Malnutrition in the Intensive Care Unit

Edward Saltzman, M.D.[1], Kris M. Mogensen, M.S., R.D.[2], Paul M. Hassoun, M.D.[3]

INTRODUCTION 1
IDENTIFYING MALNUTRITION IN THE ICU 1
CLINICAL CONSEQUENCES OF MALNUTRITION 4
Respiratory Failure 4
HIV Patients 6
Acute Renal Failure 6
Postoperative Patients 6
Obesity 6
ADEQUACY OF NUTRITIONAL SUPPORT 6
CONCLUSIONS 7
REFERENCES 7

Introduction

For decades it has been recognized that malnutrition contributes to increased risk for morbidity and mortality in hospitalized patients. In patients with acute or chronic illness, the term malnutrition has generally been used synonymously with protein energy malnutrition (PEM), but micronutrient disorders also commonly occur in this population. Some acutely ill patients will have histories or clinical findings to suggest PEM or other forms of malnutrition on admission or during the hospital stay. However, in the ICU, histories may be more difficult to obtain, and nutrition-related sequelae may occur in the absence of usual clinical signs. This is due in part to the difficulty in assessing nutritional parameters and body composition in seriously ill patients. Disorders of fluid balance may mask muscle wasting or weight changes. There is considerable overlap between the effects of malnutrition and disease itself in critically ill patients, and differentiating between the role of nutritional and non-nutritional factors in clinical outcome is often difficult or impossible.[1] Further, the provision of nutritional support may influence outcome for reasons other than its contribution to nitrogen (N) or energy balance, as is suggested by the effects of early enteral nutrition on infection risk in trauma patients, which is discussed in Chapter 20.

Identifying Malnutrition in the ICU

No general agreement exists as to how to define malnutrition in acutely ill patients.[2] When different markers of PEM are simultaneously compared in critically ill patients, inconsistent agreement between measures is often found.[3–6] This reflects the problems mentioned above, as well as the variability introduced by the wide range of diagnoses, combinations of acute and chronic comorbidities, and demographic variables that make up the population of patients with critical illness. Table 1.1 lists some of the parameters in published studies that have been used singly or in combination to define malnutrition in critically ill patients. Thus, an appropriately broad definition is that of Birmingham,[7] who describes malnutrition as "a diagnosis that includes an absolute or functional deficiency or excess of energy, protein, vitamins, or minerals, whether in combination or as isolated abnormalities." This broader definition also includes risks associated with overnutrition, either acutely, as with overfeeding, or chronically, as manifested by obesity.

Most investigators who have sought to link nutritional status to ICU outcome have assessed nutritional status at admission to the ICU, or preoperatively in the case of surgical patients. There are few published descriptions of development of malnutrition in the ICU, again, in large part due to the technical challenges of measuring changes in body composition in the ICU patient and the difficulty in differentiating the

TABLE 1.1

Criteria Used in Trials to Identify Malnutrition in Hospitalized Patients

- **Weight**
  - Weight for height
    - % ideal body weight
    - BMI (range >15, >20, >30 kg/m^2)
  - Weight loss
- **Body composition**
  - Anthropometrics
    - Skinfold thickness
    - Limb circumference
  - Bioelectrical impedance
    - Fat-free mass
    - Body-cell mass
  - Dilution techniques
    - Fat-free mass
    - Body-cell mass
    - Ratio of extracellular to intracellular water
    - Ratio of exchangeable sodium to potassium
  - In vivo neutron activation
    - Total body protein
    - Total body potassium
  - Dual energy x-ray absorptiometry
    - Fat-free mass
- **Biochemical**
  - Hepatic secretory proteins: albumin, prealbumin, transferrin, c-reactive protein
- **Hematologic: hemoglobin, lymphocyte count**
- **Urinary urea nitrogen excretion**
- **Energy intake**
- **Energy expenditure**
- **Functional indices**
  - Grip strength
  - Pulmonary function tests and pulmonary muscle strength
  - Non-volitional muscle function
- **Combinations and indices**
  - Weight loss and albumin
  - Hepatic proteins, hematologic indices and weight loss
  - Nitrogen balance by intake and UUN
  - Creatinine height/arm index
  - Measured energy expenditure and body energy losses by body composition

effects of critical illness from malnutrition. Also, for most patients, ICU stays are too short to allow measurable changes in nutritional status.

The effects of hypocaloric feeding or starvation in healthy persons differ markedly from those of malnutrition in the critically ill patient. In healthy well-nourished persons, underfeeding or starvation results in oxidation of endogenous reserves, and there is a predictable transition from glycogenolysis to gluconeogenesis, from glucose oxidation to fat oxidation, and eventually to increased ketogenesis over days to weeks. Resting energy expenditure (REE) decreases early in energy restriction, the magnitude of which depends on the degree of restriction. Further decreases in REE occur as a function of fat free mass (FFM) losses as well as energy restriction.[8] Relative sparing of body protein is facilitated by increased oxidation of ketones and free fatty acids, which decreases the need for protein-derived gluconeogenesis. The relative sparing of fat-free mass was illustrated by Keys'[9] experiment of underfeeding over 6 months. Approximately one-quarter of initial weight was lost, which was distributed as 72% fat and 27% cell mass.[8,9] Reliance on lipid as an energy substrate remains high until body fat stores are diminished to very low levels; this phenomenon is observed in profound PEM, where the depletion of body fat and hence lipid substrate is reflected by an increase in respiratory quotient.

In contrast to chronic energy restriction, the metabolic response to critical illness is characterized by increased energy expenditure (hypermetabolism), proteolysis, gluconeogenesis, and lipolysis (see Chapter 2). Severely traumatized or septic patients may expend >150%–200% of predicted energy expenditure,[10,11] while typical expenditures in critically ill medical and surgical patients are in the range of 100%–150% of predicted, and in a minority of patients, energy expenditure may be lower than predicted.[12,13] Increased energy requirements may accelerate PEM in critical illness, but meeting increased needs is often difficult for multiple metabolic, physiologic, and practical reasons (as is discussed below). Prediction of expenditure in ICU patients may be influenced by volume overload, since body weight is often used in equations to predict energy needs.[11]

Increased proteolysis leads to accelerated protein loss, which, unlike uncomplicated underfeeding, occurs despite provision of exogenous protein and non-protein substrates.[14] Negative N balance is common, and is evidenced by urinary losses often >15–20 g/d.[15,16] Nitrogen excretion is a crude indicator of the degree of catabolism, but should be interpreted in light of N balance. This is illustrated in a trial of surgical patients, where provision of nutritional support resulted in increased urinary N excretion despite improved N balance.[16] Protein loss has been demonstrated on a biochemical level by skeletal muscle biopsy in critically ill patients, which revealed a 59% reduction in total amino acids, a 72% decrease in glutamine, and an increase in aromatic amino acids of 88% in contrast to healthy controls.[17] Body composition changes in critical illness have been measured on the whole body level by techniques such as neutron activation, dilution methods to discriminate between intracellular water (ICW) and extracellular water (ECW), and dual x-ray absorptiometry (DEXA).[18,19] Hill et al.[19] measured FFM and limb muscle mass by DEXA and total body N (TBN) by in-vivo neutron activation in 13 septic patients over 21 days. After an initial gain of weight due to fluid resuscitation, over the study period loss of weight was 15% of initial, 82% of which was water. Fat-free mass loss was 19% of initial, 46% of which was limb muscle mass. Loss of TBN was 14% despite provision of nutritional support.

Critical illness results in gains of body water and perturbations of body water distribution. There is expansion of the ECW compartment relative to the ICW compartment,[5,11] which is likely to exist even when edema is not clinically apparent. Gains in body water over 10 kg are not uncommon early in critical illness. Use of medications such as diuretics that can rapidly alter body water are also common. The limited utility of body weight as a marker in the ICU is further diminished by inaccuracy of self-reported weights (if available), as demonstrated in hospitalized patients where approximately one-third of patients who had lost weight were misclassified as not having lost by use of recalled weight.[20,21]

Despite these caveats, weight is among the most easily obtained measures and has often been employed as an index of PEM. Malnutrition prevalence varies substantially among studies in ICU patients when criteria for malnutrition are based on relative weight or weight loss. In HIV patients admitted to an ICU, De Palo found that 18% of patients were <90% of ideal body weight (IBW).[22] In different studies of COPD patients with acute respiratory failure, 39% of patients weighed <90% of IBW,[23] and 24% weighed <80% of IBW.[24] In preoperative patients awaiting major surgery, a weight loss of ≥10% of usual body weight (UBW) was found in 15%.[6] In critically ill patients, Giner[25] found that 43% of patients were malnourished, as defined as <100% of weight for height and albumin <3.5 mg/dL. Thus, prevalence varies widely depending on criteria used and the population studied. Patients who are admitted with acute complications of chronic disease appear far more likely to have experienced weight loss in comparison to previously healthy patients, such as those admitted for trauma or burns.

Body mass index (BMI) is currently used to classify weight for height in healthy persons and in patients with chronic PEM, with BMI <18.5 indicative of chronic energy deficiency.[26] The survivable lower limits of BMI have been derived from patients with anorexia nervosa or starvation and are estimated to be 11 kg/m^2 for women and 13 kg/m^2 for men,[27] although there are reports of 9–10 kg/m^2 or even lower. BMI on admission has been used as an index of nutritional status, but criteria have been based on either the above definition, or arbitrary cut-offs, which have included levels of BMI such as 15, 16, 18, 20, and 25 kg/m^2. Adverse outcomes in critically ill patients have been reported at levels of 15–20 or even 25 kg/m^2 in reference to higher levels.[28–32] Obesity, as defined as BMI ≥30 kg/m^2, has also been associated with increased morbidity in the critically ill,[31–33] which is discussed below and in detail in Chapter 28.

Anthropometric measurements poorly reflect body protein and fat in critical illness. Body water gains early in critical illness primarily reflect expansion of ECW, which makes interpretation of limb circumference and skinfold thickness problematic. In patients who remain in the ICU after several days, a gradual decrease in weight has been observed, also reflecting loss of body water primarily as ECW.[11] In the short-term, changes in anthropometric measurements are more likely to reflect changes in body water and its distribution. Green and et al.[3] conducted serial measurements of midarm circumference (MAC), total body water, N balance, and muscle protein content in patients with multiorgan system failure (MOSF) over 3–30 days. No relation was found between MAC and N balance, but in those with decreases in MAC, mean body water decreased significantly by 8 L. Further, in biopsy data obtained in 6 patients, changes in MAC were not related to changes in muscle fiber area. Thus, in the critically ill population, use of anthropometrics as a measure of nutrition status appears to be of limited use.

Circulating hepatic proteins have been utilized as indicators of PEM in malnourished and ill patients. While serving as a marker of prognostic importance,[34] concentrations of albumin and other proteins also reflect disease severity and non-nutritional alterations in hepatic protein synthesis, increased catabolism, alterations in distribution, and derangements of body water.[35–37] Recent confirmatory evidence for this was found in severely septic patients followed over 3 weeks, as changes in secretory proteins did not correlate with measured changes in TBN.[11]

In preoperative and chronically ill patients, tests of voluntary[38] and involuntary muscle function[38] correlate with weight loss and PEM, and have been predictive of adverse outcome in hospitalized patients.[39] These tests may also reflect shorter-term energy balance or status of intracellular energy substrates and intracellular ions, as improvement is seen early in refeeding and precedes measurable protein accretion.[40] In the ICU, use of voluntary muscle function, such as handgrip strength or respiratory muscle strength, is potentially complicated by altered levels of consciousness induced by illness or sedation, critical illness-associated neuropathy or myopathy, and discomfort induced by the presence of invasive catheters or devices. Measures of involuntary muscle function, such as adductor pollicis contraction and relaxation characteristics, are subject to some of the same constraints and may induce temporary discomfort.[18] While some investigators have successfully employed involuntary muscle function testing in critically ill patients,[40] others have reported that its use in trauma and sepsis patients was technically difficult and of limited value in predicting loss of body protein.[18]

Micronutrient deficiency or excess is common in the ICU setting and may occur as a result of acute or chronic disease, changes in hydration status, treatment or medication use, refeeding, or normal losses. While some measured micronutrient concentrations accurately represent whole-body or tissue depletion, several vitamin and mineral concentrations are abnormal in critical illness but are not necessarily indicative of tissue or body stores (as is discussed in Chapters 6, 7, and 8). Thus, for several vitamins and minerals, use of confirmatory or functional tests, or subsequent measurement when disease acuity has remitted, is necessary. Hypophosphatemia, hypomagnesemia, and hypokalemia are common in critical illness[41–44] and may contribute to respiratory, neuromuscular, and cardiac compromise, and are discussed below. Decreased concentrations of several antioxidant vitamins have been reported, prompting some to suggest that such deficiencies contribute to oxidative damage or to immune dysfunction;[45–47] the clinical significance in the setting of critical illness of decreased concentration of antioxidants, as well as the potential benefits of supplementation, are as yet unknown.

Clinical Consequences of Malnutrition

Malnutrition diagnosed on admission to the ICU has been associated with a variety of adverse outcomes. Outcome measures have frequently been labeled "nutrition-related," but differentiating between the effects of nutrition and disease is often difficult or impossible. Supportive evidence for a detrimental role of malnutrition in ICU outcome is suggested by the fact that PEM in the settings of starvation and chronic illness is associated with immune dysfunction and increased infection risk,[48–50] impaired skeletal and respiratory muscle strength,[38,51–56] and increased mortality risk.[57–61] In acutely (but not necessarily critically) ill medical patients, PEM and weight loss have been associated with increased risk for infectious and non-infectious complications, longer hospital stays, and increased rates of in-hospital and post-discharge mortality.[29,31,62,63] In surgical patients, indicators of PEM, preoperative weight loss (e.g. >10% UBW), and decreased handgrip or respiratory muscle strength have been associated with increased postoperative complications such as pneumonia, wound infection, length of hospital stay, and mortality.[38,39,64–66]

While critical illness can seldom be categorized by a single disease state or dysfunction of a single organ system, attempts have been made to determine effects of malnutrition in specific primary diseases. The sections below review nutrition-related issues in specific illnesses or clinical scenarios.

Respiratory Failure

Loss of body weight is accompanied by loss of diaphragmatic mass and diminutions in respiratory muscle strength, maximal voluntary ventilation, and vital capacity, as well as respiratory drive.[24,54,67,68] The consequences of decreased respiratory strength and decreased ventilatory drive are numerous in the critically ill patient. Decreased respiratory strength may lead to decreased cough, atelectasis, and subsequent pneumonia. Decreased ventilatory drive may prolong mechanical ventilation in patients who are otherwise candidates for being liberated from ventilation.[69]

Malnutrition associated with lung disease, in particular chronic obstructive lung disease (COPD) but also other forms of advanced lung disease, has been termed the "pulmonary cachexia syndrome." This syndrome is characterized by a progressive reduction in lean body mass that is multifunctional in origin; lack of exercise due to respiratory limitation, chronic tissue hypoxia, medications (e.g., steroids), and hypermetabolism (due to increased work of breathing) are all contributory factors. Recent estimates suggest that up to 50% of COPD patients may be <90% of IBW.[70] Despite increases in energy expenditure from respiratory muscle overfunction, COPD patients often have a reduced dietary intake due to alteration in appetite and intercurrent infectious etiologies.

As recently reviewed, both COPD itself and PEM independently (or even synergistically) compromise respiratory function.[69,71] In addition to the anatomic and functional manifestations, PEM in COPD has been associated with reduction in intramuscular high-energy phosphates as measured by nuclear magnetic resonance, indicating a deficit of intracellular energy substrates.[71]

Alterations in body water and electrolytes, as well as increased metabolic demands in the critically ill, may lead to respiratory compromise in the absence of pre-existing lung disease. Impaired gas exchange may result from expansion of ECW, resulting in interstitial edema, while hypoalbuminemia may contribute to pulmonary edema. Hypophosphatemia has been shown to reduce diaphragmatic contractility as measured by trans-diaphragmatic pressures in mechanically ventilated patients with acute respiratory failure.[72] Thus it is not surprising that hypophosphatemia is associated with respiratory muscle weakness, may precipitate respiratory failure, and can impair weaning from mechanical ventilation.[72] Further tissue oxygenation may be impaired in hypophosphatemia by reduction of red blood cell 2,3-DPG.[42] Respiratory muscle weakness may also result from hypomagnesemia and hypokalemia, and improvements in pulmonary function have been observed with appropriate repletion.[41] Hypocalcemia could also theoretically influence diaphragmatic contractility and respiratory muscle strength.[73] Hypocalcemia appears to be quite common in the critically ill, occurring in 15% to 50% of patients.[74] More prevalent in certain diseases such as pancreatitis, sepsis, and major trauma, hypocalcemia correlates with disease severity and increased mortality.[75–77] Whereas correction of hypocalcemia may lead to transient improvement in hemodynamics,[78] long-term effects of replacement on pulmonary function and clinical outcome, if any, are not known.

Trials of renutrition on critically ill patients with lung disease have shown inconsistent results on repletion of body weight and respiratory function. Extrapolation from studies obtained on patients with anorexia nervosa suggests that diaphragm contractility (severely depressed in these patients) may improve with adequate nutrition.[68] In COPD patients with acute exacerbations, nutritional support may increase muscle strength, which should theoretically improve clinical outcome. However, only small gains (about 8% improvement) in forced vital capacity were found in one study, in which patients with an acute exacerbation of COPD were provided supplemental oral nutritional support as opposed to regular hospital care for the control patients.[79] Several retrospective studies have suggested that weaning from mechanical ventilation can be facilitated by supplemental nutrition.[80,81] However, until adequate prospective, randomized, controlled studies are performed, the exact role of nutrition in the management of the critically ill with respiratory failure is unclear.

Nutritional support, in particular high carbohydrate (CHO) loads, may worsen hypercapnia in patients with acute respiratory failure,[82] occasionally leading to delayed weaning from mechanical ventilation.[83] However, total calories rather than percentage of carbohydrates in the diet may be the predominant determinant of carbon dioxide production ($\dot{V}CO_2$), as suggested by a study in which increments of CHO did not lead to increases in $\dot{V}CO_2$ for isocaloric regimens, as opposed to significant increments in $\dot{V}CO_2$ when the nutritional regimens were 1, 1.5, and 2 times REE.[84]

Several trials have attempted to define nutritional predictors of outcome in acute respiratory failure. In elderly patients admitted with respiratory failure and treated with mechanical ventilation, admission BMI and MAC did not predict mortality while in the ICU.[85] However, in that trial patients were followed after discharge and mortality at 6 months was observed in 35% of those with MAC ≤10th percentile, in contrast to 11% mortality in those with MAC >10th percentile. Laaban et al.[23] assessed anthropometric and biochemical parameters in COPD patients admitted with acute respiratory failure, and found that 39% weighed ≤90% IBW, but use of a combined index of nutritional status (weight, MAC, triceps skinfold, creatinine height index, albumin, and prealbumin) classified 60% of patients as malnourished. In comparison to those classified as well-nourished, need for mechanical ventilation was significantly higher (74% vs. 43%) in the malnourished group. In another trial of COPD patients with acute respiratory failure, bioelectrical impedance (BIA) was contrasted with anthropometric and biochemical measures of nutritional status at admission.[5] Patients requiring intubation had lower cell mass by BIA, greater ECW:ICW, and lower albumin and prealbumin in comparison to patients who did not require intubation. In contrast, BMI and fat mass (both by anthropometry and by BIA) were significantly greater in the intubated group. Agreement between anthropometric measurements and cell mass was poor, and only low concentrations of albumin and prealbumin were associated with significantly lower cell mass. ICU mortality was associated with cell mass ≤40.6% of body weight, albumin <3.0 mg/dL, and MAC ≥80% predicted. The authors suggest that the deleterious effects of low cell mass indicated a greater loss of muscle mass, and that the increased ECW:ICW spuriously resulted in elevations of BMI and MAC in the ventilated group.

HIV Patients

In HIV patients admitted to an ICU, in-hospital and subsequent mortality has been predicted by prior weight loss in two trials. In one trial, ICU mortality was significantly correlated with reported weight loss prior to admission; in those who were discharged home, a reported weight loss of >12% of UBW at the initial hospitalization was associated with a 4-fold decrease in survival time after discharge.[86] In another report, HIV patients who weighed <90% of IBW at ICU admission demonstrated an in-hospital mortality rate of 92% vs. 42% in those who weighed ≥90% IBW.[22]

Acute Renal Failure

In contrast to the relationship between nutrition and chronic renal disease, the role of malnutrition in the development of acute renal failure (ARF) has received little attention. ARF may exacerbate malnutrition by limiting ability to deliver nutritional support due to volume restriction, as well as by effects of azotemia and acid/base disturbances on protein metabolism. In hospitalized patients who were admitted to a specialized nephrology ward with ARF, the subjective global assessment (SGA) score at admission predicted the in-hospital complication rate as well as mortality.[87] In comparison to other patients, the 42% of patients with SGA class C (the highest degree of malnutrition) had greater rates of prior chronic illness, had greater severity of illness, and had significantly greater rates of concomitant acute comorbidities (including heart failure, hepatic failure, respiratory failure, sepsis, and the systemic inflammatory response syndrome). In addition, these patients subsequently developed significantly greater rates of sepsis, hemorrhage, GI bleeding, cardiogenic shock, cardiac dysrhythmia, and need for mechanical ventilation. In-hospital mortality was markedly increased in SGA class C patients (OR 7.21, 95% CI 4.08-12.73). In regression analysis controlling for acute comorbidities, development of complications, and chronic illness, SGA class remained a highly significant predictor of mortality (OR 2.12 95% CI 1.61-2.89).

Postoperative Patients

A number of investigators have evaluated preoperative nutritional status in patients typically requiring postoperative ICU care. In patients undergoing cardiac surgery, low preoperative BMI has been associated with increased risk for prolonged mechanical ventilation, ARF, need for reoperation, and mortality in many,[32,88] but not all,[89] trials. The effects of nutritional status in patients undergoing major abdominal surgery or cancer resection are well documented and reviewed elsewhere.[38,67,90,91] In surgical patients who develop MOSF, PEM is associated with increased risk for infection and mortality.[92,93] Recent data in transplantation patients also suggest an influence of pre-transplantation nutritional status. Figueiredo et al.[4] assessed anthropometrics, SGA, handgrip strength, biochemical indices and body composition by isotope dilution in liver transplant patients, and found that only handgrip strength and low FFM predicted longer ICU stay, while no nutritional variable predicted infection or mortality; however, this trial may have been underpowered to detect effects of malnutrition since only 9% of patients were classified as severely malnourished by SGA. In another report, low body cell mass prior to liver transplant was associated with increased long-term mortality.[94] In lung transplant recipients, BMI did not predict mortality in patients with ICU stays of <5 days, but in those with longer stays, low BMI was associated with increased mortality.[95]

Obesity

The marked increase in obesity prevalence is now readily apparent in the ICU. Obese patients, like leaner patients, are hypermetabolic and catabolic, and despite increased stores of body protein and energy suffer the ill effect of malnutrition.[96] Following cardiovascular surgery, patients with BMI ≥30 kg/m^2 have been observed to have increased rates of pulmonary dysfunction[89] and wound infection,[32] and obesity is associated with increased mortality following heart transplantation.[97] Obese patients with pancreatitis experience increased rates of complications such as abscess formation, pancreatic necrosis, MOSF, and mortality.[98–100] Increased infection rate and need for mechanical ventilation has been reported in obese burn patients.[101]

Adequacy of Nutritional Support

Inadequate provision of energy, protein, and other nutrients is common in the ICU and can thus contribute to malnutrition. Inadequate delivery commonly occurs due to inadequacy of orders to meet needs, or due to disruption of infusions. McClave et al.[90] studied 44 medical and surgical ICU patients receiving enteral nutrition. The daily mean volume of enteral nutrition ordered by physicians was 65.6% (range 11%–102%)

of the estimated energy needs, and patients received only 78.1% (range 36%–123%) of what was ordered. De Jonghe et al.[102] studied 51 medical ICU patients receiving enteral and/or parenteral nutrition and found similar results, with orders meeting approximately 78% of estimated energy requirements, and that patients who were fed enterally received a significantly lower proportion of prescribed energy than patients receiving parenteral nutrition. In another study of 193 medical and surgical ICU patients, 76% of the prescribed enteral feeding was infused.[103]

Enteral feedings are interrupted for a variety of reasons including diagnostic or therapeutic procedures, gastrointestinal intolerance, airway management, tube displacement, mechanical problems, administration of incompatible medications, and routine nursing care.[90,102–104]

While deliberate underfeeding has become a popular strategy to minimize the metabolic or infectious risks of nutritional interventions, hypocaloric feeding will eventually result in weight loss and PEM. This was confirmed in a trial where correlations between changes in weight and visceral proteins and degree of underfeeding were observed.[90]

Conclusions

Malnutrition is likely to contribute to ICU morbidity across a spectrum of diagnoses. The scope of malnutrition extends beyond PEM to include overnutrition and micronutrient abnormalities, which are prevalent in critically ill patients. Differentiating between the effects of malnutrition and critical illness is difficult, making definition and diagnosis problematic. While better definition is needed, the distinction between nutritional and non-nutritional etiologies may be of little consequence if nutritional support in the ICU is demonstrated to improve clinical outcome.

References

1. Weinsier RL, Heimburger DC. Distinguishing malnutrition from disease: the search goes on. *Am J Clin Nutr.* 1997;66:1063–1064.
2. Souba WW. Nutritional support. *New Engl J Med.* 1997; 336:41–48.
3. Green CJ, Campbell IT, McClelland P, et al. Energy and nitrogen balance and changes in midupper-arm circumference with multiple organ failure. *Nutrition.* 1995;11:739–746.
4. Figueiredo F, Dickson ER, Pasha T, et al. Impact of nutritional status on outcomes after liver transplantation. *Transplantation.* 2000;70:1347–1352.
5. Faisy C, Rabbat A, Kouchakji B, et al. Bioelectrical impedance analysis in estimating nutritional status and outcome of patients with chronic obstructive pulmonary disease and acute respiratory failure. *Intensive Care Med.* 2000;26:518–525.
6. Klidjian AM, Foster KJ, Kammerling RM, et al. Relation of anthropometric and dynamometric variables to serious postoperative complications. *BMJ.* 1980;281:899–901.
7. Birmingham CL. Total parenteral nutrition in the critically ill patient. *Lancet.* 1999;353:1116–1117.
8. Shetty PS. Adaptation to low energy intakes: the responses and limits to low intakes in infants, children and adults. *Eur J Clin Nutr.* 1999;53:S14–33.
9. Keys A, Brozek J, Henschel A, et al. The biology of human starvation. Minneapolis: University of Minnesota Press; 1950.
10. McClave SA, Snider HL. Use of indirect calorimetry in clinical nutrition. *Nutr Clin Prac.* 1992;7:207–221.
11. Plank LD, Connolly AB, Hill GL. Sequential changes in the metabolic response in severely septic patients during the first 23 days after the onset of peritonitis. *Ann Surg.* 1998;228:146–158.
12. Frankenfield DC, Smith JS Jr., Cooney RN, et al. Relative association of fever and injury with hypermetabolism in critically ill patients. *Injury.* 1997;28:617–621.
13. Weissman C, Kemper M, Askanazi J, et al. Resting metabolic rate of the critically ill patient: measured versus predicted. *Anesthesiology.* 1986;64:673–679.
14. Wolfe RR, Martini WZ. Changes in intermediary metabolism in severe surgical illness. *World J Surg.* 2000;24: 639–647.
15. Jeevanandum M, Young DH, Schiller WR. Obesity and the metabolic response to severe multiple trauma in man. *J Clin Invest.* 1991;87:262–269.
16. Sandstrom R, Drott C, Hyltander A, et al. The effect of postoperative intravenous feeding (TPN) on outcome following major surgery evaluated in a randomized study. *Ann Surg.* 1993;217:185–195.
17. Gamrin L, Essen P, Forsberg AM, et al. A descriptive study of skeletal muscle metabolism in critically ill patients: free amino acids, energy-rich phosphates, protein, nucleic acids, fat, water, and electrolytes. *Crit Care Med.* 1996;24:575–583.
18. Finn PJ, Plank LD, Clark MA, et al. Assessment of involuntary muscle function in patients after critical injury or severe sepsis. *J Parenter Enteral Nutr.* 1996;20:332–337.
19. Hill AA, Plank LD, Finn PJ, et al. Massive nitrogen loss in critical surgical illness: effect on cardiac mass and function. *Ann Surg.* 1997;226:191–197.
20. Morgan DB, Hill GL, Burkinshaw L. The assessment of weight loss from a single measurement of body weight: the problems and limitations. *Am J Clin Nutr.* 1980;33: 2101–2105.
21. Pirie P, Jacobs D, Jeffery R, et al. Distortion in self-reported height and weight. *J Am Diet Assoc.* 1981;78:601–606.

22. De Palo VA, Millstein BH, Mayo PH, et al. Outcome of intensive care in patients with HIV infection. *Chest.* 1995; 107:506–510.
23. Laaban JP, Kouchakji B, Dore MF, et al. Nutritional status of patients with chronic obstructive pulmonary disease and acute respiratory failure. *Chest.* 1993;103:1362–1368.
24. Pingleton SK, Harmon GS. Nutritional management in acute respiratory failure. *JAMA.* 1987;257:3094–3099.
25. Giner M, Laviano A, Meguid MM, et al. In 1995 a correlation between malnutrition and poor outcome in critically ill patients still exists. *Nutrition.* 1996;12:23–29.
26. James WP, Ferro-Luzzi A, Waterlow JC. Definition of chronic energy deficiency in adults. Report of a working party of the International Dietary Energy Consultative Group. *Eur J Clin Nutr.* 1988;42:969–981.
27. Henry CJ. Body mass index and the limits of human survival. *Eur J Clin Nutr.* 1990;44:329–335.
28. Fife C, Otto G, Capsuto EG, et al. Incidence of pressure ulcers in a neurologic intensive care unit. *Crit Care Med.* 2001;29:283–290.
29. Potter JF, Schafer DF, Bohi RL. In-hospital mortality as a function of body mass index: an age-dependent variable. *J Gerontol.* 1988;43:M59–63.
30. Galanos AN, Pieper CF, Kussin PS, et al. Relationship of body mass index to subsequent mortality among seriously ill hospitalized patients. SUPPORT Investigators. The study to understand prognoses and preferences for outcome and risks of treatments. *Crit Care Med.* 1997;25: 1962–1968.
31. Landi F, Onder G, Gambassi G, et al. Body mass index and mortality among hospitalized patients. *Arch Intern Med.* 2000;160:2641–2644.
32. Engelman DT, Adams DH, Byrne JG, et al. Impact of body mass index and albumin on morbidity and mortality after cardiac surgery. *J Thorac Cardiovasc Surg.* 1999;118: 866–873.
33. Gloor B, Muller CA, Worni M, et al. Late mortality in patients with severe acute pancreatitis. *Br J Surg.* 2001;88: 975–979.
34. Herrmann FR, Safran C, Levkoff SE, et al. Serum albumin level on admission as a predictor of death, length of stay, and readmission. *Arch Intern Med.* 1992;152:125–130.
35. Klein S. The myth of serum albumin as a measure of nutritional status. *Gastroenterology.* 1990;99:1845–1846.
36. Fleck A, Raines G, Hawker F, et al. Increased vascular permeability: a major cause of hypoalbuminaemia in disease and injury. *Lancet.* 1985;1:781–784.
37. Rothschild MA, Oratz M, Schreiber SS. Albumin synthesis. *N Engl J Med.* 1972;286:816–821.
38. Windsor JA, Hill GL. Weight loss with physiologic impairment: a basic indicator of surgical risk. *Ann Surg.* 1988;207:290–296.
39. Webb AR, Newman LA, Taylor M, et al. Hand grip dynamometry as a predictor of postoperative complications reappraisal using age standardized grip strengths. *J Parenter Enteral Nutr.* 1989;13:30–33.
40. Jeejeebhoy KN. Rhoads lecture—1988. Bulk or bounce—the object of nutritional support. *J Parenter Enteral Nutr.* 1988;12:539–549.
41. Dhingra S, Solven F, Wilson A, et al. Hypomagnesemia and respiratory muscle power. *Am J Resp Dis.* 1984;129: 497–498.
42. Weisinger JR, Bellorin-Font E. Magnesium and phosphorus. *Lancet.* 1998;352:391–396.
43. Polderman KH, Bloemers FW, Peerdeman SM, et al. Hypomagnesemia and hypophosphatemia at admission in patients with severe head injury. *Crit Care Med.* 2000;28: 2022–2025.
44. Haglin L, Burman LA, Nilsson M. High prevalence of hypophosphataemia amongst patients with infectious diseases. A retrospective study. *J Intern Med.* July 1999;246: 45–52.
45. Story DA, Ronco C, Bellomo R. Trace element and vitamin concentrations and losses in critically ill patients treated with continuous venovenous hemofiltration. *Crit Care Med.* 1999;27:220–223.
46. Schorah CJ, Downing C, Piripitsi A, et al. Total vitamin C, ascorbic acid, and dehydroascorbic acid concentrations in plasma of critically ill patients. *Am J Clin Nutr.* 1996; 63:760–765.
47. Kharb S, Ghalaut VS, Ghalaut PS. Alpha tocopherol concentration in serum of critically ill patients. *J Assoc Physicians India.* 1999;47:400–402.
48. Lipschitz DA, Mitchell CO. The correctability of the nutritional, immune, and hematopoietic manifestations of protein calorie malnutrition in the elderly. *J Am Coll Nutr.* 1982;1:17–25.
49. Coodley GO, Loveless MO, Merrill TM. The HIV wasting syndrome: a review. *J Acquir Immune Defic Syndr.* 1994;7:681–694.
50. Chandra RK. 1990 McCollum Award lecture. Nutrition and immunity: lessons from the past and new insights into the future. *Am J Clin Nutr.* 1991;53:1087–1101.
51. Payette H, Hanussaik N, Boutier V, et al. Muscle strength and functional mobility in relation to lean body mass in free-living frail elderly women. *Eur J Clin Nutr.* 1998;52: 45–53.
52. Russell DM, Prendergast PJ, Darby PL, et al. A comparison between muscle function and body composition in anorexia nervosa: the effect of refeeding. *Am J Clin Nutr.* 1983;38:229–237.
53. Vaz M, Thangam S, Prabhu A, et al. Maximal voluntary contraction as a functional indicator of adult chronic undernutrition. *Br J Nutr.* 1996;76:9–15.
54. Arora NS, Rochester DF. Effect of body weight and muscularity on human diaphragm muscle mass, thickness, and area. *J Appl Physiol.* 1982;52:64–70.
55. Geerling BJ, Badart-Smook A, Stockbrugger RW, et al. Comprehensive nutritional status in patients with long-standing Crohn disease currently in remission. *Am J Clin Nutr.* 1998;67:919–926.

56. Jensen GL, Kita K, Fish J, et al. Nutrition risk screening characteristics of rural older persons: relation to functional limitations and health care charges. *Am J Clin Nutr.* 1997;66:819–828.

57. Boult C, Krinke UB, Urdangarin CF, et al. The validity of nutritional status as a marker for future disability and depressive symptoms among high-risk older adults. *J Am Geriatr Soc.* 1999;47:995–999.

58. Kopple JD, Zhu X, Lew NL, et al. Body weight-for-height relationships predict mortality in maintenance hemodialysis patients. *Kidney Int.* 1999;56:1136–1148.

59. Landi F, Zuccala G, Gambassi G, et al. Body mass index and mortality among older people living in the community. *J Am Geriatr Soc.* 1999;47:1072–1076.

60. Omran ML, Morley JE. Assessment of protein energy malnutrition in older persons, part I: history, examination, body composition, and screening tools. *Nutrition.* 2000; 16:50–63.

61. Vellas B, Guigoz Y, Garry PJ, et al. The Mini Nutritional Assessment (MNA) and its use in grading the nutritional state of elderly patients. *Nutrition.* 1999;15:116–122.

62. Naber TH, Schermer T, de Bree A, et al. Prevalence of malnutrition in nonsurgical hospitalized patients and its association with disease complications. *Am J Clin Nutr.* 1997;66:1232–1239.

63. Dewys WD, Begg C, Lavin PT, et al. Prognostic effect of weight loss prior to chemotherapy in cancer patients. *Am J Med.* 1980;69:491–497.

64. Hunt DR, Rowlands BJ, Johnston D. Hand grip strength—a simple prognostic indicator in surgical patients. *J Parenter Enteral Nutr.* 1985;9:701–704.

65. Windsor JA. Underweight patients and the risks of major surgery. *World J Surg.* 1993;17:165–172.

66. Studley HO. Percentage of weight loss. A basic indicator of surgical risk in patients with chronic peptic ulcer disease. *JAMA.* 1936;106:458–460.

67. Hill GL. Body composition research: implications for the practice of clinical nutrition. *J Parenter Enteral Nutr.* 1992; 16:197–218.

68. Murciano D, Rigaud D, Pingleton S, et al. Diaphragmatic function in severely malnourished patients with anorexia nervosa. Effects of renutrition. *Am J Resp Crit Care Med.* 1994;150:1569–1574.

69. Pingleton SK. Nutrition in chronic critical illness. *Clin Chest Med.* 2001;22:149–163.

70. Farber MO, Mannix ET. Tissue wasting in patients with chronic obstructive pulmonary disease. *Neurol Clin.* 2000; 18:245–262.

71. Wouters EF. Nutrition and metabolism in COPD. *Chest.* 2000;117:274S–280S.

72. Aubier M, Murciano D, Lecocguic Y, et al. Effect of hypophosphatemia on diaphragmatic contractility in patients with acute respiratory failure. *N Engl J Med.* 1985;313: 420–424.

73. Aubier M, Viires N, Piquet J, et al. Effects of hypocalcemia on diaphragmatic strength generation. *J Appl Physiol.* 1985;58:2054–2061.

74. Zaloga GP. Hypocalcemia in critically ill patients. *Crit Care Med.* 1992;20:251–262.

75. Carlstedt F, Lind L, Rastad J, et al. Parathyroid hormone and ionized calcium levels are related to the severity of illness and survival in critically ill patients. *Eur J Clin Invest.* 1998;28:898–903.

76. Desai TK, Carlson RW, Geheb MA. Prevalence and clinical implications of hypocalcemia in acutely ill patients in a medical intensive care setting. *Am J Med.* 1988;84:209–214.

77. Desai TK, Carlson RW, Thill-Baharozian M, et al. A direct relationship between ionized calcium and arterial pressure among patients in an intensive care unit. *Crit Care Med.* 1988;16:578–582.

78. Vincent JL, Bredas P, Jankowski S, et al. Correction of hypocalcaemia in the critically ill: what is the haemodynamic benefit? *Intensive Care Med.* 1995;21:838–841.

79. Saudny-Unterberger H, Martin JG, Gray-Donald K. Impact of nutritional support on functional status during an acute exacerbation of chronic obstructive pulmonary disease. *Am J Respir Crit Care Med.* 1997;156:794–799.

80. Bassili HR, Deitel M. Effect of nutritional support on weaning patients off mechanical ventilators. *J Parenter Enteral Nutr.* 1981;5:161–163.

81. Larca L, Greenbaum DM. Effectiveness of intensive nutritional regimes in patients who fail to wean from mechanical ventilation. *Crit Care Med.* 1982;10:297–300.

82. Covelli HD, Black JW, Olsen MS, et al. Respiratory failure precipitated by high carbohydrate loads. *Ann Intern Med.* 1981;95:579–581.

83. Dark DS, Pingleton SK, Kerby GR. Hypercapnia during weaning. A complication of nutritional support. *Chest.* 1985;88:141–143.

84. Delafosse B, Bouffard Y, Viale JP, et al. Respiratory changes induced by parenteral nutrition in postoperative patients undergoing inspiratory pressure support ventilation. *Anesthesiology.* 1987;66:393–396.

85. Dardaine VMD, Dequin P-FMD, Ripault HMD, et al. Outcome of older patients requiring ventilatory support in intensive care: impact of nutritional status. *J Am Geriatr.* Soc 2001;49:564–570.

86. Casalino E, Mendoza-Sassi G, Wolff M, et al. Predictors of short- and long-term survival in HIV-infected patients admitted to the ICU. *Chest.* 1998;113:421–429.

87. Fiaccadori E, Lombardi M, Leonardi S, et al. Prevalence and clinical outcome associated with preexisting malnutrition in acute renal failure: a prospective cohort study. *J Am Soc Nephrol.* 1999;10:581–593.

88. Schwann TA, Habib RH, Zacharias A, et al. Effects of body size on operative, intermediate, and long-term outcomes after coronary artery bypass operation. *Ann Thorac Surg.* 2001;71:521–530.

89. Rady MY, Ryan T, Starr NJ. Clinical characteristics of preoperative hypoalbuminemia predict outcome of cardiovascular surgery. *J Parenter Enteral Nutr.* 1997;21:81–90.

90. McClave SA, Sexton LK, Spain DA, et al. Enteral tube feeding in the intensive care unit: factors impeding adequate delivery. *Crit Care Med.* 1999;27:1252–1256.

91. McClave SA, Snider HL, Spain DA. Preoperative issues in clinical nutrition. *Chest.* 1999;115:64S–70S.

92. Tran DD, Cuesta MA, van Leeuwen PA, et al. Risk factors for multiple organ system failure and death in critically injured patients. *Surgery.* 1993;114:21–30.

93. Tran DD, Van Onselen EB, Wensink AJ, et al. Factors related to multiple organ system failure and mortality in a surgical intensive care unit. *Nephrol Dial Transplant.* 1994; 9:172–178.

94. Selberg O, Bottcher J, Tusch G, et al. Identification of high- and low-risk patients before liver transplantation: a prospective cohort study of nutritional and metabolic parameters in 150 patients. *Hepatology.* 1997;25:652–657.

95. Plochl W, Pezawas L, Artemiou O, et al. Nutritional status, ICU duration and ICU mortality in lung transplant recipients. *Intensive Care Med.* 1996;22:1179–1185.

96. Ireton-Jones CS, Francis C. Obesity: nutrition support practice and application to critical care. *Nutr Clin Prac.* 1995;10:144–149.

97. Grady KL, Constanzo MR, Fisher S, et al. Preoperative obesity is associated with decreased survival after heart transplantation. *J Heart Lung Transplant.* 1996;15:863–871.

98. Funnell IC, Bornman PC, Weakley SP, et al. Obesity: an important prognostic factor in acute pancreatitis. *Br J Surg.* 1993;80:484–486.

99. Tsai CJ. Is obesity a significant prognostic factor in acute pancreatitis? *Dig Dis Sci.* 1998;43:2251–2254.

100. Suazo-Barahona J, Carmona-Sanchez R, Robles-Diaz G, et al. Obesity: a risk factor for severe acute biliary and alcoholic pancreatitis. *Am J Gastroenterol.* 1998;93:1324–1328.

101. Gottschlich MM, Mayes T, Khoury JC, et al. Significance of obesity on nutritional, immunologic, hormonal, and clinical outcome parameters in burns. *J Am Diet Assoc.* 1993;93:1261–1268.

102. De Jonghe B, Appere-De-Vechi C, Fournier M, et al. A prospective survey of nutritional support practices in intensive care unit patients: what is prescribed? What is delivered? *Crit Care Med.* 2001;29:8–12.

103. Adam S, Batson S. A study of problems associated with the delivery of enteral feed in critically ill patients in five ICUs in the UK. *Intensive Care Med.* 1997;23:261–266.

104. Montejo JC. Enteral nutrition-related gastrointestinal complications in critically ill patients: a multicenter study. The Nutritional and Metabolic Working Group of the Spanish Society of Intensive Care Medicine and Coronary Units. *Crit Care Med.* 1999;27:1447–1453.

CHAPTER 2

The Metabolic Response to Stress and Alterations in Nutrient Metabolism

Robert G. Martindale, M.D., Ph.D., F.A.C.S., Scott A. Shikora, M.D., F.A.C.S., Reid Nishikawa, Pharm.D., F.C.S.H.P., B.C.N.S.P., John K. Siepler, Pharm.D., B.C.N.S.P.

Introduction 11
An Overview of the Stress Responses 11
The Mediators of the Response 13
Nutrient Alterations During the Stress Response 14
Protein Metabolism 15
Carbohydrate Metabolism 15
Lipid Metabolism 16
Fluid and Electrolytes 17
Vitamins and Minerals 17
Conclusions 17
References 18

Introduction

The metabolic response to severe injury, illness, and sepsis has been extensively studied since the pioneering work by Cuthbertson et al.[1–3] In general, it represents significant physiologic alterations from normal metabolic homeostasis designed to enhance the likelihood of survival. These stress responses are generally characterized by hypermetabolism, hypercatabolism, persistent lean body mass wasting, hyperglycemia, and fluid accumulation. Should the insult be short lived, the patient will usually recover as a result of these processes. However, with prolonged illness, protein-calorie malnutrition and its consequences are inevitable.

The metabolic response to stress or injury is a complex interaction of numerous mediators, including nervous system input, hormones, and cytokine messengers. Although the effects on the organism are relatively well described, the events that take place at the nuclear level have only recently begun to be unraveled. Recent data showing changes in transcription rates of messenger RNA and the production of substances like heat shock protein may in fact alter the outcome and modulate the hyperdynamic response to insults. These in addition to the complex metabolic responses already described make this elaborate system even more difficult to fully comprehend.

The importance of nutritional intervention for the metabolically stressed patient cannot be overstated. For the past 3 decades, physicians have begun to understand the molecular and biological effects of nutrients in supporting the response and maintaining homeostasis in the metabolically stressed population. Since the work by Studley,[4] investigators have acknowledged the adverse effects of malnutrition and the importance of nutritional support in optimizing intensive care unit and surgical outcome, but only recently have these assumptions been verified with well-designed clinical studies. However, nutritional intervention can be difficult to provide for this patient population because of alterations in nutrient utilization and limitations of nutrient delivery associated with critical illness. This chapter will briefly review the metabolic response to stress and its effects on nutrient metabolism. Proper macronutrient and micronutrient provision will be covered in subsequent chapters.

An Overview of the Stress Responses (Tables 2.1 and 2.2)

As previously stated, the stress responses to any injurious event such as trauma, sepsis, or surgery are a characteristic network of physiologic responses employed by the organism in an effort to survive. These pro-

TABLE 2.1

Physiologic Changes Associated with Stress Response		
Response	**Physiologic Benefit**	**Potential Physiologic Risk**
Protein catabolism	Ensure adequate substrate for acute phase response, gluconeogenesis, wound healing, immune function	Functional tissue loss Hypoalbuminemia
Hyperglycemia	Ensure substrate availability	Hyperglycemia Immune dysfunction Osmotic diuresis Hyperosmolarity Protein glycosylation
Sodium and water retention	Maintain intravascular volume	Hyponatremia Hypervolemia Pulmonary edema Congestive heart failure Hypokalemia Hypomagnesemia
Increase heart rate and cardiac output	Maintain organ perfusion	Increase cardiac work Increase myocardial ischemia Arrhythmias
Hypercoagulability; Increased platelet aggregation	Hemostasis	Microvascular thrombosis Deep venous thrombosis Pulmonary embolus
Increase sympathetic tone	Increase cardiac output Increase substrate availability (glycogenolysis, lipolysis)	Increase myocardial irritability Hyperglycemia Inhibits insulin Shunting of blood flow to central organs, away from gut

TABLE 2.2

The Metabolic Alterations of the Stress Response	
Metabolic Parameters	**Rate Compared to Normal**
Resting energy expenditure	I
Oxygen consumption	I
Carbohydrate metabolism	
Blood sugar concentration	I
Gluconeogenesis	I
Glycogenolysis	I
Tissue glucose uptake/oxidation	I
Fat metabolism	
Ketogenesis	N/D
Lipolysis	I
Tissue uptake/oxidation	I
Protein metabolism	
Net synthesis	D
Net breakdown	I
Hepatic synthesis	I
Muscle synthesis	D
Ureagenesis	I

I = Increased
D = Decreased
N = No change from normal

cesses were first described by Cuthbertson over 50 years ago and have been extensively studied since. In simplest terms, these responses are activated to liberate stored nutrients and substrates to support the healing process and endogenously nourish the organism. These nutrients are utilized as oxidative fuels and for the synthesis of building blocks essential for the stabilization of organ function, maintenance of immunocompetency, and repair of injured tissue.[5,6] The byproducts of these efforts are the commonly encountered derangements of critical illness including fluid and sodium overload, hypermetabolism, hypercatabolism, and glucose intolerance.

The duration and severity of these responses are quite variable. Numerous factors will determine the extent of the metabolic responses. These include the degree of insult, the persistence of the insult, the host response, the nutritional status of the host, and the timing in relation to previous insults. For simplicity, the metabolic responses to infection, injury, and catabolic illness can be divided into local responses and systemic responses. The local responses to insult yield a predictable neurohormonal response that increases metabolic activity and increases local cellular work. The increases in energy consumption by the inflammatory cells and fibroblasts allow for collagen synthesis, matrix protein synthesis, and wound repair. The systemic response is manifested by the elevation of the "counter-regulatory hormones" such as cortisol, epinephrine, and glucagon, as well as the elaboration of the cytokine cascade. This systemic response results in a myriad of effects including altered protein synthesis, increased nitric oxide synthase, and an increase in leucocyte endothelial cell adhesion molecules.[7] When the systemic insult becomes overwhelming, distinct remote organ and tissue injury can occur.[8] In addition to the hormonal and cytokine response, other mediators propagate the responses including reactive oxygen metabolites, nitric oxide, and archidonic acid products.[9]

The classical description of the stress response by Cuthbertson employed a two-phase theory.[1] The ebb phase occurs immediately after injury and lasts approximately 24 to 48 hours. During this short-lived period, there is an increase in sympathetic activity and a stimulation of the hypothalamic-pituitary axis.[10] This period is characterized by marked hypometabolism and decreased oxygen consumption.[10] It is now recognized that these findings are primarily the result of hypovolemia leading to decreased cardiac output and inadequate oxygen transport to the tissues.[11] In contrast to the ebb phase, the second phase, called the acute or flow phase, is one of hypermetabolism, catabolism, and increased oxygen consumption.[12] These mechanisms are known to be mediated by cytokines, hormones, and the afferent nervous signals from the injured tissues.[13] It is during this phase that there is an active liberation of endogenous substrates such as glycogen-derived glucose, skeletal muscle-derived and labile amino acids, and adipose tissue fatty acids.[5,6,14,15] Since glycogen stores are limited, this source of glucose is rapidly depleted.[5] The need for readily available glucose will then be met by enhanced muscle protein breakdown to provide amino acids for hepatic gluconeogenesis.[5,6,10]

The net effect of these metabolic pathways is the liberation of peripherally stored substrates to meet the energy and substrate requirements of the major organ systems. Each substrate plays a vital physiologic role in the stress response. Glucose is an important fuel for the central nervous system, the wound, and the immune system, all of which are metabolically active during stress.[5,6,12] The fatty acids provide a readily available energy source for cardiac and skeletal muscle, the liver, and many other tissues.[5,6,12] Although some liberated amino acids are utilized for gluconeogenesis, the majority are required for the synthesis of the acute phase proteins, for thermogenesis, and as the precursors for tissue repair.[5,6,12,15]

Recovery, should it occur, leads to a decrease in the metabolic rate, a replenishing of the depleted body energy stores, and a rebuilding of the lost lean body mass. Catabolic, metabolic rates, fluid status and insulin sensitivity all return to pre-injury levels and homeostasis is renewed. Anabolism becomes the predominant event.

The Mediators of the Response

The stress responses to illness are mediated by a number of different hormones, protein messengers, and nervous activity that work in concert. There is tremendous synergy of function and influence on other factors. While much has been learned of the major players in this response, much still needs to be elucidated.

The counter-regulatory hormones

These are the "fight or flight" hormones such as glucagon, catecholamines, and the glucocorticoids. They are found to be markedly elevated during surgical stress, trauma, sepsis, and critical illness.[16,17] The net result of their elevation is increased protein mobilization, hyperglycemia, insulin resistance, and increased lipolysis. Glucagon stimulates gluconeogenesis, cortisol increases net protein catabolism, and the catecholamines result in glucose intolerance.[16,18]

Cytokines and other mediators

Cytokines are peptide messengers secreted by mononuclear cells (macrophages) as a normal part of the inflammatory response during surgical stress and critical illness.[19–20] Cytokines act as hormonal regulators of the immune system. During sepsis and trauma, elevated levels of cytokines have been reported.[20–22] Important cytokines include tumor necrosis factor (TNF)/cachectin, interleukin-1 (IL-1), and interleukin-6 (IL-6). The levels of interleukin-10 (IL-10), interleukin-8 (IL-8), and transforming growth factor β (TGF-β), are also elevated during trauma or injury; however, their ultimate roles remain to be defined.[23] Correlations have been reported between the degree of up regulation of cytokine production and severity of illness and also the probability of death.[24] A study was conducted in 338 critically ill patients with a Physiologic State Classification system. The mean "injury severity score" (ISS) was 27.6. IL-1, IL-6, IL-8, and TNF levels were measured by enzyme-linked immunosorbent assay (ELISA). This Physiologic State Classification system allowed for classification of the physiologic and cytokine mediator response to trauma and permitted stratification of severity in post trauma illness.[24]

TNF induces a net catabolic state by (1) mediating increased catabolism at the level of the specific tissues, (2) causing anorexia, and (3) activating the hypothalamic-pituitary-adrenal axis.[20,21] The effects of TNF are dose related and can potentially result in catastrophic tissue injury and lethal shock.

IL-1 is a key mediator of the acute phase response. In low concentrations, IL-1 is beneficial to the host and stimulates defense mechanisms. However, during critical illness and surgical stress, it has been reported to be associated with the development of fever, hypotension, inflammation, and accelerated protein breakdown.[25–27]

IL-6 is associated with stimulation of the release of hepatic acute phase reactants.[28,29] C-reactive protein, fibronectin, antitrypsin, ceruloplasmin, and 1-acid glycoprotein are considered acute phase reactants. Trace elements including zinc, selenium, and iron decrease while copper increases in response to IL-6.[30]

The release of acute phase reactants is part of the Systemic Inflammatory Response Syndrome (SIRS), a normal host response to an inflammatory process, infection, trauma, pancreatitis, or any surgical stress. It is characterized by generalized activation of the vascular endothelium and polymorphonuclear cells. The net result is the mobilization of endogenous substrates for tissue repair, energy, and support of the immune system. SIRS is induced by cytokine production, where TNF, IL-6, and IL-1 play a major role.[31] Cytokines may demonstrate a synergistic effect in producing the adverse effects on substrate metabolism, such as the combination of IL-1 and TNF.

Cytokines or counter regulatory hormones alone cannot fully explain the effect on skeletal muscle proteolysis during sepsis. Antagonists to TNF, IL-1, and IL-6 have demonstrated reduction but not normalization of protein breakdown rates.[32,33] In addition, cytokine-mediated metabolic alterations can explain the inability of adequate nitrogen and energy substrates to effectively result in complete lean tissue repletion.[34,35]

Nutrient Alterations During the Stress Response

The alteration in nutrient homeostasis elicited following metabolic stress has presumably evolved to enhance the chances for survival. However, it is well described that the host response itself at times becomes maladaptive.[8] When reviewing nutrient metabolism, one must consider total body energy stores.[36] Adipose tissue triglyceride storage in the average 70 kg male consists of approximately 140,000 calories. Muscle contains approximately 24,000 calories of protein, 2,000 calories of glycogen and approximately 3,000 calories from triglyceride. The liver contains 300 calories of glucose in the form of glycogen and 500 calories available from triglyceride.

During unstressed starvation, the body mainly relies on mobilization of endogenous adipose stores for its calorie requirements. Adipose utilization follows a brief period in which glycogen stores are mobilized. In situations of unstressed starvation, most glycogen stores are depleted within 18 to 24 hours. During the initial 24 to 48 hours of unstressed starvation, the basic energy needs are supplied by glycogen and protein with some contribution from fat stores. Following the initial 48 to 72 hours of unstressed starvation, there is a relative increase in the utilization of fat stores in most tissues, with the exception of tissues that have an obligate glucose requirement, such as red cells, white cells, and renal medulla.

The brain also has an initial obligate glucose requirement; however, over 3 to 5 days will transition to the utilization of fatty acids for energy.[37] During unstressed starvation, there is a general decrease in energy expenditure and a change in the insulin-to-glucagon ratio to favor mobilization of stored fuels and minimize the loss of lean body tissue. Protein catabolism is kept at a minimum. However, it is important to realize that there is very little protein storage per se, and that any protein utilized for gluconeogenesis and acute phase protein synthesis should be considered as loss of functional myofibrillar protein.

The adequately nourished human body stores approximately 100 gm of labile protein nitrogen and is designed to withstand about one week of limited stress without supplementation.[38] However, patients with limited protein reserves or a more intense stress response may be metabolically compromised in less time. Using sophisticated neutron activation analysis to measure body composition, Hill has been able to accurately identify the degree of wasting.[39] He demonstrated that most physiologic functions become impaired when 20% of body protein is depleted. Wasting has been shown to impair most organ systems, including respiratory,[40] cardiac,[41,42] and the immune system.[43]

As opposed to unstressed starvation, hypermetabolism associated with major catabolic illness, surgery, or trauma results in significant alterations in nutrient homeostasis. As mentioned earlier, systemic hormonal responses to the metabolic insult results in increased ACTH, epinephrine, glucagon, and cortisol production, as well as a host of proinflammatory cytokines such as IL-1, IL-2, IL-6, and TNF in addition to other systemic mediators. These factors, as well as localized tissue ischemia and acidosis, will amplify the catabolic response. Similar to unstressed starvation, glycogen stores are exhausted within 12 to 24 hours. In contrast to unstressed starvation, hypermetabolism and gluconeogenesis continue at an accelerated rate.[44] Gluconeogenesis yields the majority of the carbohydrate source to the tissues that require glucose. Muscle protein, in addition to providing the carbon skeleton for gluconeogensis, serves as a substrate for acute phase protein synthesis by providing the necessary amino acids. As a result of the catabolic insult, the liver reprioritizes its protein synthesis from the production of visceral protein to acute phase proteins.[45] Glutamine and alanine are released from the muscle, delivering glutamine to the gastrointestinal tract and kidney and alanine to the liver for gluconeogenesis.

Hyperglycemia is a common occurrence during the hypermetabolic state and is thought to result from an accelerated gluconeogenesis and the relative peripheral insulin resistance. This hyperglycemia associated with hypermetabolic stress is seen despite the usual compensatory increase in insulin release commonly noted in ICU patients. The main site of insulin resistance during stress is at the peripheral tissue level.[46] The specific defect in the hyperdynamic state has been recently reported to be in GLUT 4 (intracellular glucose transport protein 4).[45] One recent paper evaluated postoperative insulin resistance and showed it to be an independent risk factor predicting the postoperative length of stay.[46]

Protein Metabolism

The critically ill patient is generally hypercatabolic secondary to marked proteolysis that exceeds protein synthesis.[47–49] This was confirmed by Wolfe and associates who using stable isotopes to measure whole body protein anabolism, determined that there was an increase in whole body protein anabolism despite a net body protein loss from massive catabolic activity.[50] This is in stark contrast to the catabolism of starvation, where the net protein loss is secondary to decreases in protein synthesis. The increased protein breakdown of critical illness is a result of large increases in protein degradation. Marked skeletal muscle catabolism is necessary to provide a substrate for immune function, tissue repair, and inflammation.[51] These processes result in an increase in urea excretion in the urine, which reflects the increased net protein catabolism. The net result is a significant decrease in the lean body mass.

It is not clear that this apparent obligatory protein catabolism is always associated with a negative outcome. In addition, it appears that protein catabolism persists despite the provision of apparently adequate nutrition support. The increased rate of net protein catabolism occurs in patients who have trauma, sepsis, and other critical illnesses. In fact, a loss of 10% to 20% of body protein is not uncommon in a critically ill patient whose illness persists for more than 5 to 7 days. Much of this loss is due to the depletion of skeletal muscle. The importance of this protein loss as it relates to commonly measured outcome parameters, such as length of time on mechanical ventilation, length of intensive care unit stay, and length of hospital stay is questionable. The influence of catabolism on the quality of life after discharge may be significant, but has not been clearly elucidated.[48]

Compared to those patients with simple starvation, the protein needs of critically ill and hyperdynamic patients are significantly increased. In concert with muscle proteolysis from the metabolic stress are increased ureagenesis, increased hepatic synthesis of acute phase proteins, increased urinary nitrogen losses, and the increased use of amino acids as oxidative substrate for energy production. Although the accelerated catabolic rate is not reversed by provision of glucose lipid or protein,[52] the protein synthetic rate is at least partially responsive to amino acid infusions. In many cases, nitrogen balance is attained through the support of protein synthesis.[53,54] Current recommendations for stressed patients are for 15% to 20% of the total nutrient intake to be provided as protein or 1.5 to 2.0 g/kg/d.[55,56] Protein administration in quantities greater than 2.0 g/kg/d has not been shown to be beneficial and in fact often results in azotemia. If provided with excess calories, it may also increase carbon dioxide production, further compromising patients with respiratory insufficiency.[57,58]

Carbohydrate Metabolism

Glucose, at least initially, is the primary fuel for the central nervous system (CNS), bone marrow, RBC, and injured tissue. A minimum of about 100 g/d is necessary to maintain CNS function as well as providing substrate to drive the Krebs cycle. In the metabolically stressed adult, the maximum rate of glucose oxidation is 4–6 mg/kg/min,[51] roughly equivalent to 400–600 g/d in a 70 kg person. Provision of glucose greater than this rate usually results in lipogenesis, hepatic steatosis, and hyperglycemia. In the hypermetabolic patient, a significant portion of the oxidized glucose will be derived from endogenous amino acid substrates via gluconeogenesis and from the Cori cycle.[59] In the severely stressed patient, up to one-half of the glucose oxidized may be provided via gluconeogenesis. In the hypermetabolic patient, this endogenous glucose production is not suppressed by exogenous glucose administration.[14]

In fact, providing additional glucose in these situations can lead to significant hyperglycemia with its associated complications. Further exacerbating this situation is the infusion of concentrated dextrose solutions such as with parenteral nutrition, medications, and resuscitative fluids. In addition, other therapies, such as peritoneal dialysis, may provide an occult source of significant dextrose.[60] Exogenous insulin delivery to offset the elevated serum glucose levels tends to be ineffective in increasing cellular glucose uptake in critically ill patients, since the rate of glucose oxidation is already maximized and because endogenous insulin concentrations are already elevated.

Several investigators have found that there is a sustained increase in plasma glucose in models simulating critical illness.[59] These authors and others demonstrated a sustained hyperglycemia associated with increased glucose production accompanied by elevated insulin levels. The increased glucose production was greater when glucagon, epinephrine, and cortisol were all given together. When this occurred, urinary nitrogen excretion was also increased. In studies simulating stress in dogs, peripheral glucose uptake was not increased over controls, also suggesting that the hyperglycemia seen is the result of increased glucose production.[61] Thus it is clear that both glucose oxidation and hepatic glucose production are increased in critically ill patients. The result of this and an unchanged peripheral uptake is a persistent hyperglycemia.

Complications of excess glucose administration include hyperglycemia, protein glycosylation, hyperosmolar states, immunosuppression, excessive carbon dioxide production associated with increased work of breathing, and hepatic steatosis.[14,62–66] Therefore it is recommended that glucose be provided at a rate ≤5 mg/kg/min or roughly 50% to 60% of total energy requirements in critically ill patients. Even when limiting the glucose load, patients need to be monitored closely for hyperglycemia.

Lipid Metabolism

In critically ill patients there is an increased rate of fatty acid oxidation. Plasma linoleic and arachidonic acid decrease, while oleic acid increases.[67] This occurs as a result of increased lipolysis that is associated with epinephrine-induced β_2-adrenergic stimulation.[68] Free fatty acids are released into the plasma at a rate far exceeding their oxidation. Excess fatty acids undergo hepatic re-esterification, with resultant accelerated hepatic triglyceride formation.[69] The resultant fatty acid profile is consistent with apparent essential fatty acid depletion. In addition, due to the hyperglycemia that often occurs, the elevated insulin levels can reduce lipid mobilization from body fat stores. Thus, in the absence of nutritional fat delivery, a clinical picture of essential fatty acid deficiency can develop earlier than occurs with starvation.

Goodenough and Wolfe studied free fatty acid and energy metabolism in six severely burned patients who were provided parenteral nutritional support.[70] A mixed caloric fuel source was used containing dextrose, fat, and amino acids. A stable isotope methodology using 1,2-13C-palmitate bound to albumin was continuously infused to determine free fatty acid turnover and oxidation. The findings of suppression of the endogenous fatty acid turnover and oxidation were identified by the infusion of parenteral nutritional support. This was thought to occur as a result of the relative increased insulin levels. Fat emulsion contributed approximately 25% of the energy released during parenteral feeding, with endogenous FFA oxidation as the major component. This study suggests that direct oxidation of intravenous fat emulsion does not contribute to the energy required for substrate utilization; rather it serves mainly to preserve endogenous fat stores.[70]

Although lipids have their limitations, they remain an important exogenous substrate in critically ill patients as they can facilitate protein sparing, decrease the risk of excess carbohydrate, limit volume delivery by their high caloric density, and provide essential fatty acids. Daily fat when given in moderation can be provided without adverse effects, as critically ill patients efficiently metabolize moderate amounts of exogenous lipids.[71] Fat may comprise between 10% to 30% of total energy requirements. If delivered parenterally, a minimum of 3% to 5% should be given as essential fatty acids to prevent deficiency.[55] If delivered enterally, the amount of essential fats given will depend on the patient's ability to absorb and digest the lipid. Hypermetabolic patients should be monitored for tolerance of lipid delivery, especially if levels are provided in excess of the usual 10% to 30%, as it may cause metabolic complications such as hyperlipidemia, coagulopathies, impaired immune function by several mechanisms, and hypoxemia resulting from impaired diffusing capacity and ventilation/perfusion abnormalities.[58,72] These complications are associated with intravenous infusions and are not only due to the quantity of lipid provided, but also result from the rate of delivery.[73] The rate of infusion should not exceed 0.1 g/kg/h. The complications of lipid infusion may be minimized by infusing lipids over longer periods of time, commonly 18 to 24 hours while monitoring serum triglyceride levels and liver function tests to assure tolerance.[62] As with glucose, some standard critical care treatment interventions may also function as occult sources of lipid infusion. Examples include lipid-based medications such as propofol.

Fluid and Electrolytes

Critically ill patients have significant gains in total body water compared to normal unstressed individuals. Much of this occurs when the patient is being resuscitated following the injury or illness that precipitates the critical illness. However, the hypermetabolic responses to stress also cause avid fluid and salt retention. There is a 15% to 20% increase in the expansion of the extracellular fluid space. The extent of the increase in total body water is not only related to the severity of the injury or insult, but is also affected by patient age and the quantity of intravenous fluids given after the injury. Total body water has been measured in patients after sepsis and trauma who were found to have a positive fluid balance of an average of 9–13 liters when compared with controls. Even after completion of resuscitation, body water remains about 5–8 liters elevated above normal.[44] The bulk of this increase is extracellular water. It also appears that older patients take a longer time to resolve the positive fluid balance following injury.[74]

Fluid and electrolyte provision can vary greatly in the critically ill. Altered electrolyte levels can impair organ function and are usually manifested by cardiac dysrhythmias, intestinal ileus, and impaired mentation. Fluid and electrolytes should be provided to maintain adequate urine output and normal serum electrolyte concentrations, with emphasis on the intracellular electrolytes, potassium, phosphorus, and magnesium. Optimal levels are required to maximize protein synthesis and the attainment of nitrogen balance. Standard fluid requirements are estimated at 35 mL/kg with increased requirements for those with increased losses (e.g., high output fistulas, ostomies, drains, significant burns or open wounds) and increased renal solute loads, or decreased for those with fluid restrictions (e.g., kidney, liver, heart failure). Once nutrition support is initiated, fluid balance, body weight, and electrolytes should be monitored closely as they may change rapidly once adequate protein and calories have been provided and the patient shifts from catabolism to anabolism.

Vitamins and Minerals

Currently there are no specific guidelines regarding vitamin and mineral requirements in the critically ill. This controversy is addressed in Chapter 7. It is estimated that micronutrient requirements are increased during stress and sepsis due to increased metabolic demands; however, consistent objective data to support universal supplementation are lacking.

Studies currently in progress are addressing supplementation at various levels and combinations. The routine practice of providing more than therapeutic doses of single vitamins or minerals in various metabolic situations may be detrimental by upsetting the delicate balance of metabolic pathways.[62] Therefore, current recommendations are to provide the recommended dietary allowance for vitamins and minerals in the critically ill until further research definitely defines optimal dosing.[55] Most currently available complete enteral formulations contain these recommended levels when they are provided at specified volumes. If adequate volumes are not tolerated over several days, patients should be supplemented intravenously.

Conclusions

Critically ill or traumatized patients present a unique array of problems for the clinician. As a result of their injury, they are hypermetabolic and hypercatabolic. In addition, there are metabolic alterations to the normal packaging and utilization of nutrients. Nutritional support of these metabolically stressed populations should complement this evolutionary response and should have the objectives of attempting to preserve lean body mass, maintain or up regulate the immune function, and sustain vital organ function while minimizing or averting metabolic complications. A litany of novel feeding approaches is now undergoing evaluation, such as preoperative carbohydrate loading, designer enteral formulas, biological mediators such as monoclonal antibodies, and anabolic agents. However, the basics of nutritional and metabolic support must be addressed before any new and novel approaches are attempted. These basics include early enteral feeding, adequate fluid resuscitation, appropriate protein, calorie, and micronutrient administration, minimally invasive surgery, epidural and regional anesthesia, pain control, coverage of open wounds, minimization of blood loss, and temperature control. Only through the use of sound critical care and intelligent nutritional support can we hope to maximize the potential for survival for the critically ill patient population.

References

1. Cuthbertson D. The physiology of convalescence after injury. *Br Med Bull.* 1945;3:96–102.
2. Moore FD. *Metabolic Care of the Surgical Patient.* Philadelphia: WB Saunders; 1959.
3. Kinney J. Metabolic responses of the critically ill patient. *Crit Care Clin.* 1995;11:569–574.
4. Studley HO. Percentage of weight loss a basic indicator of surgical risk in patients with chronic peptic ulcer. *JAMA.* 1936;458–460.
5. Blackburn GL. Nutrition in surgical patients. In: Hardy JD, Kukora JS, Pass HI, eds. *Hardy's Textbook of Surgery.* 2nd ed. Philadelphia: JB Lippincott; 1988:86–104.
6. Hensle TW, Askanazi J. Metabolism and nutrition in the perioperative period. *J Urol.* 1988;139:229–239.
7. Fischer J. Metabolism in surgical patients: protein, carbohydrate, and fat utilization by oral and parenteral routes. In: Sabiston D, ed. *Textbook of Surgery.* 16th ed. Philadelphia: WB Saunders; 2001:90–130.
8. Meldrum DR, Cleveland JC, Moore EE, et al. Adaptive and maladaptive mechanism of cellular priming. *Ann Surg.* 1997;226:587–598.
9. Hasselgren PO. Pathways of muscle protein breakdown in injury and sepsis. *Curr Opin Clin Nutr Metab Care.* 1999;2:155–160.
10. Douglas RG, Shaw JHF. Metabolic response to sepsis and trauma. *Br J Surg.* 1989;76:115–122.
11. Bessey PQ, Downey RS, Monafo WW. Metabolic response to injury and critical illness. In: Civetta JM, Taylor RW, Kirby RR, eds. *Critical Care.* 2nd ed. Philadelphia: JB Lippincott; 1992:427–440.
12. Wilmore DW, Aulick LH. Systemic responses to injury and the healing wound. *J Parenter Enteral Nutr.* 1980;4:147–151.
13. Cerra FB, Upson D, Angelico R, et al. Branch chains support postoperative protein synthesis. *Surgery.* 1982;92:192–198.
14. Cerra FB. Hypermetabolism, organ failure, and metabolic support. *Surgery.* 1987;92:1–14.
15. Rennie MJ, Harrison R. Effects of injury, disease, and malnutrition on protein metabolism in man: unanswered questions. *Lancet.* 1984;5:323–325.
16. Bessey PQ, Watters JM, Aoki TT, et al. Combined hormonal infusion simulates the metabolic response to injury. *Ann Surg.* 1984;200:264–281.
17. Bessey PQ, Low KA. Early hormonal changes affect the catabolic response to trauma. *Ann Surg.* 1993;218:476–489.
18. Brillon DJ, Zheng B, Campbell RG, et al. Effect of cortisol on energy expenditure and amino acid metabolism in humans. *Am J Physiol.* 1995;268:E501–E513.
19. Fong Y, Moldawer LL, Shires GT, et al. The biology of cytokines: implications in surgical injury. *Surg Gynecol Obstet.* 1990;170:363–378.
20. Starnes HF, Warren RS, Jeevanadam M, et al. Tumor necrosis factor and the acute metabolic response to injury in man. *J Clin Invest.* 1988;82:1321–1325.
21. Tracey KJ, Wei H, Manogue KR, et al. Cachectin/tumor necrosis factor induces cachexia, anemia, and inflammation. *J Exp Med.* 1988;167:1211–1227.
22. Hack CE, De Groot E, Felt-Berama RJ, et al. Increased plasma levels of interleukin-6 in sepsis. *Blood.* 1989;74:1704–1710.
23. Hill AG. Initiators and propagators of the metabolic response to injury. *World J Surg.* 2000;24:624–629.
24. Rixen D, Siegel JH, Friedman HP. "Sepsis/SIRS," physiologic classification, severity stratification, relation to cytokine elaboration and outcome prediction in post trauma critical illness. *J Trauma.* 1996;41:581–598.
25. Dinarello CA, Wolff S. The role of interleukin-1 in disease. *N Engl J Med.* 1993;328:106–113.
26. Dinarello C. The proinflammatory cytokines interleukin-1 and tumor necrosis factor and treatment of the septic shock syndrome. *J Infect Dis.* 1991;163:1177–1184.
27. Hill AG, Siegel J, Rounds J, et al. Metabolic responses to interleukin-1. *Ann Surg.* 1997;225:246–251.
28. Gabay C, Kushner I. Acute-phase proteins and other systemic responses to inflammation. *N Engl J Med.* 1999;340:448–454.
29. Tang GJ. Similarity and synergy of trauma and sepsis: role of tumor necrosis factor-alpha and interleukin-6. *Acta Anaesthesiol.* 1996;34:141–149.
30. Shenkin A. Trace elements and inflammatory response: implications for nutritional support. *Nutrition.* 1995;11:100–105.
31. Hirota M, Ogawa M. Immune response induced by surgical trauma. *Nippon Geka Gakkai Zasshi.* 1996;97:721–725.
32. Chang HR, Bistrian B. The role of cytokines in the catabolic consequences of infection and injury. *J Parenter Enteral Nutr.* 1998;22:156–166.
33. Kim PK, Deutschman CS. Inflammatory responses and mediators. *Surg Clin North Am.* 2000;80:885–894.
34. Tracey KJ, Beutler B, Lowry SJ, et al. Shock and tissue injury induced by recombinant human cachectin. *Science.* 1986;234:470–474.
35. Espat NJ, Moldawer LL, Copeland EM. Cytokine-mediated alterations in host metabolism prevent nutritional repletion in cachectic cancer patients. *J Surg Oncol.* 1995;58:77–82.
36. Cahill GF. Starvation in man. *N Engl J Med.* 1970;668:282–286.
37. Amaral JF, Caldwell MD. Metabolic response to starvation, stress, and sepsis. In: Thomas Miller, ed. *Modern Surgical Care Physiologic Foundations and Clinical Applications.* St. Louis, MO: Quality Medical Publishing, Inc.; 1998:1–37.
38. Shikora SA, Blackburn GL. Nutritional consequences of major gastrointestinal surgery. Patient outcome and starvation. *Surg Clin North Am.* 1991;71:509–521.

39. Hill GL. Body composition research. Implications for the practice of clinical nutrition. *J Parenter Enteral Nutr.* 1992; 16:197–218.
40. McMahon MM, Benotti PN, Bistrian BR. A clinical application of exercise physiology and nutritional support for the mechanically ventilated patient. *J Parenter Enteral Nutr.* 1990;14:538–542.
41. Abel RM, Grimes JB, Alonso D, et al. Adverse hemodynamic and ultrastructural changes in dog hearts subjected to protein-calorie malnutrition. *Am Heart J.* 1979;97:733–744.
42. Heymsfield SB, Bethel RA, Ansley JD, et al. Cardiac abnormalities in cachetic patients before and during repletion. *Am Heart J.* 1978;95:584–594.
43. Haw MP, Bell SJ, Blackburn GL. Potential of parenteral and enteral nutrition in inflammation and immune dysfunction: a new challenge for dietitians. *J Am Diet Assoc.* 1991;91:701–706.
44. Plank LD, Hill GL. Sequential metabolic changes following induction of systemic inflammatory response in patients with severe sepsis or major blunt trauma. *World J Surg.* 2000;24:630–638.
45. Leverve XM. Inter-organ substrate exchanges in critically ill. *Curr Opin in Clin Nutr and Metabolic Care.* 2001;4:137–142.
46. Nygren J, Thorell A, Efendic S, et al. Site of insulin resistance after surgery: the contribution of hypocaloric nutrition and bed rest. *Clin Sci (Colch).* 1997;93:137–146.
47. Bistrian B, Babineau T. Optimal protein intake in critical illness? *Crit Care Med.* 1998;26:1476–1477.
48. Wilmore DW. Does loss of body protein determine outcome in patients who are critically ill? *Ann Surg.* 1998;228: 143–145.
49. Wolfe RR, Goodenough RD, Burke JF, et al. Response of protein and urea kinetics in burn patients to different levels of protein intake. *Ann Surg.* 1983;197:163–171.
50. Nelson KM, Long CL. Physiologic basis for nutrition in sepsis. *Nutr Clin Pract.* 1989;4:6–15.
51. Wolfe RR, Allsop J, Burke J. Glucose metabolism in man: response to intravenous glucose infusion. *Metabolism.* 1979;28:210–220.
52. Elwyn DH. Nutritional requirements of adult surgical patients. *Crit Care Med.* 1980;8:9–20.
53. Cerra FB, Siegel JH, Coleman B, et al. Septic autocatabolism, a failure of exogenous nutritional support. *Ann Surg.* 1980;192:570–580.
54. Shaw J, Wildbore M, Wolfe R. Whole body protein kinetics in severely septic patients. *Ann Surg.* 1987;205:288–294.
55. Cerra F, Benitez M, Blackburn G, et al. Applied nutrition in ICU patients. *Chest* 1997;111:769–778.
56. A.S.P.E.N. Board of Directors. Practice Guidelines. *J Parenter Enteral Nutr.* 2002;26(Suppl) (in Press).
57. Hill GL. Implications of critical illness, injury, and sepsis on lean body mass and nutritional needs. *Nutrition.* 1998; 14:557–558.
58. Klein C, Stanek G, Wiles C. Overfeeding macronutrients to critically ill adults: metabolic complications. *J Am Diet Assoc.* 1998;98:795–806.
59. Heise T, Heinemann L, Starke AA. Simulated post aggression metabolism in healthy subjects: metabolic changes and insulin resistance. *Metabolism.* 1998;47:2363–2368.
60. Manji N, Shikora S, McMahon M, et al. Peritoneal dialysis for acute renal failure: overfeeding resulting from dextrose absorbed during dialysis. *Crit Care Med.* 1990;18:29–31.
61. McGuinness OP, Fugiwara T, Murrel S, et al. Impact of chronic stress hormone infusion on hepatic carbohydrate metabolism in the conscious dog. *Am J Physiol.* 1993;265: E314–E322.
62. Cresci GA, Martindale RG. Nutrition support in trauma. In: Gottschlich, MM, ed. *The Science and Practice of Nutrition Suppor.* 3rd ed. Dubuque, IA: Kendall/Hunt; 2001: 445–464.
63. McMurray JF. Wound healing with diabetes mellitus. Better glucose control for better wound healing in diabetes. *Surg Clin North Am.* 1984;64:769–778.
64. Bagdade JD, Stewart M, Walters E. Impaired granulocyte adherence. A reversible defect in host defense in patients with poorly controlled diabetes. *Diabetes.* 1978;27:677–681.
65. Jones RL, Peterson CM. Hematologic alterations in diabetes mellitus. *Am J Med.* 1981;70:339–352.
66. Hostetter MK. Handicaps to host defense. Effects of hyperglycemia on C3 and Candida Albicans. *Diabetes.* 1990; 39:271–275.
67. Barton RG. Nutrition support in critical illness. *Nutr Clin Pract.* 1994;9:127–139.
68. Demling RH, Seigne P. Metabolic management of patients with severe burns. *World J Surg.* 2000;24:673–680.
69. Wolfe RR. Substrate utilization/insulin resistance in sepsis/trauma. *Clin Endocrinol Metab.* 1997;11:645–657.
70. Goodenough RD, Wolfe RR. Effect of total parenteral nutrition on free fatty acid metabolism in burned patients. *J Parenter Enteral Nutr.* 1984;8:357–360.
71. Nordenstrom J, Carpentier Y, Askanazi J, et al. Free fatty acids mobilization and oxidation during total parenteral nutrition in trauma and infection. *Ann Surg.* 1983;198: 725–735.
72. Wan JM-F, Teo TC, Babayan VK, et al. Invited comment: Lipids and the development of immune dysfunction and infection. *J Parenter Enteral Nutr.* 1988;12(Suppl):43s–52s.
73. Jensen GL, Mascioli EA, Seidner DL. Parenteral infusion of long- and medium-chain triglycerides and reticuloendothelial system function in man. *J Parenter Enteral Nutr.* 1990;14:467–471.
74. Streat SJ, Plank LD, Hill GL. Overview of modern management of patients with critical injury and severe sepsis. *World J Surg.* 2000;24:655–663.

CHAPTER

3

Nutrition Assessment and Monitoring

Gail A. Cresci, M.S., R.D., L.D., C.N.S.D.

INTRODUCTION 21
CLINICAL ASSESSMENT 21
PHYSICAL EXAMINATION 22
CLINICAL ASSESSMENT OF BODY COMPOSITION 24
BIOCHEMICAL MEASUREMENTS 26
Immune Competence 26
Nitrogen Balance Studies 26
Serum Proteins 26
ENERGY AND PROTEIN REQUIREMENTS 27
FLUID REQUIREMENTS 28
MONITORING NUTRITION SUPPORT 28
CONCLUSIONS 29
CASE STUDY 29
Assessment 29
REFERENCES 29

Introduction

It is estimated that over 50% of hospitalized patients are malnourished upon hospital admission as well as upon discharge.[1–4] Despite the theoretical ability to adequately meet the nutritional needs of every hospitalized patient, this incidence of malnutrition is strikingly similar to the prevalence first documented in the late 1970s by Bistrian et al.[5] Preexisting malnutrition is thought to contribute to the advancement of disease in the elderly population.[6] Additionally, chronic illness, radiation, chemotherapy, nausea and vomiting, dysphasia, and constipation may further depress nutrient intake before the patient is even in the acute phase of critical illness. Malnutrition is associated with increased morbidity and mortality.[7] Therefore a nutritional assessment in the critically ill is essential to identify those who are malnourished or at risk of malnutrition, to quantify a patient's risk of developing malnutrition-related medical complications, and to monitor the adequacy of nutritional therapy.[7] Patients most likely to benefit from nutritional support are those with baseline malnutrition in whom a protracted period of starvation would otherwise occur. In well-nourished persons with short (<1 week) anticipated duration of nil *per os* status, it is very difficult to demonstrate improvement in outcome with nutrition support.[8]

Several formal approaches evaluate nutritional status linking nutrition assessment with clinical outcome. These methods utilize clinical, anthropometric, and body composition, and biochemical assessments.

Clinical Assessment

Patients in intensive care requiring nutrition intervention typically fall into three main groups: postoperative major elective surgery, major trauma, and serious sepsis. The patients grouped as major elective surgery are often moderately depleted of body protein preoperatively, and without nutrition support lose approximately another 5% or 43 gm/day body protein the first 2 weeks postoperatively.[9] Most trauma patients are young and presumed in good health prior to injury. Intensive care patients with major trauma typically are not protein depleted initially, but despite moderate nutrition support, lose a large amount of body protein in the first 10 days after trauma (~110 gm/day).[9] ICU patients with serious sepsis are usually elderly and some may have preexisting nutrition depletion as a result of cancer, medical conditions (e.g., diabetes mellitus, renal failure, hepatic failure), multiple operations, or semi-starvation. Great losses of total body protein (~150 gm/day) occur in septic patients despite aggressive nutrition support sufficient to result in a gain in total body fat.[9]

Ideally a nutrition screen is completed on all patients admitted to the hospital. A screen involves minimal nutrition information such as measurement of height and weight with weight changes noted, a health history regarding conditions that influence adequate nutrient intake, and assessment of routine laboratory values (Table 3.1). Patients admitted to the intensive care unit typically require a more detailed nutrition assessment that should be completed within 48 hours of admission.

Nutrition assessment begins with a thorough history that reviews previous medical conditions, dietary habits, allergies and food intolerance, recent weight changes, medications that may affect appetite, and gastrointestinal function. In the critically ill patient it is often necessary to obtain this information from the patient's family members or caretakers.

Physical Examination

A thorough nutrition-focused physical examination remains a primary nutritional-assessment tool. This assessment predominantly relies on subjective and descriptive information. Although not quantitative, a physical examination may still influence the nutritional management of a patient (Table 3.2). The main objective of a physical examination is to establish signs and symptoms of nutrient deficiencies or toxicities, and tolerance of current nutritional support.[10] A systems approach should be applied using the examination techniques of inspection, palpation, percussion, and auscultation. The physical examination should include:

- Assessment of muscle mass and subcutaneous fat stores. Protein stores may be assessed by inspection and palpation of a number of muscle groups. The temporalis muscles, deltoids, suprascapular and infrascapular muscles, the bellies of biceps and triceps, and the interossei of the hands should be examined and palpated. The long muscles in particular are considered to be profoundly protein depleted when the tendons are prominent to palpation. Body composition studies have shown that when the tendons are prominent to palpation, more than 30% of total body protein stores have been lost.[9] Gross loss of body fat can be observed not only from the patient's appearance, but also by palpating a number of skinfolds between the finger and thumb. When the dermis can be felt between the finger and thumb when pinching the triceps and biceps skinfolds, then body mass is estimated to be composed of less than 10% to 13% fat.[9]
- Inspection and palpation for edema and ascites. These two conditions are important physical indicators of diminished visceral protein levels and hepatic dysfunction.
- Inspection and evaluation for signs and symptoms of vitamin and mineral deficits, such as dermatitis, glossitis, cheilosis, neuromuscular irritability, and coarse, easily pluckable hair (Table 3.3).

TABLE 3.1

Nutrition Screening Criteria
Diagnosis and past medical history associated with increased nutritional risk
Diagnosis and current clinical condition
Past surgical history
Preexisting medical conditions
Diet information
History of poor nutrient intake
Recent changes in intake
Restrictive dietary habits
Tolerance of diet
Physical assessment
Obvious muscle wasting, excessive body fat
Cachexia
Edema, ascites
Abdominal assessment
Anthropometric data
Height
Current weight
Weight changes and time frame
Laboratory data (if available)
Visceral proteins (albumin, prealbumin, transferrin)
Liver function tests
Lymphocyte count
Hemoglobin

TABLE 3.2

Physical Examination[10]
Nasal, esophageal, mucosal ulceration
Palatability—taste fatigue
Stoma—functional
Urine—output, color
Gastric output—amount, color
Temperature
Nausea/vomiting
Abdominal distension
Appetite—anorexia, hungry, dry mouth, mouth sores
Nutrient intake versus prescribed or estimated required intake
Intravenous site intact (uninfected or inflamed)
Enteral feeding site—unobstructed, uninfected or inflamed
Bowel function—stool frequency, consistency, color
Medications—potential drug-nutrient interactions, GI side effects

TABLE 3.3

Nutrient Deficiencies Revealed by Physical Examination	
Deficient Nutrient	**Findings**
General Exam	
Protein, calories	Weight loss, muscle mass, or fat stores; growth retardation; infection; poor wound healing
Protein, thiamine	Edema (ankles and feet; rule out sodium and water retention, pregnancy, protein-losing enteropathy)
Obesity	Excessive fat stores
Vitamin A	Poor growth
Iron	Anemia, fatigue
Skin	
Protein, vitamin C, zinc	Poor wound healing, pressure ulcers
Fat, vitamin A	Xerosis (rule out environmental cause, lack of hygiene, aging, uremia, hypothyroidism), follicular hyperkeratosis, mosaic dermatitis (plaques of skin in center, peeling at periphery on shins)
Vitamin C	Slow wound healing
Niacin	Red, swollen skin lesions
Zinc	Delayed wound healing, acneiform rash, skin lesions, hair loss
Vitamin K or C	Excessive bleeding, petechiae, ecchymoses; small red, purple, or black hemorrhagic spots
Dehydration (fluid)	Poor skin turgor
Nails	
Iron	Koilonychia (rule out cardiopulmonary disease)
Protein deficiency	Dull, lusterless with transverse ridging across nail plate
Vitamin A, C	Pale, poor blanching, irregular, mottled
Protein, calories	Bruising, bleeding
Vitamin C	Splinter hemorrhages
Hair	
Protein	Hair lacks shine, luster (cause may be environmental or chemical)
Protein, copper	Dyspigmentation (lightening of normal hair color, consider if hair is bleached or dyed)
Copper	Corkscrew hair (Menkes' syndrome)
Face	
Protein	Diffuse pigmentation, swelling
Calcium	Facial paresthesias
Eyes	
Iron, folate, or vitamin B_{12}	Pale conjunctivae (anemia)
Vitamin A	Bitot's spots (more common in children), conjunctival xerosis (rule out chemical or environmental irritation), corneal xerosis, keratomalacia
Pyridoxine, niacin, riboflavin	Angular palpebritis
Hyperlipidemia	Corneal arcus, xanthelasma
Nose	
Riboflavin, niacin, pyridoxine	Seborrhea on nasolabial area, nose bridge, eyebrows, and back of ears (rule out poor hygiene)
Lips and mouth	
Niacin, riboflavin	Cheilosis, angular scars
Riboflavin, pyridoxine, niacin, iron	Angular stomatitis
Tongue	
Niacin, riboflavin, folic acid, iron	Atrophic filiform papillae
Vitamin B_{12}	Glossitis
Zinc	Taste atrophy
Riboflavin	Magenta tongue
Teeth	
Excess sugar, vitamin C	Edentia, caries
Fluorosis	Mottled

(continued)

TABLE 3.3

Nutrient Deficiencies Revealed by Physical Examination (CONTINUED)	
Deficient Nutrient	**Findings**
Gums	
Vitamin C	Spongy, bleeding, receding
Neck	
Iodine	Enlarged thyroid gland
Protein, bulimia	Enlarged parotid glands (bilateral)
Excess fluid	Venous distention, pulsations
Thorax	
Protein, calories	Decreased muscle mass and strength, shortness of breath, fatigue, decreased pulmonary function
Cardiac System	
Thiamine	Heart failure
Gastrointestinal System	
Protein, calories, zinc, vitamin C	Poor wound healing
Protein	Hepatomegaly
Urinary Tract	
Dehydration	Dark, concentrated urine
Overhydration	Light, dilute urine
Musculoskeletal System	
Vitamin D, calcium	Rickets, osteomalacia
Vitamin D	Persistently open anterior fontanel (after age 18 months), craniotabes (softening of skull across back and sides before age 1 year); epiphyseal enlargement (painless) at wrist, knees, and ankles; pigeon chest and Harrison's sulcus (horizontal depression on lower chest border)
Protein	Emaciation, muscle wasting, swelling, pain, pale hair patches
Vitamin C	Swollen, painful joints
Thiamine	Pain in thighs, calves
Nervous System	
Protein	Psychomotor changes (listless, apathetic), mental confusion
Thiamine, vitamin B_6	Weakness, confusion, depressed reflexes, paresthesias, sensory loss, calf tenderness
Niacin, vitamin B_{12}	Dementia
Calcium, magnesium	Tetany

The patient's prescribed medication should be examined for potential drug-nutrient interactions, increased macro- or micronutrient requirements, and nutritionally related side effects such as constipation, diarrhea, nausea, vomiting.

Clinical Assessment of Body Composition

All patients' height and weight should be measured upon admission to the ICU. However, in critically ill patients, body weight typically fluctuates erratically. Such patients often require large amounts of fluid for ongoing resuscitation, or may have edema or ascites that may result in a retention of several liters of fluid, sometimes as much as 10 to 15 liters. Therefore accurate determination of dry weight in the ICU is difficult to obtain. Additionally, malnutrition is associated with fluid shifts from the intravascular space to extravascular space with a concurrent decline in lean body mass. Hence, loss of lean body mass may be masked with little obvious change in body weight. However, these are valuable points of baseline information and remain a practical and simple measure of the total body compartments.

It may be necessary to obtain a pre-injury body weight from a family member or the patient (e.g., identification card). Dry weight and height are used to calculate the ideal body weight, the percentage of ideal body weight, and the body mass index (BMI) (Table 3.4). Survival of a BMI below 14 is very unusual. The percentage recent weight change with respect to the

TABLE 3.4

Ideal Body Weight and Body Mass Index	
Ideal Body Weight (IBW)	
Men: 106 lb for 5 feet in height plus 6 lb for each additional inch	
Example: 5 feet 10 inches	
IBW = 106 + (10 × 6 lbs) = 166 lbs	
Women: 100 lb for 5 feet in height plus 5 lb for each additional inch	
Example: 5 feet 5 inches	
IBW = 100 + (5 × 5) = 125 lbs	
Small frame, subtract 10%	
Large frame, add 10%	
Body Mass Index (BMI)	
BMI = weight (kg) ÷ height^2 (m^2)	1 kg = 2.2 lbs 1 inch = 2.54 cm
Normal BMI = 19 - 25 kg/m^2	1 meter = 100 cm
Example: 160 lb, 5 feet 10 inches (70 inches)	
160 lbs ÷ 2.2 lbs/kg = 72 kg	
70 inches × 2.54 cm/inch = 178 cm	
178 cm ÷ 100 = 1.78 meters	
1.78 × 1.78 = 3.17 m^2	
BMI = 72 kg ÷ 3.17 m^2 = 22.7 kg/m^2	

usual body weight is used most commonly and correlates best with acute morbidity and mortality[11] (Table 3.5).

The key is to estimate weight loss properly and assess its impact on physiological function. Any unintentional weight loss, whether in obese or normal-weight individuals, greater than 5% over the preceding month or greater than 10% over the past 6 months is important and suggestive of nutritional risk.[12] The overall impact of weight loss on physiological function is assessed from the history and by examination. Organomegaly or massive tumor growth may mask progressive loss of lean body weight, while rapid weight gain usually reflects fluid retention or fat weight gain. Weight should preferably be measured weekly, noting that acute weight changes are most likely due to fluid shifts. A standardized weight measuring protocol should be followed.

Anthropometric data (skinfold thickness and arm muscle circumference) as well as creatinine height index (the urinary creatinine level according to height), while useful in ambulatory patients, are significantly

TABLE 3.5

Degree of Malnutrition as Determined by Body Weight[10,11]

$$\%\ \text{Usual body weight} = \frac{\text{actual weight}}{\text{usual weight}} \times 100$$

$$\%\ \text{Recent weight change} = \frac{(\text{usual weight} - \text{actual weight})}{\text{usual weight}} \times 100$$

Degree of malnutrition	% usual body weight
Mild	85–95
Moderate	75–84
Severe	<74

Time Period	Significant weight loss, %	Severe weight loss, %
1 week	1-2	>2
1 month	5	>5
3 months	7.5	>7.5
6 months or more	10	10

less accurate measures of malnutrition in the critically ill patient, particularly in those who have fluid overload, tissue edema, or renal dysfunction.[8] Measurements obtained are compared to various standards in which no standard tables are available for hospitalized patients. Other problems from skinfold measurements and values derived from them include errors in measurement, individual differences in fat and muscle distribution, inter-observer errors, and the time frame required to see changes in measurements.[14]

Bioelectric impedance (BIA) measures fat-free mass by determining differences in electrical conductivity between fat and fat-free mass. This technique is safe, noninvasive, inexpensive, and requires little patient cooperation. BIA use is not recommended in individual patients, but rather for population studies. Furthermore, it may not be useful in critically ill patients with significant alterations in fluid and electrolyte status, as edema and dehydration lead to alterations in resistance measurements.[14] Other techniques for measuring body composition include duel-energy x-ray absorptiometry, computed tomography, ultrasonography, magnetic resonance imaging, total body potassium counting, neutron activation analysis, and isotope dilution techniques. These techniques are not readily available for clinical use and no body composition measurement has been shown to consistently predict clinical outcome.[7]

Subjective global assessment (SGA) evaluates nutritional status and malnutrition based on historical factors (weight change, dietary intake change, gastrointestinal symptoms that have persisted for greater than 2 weeks, functional capacity, underlying disease and effect on metabolic stress) and physical findings (loss of subcutaneous fat, muscle wasting, ankle edema, sacral edema and ascites). Patients are rated as being well nourished, or moderately or severely malnourished.[11] SGA is considered a relatively reliable indicator for nutritional support, but may not be sensitive enough to reflect a patient's early response to nutrition support, therefore limiting its use in critical care.

Biochemical Measurements

Immune Competence

Immune competence as measured by delayed cutaneous hypersensitivity (DCH) and total lymphocyte count (TLC) is reduced in malnutrition. The following factors nonspecifically alter DCH in the absence of malnutrition: infection, uremia, cirrhosis, hepatitis, trauma, burns, hemorrhage, steroids, immunosuppressants, cimetidine, coumadin, general anesthesia, and surgery.[15] Non-nutritional factors that affect TLC include hypoalbuminemia, metabolic stress, infection, cancer, and chronic diseases. Therefore, critically ill patients have multiple factors that can alter DCH and TLC, making them valueless in assessing nutritional risk and status.

Nitrogen Balance Studies

Nitrogen balance studies are commonly used in the critical care setting to determine protein turnover and whether the patient is in a state of anabolism or catabolism. Nitrogen is released as the result of catabolism of amino acids in proteins and is excreted in the urine in the form of urea. Nitrogen balance is calculated by subtracting the excreted nitrogen (24-hour urine urea nitrogen [UUN]) collection plus insensible losses) from the nitrogen intake provided in the nutrition support regimen:

$$\text{Nitrogen balance g/d} = (\text{protein or amino acid intake}/6.25) - (\text{UUN} + 4)$$

A positive nitrogen balance in the range of 2 to 4 grams of nitrogen per day, indicating an anabolic state, is desired, but often difficult to achieve in the critically ill. Measurement of nitrogen balance does not indicate gains or losses of individual organs, since nitrogen balance is the sum total of body gains and losses. Validity of nitrogen balance is affected by severe nitrogen retention disorders (e.g., creatinine clearance <50 mL/min or severe hepatic failure), massive diuresis, accuracy of the 24-hour urine collection, abnormal nitrogen losses through diarrhea or large draining wounds, skin exfoliation as in burns, and completeness of protein or amino acid intake data.[13]

Serum Proteins

Because of flaws with nitrogen balance studies, monitoring of serum protein levels is often used to help assess a patient's nutritional status. Serum albumin, transferrin, thyroxine-binding prealbumin, and retinol-binding protein are most commonly used in the clinical setting (Table 3.6). All of these proteins have transport functions separate from their use in nutrition assessment. The use of serum proteins for nutrition assessment assumes that decreased levels are solely caused by malnutrition. When evaluating serum protein concentration determinants such as synthesis, degradation, and distribution, all must be considered to produce a valid interpretation. Serum proteins are produced by the liver; therefore, several factors can affect their synthesis, including hepatic function and amino acid availability.

The use of these transport proteins in the critically ill to assess nutrition status is less clear. Following a metabolic insult, inflammatory cytokines (tumor necrosis factor [TNF], interleukin-1 [IL-1]) are released in response to the injury. With resultant cytokine release, hepatic reprioritization occurs, leading to upregulation of acute phase reactant (C-reactive protein, fibrinogen, ceruloplasmin, α_1-antitrypsin) synthesis and downregulation of transport protein synthesis.[16–20] This results in a rapid decrease in serum protein levels. This reprioritization of protein synthesis by the hepatocyte returns toward normal within several days unless complications, such as sepsis, ensue. These changes have been described in many clinical situations such as severe multiple trauma, post-operative course, sepsis, and burn injury.[16] Therefore it is not uncommon to find depleted transport protein levels within the first few days of a critically ill patient's hospital stay. These initially low levels are more reflective of illness severity than nutritional status. In addition, due to the long half-life of serum albumin and its depletion with large fluid volumes, it is not recommended to rely on albumin levels as a nutritional marker during critical illness. However, in spite of this lack of specificity, critically ill patients are at high risk for developing nutritional deficiencies, and decreased

TABLE 3.6

Serum Transport Proteins Features in Nutrition Assessment[11,13]				
Serum Protein	**Normal Value**	**Half-Life**	**Function**	**Clinical Significance and Other Comments**
Albumin	3.5-5.0 g/dL <2.1 severe depletion 2.1-2.8 moderate depletion 2.8-3.5 mild depletion	21 days	Maintain plasma oncotic pressure, carrier for amino acids, zinc, magnesium, calcium, free fatty acids, drugs	Routinely available Useful in long-term nutritional assessment Limited value in short-term nutrition indicator due to long half-life, and other variables (albumin infusion, hydration status) Reliable prognostic indicator of morbidity and mortality Synthesized in liver (low levels with hepatic disease) + 60% total body albumin found extravascular
Transferrin	200-400 mg/dL <100 severe depletion 100-150 moderate depletion 150-200 severe depletion	8-10 days	Binds iron in plasma and transports to bone	Strongly influenced by iron status Synthesized in liver and found primarily extravascular Increased levels with pregnancy, estrogen & iron therapy, acute hepatitis, iron deficiency anemia, chronic blood loss and dehydration Decreased levels with hepatic disease, protein losing states (nephrotic syndrome), hemolytic anemia, metabolic stress
Prealbumin	10-40 mg/dL <5 severe depletion 5-10 moderate depletion 10-15 mild depletion	2-3 days	Binds thyroxin, carrier or RBP	Useful as short term nutritional index Better index of visceral protein especially in acute states of protein-calorie malnutrition Synthesized in the liver Increased levels with renal dysfunction Decreased levels with acute catabolic states, post-surgery, hyperthyroidism, liver disease, protein-calorie malnutrition
Retinol-binding protein (RBP)	2.7-7.6 mg/dL	12 hours	Transports vitamin A in plasma, binds to prealbumin	Reflects acute changes in protein malnutrition and changes in dietary intake Limited use in renal failure because it is metabolized by the proximal tubular cells Increased levels in chronic renal failure and in patients on oral contraceptives Decreased levels with vitamin A deficiency, protein-calorie malnutrition, acute catabolic states, post-surgery, hyperthyroidism, liver disease

transport protein levels may assist in rapid identification of the potential nutritional risk and otherwise unidentified inflammatory process.[14,20]

Energy and Protein Requirements

In the critically ill patient, the goal of nutritional support is maintenance, not repletion and should serve as an adjunct to other critical therapies. Numerous factors limit the effectiveness of exogenously administered nutritional substrates in preventing catabolism regardless of the level of support. The conversion of a catabolic septic patient into an anabolic state should not be expected. Many undesirable metabolic complications can occur in attempting to do so, such as hypercapnia, hyperglycemia, hypertriglyceridemia, hepatic steatosis.[21–23] Once the hypermetabolic process is corrected, anabolism is favored and repletion can occur. Multiple methods are used to determine energy requirements in the critically ill, which are discussed in detail in Chapter 4.

Protein requirements in the critically ill are elevated compared to nonstressed patients. Stressed critically ill patients require protein in the range of 1.5 to 2.0 g/kg/d.[24] Achieving positive nitrogen balance is nearly impossible immediately after the metabolic insult, but after the primary insult is controlled or resolved, positive nitrogen balance is feasible. Protein requirements do not decrease with increasing age. Reduction in lean-body mass and obligatory loss of protein during physiologic stress increase protein requirements for the critically ill older patient as well as for the younger patient.[25] Protein tolerance as opposed to protein requirement often determines the amount of protein delivered. The onset of azotemia, impaired renal or hepatic function signals the need to reduce protein delivery. Most studies examining graded protein intakes in septic, injured, or burned patients have found no protein-sparing benefit to giving protein in excess of the above recommendations.[26]

Fluid Requirements

Fluid requirements will vary depending upon the status of the critically ill patient. The primary goal is to maintain adequate urinary output and serum electrolyte levels. Typically, fluid requirements for nonfebrile patients include 35 mL/kg/d. Insensible fluid losses increase with fever. However, many critically ill patients are at risk for fluid overload with large amounts of fluids administered for fluid resuscitation, antibiotics, and other medications. In many situations, nutrition support regimens in critically ill patients are concentrated due to other obligatory fluid delivery.

Monitoring Nutrition Support

Although much emphasis is placed on initiating nutrition support in the critically ill, it is equally important to monitor the nutrition-support regimen and prevent adverse effects, and to ensure adequate nutrient delivery and tolerance. Several reviews have noted that despite strict protocols and defined nutrition targets, many other management decisions or procedures influence delivery such that underfeeding is the norm.[27] Several reviews of intensive care patients have revealed that on average only 75% of the quantity of feed prescribed was actually delivered to the patient,[28] with only half of the patients reaching 80% of the target energy and 70% of target nitrogen intakes.[29] The main problems preventing delivery of feed were gut dysfunction and elective stoppage for procedures. ICUs with well-defined feeding protocols delivered significantly greater volumes of feed than those without.[28]

A broad range of interrelated metabolic derangements can occur during the refeeding state of an individual at risk. Changes in phosphorus, potassium, magnesium, and glucose metabolism; occurrence of vitamin deficiency; and need for fluid resuscitation may all have a significant bearing on the metabolic milieu of the critically ill patient.[30] Systemic abnormalities may also occur, including neurological dysfunction, muscular dysfunction, hematologic disorders, and diminished cardiac performance. Attention to each of these abnormalities will allow proper recognition and treatment of the refeeding syndrome.

Optimal treatment guidelines do not exist, but recommendations can be made (Table 3.7). When utilizing serum protein levels to assess the patient's response to the nutrition therapy, analysis of trends in protein concentrations, with attention to the direction of change, is more important than assessment of a single level. If positive trends in serum proteins are desired but not revealed, then monitoring an acute phase reactant (e.g., C-reactive protein) along with a short turnover serum protein (e.g., prealbumin) can be helpful. This will aid in determining if the diminished protein value is due to hepatic reprioritization of protein synthesis or a lack of nutrient provision. As the inflammatory process is detected and treated, the acute phase reactants should decrease and the serum protein levels increase if nutrient provision is adequate.[16,17]

Although enteral nutrition is the preferred route of nutrient provision in the critically ill, many times patients do not tolerate it. Intolerance can be identified as increased abdominal distention after the initiation of feedings, formula reflux, increased gastric re-

TABLE 3.7

Recommendations for Initiating and Monitoring Nutrition Support[31]

Nutrient	Guidelines
Calories	Initiate with ≤20 kcal/kg or 1000 npc; maintain for ~2-5 days; increase as tolerated per patient
Protein	1.2-1.5 gm/kg/day; increase as tolerated monitoring BUN and creatinine, LFT's
Carbohydrate	150-200 gm/day; increase based upon glycemic control and insulin requirement
Lipid	≤1 gm/kg/day; infuse over 18-24 hours; monitor serum triglyceride levels for tolerance
Fluid	Usually maximal concentration desired; monitor intake and output, weight changes, peripheral edema, and tachycardia for fluid balance and signs for fluid overload
Blood work	*Monitor daily:* phosphorus, magnesium, glucose, potassium, sodium, chloride, bicarbonate, BUN, creatinine, ionized calcium, hemoglobin, pCO_2
	Monitor bi-weekly: LFTs, prealbumin, CRP, triglyceride

BUN: blood urea nitrogen; LFT: liver function tests; CRP: C-reactive protein

siduals (≥250 mL of formula), nausea, vomiting, diarrhea, and abdominal pain. If intolerance of enteral nutrition continues for ≥72 hours, potential nutrition should be considered.

Other indices to monitor to determine adequacy of the nutrition support regimen include rate of wound healing. If wounds are not demonstrating optimal healing, such as good granulation tissue, this signals the need to reassess nutrient requirements for calories, protein, and micronutrients. It is also helpful to monitor the patient's functional status and ability to tolerate ventilator-weaning strategies and overall stamina to work with other therapies, such as physical and speech therapy to help determine if the patient is receiving adequate energy needs.

Conclusions

Many methods of nutrition assessment have been developed and formulated. It is generally accepted that no single parameter can be considered as an indicator of nutritional status. Reviewing the complete patient presentation and making a clinical rational assessment is of most value. This includes obtaining the patient's previous medical and nutritional history, evaluating the physical exam, and understanding the severity of the illness and its medical treatment plan. Completing all components is necessary in the critically ill patient so that an optimal nutrition plan can be implemented and monitored.

Case Study

The patient is a 55-year-old male injured in a motor vehicle accident. His injuries include a closed head injury (Glasgow coma scale of 8T), a sacral fracture, and a mild liver laceration. He is in the intensive care unit, chemically paralyzed, sedated and on the respirator. Currently he is receiving intravenous fluids of one-half normal saline at 120 mL/hr. He has a nasogastric tube to wall suction that is removing 700 mL bilious fluid/d. Over the past 48 hours he has received 5 liters of fluid in excess of his outputs. He currently weighs 105 kg. Remarkable laboratory values include: glucose: 220 mg/dL, albumin: 2.2 g/dL, prealbumin: 12.0 mg/dL, c-reactive protein: 19 mg/dL. His past medical history includes type II diabetes mellitus and hypertension.

Assessment

Since the patient is not able to provide a nutrition history, his family members are interviewed. They state that his normal weight is 210 lbs (95 kg) and he is about 6 feet tall. He has had diabetes for 10 years and takes an oral hypoglycemic agent for control and blood pressure medication; he eats a regular diet and has a good appetite. He does not take any vitamin or nutritional supplements.

Physical exam reveals the patient to be edematous and to have a distended abdomen with no active bowel sounds. He otherwise appears to have good muscle and fat stores and no visible vitamin or nutrient deficiencies or chronic wounds.

This patient is presumed to be in good health; elevated weight above usual weight is due to resuscitative fluids. His abnormal serum protein levels are most likely due to fluid overload (albumin) and the inflammatory process (elevated CRP, decreased prealbumin). His hyperglycemia is due to his underlying diabetes and stress hyperglycemia.

The patient's nutrition needs are assessed using his ideal body weight of 88 kg (for large frame). He is estimated to require 2200 to 2640 kcal/d (25–30 kcal/kg) and 132–175 gm protein/day (1.5–2 g/kg). His fluid requirements are approximately 3000 mL/d (35 mL/kg), which he is already receiving with IVF and medications. Therefore, when the nutrition support regimen is started, IVF should be decreased accordingly so as to not over-hydrate him. Enteral feeding is the preferred route of nutrition intervention, beginning cautiously in the small bowel due to the distended abdomen and absence of bowel sounds. Feedings should be advanced slowly (~10 mL every 4 to 6 hours), monitoring for GI tolerance (reflux, further distention). His laboratory values should be monitored daily, with blood glucose levels checked every 4 hours with an order for sliding scale insulin to maintain glucose levels ≤180 mg/dL. Serum protein levels and inflammatory markers (prealbumin, c-reactive protein) can be monitored twice a week for adequacy of nutrition therapy. Other laboratory measurements can be monitored weekly (liver function tests, triglyceride). If the patient is not able to tolerate ≥60% of his nutrient needs via the enteral feeds for ≥72 hours, then supplemental TPN should be considered.

References

1. Vitello J. Prevalence of malnutrition in hospitalized patients remains high. *J Am Coll Nutr.* 1993;12:589.
2. Naber T, Schermer T, de Bree A, et al. Prevalence of malnutrition in nonsurgical hospitalized patients and its association with disease complication. *Am J Clin Nutr.* 1997; 66:1232–1239.

3. Coats K, Morgan S, Bartolucci A, et al. Hospital-associated malnutrition: a reevaluation 12 years later. *J Am Diet Assoc.* 1993;93:27–33.
4. Kelly I, Tessier A, Cahill SE, et al. Still hungry in hospital: identifying malnutrition in acute hospital admissions. *Q J Med.* 2000;93:93–98.
5. Bistrian B, Blackburn G, Hallowell E, et al. Protein status of general surgical patients. *J Am Med Assoc.* 1979;239: 858–860.
6. Mowe M, Bohmer T, Kindt E. Reduced nutritional status in an elderly population (>70 years) is probable before disease and possibly contributes to the development of disease. *Am J Clin Nutr.* 1994;39:317–324.
7. Klein S, Kinney J, Jeejeebhoy K, et al. Nutrition support in clinical practice: review of published data and recommendations for future research directions. *J Parenter Enteral Nutr.* 1997;21:133–156.
8. Chan S, McCowen K, Blackburn G. Nutrition management in the ICU. *Chest.* 1999;115(Suppl):145S–148S.
9. Hill GL. Body composition research: implications for the practice of clinical nutrition. *J Parenter Enteral Nutr.* 1992; 16:197–218.
10. Hammond K. History and physical examination. In: Matarese LE, Gottschlich MM, eds. *Contemporary Nutrition Support Practice.* Philadelphia: WB Saunders Co; 1998: 25–26.
11. Downs J, Haffejee. Nutritional assessment in the critically ill. *Curr Opin Clin Nutr Metab Care.* 1998;1:275–279.
12. Windsor JA, Hill GL. Weight loss with physiological impairment—basic indicator of surgical risk. *Ann Surg.* 1988; 207:290–6.
13. Shronts EP, Fish JA, Pesce-Hammond K. Nutrition assessment. In: Merritt RJ, ed. *The ASPEN Nutrition Support Practice Manual.* Silver Spring, MD: The American Society for Parenteral and Enteral Nutrition; 1998:1–17.
14. Charney P. Nutrition assessment in the 1990s: where are we now? *Nutr Clin Pract.* 1995;10:131–139.
15. Jeejeebhoy K, Detsky A, Baker J. Assessment of nutritional status. *J Parenter Enteral Nutr.* 1990;14(Suppl):193S–196S.
16. Manelli J, Badetti C, Botti G, et al. A reference standard for plasma proteins is required for nutritional assessment of adult burn patients. *Burns.* 1998;24:337–345.
17. Sganga G, Siegel J, Brown G, et al. Reprioritization of hepatic plasma protein release in trauma and sepsis. *Arch Surg.* 1995;120:187–199.
18. Kudsk K, Minard G, Wijtysiak S, et al. Visceral protein response to enteral versus parenteral nutrition and sepsis in patients with trauma. *Surgery.* 1994;116:516–523.
19. Gabay C, Kushner I. Acute-phase proteins and other systemic responses to inflammation. *NEJM.* 1999;340:448–454.
20. Boosalis M, Ott L, Levine A, et al. Relationship of visceral proteins to nutritional status in chronic and acute stress. *Crit Care Med.* 1989;17:741–747.
21. Klein C, Stanek G, Willes C. Overfeeding macronutrients to critically ill adults: metabolic complications. *J Am Diet Assoc.* 1998;98;795–806.
22. Pomposelli JJ, Baxter JK, Babineau TJ, et al. Early postoperative glucose control predicts nosocomial infection rate in diabetic patients. *J Parenter Enteral Nutr.* 1998;22:77–81.
23. Pomposelli JJ, Bistrian BR. Is total parenteral nutrition immunosuppressive? *New Horiz.* 1994;2:224–229.
24. A.S.P.E.N. Board of Directors. Guidelines for the use of parenteral and enteral nutrition in adult and pediatric patients. *J Parenter Enteral Nutr.* 1993; 17(Suppl):20SA–21SA.
25. Campbell W, Crin M, Dallal G, et al. Increased protein requirements in elderly people: new data and retrospective reassessments. *Am J Clin Nutr.* 1994;60:501–509.
26. Dabrowski G, Rombeau J. Practical nutritional management in the trauma intensive care unit. *Surg Clin N Am.* 2000;80:922–932.
27. Griffiths R. Feeding the critically ill—should we do better? *Int Care Med.* 1997;23:246–247.
28. Adam S, Batson S. A study of problems associated with the delivery of enteral feed in critically ill patients in five ICUs in the UK. *Int Care Med.* 1997;23:261–266.
29. Green CJ, Campbell IT, McClelland P, et al. Energy and nitrogen balance and changes in mid upper-arm circumference with multiple organ failure. *Nutrition.* 1995;11: 739–746.
30. Solomon S, Kirby D. The refeeding syndrome: a review. *J Parenter Enteral Nutr.* 1990;14:90–97.
31. Patino J, Echeverri de Pimiento S, Vergara A, et al. Hypocaloric support in the critically ill. *W J Surg.* 1999;23:553–559.

CHAPTER

4

Estimating Energy Requirements

Carol S. Ireton-Jones, Ph.D., R.D., L.D., C.N.S.D., F.A.C.N.

COMPONENTS OF DAILY ENERGY EXPENDITURE 31
MEASUREMENT OF ENERGY EXPENDITURE: INDIRECT CALORIMETRY 32
ENERGY EQUATIONS 33
ENERGY EXPENDITURE ASSESSMENT IN OBESITY 34
HYPOCALORIC FEEDING 35
GOALS OF NUTRITION SUPPORT 35
CONCLUSIONS 36
REFERENCES 36

One of the most important decisions in providing nutrition support to patients is calculating the number of calories. Determining energy requirements is one of the first steps in the development of the nutrition care plan. After energy/calorie requirements have been identified, individual nutrient prescriptions for protein, carbohydrate, and fat can be formulated. This chapter will review the components of energy expenditure and methods of determining energy expenditure and energy requirements. The information is focused on the intensive care unit (ICU) patient, but can be applied across the healthcare continuum—hospital, home, or long-term care.

Components of Daily Energy Expenditure

The factors associated with energy expenditure in normal individuals are illustrated schematically in Figure 4.1. Stature and size, race, gender, height, and body composition all affect basal energy expenditure (BEE). Males typically have higher metabolic rates than do females because energy expenditure is proportionate to the body surface area and to the percentage of lean body mass.[1] In the ill or injured person, the factors that determine energy expenditure apply; however, physical activity is replaced with the energy cost of the disease or injury, as demonstrated in Figure 4.2. Some studies have been done to estimate the energy costs of illness and disease. It has been demonstrated that traumatic injuries, burns, and head injuries raise metabolic rate and therefore energy requirements.[2–4] Treatment regimens, age, and body composition also affect an individual's response to injury and illness. In response to a traumatic injury, for example, a debilitated elderly person may not experience an increase in energy expenditure as significant as that of a well-nourished, formerly active person.[5]

Once the components of energy expenditure are defined, the choice of the appropriate method for determining energy expenditure can be made. There are two methods of determining an individual's energy requirements: measurement of energy expenditure or the use of predictive equations.

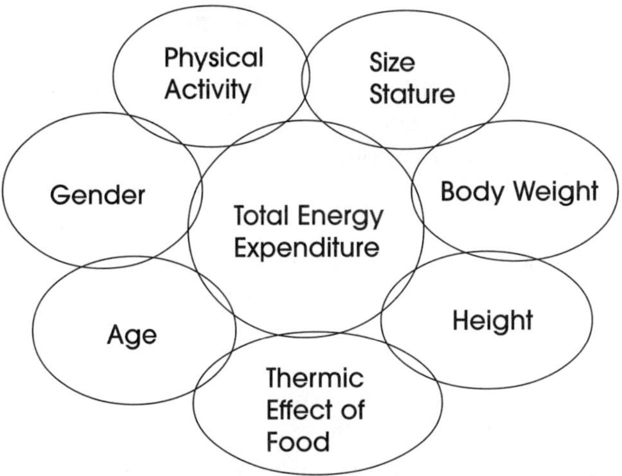

Figure 4.1

Components of Daily Energy Expenditure for the Normal Individual

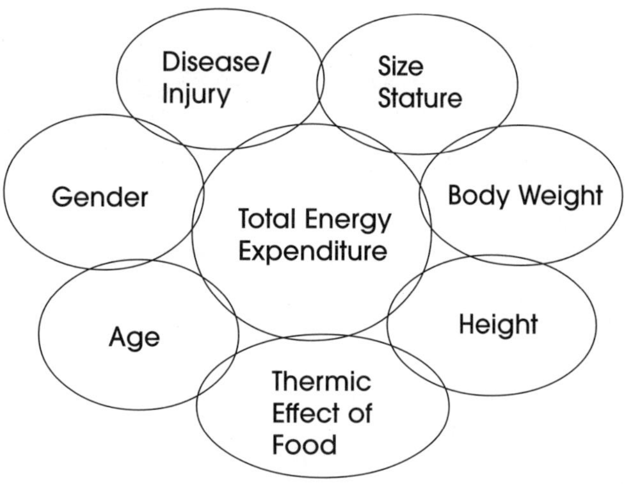

Figure 4.2

Components of Daily Energy Expenditure for the Ill or Injured Individual

Measurement of Energy Expenditure: Indirect Calorimetry

Indirect calorimetric determinations of energy expenditure are accomplished by measuring the oxygen consumption and carbon dioxide production during respiratory gas exchange.[6,7] Indirect calorimetry is based on the premise that the energy released by oxidative processes and by anaerobic glycolysis is ultimately transformed into heat or external work.[6,8] In addition to energy expenditure, respiratory quotient (RQ) may be calculated from the ratio of carbon dioxide produced ($\dot{V}CO_2$) to oxygen consumed ($\dot{V}O_2$) and reflects net substrate utilization ($\dot{V}CO_2/\dot{V}O_2$).[9] The amounts of oxygen consumed and carbon dioxide produced are characteristic and constant for protein, carbohydrate, and fat. Oxidation of each major nutrient class occurs at a known RQ, ranging from 0.7 for fat oxidation to 1.0 for glucose oxidation (Table 4.1). Net fat synthesis is demonstrated by the occurrence of an RQ greater than 1.0.[9,10] RQs greater than 1.0 can occur when carbohydrate (glucose) intake or total caloric intake is excessive. The effect is probably a function of excessive glucose intake.[10,11]

Measurement of energy expenditures for both ventilator-dependent and spontaneously breathing patients can be done using a portable indirect calorimeter.[12,13] Patients with tracheotomies can be measured as long as the endotracheal tube cuff is inflated, assuming no inspiratory or expiratory air leaks.[14] In the ICU patient, a system for measuring energy expenditure via indirect calorimetry may be an integrated component of the mechanical ventilator. This allows for continuous measurement of energy expenditure without the need for another piece of equipment or a skilled person to perform the measurement.

Careful attention must be given to maintaining standard measurement conditions to assure that the results of the indirect calorimetric measurement of energy expenditure (MEE) are useful and accurate in acutely and chronically ill patients (Table 4.2).[8,15–18] Gottschlich et al.[19] measured energy expenditures of burned patients over 24 hours and found very little variation in energy expenditure throughout the day, indicating that measurement of energy expenditure can be accurately determined at any time. Smyrnios et al.[20] analyzed measurement data over a continuous period of 24 hours and correlated this with individual 30-minute measurements of energy expenditure. These researchers found that the data obtained under standard conditions for 30 minutes were not significantly different from those obtained from a 24-hour measurement. In addition, researchers suggested that patient measurements be conducted between the hours of 3 p.m. and 11 p.m., when heart rate, systolic blood pressure, and breath rate are near the day's average, or in other words, when the least variability in energy expenditure occurs.[20]

TABLE 4.1

Respiratory Quotient (RQ)

Energy Source	RQ
Fat	0.70
Protein	0.80
Carbohydrate (Glucose)	0.95–1.00
Mixed Diet	0.85
Net Fat Synthesis	>1.01
Hyperventilation	>1.10
Ketosis	<0.60

TABLE 4.2

Standard Testing Conditions for Accurately Measuring Energy Expenditure

- Patients should be measured when they are awake but at rest and in a supine position.
- Patients should be measured 2 hours after a meal unless they are on continuous nutritional support.
- Measurements should be taken at least 60 minutes following strenuous activity such as a dressing change, chest physiotherapy, or physical therapy.

TABLE 4.3

Situations That May Cause Measurements of Energy Expenditure to be Unreliable

- Patients measured while receiving high frequency mechanical ventilation
- Patients with chest tubes that leak air
- Patients receiving mechanical ventilation with fractional expired oxygen concentrations >60% when open circuit measurement systems are used
- Patients in whom the tracheotomy tube has an incompetent or non-existent tracheal cuff
- Patients receiving inconsistent sources of inspired oxygen (variable levels of inspired oxygen)
- Unskilled personnel conducting the metabolic measurement

TABLE 4.4

The Harris-Benedict Energy Equations

Males: EE = 66 + 13.8 (W) + 5 (H) - 6.8 (A)

Females: EE = 655 + 9.6 (W) + 1.8 (H) - 4.7 (A)

Where:

EE = Energy Expenditure (kcal/d)

W = Weight in kg

H = Height in cm

A = Age in years

There are some limitations to indirect calorimetry due to both physiological and mechanical factors (Table 4.3).[12,21] While indirect calorimetry is accurate, it is expensive to obtain and maintain the equipment and personnel necessary to provide accurate measurements of energy expenditure, necessitating an alternate method.

Energy Equations

Most clinicians use energy expenditure equations to predict the energy expenditure of patients either prior to or instead of indirect calorimetry. Over 200 equations have been developed for estimating energy expenditure, although few of these are designed for acutely ill or chronically ill patients.[22] Any equation used for estimating energy expenditure should be evaluated by the clinician for applicability and accuracy in the patient population for which it is to be used. To evaluate an energy expenditure equation, the original published data must be obtained in order to evaluate the study population, study conditions, age of subjects, body weight, body mass index (BMI), diagnosis, activity level, and methodology for determining energy expenditure and statistical analysis.[23]

For example, the Harris-Benedict equations (HBEE) were developed from indirect calorimetric measurements of energy expenditure in normal-weight, healthy adults in the early 1900s and are used to predict resting energy expenditure (Table 4.4).[24] A study by Garrel et al.[25] found that the Harris-Benedict equations are less accurate in predicting the energy expenditures of normal subjects than are several other similar equations, and that they are more inaccurate in females than males. Stress factors or correction factors are often added to the HBEE so that these equations can be utilized to predict energy expenditures of critically ill or injured patients.[4] These factors range from an addition of 30% to 50% above resting energy expenditure.[26–30] Jeevanandum recommends an addition of 40% to the HBEE for patients with severe catabolic trauma.[5] Another way to estimate energy expenditures of patients is the calorie per kilogram of body weight (kcal/kg) method, using a range of calories from 25–40 kcal/kg based on clinical judgment.[29] A consensus statement of the American College of Chest Physicians suggested that providing 25 kcal/kg of usual body weight is adequate to promote anabolic functions for patients in the intensive care unit.[31]

Energy equations have been developed recently for estimating the energy expenditures of ill and injured patients in critical care units as well as less acute settings.[15] These equations, referred to in the literature as the Ireton-Jones Equations (IJEE), were developed from indirect calorimetry measurements of energy expenditure of hospitalized patients correlated through multivariate regression analysis with easily measured variables including height, weight, age, gender, diagnosis, presence of obesity, and ventilatory status. For the variable of obesity, a body weight greater than 130% of ideal or a body mass index of greater than 27 was used to indicate the presence of obesity. No patient with a body mass index (BMI) >40 was included in the study. For diagnosis, patients were designated as burn, non-burn trauma, or other. Statistical correlation of data was found only when patients were stratified by ventilatory status, indicating that there was a significant difference in energy expenditure between ventilator-dependent patients and spontaneously breathing patients.[15] Two equations were developed and subsequently revised to provide statistically significant equations for estimating energy expenditure in patients whom nutrition-support clinicians are most likely to encounter in practice (Table 4.5).[15,32]

TABLE 4.5

The Ireton-Jones Energy Equations
Spontaneously breathing patients:
EEE(s) = 629 - 11(A) + 25(W) - 609(O)
Ventilator-dependent patients:
EEE(v) = 1784 - 11(A) + 5(W) + 244(G) + 239(T) + 804(B)
Where:
EEE = Estimated Energy Expenditure (kcal/day)
s = spontaneously breathing
v = ventilator-dependent
A = Age (years)
W = Weight (kg)
O = Presence of obesity: >30% above ideal body weight or BMI >27 (0 = absent, 1 = present)
G = Gender (0 = female, 1 = male)
T = Trauma diagnosis (0 = absent, 1 = present)
B = Burn diagnosis (0 = absent, 1 = present)

The IJEE were developed using a similar methodology as the Harris-Benedict equations but from measurements of energy expenditure of patients requiring enteral and parenteral nutrition support. The IJEE include considerations for diagnosis, obesity, and ventilatory status, so they are applicable to a wide range of patients. Furthermore, these equations have been validated in similar patient populations after development and by Wall, Gagliardi, and Amato.[33–35]

A comparison was done between the IJEE and the HBEE × 1.3 method for a group of 300 hospitalized patients.[36] Of these patients, 201 were spontaneously breathing and 99 were ventilator-dependent. The IJEE showed a stronger correlation to measured energy expenditure than did HBEE × 1.3. The IJEE also predicted energy expenditure more accurately (in 55% of the patients) than HBEE × 1.3. This is attributed to the inputs used in the IJEE that compensate for specific conditions affecting energy expenditure (such as ventilator dependence, diagnoses, and obesity), which are not used in HBEE × 1.3. A fixed correction factor of 1.3 for HBEE is a compromise that attempts to meet the average needs of a diverse patient group. However, this tends to overestimate the energy expenditure of obese or spontaneously breathing patients, but underestimates the energy expenditure for ventilator-dependent patients. Therefore, the IJEE is recommended because it was developed specifically for estimating energy expenditures of ventilator-dependent and spontaneously breathing patients requiring nutrition support.

Energy Expenditure Assessment in Obesity

Predicting energy expenditures of obese patients is a challenge for clinicians because weight is a factor in most equations. In previous studies, actual body weight has been demonstrated to correlate better with measured energy expenditure than ideal body weight.[30,37] A recent study evaluated energy requirements in ventilator-dependent, critically ill patients and attempted to correlate measured energy expenditure with a modification of the body weights of obese patients.[27] The study demonstrated that standard energy estimations for kcal/kg (30–35 kcal/kg) could be utilized in obese patients when body weight was adjusted down to account for adiposity. When actual body weight was used, measured energy expenditures of obese patients were approximately 21 kcal/kg. Using a weight other than actual body weight introduces potential error to the equation.

It is difficult to predict the energy expenditures of obese patients, and most researchers suggest the use of indirect calorimetry when it is available. However, the IJEE can be used to estimate the energy expenditures of obese patients because obesity was a variable in the development of both the spontaneously breathing and ventilator-dependent equations. The presence of obesity (BMI >27) is only a factor in the spontaneously breathing equation even though it was evaluated in the ventilator-dependent equation. Inherent in the two equations are different multiplication factors for actual body weight; however, the other factors in the ventilator-dependent equation clearly dominate the energy expenditure prediction making a correction factor for obesity unnecessary.

There is limited evidence suggesting the metabolic response to injury in obese patients is different from that of normal-weight people. Jeevanandam[5] found decreased growth-hormone levels in the catabolic phase of severe injury in a group of obese trauma patients as compared to normal-weight trauma patients. This decreased level seems to be a defense mechanism to facilitate the maintenance of the hypercatabolic state needed to provide amino acids for hepatic gluconeogenesis. The traumatized obese patients mobilized relatively more protein and less fat as compared with non-obese subjects. A block in both lipolysis and fat oxidation occurred in the obese patients, which resulted in a shift to the preferential use of proteins and carbohydrates, indicating that obese patients are unable to utilize their abundant fuel stores of fat due to a limited capacity to oxidize fat and have to depend on other fuel sources such as body protein stores. Growth-hormone levels do not increase in the obese patients in response to feeding as they do in non-obese trauma patients, negatively affecting response to nutritional support.[5]

For the morbidly obese patient, prediction of energy expenditures is a moot point. Typically, these patients have altered cardiac function, fluid tolerance problems, altered immune response, and altered glucose metabolism.[38] Because of these complications, the caloric prescription may not equal the patient's energy expenditure. Clinical status is of the utmost importance in determining the obese patient's energy requirements, with the goal of nutrition support being preservation of lean body mass.

Hypocaloric Feeding

Because of the challenges of hyperglycemia and other metabolic complications seen in critically ill patients, hypocaloric feeding has been utilized as a means of providing energy and protein substrate at a minimum level so as not to negatively affect the metabolic adaptive response to injury.[39] This has been studied in patients receiving total parenteral nutrition. The hypocaloric feeding regimen or "protein sparing" regimen, as it has been called, focuses on decreasing the dextrose administration, which results in a lowered blood glucose and a concomitant decrease in insulin secretion.[40] Patino[39] recommends a feeding regimen for critically ill patients providing approximately 50% of the estimated energy requirements as glucose (100 to 200 gm) and 100% of the protein requirements (1.5 to 2.0 gm protein per kg ideal body weight) during the first few days of the stress situation. This avoids the potential complications associated with parenteral nutrition regimens containing high glucose loads, which result in higher CO_2 production and hyperglycemia. McCowen[41] compared a hypocaloric feeding regimen to a standard regimen (25 kcal/kg) in hospitalized patients fed intravenously. Average blood glucose, frequency of hyperglycemia, and infection rates were found to be similar for both groups of patients, leading these researchers to recommend 25 kcal/kg with 1.5 g of protein/kg as the optimal nutrition support regimen for patients requiring parenteral nutrition.

Hypocaloric feeding regimens are more often utilized in obese and morbidly obese patients who require total parenteral nutrition. Dickerson et al[42] examined the energy expenditures of obese patients in relation to protein metabolism. The goal of this study was to evaluate the clinical efficacy of hypocaloric, high-protein parenteral feedings in obese stressed patients with surgical complications. Researchers studied thirteen obese patients with postoperative complications of sepsis and anastomotic leaks, abscesses, or fistulae. Energy expenditures were measured, and nonprotein calories of approximately 52% of the MEE were provided. Protein intakes averaged 2 g/kg body weight, which would calculate to be about 1.2 g of protein/kg actual weight. The obese patients lost an average of 2 kg/wk. Serum albumin increased over the study period, which ranged from 12 to 119 days. Nitrogen balance was achieved after 24 days of hypocaloric feeding. All patients' wounds healed with the average hospital stay of 60 days. The theory proposed by these authors is that morbidly obese patients should not need excess caloric supply. If adequate protein is supplied and obligatory glucose requirements are met, endogenous fat stores will be used for energy; however, these authors further state that this occurred in their study population of mild to moderately stressed obese patients.

Goals of Nutrition Support

The final determination of energy requirements for any patient should be based on the goal of nutrition support—maintenance or repletion. Many questions arise as to the provision of calories based on the predicted or the measured energy expenditure. The IJEE and the measured energy expenditure by using indirect calorimetry are essentially equivalent. Measured energy expenditure can be translated to the number of calories a patient is expending. This does not necessarily mean that the patient's energy expenditure is the same as his or her energy requirements, but there should be a relationship. Clinical judgment may lead to the addition of calories to account for repletion or anabolism, as a subtraction of calories may be necessary to account for glucose intolerance, substrate or fluid tolerances, or weight loss goals.[23] Energy requirements are individualized and based on more than just a number derived from indirect calorimetry or any equation. A patient in the ICU may not be able to become anabolic and replete or gain true weight until the inflammatory response has subsided. Using the predicted or measured energy expenditure as a guide, the clinician must determine the individual patient's energy requirements based on the patient's ability to tolerate more calories (i.e., use these calories and not become over-fed as evidenced by high CO_2, hyperglycemia, etc.) or tolerate fewer calories (i.e., not be undernourished).

Conclusions

Nutrition is not an exact science because of the many individual variations among people in size, stature, intake, output, and race, without regard to the overlying effects of illness or injury. Energy expenditure is not necessarily equivalent to energy requirement. Energy requirement may be greater or less than energy expenditure, whether it is predicted using an energy equation or measured using indirect calorimetry. Clinical issues such as fluid balance, substrate tolerance, and metabolic status will affect the provision of nutrients to a patient.

While determination of energy requirement is the first step in the nutrition support process, evaluation of clinical status and expected or desired outcomes such as positive nitrogen balance and healing must also be considered as factors affecting energy requirements. In the end, the clinician is the most valuable asset in the determination of energy requirements of nutrition support patients. Clinical judgment and expertise should be used in the development of the nutrition support regimen and goals of therapy to ensure that an optimal outcome is obtained. These goals are to support the lean body mass, minimize nutritional risk, and promote rapid recovery.

References

1. James W, Davies H, Bailes J, et al. Elevated metabolic rates in obesity. *Lancet*. 1978;1122–1125.
2. Turner WW, Ireton CS, Hunt JL, et al. Predicting energy expenditures in burned patients. *J Trauma*. 1985;25:11–17.
3. Turner WW. Nutritional considerations in the patient with disabling brain disease. *Neurosurgery*. 1985;16:707–713.
4. Long CL, Schaffel N, Geiger JW, et al. Metabolic response to injury and illness: estimation of energy and protein needs from indirect calorimetry and nitrogen balance. *J Parenter Enteral Nutr*. 1979;3:452–459.
5. Jeevanandam M, Ramias L, Shamos RF, et al. Decreased growth hormone levels in the catabolic phase of severe injury. *Surgery*. 1992;111:496–502.
6. Westerterp KR. Energy expenditure. In: Westerterp MS, Fredrix EWHM, Steffens AB, eds. *Food Intake and Energy Expenditure*. Boca Raton: CRC Press;1994:237–257.
7. Douglas CG. A method for determining the total respiratory exchange in man. *J Physiol* (London). 1911;42:xvii–xxvi.
8. Jequier E. Measurement of energy expenditure in clinical nutritional assessment. *J Parenter Enteral Nutr*. 1987;11:86S–89S.
9. Ireton-Jones CS, Turner WW. The use of respiratory quotient to determine the efficacy of nutritional support regimens. *J Am Diet Assoc*. 1987;87:180–183.
10. Elia M, Livesey G. Theory and validity of indirect calorimetry during net lipid synthesis. *Am J Clin Nutr*. 1988;47:591–607.
11. Askanazi J, Rosenbaum SH, Hyman AI, et al. Respiratory changes induced by the large glucose loads of total parenteral nutrition. *JAMA*. 1980;243:1444–1447.
12. Ireton-Jones C. Indirect Calorimetry. In: Skipper A, ed. *The Dietitian's Handbook of Enteral and Parenteral Nutrition*. 2nd ed. Gaithersburg, MD: Aspen Publishers;1998.
13. Ireton-Jones CS, Borman KR, Turner WW. Nutrition considerations in the management of ventilator-dependent patients. *Nutr Clin Prac*. 1993;8:60–64.
14. Dietrich KA, Romero MD, Conrad SA. Effects of gas leak around endotracheal tubes on indirect calorimetry measurements. *J Parenter Enteral Nutr*. 1990;14:408–413.
15. Ireton CS, Turner WW, Hunt JL, et al. Evaluation of energy expenditures in burn patients. *J Am Diet Assoc*. 1986;86:331–333.
16. Ireton-Jones CS, Turner WW, Liepa GU, et al. Equations for estimation of energy expenditures in patients with burns with special reference to ventilatory status. *J Burn Care Rehab*. 1992;13:330–333.
17. Porter C, Cohen N. Indirect calorimetry in critically ill patients: role of the clinical dietitian in interpreting results. *J Am Diet Assoc*. 1996;96:49–57.
18. McClave SA, Snider HL. Use of indirect calorimetry in clinical nutrition. *Nutr Clin Prac*. 1992;7:208–221.
19. Gottschlich MM, Jenkins M, Mayes T, et al. Lack of effect of sleep on energy expenditure and physiologic measures in critically ill burn patients. *J Am Diet Assoc*. 1997;97:131–139.
20. Smyrnios N, Curley F, Shaker KG. Accuracy of 30 minute indirect calorimetry (IC) studies in predicting 24 hour energy expenditure (EE) in critically ill patients. *J Parenter Enteral Nutr*. 1997;21:168–174.
21. Shronts EP, Lacy JA. Metabolic support. In: Gottschlich MM, Matarese LE, Shronts EP, eds. *Nutrition Support Dietetics Core Curriculum*. Silver Spring, MD:American Society for Parenteral and Enteral Nutrition;1993:356.
22. Foster GD, Knox, LS, Dempsey, DT, et al. Caloric requirements in total parenteral nutrition. *J Am Coll Nutr*. 1987;6:231–253.
23. Ireton-Jones C, Jones JD. Predictive equations should be used. *Nutr Clin Prac*. 1998;13:141–146.
24. Harris, JA, Benedict FG. *Biometric Studies of Basal Metabolism in Man. Carnegie Institution of Washington*, publication no. 270; 1919.
25. Garrel DR, Jobin N, De Jonge LHM. Should we still use the Harris and Benedict equations? *Nutr Clin Prac*. 1996;11:99–103.
26. Cortes V, Nelson L. Errors in estimating energy expenditure in critically ill surgical patients *Arch Surg*. 1989;124:287–290.
27. Cutts ME, Dowdy RP, Ellersieck MR, et al. Predicting energy needs in ventilator-dependent critically ill patients: effect of adjusting weight for edema or adiposity. *Am J Clin Nutr*. 1997;66:1250–6.

28. Van Lanschot J, Feenstra B, Vermeij C, et al. Calculation versus measurement of total energy expenditure. *Crit Care Med.* 1986;14:981–985.

29. Hopkins B. Assessment of nutritional status. In: Gottschlich M, Matarese L, Shronts E, eds. *Nutrition Support Dietetics Core Curriculum.* 2nd ed. Silver Spring, MD: American Society for Parenteral and Enteral Nutrition, 1993:15–70.

30. Ireton-Jones C. Comparison of the metabolic response to burn injury in obese and nonobese patients. *J Burn Care and Rehab.* 1997;18:82–85.

31. Cerra FB, Benitez MR, Blackburn GL, et al. Applied nutrition in ICU patients—a consensus statement of the American College of Chest Physicians. *Chest.* 1997;111: 769–778.

32. Ireton-Jones CS, Jones JD. Why use predictive equations for energy expenditure assessment? *J Am Diet Assoc.* 1997;97:A-44.

33. Wall JO, Wall PT, Ireton-Jones CS, et al. Accurate prediction of the energy expenditures of hospitalized patients. *J Am Diet Assoc.* 1995;95:A–24.

34. Gagliardi E, Brathwaite LEM, Ross SE. Predicting energy expenditure in trauma patients. Validation of the Ireton-Jones equation. *J Parenter Enteral Nutr.* 1995;19:22S.

35. Amato P, Keating KP, Quercia RA, et al. Formulaic methods of estimating calorie requirements in mechanically ventilated obese patients: a reappraisal. *Nutr Clin Prac.* 1995;10:229–232.

36. Ireton-Jones C, Jones J. Improved equations for predicting energy expenditure in patients: the Ireton-Jones equations. *Nutr Clin Prac.* (submitted).

37. Ireton-Jones CS, Turner WW. Actual or ideal body weights: which is more accurate to estimate energy expenditure? *J Am Diet Assoc.* 1990;90:193–195.

38. Choban P, Burge J, Flaucbaum L. Nutrition support of the obese hospitalized patient. *Nutr Clin Prac.* 1997;4:149–154.

39. Patino JF, de Pimiento SE, Vergara A, et al. Hypocaloric support in the critically ill. *World J Surg.* 1999;23:553–559.

40. Scott RL, Albina JE, Caldwell MD. Effects of hypocaloric dextrose and amino acids on body composition and nitrogen balance in rats. *J Parenter Enteral Nutr.* 1982;6:489–495.

41. McCowen KC, Friel C, Sternberg J, et al. Hypocaloric total parenteral nutrition: effectiveness in prevention of hyperglycemia and infectious complications—a randomized clinical trial. *Crit Care Med.* 2000;28:3606–3611.

42. Dickerson RN, Rosato, EF, Mullen, JL. Net protein anabolism with hypocaloric parenteral nutrition in obese stressed patients. *Am J Clin Nutr.* 1986;44:747–755.

CHAPTER

5 Parenteral Nutrition (Macronutrient Fuels)

David F. Driscoll, Ph.D., Bruce R. Bistrian, M.D., Ph.D.

INTRODUCTION 39

MACRONUTRIENT BIOCHEMISTRY 40
- Protein 40
- Carbohydrate 41
- Lipids 42

NUTRITION-RELATED COMPLICATIONS 43
- Under-Nutrition 43
- Over-Nutrition 45

DESIGNING THE MACRONUTRIENT REGIMEN 45
- Feeding Weight 45
- Caloric Intake 46
- Volume 46

DEVISING THE FINAL TPN FORMULATION: APPLYING THE ASPEN GUIDELINES 47
- The Initial Critical Care PN Regimen 47
- The Weight-Based Eucaloric PN Regimen 47

CONCLUSIONS 47

REFERENCES 48

Introduction

Parenteral nutrition (PN) therapy is unquestionably one of the major advances of the 20th century in the medical and surgical management of patients with significant gastrointestinal disease or impaired gastrointestinal function. It is also a therapy that has sometimes been unfairly criticized for producing more harm than good in certain clinical situations, especially during critical illness. Clearly, if PN therapy is inappropriately applied, it has the potential to cause significant morbidity and even mortality. As nutrition support has evolved over the last 30 to 35 years, many therapy-refining lessons have been learned. The term hyperalimentation clearly describes the early therapy where excessive nutrition was routinely and consciously supplied, often in quantities exceeding 4000 calories per day, and in nearly equal volumes (mLs) of fluid. From these early days of excessive feeding to a period where "hyperalimentation" therapy became more widely applied, "standardized" nutrition support regimens evolved in order to minimize variations in clinical application. Although the total amounts of nutrition support administered to the patient began to decrease, the initial attempts at standardizing the approach to parenteral feeding was oversimplified. A single common formula, consisting of final concentrations of amino acids of 4.25% (42.5 g/L) and 25% (250 g/L) dextrose, was prescribed in varying final volumes per day. This regimen provided a 125:1 calorie-to-nitrogen ratio. Such proportions often resulted in suboptimal protein intakes in most fluid-restricted, critically ill patients and excessive carbohydrate intakes at reasonable protein intakes in patients not fluid-restricted. Furthermore, some clinicians opted even to standardize the volume for all patients at 2000 mL, which consisted of 1000 mL of 8.5% stock amino acids and 1000 mL of dextrose 50%, to yield the aforementioned final concentrations, and only adjusted the infusion rate to the patient. In so doing, the infusion was either prolonged beyond 24 hours or the remaining volume at the end of the day was discarded. In either case, attempts to standardize the practice of intravenous nutrition support were flawed on clinical, pharmaceutical, and economic grounds.

In the intensive care unit setting, a patient-specific approach is often warranted. Moreover, the amounts of protein and energy provided may often be a fraction of the quantities normally given to achieve eucaloric nutrition support. This is largely a consequence of severe metabolic stress that limits the amount of macronutrients and volume that may be supplied during the early phases of critical illness. The nutrition support clinician must be cognizant of these limitations and work with the primary care team to provide optimal clinical care.

Macronutrient Biochemistry

Protein

Early in the development of PN therapy, hydrolysate mixtures from dairy protein sources, such as casein, or beef blood as fibrin were the principal forms of protein for intravenous nutrition.[1] Unfortunately, although rich in peptides as well as individual amino acids, these mixtures served as an excellent nutrient source for microbial growth, particularly if inadvertent contamination occurred during either their extemporaneous preparation or infusion in the clinical setting. The early literature is replete with iatrogenic infections emanating from these mixtures. Furthermore, the more complex oligopeptides could not be assimilated and were excreted in the urine. By the early 1970s, newer sources of protein were developed using synthetic crystalline amino acids that provided improved nitrogen balance and did not support the growth of nosocomial pathogens.[2] As research in the field of amino acids advanced, further refinements in the ratios of individual amino acids were developed, particularly for patients with nitrogen accumulation disorders. Special emphasis was placed on the essential amino acids for patients with renal failure, while the importance of branched-chain amino acids was heralded for patients with end-stage liver disease and critical illness. Although the early metabolic and clinical data were promising in these conditions, subsequent studies showed little measurable clinical benefit from these therapies.[3,4] Moreover, in some cases the limitation or exclusion of other amino acids in these conditions was problematic, producing a spectrum of clinical issues. These issues ranged from an individual amino acid being rate-limiting in terms of achieving nitrogen balance, to actually producing clinically significant adverse events (hyperammonemia), when these unbalanced formulations attempted to provide adequate-to-optimal levels of protein intakes.[5]

It is generally recognized that, under most conditions, conventional amino acid formulations, rather than the specialized ones, are the optimal form of intravenous amino-acid therapy. If mild to moderate pathological retention of nitrogen is present, whether of renal (urea) or hepatic (ammonium) origin, reducing conventional protein intake to between 0.8–1.2 g/kg/d provides adequate nutrition for a brief period (7 to 10 days) until the stress response remits, or there is a significant change in the clinical condition. For moderate to severe kidney or liver disease, where the retention of nitrogen may be clinically significant, the short-term use of these specialized amino acid formulations may be considered, even though the only clear demonstrable impact has been improved protein utilization. This means that more protein can be provided for a given urea or ammonium level, which would be theoretically important if only marginal levels of total amino acids (0.8 g/kg/d or less) could otherwise be provided.

One example would be in a patient with hepatic encephalopathy who is amino acid responsive (usually due to chronic disease) and is not a candidate for nasogastric feeding. Under these conditions, the use of branched-chain enriched amino acids in the TPN admixture may be indicated. This, of course, should be adjunctive therapy to other aggressive medical maneuvers to reduce the nitrogen burden, such as lactulose therapy.

Alternatively, if a patient is severely azotemic (BUN >100–150 mg%) and there is an increased risk of uremic complications (i.e., bleeding), then short-term branched chain-enriched amino acid therapy is also reasonable, when used along with other methods to manage renal failure, such as dialysis. Essential amino acid therapy is no longer used, because the total protein intake that can be safely provided is too low for the critically ill. Thus, the use of these specialized amino acid formulations, which are enriched with branched chain amino acids either with or without a reduction in aromatic amino acids, and are considerably more expensive than conventional products, may be indicated for short-term use in the critically ill.

The use of novel amino acid therapies, such as glutamine supplementation, is still considered innovative clinical care and therefore the benefits are yet to be completely defined. Moreover, in the United States, the addition of glutamine requires the product to be extemporaneously prepared by the pharmacy under aseptic conditions and often for immediate use. In other centers, batches are made and stored for use over several weeks. However, the stability of glutamine is limited to between 4 and 6 weeks, and this degree of pharmacy preparation requires a much higher level of practice and environmental conditions than are available in most institutions. Even when such compounding conditions are met in accordance with professional guidelines, this practice is considered manufacturing, not extemporaneous compounding, and requires a batch record for each lot made. The batch record should include specific information, such as content analysis (glutamine concentration), sterility and pyrogen testing, controlled temperature and storage conditions, among other requirements typically necessary to comply with good manufacturing practices (GMPs) that are normally expected of the pharmaceutical manufacturer. It is unacceptable for a pharmacy to make such batches without an appropriate quarantine period until the results of these quality assurance tests are completed and recorded into each and every batch record. These stringent requirements leave this therapy largely unavailable in the United States until glutamine peptides, *available* in much of the European community, are approved in this country.

For acutely ill patients who are candidates for parenteral nutrition and are free of significant nitrogen accumulation disorders, usual protein intake during metabolic stress is approximately double the recommended dietary allowance for protein under unstressed conditions. For example, 0.8 g/kg/d is the RDA for normal protein intake, whereas during acute metabolic stress, the amounts that should be given are up to approximately 1.5 g/kg/d, a level that provides maximal utilization. This is due to the metabolic inefficiencies that occur with respect to protein utilization. During moderate to severe metabolic stress, as encountered in the intensive care unit, a greater percentage of parenteral and enteral protein intake is catabolized. However, limits to the amounts of protein that can be given, where no further improvement in utilization occurs, have been estimated to be approximately 1.5–1.75 g/kg/d.[6,7] This may not, however, apply for those patients with protein-losing conditions such as an open wound, major thermal burns, or high-output gastrointestinal fistula. Providing amounts greater than this only increases the rate of ureagenesis, which appears in the 24-hour urine in those with adequate renal function or, worse, accumulates in those with deteriorating end-organ function, eventually producing additional clinical problems.

Carbohydrate

Glucose is the only carbohydrate source available for parenteral administration in the United States. It is a highly efficient source of energy and essential for some tissues (i.e., brain, renal medulla, white [facultatively] and red blood cells.). During severe metabolic stress, glycogen stores are rapidly depleted, often within 24 hours of the injury or stress. In the absence of exogenous provision of this fuel, the body will make glucose from amino acid precursors, particularly alanine and glutamine, through skeletal muscle proteolysis initiated through a series of neurohumoral signals coincident with the injury response,[8] as well as from lactate from the Cori Cycle and glycerol from adipose tissue released during lipolysis. This occurs in order to provide a basal amount of glucose to obligate tissues of the body. Although this is a life-saving metabolic adaptation, it occurs at the expense of lean body mass, and if sustained, particularly in patients with pre-existing malnutrition, can lead to significant morbidity and mortality. Even in the well-nourished, if the stress response continues without nutrition support for prolonged periods (typically more than 10 days), or if the initial stress is very large (i.e., major burns, sepsis, trauma, head injury), complications due to inadequate feeding can also occur. The difference, of course, relates to the initial lean body mass reserves and the severity and duration of the systemic inflammatory response, which will dictate the rapidity with which complications develop that can lead to poor wound healing and increased susceptibility to infection, organ failure, and death.

Conversely, providing exogenous glucose must be carefully undertaken in the presence of ongoing metabolic stress. The amounts of glucose that can be safely given are a function of its oxidation. When the rate of glucose infusion rate exceeds its oxidation rate (and in parenteral glucose infusion this occurs at rates of even 100 g/24 hours) it is the subsequent non-oxidative disposal that may produce clinical problems.[9] Therefore, the clinician must be cognizant of the significance of glucose-infusion rate to avoid iatrogenic feeding complications. First, as alluded to above, there is a basal amount of glucose necessary to meet the metabolic demands of the obligate tissues, as well as an optimal fuel for other tissues. Based on studies performed over 30 years ago during starvation in man,[10] the basal amount of glucose produced is estimated to be approximately 2 mg/kg/min or roughly 200 g/24 h in the 70 kg reference individual. Providing these levels will lessen the burden of glucose production from lean body mass and in the normal individual but not the critically ill, will largely prevent gluconeogenesis. Generally, this amount is a reasonable starting point for critically ill patients when initiating PN therapy. The important difference between normal subjects and critically ill patients is that the systemic inflammatory response increases insulin resistance leading to impaired uptake of glucose by muscle, acceleration of glucose production by the liver, and limited suppression of gluconeogenesis by exogenous *glucose* infusion. Thus, providing 200 g of glucose to critically ill patients may cause a total appearance of as much as 500 g/24 h, since an enhanced state of gluconeogenesis of 300 g/24 h is not suppressed. Furthermore, if the patient is glucose intolerant or has a history of diabetes, then the initial glucose infusion rate during the early critical care period should be a fraction of the basal glucose infusion rate that does not worsen present glucose homeostasis. A progressive schedule of representative daily glucose infusion rates in adults (via PN therapy) up to the basal requirements is shown in Table 5.1. Although the final amounts in Table 5.1 are specifically calculated, they can be rounded to the nearest 10 g. Alternatively, these quantities can be easily delivered and are within the capability of most automated TPN compounding devices. Presently, over 65% of health care institutions use automated compounding devices to provide PN therapy.[11]

TABLE 5.1

Glucose Infusion Rates Up to Basal Requirements in Adults in the Intensive Care Unit

Weight	1 mg/kg/min	1.5 mg/kg/min	2 mg/kg/min
40 kg	57.6 g	86.4 g	115.2 g
50 kg	72.0 g	108.0 g	144.0 g
60 kg	86.4 g	129.6 g	168.0 g
70 kg	100.8 g	151.2 g	201.6 g
80 kg	115.2 g	172.8 g	230.4 g

LIPIDS

Intravenous lipid emulsions (IVLEs) are an alternative or complementary fuel to glucose. The first triacylglycerol fats that were successfully introduced into clinical use comprised long-chain fatty acids derived from soybean oil alone or in equal combination (by weight) with safflower oil. For soybean oil-based emulsions, they included, in descending order of concentration, linoleic acid, oleic acid, alpha-linolenic acid, palmitic acid, stearic acid, and small quantities of other neutral fatty acids. The 1:1 w/w mixture of soybean and safflower oils has a similar mixture of fatty acids as above, but approximately 50% more linoleic acid and a corresponding decrease in alpha-linolenic acid, as safflower oil contains very little linolenic acid. The fatty acid profiles of representative IVLEs that are commercially available around the world are shown in Table 5.2.

At the present time in the United States, only long-chain triglyceride mixtures as described above are commercially available. The clinical indications for IVLE include prevention of essential fatty acid deficiency (EFAD) and as a daily caloric source substituting for glucose calories. The syndrome of EFAD is usually a consequence of intestinal failure where there is malabsorption of essential lipid nutrients, linoleic

TABLE 5.2

Principal Fatty Acid Profiles* in Commercial IVLEs (per 10 g of lipid emulsion mixture)

			Amounts per Product* (g/10 g of oil)						
Fatty Acid	*Carbon No.*	*Notation*	*A*	*B*	*C*	*D*	*E*	*F*	*G*
Caprylic	C-8	c8:0		2.52		3.5	3.5	5.25	
Capric	C-10	c10:0		1.08		1.5	1.5	2.25	
Myristic	C-14	c14:0	0.01	0.006	0.01	0.005	0.004	0.002	0.002
Palmitic	C-16	c16:0	1.1	0.70	0.87	0.55	0.613	0.27	1.18
Palmitoleic	C-16	c16:1ω7	0.01	0.006	0.005	0.005	0.09	0.002	0.082
Stearic	C-18	c18:0	0.4	0.25	0.32	0.20	0.18	0.1	0.24
Oleic	C-18	c18:1ω9	2.34	1.49	1.82	1.17	1.06	0.58	6.22
Linoleic	C-18	c18:2ω6	5.32	3.40	6.54	2.66	2.14	1.33	1.94
α-linolenic	C-18	c18:3ω3	0.78	0.49	0.39	0.39	0.32	0.19	0.236
γ-linolenic	C-18	c18:3ω6					0.001		
Arachidonic	C-20	c20:4ω6					0.008		
Eicosapentaenoic	C-20	c20:5ω3					0.128		
Docosahexaenoic	C-22	c22:6ω3					0.087		

***Products (oil composition by weight)**
A: 100% Soybean Oil
B: 64% Soybean Oil/36% MCT Oil
C: 50% Soybean Oil/50% Safflower Oil
D: 50% Soybean Oil/50% MCT Oil
E: 40% Soybean Oil/50% MCT Oil/10% Fish Oil
F: 25% Soybean Oil/75% MCT Oil
G: 20% Soybean Oil/80% Olive Oil

Reprinted with permission from *American Society for Parenteral and Enteral Nutrition, In: Nutrition in Clinical Practice* (NCP) 2001;16:215–218.

and alpha-linolenic acids, as well as fat soluble vitamins A, D, E and K. The use of lipids as a daily caloric source has been shown to be equally nitrogen-sparing with glucose after four days of continuous use.[12] IVLEs may be given as a separate infusion using the manufacturers' ready-to-use container or may be mixed with amino acids, dextrose, electrolytes, vitamins, and minerals and called an all-in-one or total nutrient admixture (TNA). Generally, when used as a daily caloric source in the critically ill, the amounts of lipids given each day are in the range of 15%–30% of the total kilocalories of nutrition support per day.[9]

Whichever option for lipid administration is chosen (separate or as a TNA), the rate of infusion is also critical to avoid iatrogenic complications. The parenteral administration of long-chain triglycerides (LCTs) exceeding a rate of 0.11 g/kg/h has been determined to underlie the vast majority of complications associated with IVLEs.[13] The risks are clearly increased when IVLEs are given by separate intravenous infusion, as this method is often accomplished as an intermittent infusion each day over several hours, whereas TNAs are generally given continuously over 24 hours. In the former case, providing IVLEs as a separate intermittent infusion each day can often exceed this toxic threshold rate. Table 5.3 shows safe infusion rates using commercially available sizes of IVLEs. It can be deduced from this table that if the toxic threshold is to be avoided, and individual IVLE bottles should not be infused for a period exceeding 12 hours, then 500 mL of 20% IVLE should not be used in any patient under 85 kg. Table 5.4 illustrates the differences between safe (50% of toxic) and unsafe intermittent IVLE infusion rates for specific TNA doses of LCTs. Alternatively, the doses calculated for each weight may be rounded to the nearest commercial size if separate IVLE administration is desired. Providing IVLEs as TNAs continuously over 24 hours in ranges of 15%–30% of total kcals per day obviates the concerns associated with excessive infusion rates of LCTs.

TABLE 5.3

Briefest* Fat Infusion Rates in Adults Using Commercially Available Sizes of IVLE

Product	Weights				
IVLE 10% (**)	*40 kg*	*50 kg*	*60 kg*	*70 kg*	*80 kg*
100 mL (10 g)	3 hours	3 hours	2 hours	2 hours	2 hours
200 mL (20 g)	6 hours	5 hours	4 hours	3 hours	3 hours
250 mL (25 g)	7 hours	6 hours	5 hours	4 hours	4 hours
500 mL (50 g)	XXX***	11 hours	9 hours	8 hours	7 hours
IVLE 20% (**)					
100 mL (20 g)	6 hours	5 hours	4 hours	3 hours	3 hours
200 mL (40 g)	11 hours	9 hours	7 hours	6 hours	6 hours
250 mL (50 g)	XXX***	11 hours	9 hours	8 hours	7 hours
500 mL (100 g)	XXX***	XXX***	XXX***	XXX***	XXX***

*Criteria: Fat Infusion Rate is <0.1 g/kg/h, rounded to nearest hour
**Grams of fat per bottle
***The safe rate would exceed a 12-hour hang time that is not recommended for individual bottles of IVLE

Reprinted with permission from *American Society for Parenteral and Enteral Nutrition, In: Nutrition in Clinical Practice* (NCP) 2001;16:215-218.

Nutrition-Related Complications

Under-Nutrition

Parenteral nutrition in the acutely ill, hospitalized patient is intended to attenuate the catabolic effects of the metabolic response to injury. It is assumed that a sustained stress response will deplete essential body protein stores that will affect recovery from acute disease. This is also assumed to be particularly important in the previously malnourished patient who has recently sustained an injury or other significant metabolic stress. These assumptions are based on a fundamental understanding of the physiologic mechanisms that affect lean body mass, and subsequently, the ability to recover from metabolic stresses such as major thoracoabdominal surgery or systemic injury, infection, or inflammation (i.e., severe pancreatitis) that are frequently complicated by organ failure. For example, every gram of nitrogen lost represents approximately 6.25 g of body protein and about 30 g of lean tissue (since body protein is hydrated at a ratio of 4 to 1).[14] The point when continued losses of nitrogen impair the host's ability to recuperate from disease and adversely affect outcome is not well-defined. However, a 10% unintentional weight loss will impair physiologic function, and a 20% weight loss will dramatically increase morbidity and mortality from stress, while a 40% weight loss is incompatible with life even without superimposed metabolic stress.

However, two significant risk factors heighten the risk of complications associated with undernutrition in the management of the acutely ill, hospitalized patient: the magnitude of the injury response and preexisting malnutrition. Contrary arguments about the need to feed acutely ill patients have arisen in light of the purported benefits of aggressive nutritional support. In particular, the lack of sufficient data in the literature to conclusively support nutritional alimentation in the acutely ill, as well as the dearth of prospective, randomized controlled trials, has fostered a prem-

TABLE 5.4

Fat Infusion Rates Up to the Toxic Threshold* for LCT Lipid Emulsions in Adults in the Intensive Care Unit						
Weight	15% of Total kcals (0.05 g/kg/h)	Safe Rate (hours)	30% of Total kcals (0.05 g/kg/h)	Safe Rate (hours)	Unsafe Rate*—(hours) (0.1 g/kg/h*)	
					15% kcals	30% kcals
40 kg	16.7 g/d	8	33.3 g/d	16	4	8
50 kg	20.8 g/d	8	41.6 g/d	16	4	8
60 kg	25.0 g/d	8	50.0 g/d	16	4	8
70 kg	29.2 g/d	8	58.4 g/d	16	4	8
80 kg	33.3 g/d	8	66.6 g/d	16	4	8

U.S. Manufacturer's Units of Use:
10% IVLE: 100 mL (10 g); 200 mL (20 g); 250 mL (25 g); 500 mL (50 g)
20% IVLE: 100 mL (20 g); 200 mL (40 g); 250 mL (50 g); 500 mL (100 g)
30% IVLE: Not for clinical use; only for pharmacy compounding procedures.
***Rates of 0.11 g/kg/hour or higher are not recommended.**

ise that no nutrition support is necessary until proven otherwise.[15]

Although claims regarding the paucity of scientific literature to conclusively support an evidence-based policy for nutrition support in acutely ill patients are superficially supportable, a more critical analysis recognizing that nutrition is unlikely to benefit the well-nourished or unstressed, nevertheless supports the efficacy of nutrition in common disorders characterized by malnutrition and moderate-to-severe metabolic stress. Furthermore, sufficient data exist about the consequences of nutritional deprivation in normal subjects that can be reasonably extrapolated to metabolically stressed patients and provide an additional rationale for the efficacy of nutrition support.[16] For example, in 1981, 10 IRA members incarcerated in a prison in Belfast, Ireland, went on a hunger strike that resulted in their deaths over a period of 45 to 73 days of fasting.[17] What is so scientifically compelling about these most unfortunate deaths was the fact that these were all young men (age 25.6 ± 0.7 years) without obvious clinical metabolic stress. The critical weight loss, derived from the final weight of the remaining four hunger strikers, was approximately 23.5 kg, or approximately 35% loss in weight. The range in days to death between strikers might be explained by the biological variations in body composition. It is known that following a brief adaptation period where nitrogen losses are accrued at a rate of 16–20 g N/day the average loss is 4–10 g N/day related to the amount of remaining adipose tissues. Thus, it can be inferred from the available data that a critical cumulative nitrogen deficit in normal unstressed individuals of between 350–500 g of nitrogen (about one third to one half of body cell mass) is incompatible with life. The body cell mass is the actively metabolizing, nitrogen-containing portion of the body (vital organs, skeletal muscle, etc.), which represents about 40% of body weight.

In the presence of acute metabolic stress, such as occurs in the intensive care unit, nitrogen deficits accrue over substantially shorter intervals. In addition, depending on the age and medical history of the patient, it is likely that many ICU patients with chronic disease are at less than their ideal body cell mass even though their weights may be normal or elevated due to excessive fluid. Thus, when malnourished patients undergo severe metabolic stress, the amount of weight loss, and specifically the nitrogen deficit that can be tolerated, is far less than normally nourished counterparts with similar levels of metabolic stress. If, for example, we conservatively assume a critical nitrogen deficit threshold to be 250 g N, then the lean patient, losing a net of 20 g of nitrogen daily, a rate seen in many moderate to severely stressed patients will be at risk of significant morbidity or even mortality in the absence of feeding within 12 to 13 days. For 30 g daily N losses, commonly seen with major burns, multiple trauma, closed head injury, and severe sepsis, this period shortens to 8 to 9 days. For patients with pre-existing severe malnutrition, the losses in body cell mass for the same degree of stress would generally be less compared to normals, and the time course may also be less. Thus, withholding nutrition support is likely to have significant consequences in terms of morbidity and mortality in the malnourished patient with moderate metabolic stress within 5 to 7 days or any patient with severe metabolic stress beyond several days.

Over-Nutrition

First, it is important to recognize that prescribing inappropriate amounts of nutrition may be detrimental to ICU patients given the clinical circumstances surrounding their condition. For example, excessive amounts of protein to patients with underlying nitrogen accumulation disorders may exacerbate central nervous system dysfunction in patients with liver disease, which might prolong the need for mechanical ventilatory assistance. Moreover, patients with renal failure may be at increased risk for uremic-associated complications such as bleeding when protein intake is excessive, although this point has not been well defined as resulting from excessive amino acid intake as opposed to protein (meat, fish, poultry) intake.

Providing inordinate amounts of calories as dextrose or fat may have similar adverse consequences. Initiating large quantities of dextrose may be harmful in ICU patients with infection, respiratory distress, liver disease, or congestive heart failure. During severe metabolic stress, glucose intolerance is common, and blood concentrations in excess of 200 mg% may impair host defenses affecting neutrophilic adhesion, chemotaxis, and phagocytosis. Glucose can also glycosylate immune proteins such as opsonins, rendering them less effective.[18] Administering even modest amounts of dextrose during this time may only serve to augment the hyperglycemic state and increase the risk of infection. For instance, providing TPN at 30–35 kcal/kg/d made more than 50% of the non-diabetic patients hyperglycemic, i.e., blood glucose >200 mg/dL.[19] Providing glucose in excess of resting energy expenditure may be especially distressing in patients with liver disease and respiratory decompensation. Following repletion of glycogen stores in normal feeding, a greater fraction of glucose is converted to fat in the liver. Such enhanced *de novo* lipogenesis occurs at all levels of glucose infusion and may not only impair vital hepatic functions, but will increase the amount of carbon dioxide produced in relation to the amount of oxygen consumed. The elevated production of carbon dioxide increases the respiratory workload, and in patients with compromised cardiopulmonary function, may precipitate respiratory decompensation and/or prolong the need for mechanical ventilatory assistance. Finally, excess dextrose administration in conjunction with 70–100 or more milliequivalents of sodium to patients with congestive heart failure or other fluid-retaining disorders (i.e., liver or kidney disease) may be dangerous. Much higher blood glucose concentrations are achieved when dextrose is delivered intravenously than when given by the enteral route, which induces a profound hyperinsulinemia. Such high concentrations of insulin produce significant antinatriuresis,[20] and thus may precipitate florid congestive heart failure if ample sodium is provided, particularly in the ICU patient with fragile cardiovascular function, where often less than 5 mEq of sodium per 24 hours is excreted in the urine.

Likewise, inappropriate administration of fat calories can be equally harmful. This is especially true when fat is given in large quantities over short intervals. Klein and Miles have concluded that IVLE of >0.11 g/kg/h for LCTs can be harmful.[13] Moreover, in ICU patients, the intermittent administration of separate infusions of 500 mL of 20% LCTs lipid emulsions over short infusion periods (i.e., 5 to 10 hours) have produced significant pulmonary gas diffusion abnormalities that worsen lung function.[21–23] In addition, hypertriglyceridemia[24] and perturbations in immune function[25] have also been associated with the inappropriate administration of long-chain triglycerides (LCTs). These and related effects have not been demonstrated when LCTs have been given continuously over 24 hours in doses up to 30% of the total calories, or when given as medium-chain triglycerides (MCT)-LCT mixtures. Moreover, quantities of fat exceeding 30% of caloric needs were found to offer no additional clinical benefit in patients with respiratory compromise.[26]

Designing the Macronutrient Regimen

Feeding Weight

When determining macronutrient requirements, ascertaining the correct weight of the patient is essential in order to avoid feeding complications associated with PN therapy. This can be achieved by using a number of tools to decide on the best feeding weight. This begins with a good medical history in order to differentiate between the hospital admission weight, the present weight, the pre-morbid weight, and the usual weight. A wide variance is often found between the weights at these various times; therefore, a detailed assessment of weight history over the last 3 to 6 months is critical. For example, the admission weight will often differ significantly from the present "hospital" weight at the time of a formal nutrition support consult. This is especially true in the critical care setting, where excessive fluid administration can rapidly increase weight.

Patients with chronic disease will often have a protracted and fluctuating weight history that may go back several years. It should be the goal of the nutrition support clinician to ascertain the usual stable weight, which is often not in concordance with ideal body weight tables. It is, however, helpful to use a variety of measures to determine the feeding weight of the patient. In addition to a detailed weight history, anthropometric measurements, subjective global assessment, standard tables of weight for height, and body mass index calculations will confirm the best feeding weight. Otherwise, if great care is not undertaken in this regard, feeding complications are more likely to occur, as the dose of macronutrients, like drugs, is predicated on a reliable body weight that reflects the metabolically active body cell mass. Table 5.5 depicts an illustrative case over a series of adult patient weights ranging from 40–80 kg.

Caloric Intake

Although early estimates of the energy requirements in critically ill patients increased with the degree of the metabolic stress, i.e., hypermetabolism, these early clinical impressions have been drastically reduced with improvements in clinical management and better measuring tools. In fact, calculated estimates as high as 50 kcal/kg/d or more[27] as originally prescribed, have since been shown to be as much as 100% higher than actual energy needs in a number of studies where energy expenditure was measured using modern indirect calorimetry and new treatment regimens. Thus, 25 kcal/kg/d is generally recommended for most acutely ill patients, where, after protein needs are determined, the remaining calories can be divided between glucose and lipid.[28] The amount of calories from glucose and fat may vary and can be solely derived from glucose if desired. However, unless a severe underlying lipid disorder exists, lipids are generally substituted for glucose calories and account for up to 15%–30% of total kcals per day. Finally, in the early critical care period, it is prudent to prescribe an initial PN regimen that provides only a fraction of the daily recommendations to ensure nitrogen and glucose homeostasis is first attained before higher levels up to eucaloric amounts of nutrition are given. It has been widely confirmed that most intensive care unit and postoperative patients (exclusive of usually younger individuals with severe stress of trauma, major burns, head injury and severe sepsis) have energy expenditures that range between 20–25 kcal/kg and rarely exceed 30 kcal/kg. Providing parenteral nutrition in such patients at 25 kcal/kg meets their energy needs and does not usually disrupt glucose homeostasis. The latter patients with the most severe degrees of stress have energy expenditures of 30–40 kcal/kg, which would be required to place them in energy balance, but this amount would severely disrupt glucose homeostasis in more than half the population. Even though patients with the most severe stress (multiple trauma, closed head injury, severe sepsis) often have measured energy expenditures of 30–40 kcal/kg, a careful reading of randomized trials in these conditions suggests that energy in the 25 kcal/kg range may be more appropriate. It has not been clearly established, but it is interesting to note that in those studies where PN produced more infections than with enteral nutrition, the enteral intake approximated 30 kcal/kg or less and the parenteral intake was significantly higher in the 35 kcal/kg range.[29–31] In a fourth study where parenteral intakes were matched to enteral intakes by prescribing higher amounts of enteral nutrition, there was no difference in infections, although these were high in both groups.[32]

TABLE 5.5

Representative Eucaloric Macronutrient Intakes for Total Nutrient Admixture Regimens in Adult Patients

Weight	Amino Acids	Glucose	Lipids	Nitrogen	~Total kcals/day
40 kg	60 g	166 g	21 g	9.6 g	1000
50 kg	75 g	208 g	26 g	12.0 g	1250
60 kg	90 g	250 g	31 g	14.4 g	1500
70 kg	105 g	290 g	37 g	16.8 g	1750
80 kg	120 g	333 g	42 g	19.2 g	2000

Based on the following conditions:

1. 24-hour supply in one bag.
2. 1.5 g/kg/d of protein.
3. 1 g Nitrogen = 6.25 g of protein.
4. caloric equivalents: protein = 4.1 kcal/g; hydrated dextrose = 3.4 kcal/g; fat = 9 kcal/g.
5. 25 kcal/kg/d—total.
6. 25% of non-protein kcals as fat.
7. 25 mL/kg/d of PN volume.
8. easily made with an automated compounding device.

Volume

During critical illness, patients invariably become fluid-overloaded, which can produce dramatic changes in the patient's actual weight as a consequence of therapeutic maneuvers frequently employed in the ICU to optimize organ function. Generally, weight increases during hospitalization, particularly in ICU patients coincident with intraoperative fluid therapy, post-operative volume resuscitation, and the parenteral administration of numerous drug therapies and associated diluents.[33] Although acute in-hospital weight typically increases 10%–20% of admission weight, this can vary and can occur in as little as 8 to 12 hours during major thoracoabdominal surgery, or over 5–7 days of severe illness in the ICU. Fluid overload is further exacerbated because of the heightened secretion of neurohumoral mediators, such as aldosterone, antidiuretic hormone, and insulin, in response to acute metabolic stress. Therefore, it would be a serious mistake to misinterpret the current morbid weight as the feeding weight, as such increases reflect extreme changes in water metabolism and are not representative of the metabolically active body cell mass. Under these circumstances, certain conventional measures of weight assessment, such as anthropometry, may be distorted by the acute increase in total body water, and therefore necessitate alternative methods to determine the feeding weight. Often, this information may be determined by a detailed weight history and/or indirect calorimetry, or, as a contingency, the use of ideal body weight. Usually the best estimate for feeding weight for energy purposes is the pre-hospitalization weight and for protein purposes, the ideal body weight.

Devising the Final TPN Formulation: Applying the ASPEN Guidelines

The Initial Critical Care PN Regimen

During the early phases of critical illness, it is not advisable to advance nutrition support beyond basal levels (i.e., 150–200 g of dextrose and 1 g/kg of protein) until metabolic, particularly glucose, homeostasis is achieved. Although it is possible to provide "full" nutrition by the intravenous route, irrespective of the metabolic response to injury, the risk of major feeding-related complications outweighs any perceived benefit. Thus, it is wise to provide hypocaloric nutrition with a major emphasis on fluid, electrolyte, and acid-base management. Hypocaloric nutrition can be accomplished by providing a fixed amount of protein with a modest amount of energy in the least volume possible. Frequently, 1000 mL of total PN fluid is a reasonably conservative and adequate volume to accomplish metabolic homeostasis. In this admixture, 70 grams of conventional amino acids may be given along with initially 100–150 but optimally 200 grams of dextrose, depending on blood glucose control.[34] It is essential that blood glucose should be controlled to a level below 220 mg/dL before any increase in the basal amount of carbohydrate intake is prescribed.[35] Therefore, the major effort during this time is directed at controlling blood glucose, providing adequate electrolyte support, and acid-base and mineral balance. As hemodynamic stability is achieved and third-space fluids are mobilized so that a net daily negative fluid balance occurs, modest increases in the PN volume may be instituted, or enteral nutrition may be initiated at low rates. If the enteral route is not possible, gradual advancement (i.e., 250 mL increments) of the PN volume, at a rate that does not counter the efforts of the primary care team's goal of achieving fluid homeostasis, may begin and continue until the highest eucaloric nutrition is accomplished.

The Weight-Based Eucaloric PN Regimen

At our institution, we have devised five adult formulas based on patient weights of 40, 50, 60, 70, and 80 kg, as shown in Table 5.5. In essence, this range will cover 95% of most hospitalized patients requiring PN therapy. Thus, orders for PN are written based on the patient's established "feeding weight." The obvious exception where such formulas can not be readily applied includes those patients with severe fluid retention or during high metabolic stress with glucose intolerance. Once the severity of these conditions subsides and interim nutrition support measures are undertaken as described above, such formulas can be used. These formulations are based on providing 1.5 g/kg/d of conventional protein and a total of 25 kcal/kg/d. We have devised standard PN regimens both with and without lipid calories. For patients between these weights, the clinician may opt for the regimen closest to the patient's established feeding weight. This level of standardization allows even the novice nutrition-prescribing clinician to provide appropriate macronutrient support that conforms to the ASPEN guidelines. Finally, the admixture should also contain adequate amounts of electrolytes, vitamins, and minerals to be a complete and balanced PN formulation.[28]

Conclusions

The clinical care of the ICU patient has always been a therapeutic challenge. Providing adequate nutrition support to these patients is equally challenging but can be safely accomplished when the feeding weight is correctly determined. However, nutrition support clinicians must be cognizant of the primary care team's goals and objectives during the acute care period and assist in providing expert metabolic management, while achieving safe levels of nutrition support.

References

1. Driscoll DF, Bistrian BR. Clinical issues in the therapeutic monitoring of total parenteral nutrition. *Clin Lab Med.* 1987;7:699–714.
2. Goldmann DA, Martin WT, Worthington JW. Growth of bacteria and fungi in total parenteral nutrition solutions. *Am J Surg.* 1973;126:314–318.
3. Mirtallo JM, Schneider PJ, Mavko K, et al. A comparison of essential and general amino acid infusions in the nutritional support of patients with compromised renal function. *J Parenter Enteral Nutr.* 1982;6:109–113.
4. Nompleggi DJ, Bonkovsky HL. Nutritional supplementation in chronic liver disease: an analytical review. *Hepatology.* 1994;19:518–533.
5. Lamiell JJ, Ducey JP, Freese-Kepczyk BJ, et al. Essential amino acid-induced adult hyperammonemic encephalopathy and hypophosphatemia. *Crit Care Med.* 1990;18: 451–452.
6. Shaw JHF, Widbore M, Wolfe RR. Whole body protein kinetics in severely septic patients: The response to glucose infusion in total parenteral nutrition. *Ann Surg.* 1987;205:66–72.
7. Shaw JHF, Wolfe RR. Whole body protein kinetics in patients with early and advanced gastrointestinal cancer: The response to glucose infusion and total parenteral nutrition. *Surgery.* 1988;103:148–155.
8. Pomposelli JJ, Flores EA, Bistrian BR. Role of biochemical mediators in clinical nutrition and surgical metabolism. *J Parenter Enteral Nutr.* 1988;12:212–218.
9. Driscoll DF, Adolph M, Bistrian BR. Lipid emulsions in parenteral nutrition. In Rombeau JL, Rolandelli R, eds. *Parenteral Nutrition.* Philadelphia: W. B. Saunders Company;2000:35–59.
10. Cahill GF. Starvation in man. *N Engl J Med.* 1970;282: 668–675.
11. Driscoll DF, Sanborn MD, Giampietro K. ASHP guidelines on the safe use of automated compounding devices for the preparation of parenteral nutrition admixtures. *Am J Health-Syst Pharm.* 2000;57:1343–1348.
12. Jeejeebhoy KN, Anderson GH, Nakhooda AF et al. Metabolic studies in total parenteral nutrition in man. *J Clin Invest.* 1975;57:125–136.
13. Klein S, Miles JM. Metabolic effects of long-chain and medium-chain triglycerides in humans. *J Parenter Enteral Nutr.* 1994;18:396–397.
14. Bistrian BR, Bothe A, Blackburn GL. Complications of total parenteral nutrition. *Clin Anaesthesiol.* 1983;1:693–705.
15. Koretz RL. Nutritional supplementation in the ICU. How critical is nutrition for the critically ill? *Am J Respir Crit Care Med.* 1995;151;570–573.
16. Klein S, Kinney J, Jeejeebhoy K, et al. Nutrition support in clinical practice: Review of published data and recommendations for future research directions. *J Parenter Enteral Nutr.* 1997;21:133–156.
17. Leiter LA, Marliss EB. Survival during fasting may depend on fat as well as protein stores. *JAMA.* 1982;248: 2306–2307.
18. Khaodhiar L, McCowen K, Bistrian BR. Perioperative hyperglycemia, infection or risk? *Curr Opin Clin Nutr Metab Care.* 1999;7:79–82.
19. Rosemarin D, Wardlaw G, Mirtallo J. Hyperglycemia associated with high, continuous infusion rates of total parenteral nutrition dextrose. *Nutr Clin Pract.* 1996;11: 151–156.
20. DeFronzo RA, Cooke CR, Andres R, et al. The effect of insulin on renal handling of sodium, potassium, calcium and phosphate in man. *J Clin Invest.* 1975;55:845–855.
21. Kadowitz PJ, Spannhake EW, Levin JL, et al. Differential effects of prostaglandins on the pulmonary vascular bed. *Prostaglandin Thromboxane Res.* 1980;7:31–44.
22. Hwang TL, Huang SL, Chen MF. Effects of intravenous fat emulsions on respiratory failure. *Chest.* 1990;97:934–938.
23. Mathru M, Dries DJ, Zecca A, et al. Effect of fast vs. slow intralipid infusion on gas exchange, pulmonary hemodynamics, and prostaglandin metabolism. *Chest.* 1991;99: 426–429.
24. Carpentier YA, Richelle M, Bury J, et al. Phospholipid excess of fat emulsion slows triglyceride removal and increases lipoprotein remodeling. *Arteriosclerosis.* 1987; 7:541A.
25. Seidner DL, Mascioli EA, Istfan NW, et al. Effects of long-chain triglyceride emulsions on reticuloendothelial system function in humans. *J Parenter Enteral Nutr.* 1989;13:614–619.
26. Delafosse B, Viale JP, Tissot S, et al. Effects of glucose-to-lipid ratio and type of lipid on substrate oxidation rate in patients. *Am J Physiol.* 1994;267(5 Part 1): E775–780.
27. Shizgal HM, Martin MF. Caloric requirement of the critically ill septic patient. *Crit Care Med.* 1988;16:312–317.
28. National Advisory Group on Standards and Practice Guidelines for Parenteral Nutrition. Special Report: Safe practices for parenteral nutrition formulations. *J Parenter Enteral Nutr.* 1998;22:49–66.
29. Moore F, Moore E, Jones T, et al. TEN versus TPN following major abdominal trauma—reduced septic morbidity. *J Trauma.* 1989;29:916–922.
30. Kudsk K, Croce M, Fabian T, et al. Enteral versus parenteral feeding. Effects on septic morbidity after blunt and penetrating abdominal trauma. *Ann Surg.* 1992;215: 503–512.
31. Moore F, Feliciano D, Andrassy R, et al. Early enteral feeding, compared with parenteral, reduces postoperative septic complications. *Ann Surg.* 1992;216:172–183.
32. Adams S, Dellinger E, Wertz M, et al. Enteral versus parenteral nutritional support following laparotomy for trauma: a randomized prospective trial. *J Trauma.* 1986; 26:882–891.

33. Lowell JA., Schifferdecker, C, Driscoll DF, et al. Postoperative fluid overload: not a benign problem. *Crit Care Med.* 1990;18:728–733.

34. McCowen KC, Friel C, Sternberg J, et al. Hypocaloric total parenteral nutrition: Effectiveness in prevention of hyperglycemia and infectious complications—A randomized clinical trial. *Crit Care Med.* 2000;28:3606–3611.

35. McMahon MM, Manji N, Driscoll DF, et al. Parenteral nutrition in patients with diabetes mellitus. Theoretical and practical considerations. *J Parent Enteral Nutr.* 1989; 13:545–553.

CHAPTER

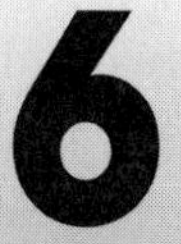

Micronutrients in Critical Illness

M. Patricia Fuhrman, M.S., R.D., L.D., F.A.D.A., C.N.S.D.,
Virginia M. Herrmann, M.D., C.N.S.P.

INTRODUCTION	51
DERANGEMENTS IN THE MICRONUTRIENT MILIEU	51
MICRONUTRIENTS	52
Selenium	52
Iron	52
Zinc	54
Copper and Manganese	54
Vitamin A	54
Vitamin C	55
Vitamin E	55
Vitamin K	55
Vitamin Cocktails	55
CONCLUSIONS	56
CASE PRESENTATIONS	57
Copper Deficiency in PN Patient with Hyperbilirubinemia	57
Micronutrient Supplementation Post Multiple Trauma	58
REFERENCES	58

Introduction

This chapter will discuss the effect of critical illness on the milieu of micronutrients in the body. There is a plethora of discussion on what should and should not be supplemented in the critically ill patient. However, there is a paucity of prospective, randomized, controlled trials providing definitive answers of what is lost and what is required during critical illness. It is often difficult to distinguish what is beneficial and what can be detrimental to patient recovery. This chapter will examine the etiologies of deficiencies and excesses as well as the indications and contraindications for supplementation. Learning objectives include the following: (1) Identify micronutrients that are affected by critical illness; (2) Examine studies that have supplemented micronutrients; and (3) Discuss benefits and caveats of supplementing micronutrients in critically ill patients.

Derangements in the Micronutrient Milieu

The acute phase response (APR), also known as the systemic inflammatory response syndrome (SIRS), manifests with elevations in counter-regulatory hormones, promotion of pro-inflammatory cytokines, and synthesis of acute phase proteins.[1] This results in cardiovascular, pulmonary, and hematological abnormalities. These changes are necessary for survival during a period of metabolic stress and trauma. Antioxidant production during this response process combats the accumulation of reactive oxygen species (ROS), which can contribute to widespread tissue injury. The proliferation of ROS is particularly noted during periods of tissue ischemia followed by reperfusion of oxygen to the tissue, which results in an oxidative burst and subsequent tissue damage. Antioxidants counter the ROS-induced tissue injury that can occur following surgical interventions, such as coronary artery bypass grafts, aortic aneurysm repair, and solid organ transplantation.

Several factors contribute to reductions and elevations in the availability of various micronutrients. During APR/SIRS there is a change in the interaction, excretion, utilization, distribution, and storage of the various micronutrients.[2] The response by the body as to whether to increase or decrease the availability of each micronutrient depends on the role the micronutrient plays in the inflammatory and recovery response. In addition, nutrient requirements will depend upon pre-existing nutritional status, losses in urine and stool, and bioavailability of the nutrient supplemented.

TABLE 6.1

Interactions of Micronutrients[4]		
Micronutrient	Increases	Decreases
Vitamin C	Vitamin E, iron	Copper
Zinc		Iron, copper, vitamin A with zinc deficiency
Iron		Zinc
Copper		Iron, zinc
Selenium	Vitamin E	
Vitamin E	Selenium, vitamin A	

The patient's past medical history will also affect utilization and requirements. Alcohol and tobacco abuse, as well as chronic inflammatory disease, malnutrition, and malabsorption can contribute to a pre-existing deficit of micronutrients that will be compounded by the current inflammatory process.[2,3] It is also important to consider the nutrient interactions that occur among the various micronutrients (Table 6.1).[4]

Micronutrients

All patients should receive a daily source of vitamins and minerals through either the oral, enteral feeding tube or parenteral route. The micronutrients provided should be consistent with the Recommended Dietary Allowance (RDA), Dietary Reference Intake (DRI), or the American Medical Association's parenteral vitamin and mineral recommendations.[5–10] Vitamins and trace elements are pivotal to metabolic homeostasis, enzymatic pathways, antioxidant activities, and tissue integrity. Insufficient micronutrient intake impairs the ability to utilize macronutrients and maintain body defense mechanisms. As clinicians, we often focus on calories and protein without sufficient attention given to the vitamin and mineral status of patients. This oversight can contribute to mortality and morbidity in critically ill patients.

Critical illness has an adverse effect on a multitude of micronutrients. However, this chapter will focus on specific nutrients that have been studied in critical illness for potential deficiencies and the effect of supplementation on recovery. These nutrients include selenium, iron, zinc, copper, manganese, vitamin A, vitamin C, vitamin E, and vitamin K. Various combinations of vitamins and minerals can be mixed into nutrient "cocktails." Table 6.2 delineates studies that have examined the effects of individual micronutrient supplementation.

Selenium

Selenium is a component of glutathione peroxidase, which is a potent antioxidant. Forceville et al[11] demonstrated that ICU patients had reduced levels of selenium and that low serum selenium levels contributed to morbidity and mortality. Serum levels were found to be at or below levels previously shown to impair glutathione peroxidase activity. It is hypothesized that the reduction in serum levels results from a redistribution from plasma into the tissue.[12] Interestingly, the patients were receiving 40 mcg of selenium daily, which is an amount commonly provided in parenteral (PN) and enteral (EN) nutrition (Table 6.3). Despite standard supplementation, serum selenium levels remained decreased for two weeks following injury. A subsequent study by Angstwurm et al[13] provided either 35 mcg selenium per day or 9 days of "loading" doses of selenium followed by a sustained dose of 35 mcg to critically ill patients. The patients who received the additional selenium (2925 mcg total over the 9 days in progressively decreased doses) demonstrated a reduction in morbidity and mortality. It therefore appears that the standard amount of selenium added to PN is not adequate to meet the requirements for selenium in critically ill patients. However, it is unclear what the optimal level of supplementation should be.

Iron

Iron functions as carrier of oxygen and is normally found in heme or bound to transferrin and ferritin. During critical illness free iron released into the bloodstream generates ROS and contributes to microorganism proliferation. In order to reduce the adverse effects of free iron availability, iron is sequestered in ferritin during APR/SIRS. Free iron levels remain decreased for 1–2 weeks following injury.[14] Iron supplementation is not recommended during an inflammatory process since iron accumulation interferes with reticuloendothelial system activity, compromises splenic function, reduces macrophage activity, increases organ damage, and promotes microorganism growth.[2,15] Circumstances justifying parenteral iron supplementation in the critically ill include documentation of iron deficiency and intolerance or inadequate absorptive capability to oral iron supplementation. However, it can be difficult to diagnose iron deficiency since ferritin increases with inflammation and transferrin decreases with protein-calorie malnutrition (PCM) and APR.

Supplementation with 100 mg oral iron per day for two weeks in healthy volunteers contributed to an increase in ROS production and increased fecal

TABLE 6.2

Studies That Have Supplemented Single Micronutrients in Humans

Author	Type of Patients	Nutrient	Amount	Outcome
Angstwurm[13]	SIRS/APACHE II≥15 n= 42	selenium 35 mcg/d	535 mcg (3d); 285 mcg (3d); 155 mcg (3d); 35 mcg/d	decreased morbidity/mortality
Braunschweig[23]	home PN n=44	zinc	30 mg × 3 d	↑ temperature
Chandra[22]	healthy n=11	zinc	150 mg bid × 6 wk	↓ immune response and HDL
Lund[16]	n=18 healthy	po iron	100 mg/d × 2 wk	↑ ROS production & fecal iron excretion
Norton[17]	long-term PN (>3 wk) n=42	IV iron	25 mg/wk 87.5 mg/wk 175 mg/wk	87.5 and 175 mg ↑ serum Fe 80% on 175 mg had Fe levels > normal after 3 weeks
Goode[31]	sepsis n=7/16	vitamin C	1000 mg	↑ free iron; ↑ free radicals in healthy
Tarng[35]	HD (↑ ferritin/HCT <30%)	vitamin C	900 mg/wk × 8 wk	responders: ↓ ferritin & EPO dose
Seeger[38]	ARDS n=14 controls n=5	vitamin E	3 g/d per g-tube 1 g/d po	delayed or no change in serum E in ARDS no effect without EN or hemodynamically stability
Novelli[39]	elective AAA repair n=6 + 6 controls	vitamin E	600 mg/d po 8 d pre-op	↓ muscle oxidative damage during ischemia and reperfusion
Houglum[40]	chronic hepatitis C n=6	vitamin E	1200 IU/d × 8 wk po	↓ hepatic fibrogenesis cascade

SIRS, systemic inflammatory syndrome; APACHE, acute physiologic and hemodynamic evaluation; PN, parenteral nutrition; HDL, high density lipoproteins; ROS, reactive oxygen species; HD, hemodialysis; AAA, abdominal aortic aneurysm; ARDS, adult respiratory distress syndrome; EPO; erythropietin; EN, enteral nutrition; HCT, hematocrit; Fe, iron.

TABLE 6.3

Micronutrients in Critical Illness[4,54]

Micronutrient	Standard Dose PN	Standard Dose EN*	Supplementation Recommendations	Enhanced EN formulas
Selenium	20-80 mcg	20-70 mcg/L	100-400 mcg/d	77-100 mcg/L
Copper	0.3 mg	1-2 mg/L	3 mg/d	1.7-2.2 mg/L
Iron	0.5-1 mg	12-20 mg/L	???	12-20 mg/L
Zinc	2.5-5 mg	11-19 mg/L	10-30 mg/d	15-24 mg/L
Vitamin A	1000 RE	800-1000 RE 2600-5200 IU/L	PN: 10,000 IU/d EN: 25,000 IU/d	4200-11985 IU/L
Beta carotene			50 mg/d	33% of vit A
Vitamin C	200 mg	125-250 mg/L	500-3000 mg/d	80-844 mg/L
Vitamin E (Alpha-tocopherol)	10 mg	25-50 IU/L	PN: 400 mg/d EN: 40-1000 mg/d	40-212 mg/L
Vitamin K	150 mcg	40-135 mcg/L		

*Standard "house" enteral formula.

iron excretion[16] (Table 6.2). The authors were concerned that routine iron supplementation could increase the risk of colon cancer in susceptible patient populations.[16] Norton et al[17] gave various doses (0, 25, 87.5 and 175 mg IV iron per wk) to patients on long-term non-lipid-containing PN and found that 87.5 mg/wk (12.5 mg/d) increased serum iron levels without exceeding normal and without an increased incidence of sepsis (Table 6.2). EN formulas generally contain 12–20 mg of iron per liter. Injectable multiple trace element preparations do not contain iron. There is controversy as to whether iron dextran should be added to PN solutions in therapeutic doses since the trivalent mineral could disrupt the lipid emulsion.[18]

However, when added to PN, the maintenance dose is 2 mg/d with lipid-containing PN and 10 mg/d in lipid-free PN.[18,19] Nutrient interactions that can affect iron availability should also be considered. Vitamin C enhances absorption of iron and hence increases free iron availability. Zinc and copper, on the other hand, inhibit iron absorption.

ZINC

Zinc levels are affected during critical illness by interleukin-1 (IL-1), tumor necrosis factor-alpha (TNF-α), and hypoalbuminemia.[20] There appears to be a compartmental shift of zinc from the serum to the tissues with inflammation. There is also a reduction in serum zinc levels because of increased uptake by the liver. Zinc levels remain decreased for four to five days in response to APR.[14] Zinc availability can also be impaired due to malabsorption with pancreatic disease, alcohol abuse, cystic fibrosis, chronic diarrhea and inflammatory bowel disease, abnormalities in vitamin D metabolism, and supplementation of calcium and iron.[20] A study reported that 30% of healthy elderly (>50 years of age) had reduced intake and absorption of zinc with subsequent mild to marginal zinc deficiency.[21] This could mean that prior to an episode of critical illness various patient populations as well as one-third of elderly patients are already at risk for zinc deficiency. The additional insult of critical illness could result in a severe zinc deficit in these susceptible patients. Enteral formulations contain 11–19 mg of zinc/L. Standard requirements may be increased by an additional 2 mg/d with catabolic illness, 12.2 mg/L of small intestinal effluent losses, and 17.7 mg/L of rectal or ileostomy output.[10] Table 6.3 provides guidelines for providing zinc with EN and PN.

Zinc deficiency reduces production of retinol-binding protein and interferes with vitamin A transport, thus compounding the micronutrient aberrations. However, keep in mind that supplementation of zinc will interfere with copper absorption and inhibit activation of macrophages. There have been reports of zinc toxicity with hyperamylasemia and pancreatitis at doses 50 times greater than recommended.[20] Healthy men, who were given 150 mg elemental zinc twice a day for 6 weeks developed elevated low density lipoproteins, reductions in high density lipoproteins and impairment of lymphocyte and neutrophil function.[22] The reduction in serum level of zinc with APR may be beneficial by contributing to a reduction in the cytokine and febrile response. A prospective, randomized, placebo-controlled study in PN patients with a mild inflammatory response reported a significant increase in febrile episodes in patients supplemented with 30 mg of zinc/d for 3 days.[23] Therefore it may not be prudent to "normalize" plasma zinc with large doses during critical illness without evidence of deficiency with large doses during critical illness unless an exaggerated cytokine response is desired, such as with HIV positive patients.[23]

COPPER AND MANGANESE

Copper and manganese will be considered together since both are elevated with APR/SIRS and both are excreted via bile. Supplementation during critical illness is generally not warranted unless a known deficiency exists. The more common concern with copper and manganese is possible excess availability with hyperbilirubinemia. Recommendations are to reduce or omit copper and manganese from PN solutions with chronic serum bilirubin elevation.[20,24,25] However, omission should be done cautiously when the patient has no other viable source of either nutrient or if the patient has extraneous losses of copper and manganese, such as with chronic diarrhea. Copper deficiency can occur with deletion from the parenteral solution and result in pancytopenia.[26] Copper deficiency contributes to iron deficiency by inhibiting the transfer of iron into stores. Copper supplementation can interfere with zinc absorption. Vitamin C supplementation can reduce the bioavailability of copper, and zinc supplementation can inhibit copper absorption.

VITAMIN A

Vitamin A, retinol, functions to enhance vision and promote wound healing. Carotenoids, primarily beta carotene, are vitamin A precursors and also function as non-enzymatic antioxidants. Serum levels of vitamins A, C, and E have been reported to be reduced post-operatively in surgical patients.[27,28] However, serum levels normalized after post-operative day seven without supplementation.[28] On the other hand, patients with reduced pre-operative levels of vitamin A, alpha-tocopherol, and gamma-tocopherol had an increased risk of infection and death.[28] Another study found that the APR was associated with a reduction in serum levels of albumin, prealbumin, lycopene, alpha-carotene, beta-carotene, and total carotenoids.[29] There are also concerns with supplementing vitamin A and beta carotene since each has potential adverse effects. An association between beta-carotene and lung cancer has been reported.[30] Vitamin A toxicity can occur in patients with renal failure secondary to reduced renal clearance of retinol-binding protein.

Vitamin C

Vitamin C functions as a non-enzymatic antioxidant and is required for wound healing and carnitine synthesis. Vitamin C levels have been reported to be decreased in critically ill and septic patients.[31–33] Nutrient interactions that can occur when vitamin C is supplemented include facilitation of iron absorption, assistance with regeneration of oxidized vitamin E, and formation of calcium oxalate kidney stones. Since 12% of Americans are in positive iron balance and 6% of the population is in negative iron balance, there is a greater potential risk of promoting the adverse effects of free iron release with vitamin C supplementation than correcting an iron inadequacy.[34] Vitamin C supplementation should not exceed 200 mg/d of ascorbic acid in patients at risk for kidney stone formation and infection.[2,35] Enteral formulations provide 60 mg/d. Injectable multivitamin preparations have recently increased from 100 mg to 200 mg per day.[36] This increase could contribute to increased risk of infections and renal stone development in susceptible patients.

Vitamin E

Vitamin E prevents peroxidation of cell membranes by ROS. Alpha-tocopherol is the most biologically active form of vitamin E and is a highly effective chain-breaking antioxidant.[3] Vitamin E protects the lung from oxidative injury.[37] Glutathione and vitamins E and C are intertwined in synergistic relationships. Ascorbic acid recycles alpha-tocopherol and glutathione reduces hepatic oxidation of vitamin E. Therefore inadequate amounts of glutathione and vitamin C can inhibit the antioxidant activity of vitamin E. However, supplementing vitamin C to maintain vitamin E could increase free iron availability and promote microorganism proliferation. It is also important to consider the effect of fat intake on absorption of oral supplementation of vitamin E. Fat-soluble vitamins require fat in the diet to facilitate absorption, and oral supplementation without adequate dietary fat can result in suboptimal effects.[38] Several studies have looked at supplementation to reduce oxidative damage.[38–40] Sawyer et al. provided vitamins E, C, n-acetylcysteine (a glutathione precursor), and selenium to patients with adult respiratory distress syndrome (ARDS) and reported increased survival in the supplemented group.[41] Excess vitamin E supplementation antagonizes vitamin A, interferes with wound healing, and contributes to platelet dysfunction.

Vitamin K

Enteral tube feeding formulations vary in the content of vitamin K, which ranges from 40–135 mcg/L. Patients who are not fed enterally and who are on antibiotics are at a potential risk of becoming deficient in vitamin K. Recently adult multivitamin preparations have been reformulated to provide 150 mcg vitamin K per day.[36] This occurred in the midst of considerable discussion over the need for vitamin K to be added to PN formulations. Intravenous lipids can contain vitamin K, but there is variability in the amount of vitamin K, with ranges of 0 to 290 mcg/L in 20% lipid emulsions.[42] Duerksen and Papineau prospectively examined the international normalized ratio (INR) in 70 hospitalized patients over a 3 week period.[43] No vitamin K was added to the solution and the lipids used provided only 7–11 mcg/L. The authors reported only mild coagulopathy in the population studied. Seven patients who developed an INR >2.4 were treated with vitamin K at the discretion of the attending physician. The authors suggested that clinicians can choose to either provide routine supplementation or monitor INR levels and treat only the small number of patients who require it. Chambrier et al. looked at serum vitamin K and prothrombin time (PT) levels in long-term PN patients and reported that the content of the vitamin K in the lipids was sufficient to maintain levels.[42] Their recommendation of 250–400 mcg/wk appears adequate to meet vitamin K requirements for most patients on PN. The intrinsic vitamin K in lipids plus the recent addition of 150 mcg of vitamin K to injectable adult multivitamins can provide a patient with more than 200 mcg/d. It is important to monitor INR and PT levels in patients receiving PN with daily lipids and a standard adult multivitamin injection. Subtle changes in the INR and PT could occur when PN is initiated, interrupted, or discontinued in patients on anticoagulation therapy.

Vitamin Cocktails

Antioxidant cocktails combine synergistic and complementary micronutrients in order to enhance the effects of supplementation.[44] Table 6.4 identifies studies that have combined various nutrients. Combinations of nutrients have been used to treat pressure ulcers or extensive wounds, adult respiratory distress syn-

TABLE 6.4

Studies That Have Supplemented Micronutrient Combinations in Humans

Author	Type of Patients	Nutrient	Amount	Outcome
Sawyer[41]	ARDS n=32 16 ARDS 16 controls	vitamin E vitamin C NAC selenium	1600 IU po/d × 48h 3 g IV/d × 48 h 24 g po/d × 48 h 200 mcg IV/d × 48 h	doubled survival at 4 weeks
Sisto[46]	CABG stable n=45 (25 controls) unstable n=36 (19 controls)	vitamin E (given 2 d or 4 wk pre-op) vitamin C allopurinol	600 mg/d po 2 g/d (2 d pre-; 1 d post-op) 600 mg/d (2 d pre-; 1 d post-op)	↓ dopamine and infarctions ↓ reperfusion injury
Maderazo[48]	blunt trauma n=46 (+ 87 controls)	vitamin E vitamin C	50 mg/d 200 or 500 mg/d	E & C significant ↑ PMN locomotion PMN locomotion improved with either vitamins E or C; best with E and C
Rabl[47]	renal transplant n=30 controls=14 treatment group=16	*Omnibionta®* vitamin C vitamin E vitamin A vitamin B complex ®Merck, Darmstadt, Germany	*2 amps* 1000 mg 12 mg 11 mg	↓ lipid peroxidation ↓ Cr and ↑ Cr Cl for 1st 6 d post-transplant
Gadek[45]	ARDS n=146 98 evaluable 47=controls 51=special formula	EPA GLA vitamin E vitamin C β-carotene	6.9 ± 0.3 g/d 5.8 ± 0.3 g/d 413 ± 18 IU/d 1127 ± 49 mg/d 6601± 258 µg/d	improved oxygenation ↓ vent days, ICU LOS and new organ failure

NAC, n-acetylcysteine; PMN, polymononuclear; EPA, eicosapentaenoic acid; GLA, γ-linolenic acid; ARDS, acute respiratory distress syndrome; CABG, coronary artery by-pass graft; Cr, creatinine; ICU, intensive care unit; LOS, length of stay.

drome,[41,45] coronary by-pass graft surgery,[46] renal transplant,[47] blunt trauma,[48] and burns.[49] Enteral nutrition formulas are being developed with micronutrient enhancement in conjunction with various combinations of arginine, glutamine, omega-3 fatty acids, and nucleotides in order to promote immunocompetence, wound healing, and antioxidant activity.[45,50] The ability to enhance parenteral solutions with various combinations of micronutrients beyond the standard vitamin and trace element components as recommended by the AMA is affected by issues of compatibility, cost, safety, and effectiveness. It is also important to consider intrinsic contamination and effects of storage, time, and temperature on micronutrient availability.[51,52] Table 6.3 contains a comparison of what is recommended in the literature and what is currently added to enteral and parenteral formulations.

Conclusions

Each micronutrient has beneficial and detrimental effects, with a narrow range of optimal supplementation between beneficial and toxic. The interactions between micronutrients, medications, and other nutrients affects the efficacy of supplementation, whether as a single nutrient or a combination of nutrients. Keep in mind that an absolute deficiency is rare except with sole dependency on PN and with inborn errors of metabolism. Although study results are intriguing, it is difficult to compare and extrapolate beyond the study population. There is often variation in how the deficiency or toxicity was induced, how the supplemental nutrients were administered, the degree and extent of deficiency or toxicity, and the time elapsed between inducing a deficiency or toxicity and treatment or exposure to a pathogen.[15] Study populations are often small and results obtained are inconclusive. Although a depleted serum level of a micronutrient is interesting and perhaps concerning, it is important to reflect on the clinical consequences, if any, of the aberration. Will supplementing the nutrient correct metabolic defects? When should supplementation be initiated and who should receive supplementation of specific micronutrients? Which micronutrients should be supplemented together, in what quantities, and for how long? These unanswered questions make definitive recommendations difficult at this time. It is important for the clinician to identify which nutrients may require

TABLE 6.5

Evaluating Laboratory Measurement of Micronutrients[11,13,42,55–57]			
Vitamin/Mineral	**Lab**	**Deficiency***	**Toxicity***
Vitamin A	serum vitamin A	<10 μg/dL	>65 μg/dL
Vitamin C	plasma ascorbic acid	<0.2 mg/dL	
Vitamin E	serum erythrocyte hemolysis	>20% hemolysis	
	serum platelet tocopherol	<0.35 μg/10^9 cells	
Vitamin K	prothrombin time (PT) international normalized ratio (INR)	>15 seconds >1.0 above baseline >2.4	
Copper	plasma copper	<50 μg/dL	>110 μg/dL** >169 μg/dL***
Manganese	intra-erythrocyte Mn level controls:	0.04 μg/g Hb (81) normal: 1.4 μg/dL M 1.7 μg/dL F	
Selenium	erythrocyte GSH peroxidase Whole blood selenium	normal: <10.5 U/mL ercs (long-term) <0.7 μmol/L (86, 87)	
Zinc	serum zinc	<70 μg/dL	

Serum levels are affected by hepatic protein status, metabolic stress, inflammation.
* Levels may vary depending on laboratory technique and ranges.
** males; *** females

supplementation in at-risk patients and monitor levels with supplementation accordingly (Table 6.5). In the meantime, it is essential that all patients receive the RDA/DRI for all micronutrients daily except when contraindicated by intolerance or disease/condition.

Case Presentations

COPPER DEFICIENCY IN PN PATIENT WITH HYPERBILIRUBINEMIA

RL is a 40-year-old female who developed short bowel syndrome following multiple enteric resections after a gunshot wound to the abdomen. After 7 months of dependency on PN she presents to the clinic with mild jaundice and a total serum bilirubin of 6 mg/dL. Her PN has provided a daily trace element preparation including chromium, copper, manganese, and zinc.

What are the possible etiologies of hyperbilirubinemia in this patient?

The patient could be developing liver impairment from long-term PN. However, it is unusual for adults to experience hyperbilirubinemia as the first sign of PN hepatic intolerance. This is seen more often in pediatric patients. Adults more often develop hepatic steatosis first. Hyperbilirubinemia also occurs with inflammation/sepsis. The patient does not appear to have an acute inflammatory process. Medications can also contribute to an elevation in the total bilirubin. The patient is on no medications known to cause this problem. Therefore, PN appears to be the contributing factor to her cholestasis.

What are the concerns with providing the trace element preparation to this patient?

There is a potential risk of manganese deposition in the brain with subsequent dysfunction when manganese is added to PN during cholestasis.[53] Copper excess can be deposited in the liver and further complicate hepatic dysfunction.

What would you recommend concerning supplementation of trace elements?

Complete removal of copper and manganese is often suggested. However this practice can lead to micronutrient deficiency. A case report demonstrated that removal of copper and manganese from PN resulted in pancytopenia and reliance on blood transfusions after 18 months.[26] The patient had a serum copper of 25 mg/dL (normal: 70–155 mg/dL). The serum copper and pancytopenia responded to copper supplementation. Our patient has diarrhea as a result of short bowel syndrome and is at risk of copper deficiency if no supplementation is given.

Therefore, serum levels of zinc and chromium should be monitored with supplementation provided two to three times a week to maintain levels without under- or over-provision. On the days when the trace element preparation is withheld, zinc and chromium should be added as separate injections to the PN solution.

MICRONUTRIENT SUPPLEMENTATION POST MULTIPLE TRAUMA

EC is a 57-year-old male who sustains massive injuries following a motor vehicle accident. His surgical procedures include splenectomy, repair of hepatic laceration, pancreatectomy, and colectomy with an ileostomy. He was in a normal state of health prior to the accident. Five days post-operative, EC became septic and developed ARDS. He has been NPO since the accident with only IV fluid and electrolyte replacement. The patient is hemodynamically unstable.

What micronutrients should be considered in this patient?

The resurgence of the inflammatory process on the heels of his primary metabolic insult will increase the demand for micronutrients (Table 6.3). Wound healing and antioxidant defenses increase the demand for selenium, zinc, vitamins A, C, and E.[13,38,41,45,48] However, vitamin C should be used cautiously with continued inflammation and increased risk of aggravating infection.

Should the micronutrients be given empirically or should serum levels be checked prior to and during supplementation?

Ideally, serum levels of these nutrients would be checked prior to initiation of supplementation with ongoing periodic monitoring during supplementation (Table 6.5).

How should micronutrients be provided?

Often micronutrients are not supplemented until macronutrients are provided with the initiation of enteral or parenteral nutrition support. However, it may be wise to provide at least 24 hours of micronutrient supplementation until the patient is stable enough to begin enteral or parenteral feeding. Micronutrients are involved in hundreds of enzyme systems and are necessary for macronutrient metabolism. Repletion prior to contributing an increased demand may improve efficiency and effectiveness of metabolic processes. Continue separate infusion until the patient is getting 100% of micronutrient recommendations via feeding modality.

The patient is given standard multivitamin and trace element IV preparations plus additional IV supplementation of vitamin C and zinc. Daily totals with all sources of supplementation are vitamin C 700 mg and zinc 30 mg. Two days after IV supplementation of micronutrients is begun, enteral tube feeding is started with a pulmonary formula enhanced with vitamin E, vitamin C, beta-carotene, and non-inflammatory fatty acids. The patient becomes febrile.

What could potentially contribute to the patient's febrile state?

The patient is receiving a fairly large dose of vitamin C, which could increase the release of free iron and contribute to microorganism proliferation and subsequent infection. In addition, the amount of zinc given has been shown to contribute to increased incidence of fever in patients with mild APR. It may be prudent to stop supplementation beyond the amounts in the standard micronutrient preparations.

The additional amounts of vitamin C and zinc are discontinued. Over the next several days, the patient's tube feeding is advanced to goal, and the intravenous multivitamin and trace element preparations are discontinued.

References

1. Gabay C, Kushner I. Acute phase proteins and other systemic responses to inflammation. *N Engl J Med.* 1999; 340:448–454.
2. Fleming R. Trace element metabolism in adult patients requiring total parenteral nutrition. *Am J Clin Nutr.* 1989; 49:573–579.
3. Kelly FJ. Vitamin E supplementation in the critically ill patient: too narrow a view? *Nutr Clin Prac.* 1994;9:141–145.
4. Demling RH, DeBiasse MA. Micronutrients in critical illness. *Crit Care Clin.* 1995;11:651–673.
5. Food and Nutrition Board, National Research Council. *Recommended Dietary Allowances.* 10th ed. Washington, DC: National Academy of Sciences; 1989.
6. Food and Nutrition Board, Institute of Medicine. *Dietary Reference Intakes for Calcium, Phosphorus, Magnesium, Vitamin D, and Fluoride.* Washington, DC: National Academy Press; 1998.

7. Food and Nutrition Board, Institute of Medicine. *Dietary Reference Intakes for Thiamin, Riboflavin, Niacin, Vitamin B6, Folate, Vitamin B12, Pantothenic Acid, Biotin, and Choline.* Washington, DC: National Academy Press; 1998.
8. Monsen ER. Dietary reference intakes for the antioxidant nutrients: Vitamin C, vitamin E, selenium, and carotenoids. *J Am Diet Assoc.* 2000;100:637–640.
9. American Medical Association Department of Foods and Nutrition. Multivitamin preparations for parenteral use: A statement by the Nutrition Advisory Group. *J Parenter Enteral Nutr.* 1979;3:258–262.
10. American Medical Association Department of Foods and Nutrition. Guidelines for essential trace element preparations for parenteral use. A statement by an expert panel. *JAMA.* 1979;241:2051–2054.
11. Forceville F, Vitoux D, Gauzit R, et al. Selenium, systemic immune response syndrome, sepsis, and outcome in critically ill patients. *Crit Care Med.* 1998;26:1536–1544.
12. Hawker FH, Stewart PM, Snitch PJ. Effects of acute illness on selenium homeostasis. *Crit Care Med.* 1990;18: 442–446.
13. Angstwurm MAW, Schottdorf J, Schopohl J, et al. Selenium replacement in patients with severe systemic inflammatory response syndrome improves clinical outcome. *Crit Care Med.* 1999;27:1807–1813.
14. Shenkin A. Trace elements and inflammatory response: Implications for nutritional support. *Nutrition.* 1995;11 (Suppl):100–105.
15. Chandra RK, Dayton DH. Trace element regulation of immunity and infection. *Nutr Res.* 1982;2:721–733.
16. Lund EK, Wharf SG, Fairweather-Tait SJ, et al. Oral ferrous sulfate supplements increase the free radical-generating capacity of feces from healthy volunteers. *Am J Clin Nutr.* 1999;69:250–255.
17. Norton JA, Peters ML, Wesley R, et al. Iron supplementation of total parenteral nutrition: A prospective study. *J Parenter Enteral Nutr.* 1983;7:457–461.
18. Kumpf VJ. Parenteral iron supplementation. *Nutr Clin Prac.* 1996;11:139–146.
19. Burns DL, Mascioli EA, Bistrian BR. Parenteral iron dextran therapy: A review. *Nutrition.* 1995;11:163–168.
20. Fleming, CR, Hodges RE, Hurley LS. A prospective study of serum copper and zinc levels in patients receiving total parenteral nutrition. *Am J Clin Nutr.* 1976;29:70–77.
21. Prasad AS, Fitzgerald JT, Hess JW, et al. Zinc deficiency in elderly patients. *Nutrition.* 1993;9:218–224.
22. Chandra RK. Excessive intake of zinc impairs immune response. *JAMA.* 1984;252:1443–1446.
23. Braunschweig CL, Sowers M, Kovacevich DS, et al. Parenteral zinc supplementation in adult humans during the acute phase response increases the febrile response. *J Nutr.* 1997;127:70–74.
24. Shils ME. Parenteral nutrition. In: Shils ME, Olson JA, Shike M, eds. *Modern Nutrition in Health and Disease*, 8th ed. Philadelphia: Lea & Febiger, 1994:1430–1458.
25. Uauy R, Olivares M, Gonzalez M. Essentiality of copper in humans. *Am J Clin Nutr.* 1998;67(Suppl):952S.
26. Fuhrman MP, Herrmann VM, Masidonski P, et al. Pancytopenia after removal of copper from total parenteral nutrition. *J Parenter Enteral Nutr.* 2000;24:361–366.
27. Louw JA, Werbeck A, Louw MEJ, et al. Blood vitamin concentrations during the acute-phase response. *Crit Care Med.* 1992;20:934.
28. Agarwal N, Norkus E, Garcia C, et al. Effect of surgery on serum antioxidant vitamins. *J Parenter Enteral Nutr.* 1996;20(Suppl):32S.
29. Boosalis MG, Snowdon DA, Tully CL, et al. Acute phase response and plasma carotenoid concentrations in older women: findings from the nun study. *Nutrition.* 1996;12: 475–478.
30. Alpha-tocopherol, B-carotene Cancer Prevention Study Group. The effect of vitamin E and B-carotene on the incidence of lung cancer and other cancers in male smokers. *N Engl J Med.* 1994;330:1029–1035.
31. Goode HF, Davies MJ, Webster NR. The effects of ascorbate loading on ascorbyl radical formation in patients with sepsis and healthy subjects. *Proc Nutr Soc* [abstract]. 1996;55(suppl):89A.
32. Borrelli E, Roux-Lombard P, Grau GE, et al. Plasma concentrations of cytokines, their soluble receptors, and antioxidant vitamins can predict the development of multiple organ failure in patients at risk. *Crit Care Med.* 1996;24:392–397.
33. Schorah CJ, Downing C, Piripitsi A, et al. Total vitamin C, ascorbic acid, and dehydroascorbic acid concentrations in plasma of critically ill patients. *Am J Clin Nutr.* 1996; 63:760–765.
34. Herbert V, Shaw S, Jayatilleke E. Vitamin C-driven free radical generation from iron. *J Nutr.* 1996;126:1213S–1220S.
35. Tarng D, Yau-Huei W, Tung-Po H, et al. Intravenous ascorbic acid as an adjuvant therapy for recombinant EPO in HD patients with hyperferritinemia. *Kid Intl.* 1999;55: 2477–2486.
36. Parenteral multivitamin products; drugs for human use; drug efficacy study implementation; amendment (21 CFR 5.70). *Federal Register.* April 20, 2000; 65:21200–21201.
37. Richard C, Lemonnier F, Thibault M, et al. Vitamin E deficiency and lipoperoxidation during adult respiratory distress syndrome. *Crit Care Med.* 1990;18:4–9.
38. Seeger W, Ziegler A, Wolf HRD. Serum alpha-tocopherol levels after high-dose enteral vitamin E administration in patients with acute respiratory failure. *Int Care Med.* 1987; 13:395, 4000.
39. Novelli GP, Adembri C, Gandini E, et al. Vitamin E protects human skeletal muscle from damage during surgical ischemia-reperfusion. *Am J Surg.* 1997;173:206–209.
40. Houglum K, Venkataramani A, Lyche K, et al. A pilot study of the effects of d-alpha-tocopherol on hepatic stellate cell activation in chronic hepatitis C. *Gastroenterology.* 1997;113:1069–1073.
41. Sawyer MAJ, Mike JJ, Chavin K, et al. Antioxidant therapy and survival in ARDS. *Crit Care Med.* 1989;17 (Suppl):S153.

42. Chambrier C, Leclercq M, Saudin F, et al. Is vitamin K_1 supplementation necessary in long-term parenteral nutrition? *J Parenter Enteral Nutr.* 1998; 22:87–90.
43. Duerksen DR, Papineau N. Is routine vitamin K supplementation required in hospitalized patients receiving parenteral nutrition? *Nutr Clin Prac.* 2000;15:18–83.
44. Goode HF, Webster NR. Free radical and antioxidants in sepsis. *Crit Care Med.* 1993;21:1770–1776.
45. Gadek J, DeMichele SJ, Karlstad MD, et al. Effect of enteral feeding with eicosapentaenoic acid, γ-linolenic acid, and antioxidants in patients with acute respiratory distress syndrome. *Crit Care Med.* 1999;27:1409–1420.
46. Sisto T, Paajanen H, Metsa-Ketela T, et al. Pretreatment with antioxidants and allopurinol diminishes cardiac onset events in coronary artery bypass grafting. *Ann Thorac Surg.* 1995;59:1519–1523.
47. Rabl H, Khoschsorur G, Columbo T, et al. A multivitamin infusion prevents lipid peroxidation and improves transplant performance. *Kid Int.* 1993;43:912–917.
48. Maderazo EG, Woronick CL, Hickingbotham N, et al. A randomized trial of replacement antioxidant vitamin therapy for neutrophil locomotory dysfunction in blunt trauma. *J Trauma.* 1991;31:1142–1148.
49. Mayes T, Gottsclich M, Warden GD. Clinical nutrition protocols for continuous quality improvements in the outcomes of patients with burn. *J Burn Care Rehabil.* 1997; 18:365–368.
50. Bower RH, Cerra FB, Bershadsky B, et al. Early enteral administration of a formula (Impact) supplemented with arginine, nucleotides, and fish oil in intensive care patients: results of a multicenter, prospective, randomized, clinical trial. *Crit Care Med.* 1995;221:327–338.
51. Pluhator-Murton MM, Fedorak RN, Audette RJ, et al. Trace element contamination of total parenteral nutrition. 1. Contribution of component solutions. *J Parenter Enteral Nutr.* 1999;23:222–227.
52. Pluhator-Murton MM, Fedorak RN, Audette RJ, et al. Trace element contamination of total parenteral nutrition 2. Effect of storage duration and temperature. *J Parenter Enteral Nutr.* 1999;23:228–232.
53. Ejima A, Imamura T, Nakamura S, et al. Manganese intoxication during total parenteral nutrition. *Lancet.* 1992; 339:426.
54. Grant JP. Nutritional support in critically ill patients. *Ann Surg.* 1994;220:610–616.
55. Teitz NW, ed. *Clinical Guide to Laboratory Tests.* 3rd ed. Philadelphia: W.B. Saunders Company; 1995.
56. Bertinet DB, Tinivella M, Balzola FA, et al. Brain manganese deposition and blood levels in patients undergoing home parenteral nutrition. *J Parenter Enteral Nutr.* 2000; 24:223–227.
57. Boosalis MG. Micronutrients. In: Gottschlich MM, ed. *The Science and Practice of Nutrition Support: A Case-Based Core Curricullum.* Dubuque, IA: Kendall/Hunt Publishers; 2000:85–106.

CHAPTER

7 Vitamins and Trace Elements in the Critically Ill Patient

Joel B. Mason, M.D.

INTRODUCTION 61

SALIENT FEATURES OF THE VITAMINS AND TRACE ELEMENTS 62
- Vitamins 62
- Trace Elements 62

IS THE MICRONUTRIENT CONTENT OF STANDARD ENTERAL AND PARENTERAL FEEDING SOLUTIONS SUFFICIENT TO MEET THE NEEDS OF THE CRITICALLY ILL PATIENT? 71

ARE THERE SITUATIONS WHERE SUPRAPHYSIOLOGIC SUPPLEMENTATION IS INDICATED? 72
- Chromium and Hyperglycemia 73
- Antioxidant Micronutrients and Critical Illness 73
- Zinc and Critical Illness 73
- Iron, B_{12} and Folate in Erythropoietin Therapy 74
- Is Iodide Supplementation Necessary for Patients on Total Parenteral Nutrition? 74

ARE THERE SITUATIONS WHERE ADMINISTERING LESS THAN CONVENTIONAL AMOUNTS OF MICRONUTRIENTS IS INDICATED? 75
- Vitamin A in Chronic Renal Insufficiency 75
- Is Iron Unsafe in the TPN of Patients Who Are Bacteremic? 75
- Vitamin K and Warfarin Therapy 75

CONCLUSIONS 76

REFERENCES 76

Introduction

Micronutrients are a highly diverse array of dietary components that are necessary to sustain health. The physiologic roles of micronutrients are as varied as their composition; some are used as either co-enzymes or as prosthetic groups in enzymes, others as biochemical substrates or hormones and, in some instances, the functions are not well defined. The unifying characteristic of micronutrients is that, under normal circumstances, the average daily dietary intake for each micronutrient that is required to sustain normal physiologic operations is measured in milligram or smaller quantities. It is in this manner that micronutrients are distinguished from macronutrients; the latter category encompassing carbohydrates, fats, and proteins, as well as the macrominerals, calcium, magnesium, and phosphorous.

For orderly homeostasis to proceed, the intake of most dietary nutrients must be in quantities that are neither too small nor too great. Disorders may arise, therefore, when this "physiologic window" is either not met or is exceeded. The size of this physiologic window varies for each micronutrient and should be kept in mind, particularly in this era when the administration of large quantities of certain micronutrients is being increasingly explored for possible therapeutic implications. The dietary requirement for a particular micronutrient is determined by many factors, only one of which is the amount needed to sustain those physiologic functions for which it is used (see Table 7.1). In the critically ill patient, particular attention needs to be paid to those factors that may impede intestinal absorption, alter normal metabolism, or enhance excretion of a nutrient and thereby increase requirements.

The U.S. National Academy of Sciences' Food and Nutrition Board regularly updates dietary guidelines that define the quantity of each micronutrient that is "adequate to meet the known nutrient needs of practically all healthy persons"; these Recommended Daily Allowances (RDAs) have undergone revision over the past 2 years and appear in Tables 7.2 and 7.3. Also established for the first time were "tolerable upper limits (TULs)" for each micronutrient, which is the maximal daily level of oral intake that is likely to pose no adverse health risks (Tables 7.2 and 7.3). The Food and Nutrition Board has not traditionally provided guidelines for parenteral administration of micronutrients; in its stead, the American Medical Asso-

TABLE 7.1

Factors That Determine the Dietary Requirement of a Micronutrient

Physiologic Factors

1. Bioavailability: the proportion of an ingested micronutrient that can be assimilated and used for physiologic purposes
2. Quantity required to fulfill physiologic roles
3. Extent to which the body can reuse the micronutrient
4. Distribution of nutrient in the body: storage compartments, etc.
5. Gender
6. Stage of life cycle: intrauterine development, infancy, childhood, adulthood, elderhood, pregnancy, etc.

Pathophysiologic and Pharmacologic Factors

1. Inborn errors of metabolism that variously affect assimilation, utilization, or excretion of micronutrients
2. Acquired disease states that alter the amounts required to sustain homeostasis (e.g., malabsorption, maldigestion, states that increase utilization)
3. Lifestyle habits, e.g., smoking, ethanol consumption
4. Drugs: may alter bioavailability and/or utilization

Adapted with permission from Mason JB. Consequences of altered micronutrient status. In: Goldman L, Bennett J, eds. *Cecil Textbook of Medicine,* 21st edition. Philadelphia: WB Saunders Co.; 2000:1171.

ciation convened a panel in 1975 that defined recommendations for parenteral delivery of micronutrients in adults (Table 7.4a: see reference 1). A decade later another panel developed recommendations for infants and children (Table 7.4b: see references 2–4). The science of micronutrients has expanded enormously, particularly since 1975, and both sets of parenteral recommendations deserve to be updated. Nevertheless, these recommendations remain valuable starting points.

The aim of this chapter is not to provide an exhaustive description of the biochemical, physiological, and nutritional features of each micronutrient; such items are instead briefly summarized in Tables 7.2 and 7.3. Other sources are available for up-to-date, comprehensive discussions of each micronutrient.[5] Rather, this chapter focuses on: (1) whether standard enteral and parenteral feeding solutions provide sufficient micronutrients for the majority of critically ill patients, and (2) identifying situations which commonly arise in critically ill patients that may impact on micronutrient requirements and therefore on our decisions regarding the appropriate amount of each nutrient to deliver. Several scenarios regularly encountered in critically ill patients, where the question of altered micronutrient delivery frequently arises, explore whether the existing scientific evidence justifies a modification in nutrient delivery. The quantities of nutrients stated in this text refer to administration in adults if not explicitly described as applicable to pediatric populations.

We begin with an overview of the salient features of the two classes of micronutrients: the vitamins and trace elements.

Salient Features of the Vitamins and Trace Elements

VITAMINS (TABLE 7.2)

Vitamins have long been categorized as either fat-soluble (A,D,E,K) or water-soluble (all the others). This remains a physiologically meaningful manner of categorization. Most of the functions of the water-soluble vitamins are as co-enzymes, and they are absorbed through an aqueous phase in the intestine. In contrast, none of the fat-soluble vitamins appear to serve as co-enzymes and intestinal absorption is primarily through a micellar route. Pathophysiologic conditions that produce selective fat malabsorption, therefore, are frequently associated with deficiencies of the fat-, but not water-soluble vitamins.

TRACE ELEMENTS (TABLE 7.3)

Fifteen trace elements have been identified as essential for health in animal studies: iron, zinc, copper, chromium, selenium, iodine, fluorine, manganese, molybdenum, cobalt, nickel, tin, silicon, vanadium and arsenic. Nevertheless, only for the first 10 of these have there been observations with compelling evidence that they are essential nutrients in humans. Cobalt seems to be essential solely as a component of vitamin B_{12}, but an isolated deficiency state has never been described. Due to the exceedingly small physiologic requirements for these elements and their ubiquitous nature in foodstuffs, essentiality of several of these elements was only recognized when long-term reliance on total paren-

TABLE 7.2

Fat-Soluble Vitamins				
	Biochemistry and Physiology	Deficiency (RDA*)	Toxicity (TUL**)	Assessment of Status
Vitamin A	Refers to a subset of the retinoid compounds, each member possessing biologic activity qualitatively similar to retinol, a member of the family. Carotenoids are structurally related to retinoids. Some carotenoids, most notably β-carotene, are metabolized into compounds with vitamin A activity and are therefore considered to be pro-vitamin A compounds. Vitamin A is an integral component of rhodopsin and iodopsins, light-sensitive proteins in rod and cone cells in the retina. Needed for the induction and maintenance of cellular differentiation in certain tissues. Serves as a signal for appropriate morphogenesis in the developing embryo and needed for maintenance of cell-mediated immunity. One microgram of retinol equivalent to 3.33 I.U. vitamin A.	Follicular hyperkeratosis and night blindness are early indicators. Conjunctival xerosis, degeneration of the cornea (keratomalacia) and de-differentiation of rapidly proliferating epithelia are later indications of deficiency. *Bitot spots* (focal areas of the conjunctiva or cornea with foamy appearance) are an indication of xerosis. Blindness, due to corneal destruction and retinal dysfunction, ensues if left uncorrected. Increased susceptibility to infection also a consequence. (F: 700 μg; M: 900 μg)	In adults, >150,000 μg may cause *acute* toxicity: fatal intracranial hypertension, skin exfoliation, and hepatocellular necrosis. *Chronic* toxicity may occur with habitual daily intake of >10,000 μg: alopecia, ataxia, bone and muscle pain, dermatitis, cheilitis, conjunctivitis, pseudotumor cerebri, hepatocellular necrosis, hyperlipidemia, and hyperostosis are common. Single, large doses of vitamin A (30,000 μg), or habitual intake of >4,500 μg per day during early pregnancy can be teratogenic. Excessive intake of carotenoids causes a benign condition characterized by yellowish discoloration of the skin. Habitually large doses of canthaxanthin, a carotenoid, has the additional capability of inducing a retinopathy. (3000 μg)	Retinol concentration in the plasma, as well as vitamin A concentrations in the milk and tears are reasonably accurate measures of adequate status. Toxicity best assessed by elevated levels of retinyl esters in plasma. A quantitative measure of dark adaptation for night vision or an electroretinogram is useful functional test.
Vitamin D	A group of sterol compounds whose parent structure is cholecalciferol (vitamin D_3). Cholecalciferol is formed in the skin from 7-dehydrocholesterol (provitamin D_3) by exposure to UV-B radiation. A plant sterol, ergocalciferol (provitamin D_2) can be similarly converted into vitamin D_2, and has similar vitamin D activity. The vitamin undergoes sequential hydroxylations in the liver and kidney at the 25 and 1 positions, respectively, producing the most bioactive form of the vitamin, 1,25-dihydroxy vitamin D. Maintains intra- and extracellular concentrations of calcium and phosphate by enhancing intestinal absorption of the two ions and, in conjunction with PTH, promoting their mobilization from bone mineral. Vitamin D retards proliferation and promotes differentiation in certain epithelia. One microgram equivalent to 40 I.U.	Deficiency results in disordered bone modeling called *rickets* in childhood and *osteomalacia* in adults. Expansion of the epiphyseal growth plates and replacement of normal bone with unmineralized bone matrix are the cardinal features of rickets; the latter feature also characterizes osteomalacia. Deformity of bone and pathologic fractures occur. Decreased serum concentrations of calcium and phosphate may occur. (5 μg, ages 19–50; 10 μg, ages 51–70; 15 μg, age >70)	Excess amounts result in abnormally high concentrations of calcium and phosphate in the serum: metastatic calcifications, renal damage, and altered mentation may occur. (50 μg)	The serum concentration of the major circulating metabolite, 25-hydroxy vitamin D, is an excellent indicator of systemic status except in chronic renal failure, where the impairment of renal 1-hydroxylation results in disassociation of the mono- and di-hydroxy vitamin concentrations. Measuring the serum concentration of 1,25-dihydroxy vitamin D is then necessary.

*Recommended Daily Allowance (RDA) established for female (F) and male (M) adults by the U.S. Food and Nutrition Board, 1999–2001. In some instances insufficient data exist to establish an RDA, in which case the Adequate Intake (AI) established by the board is listed.

**Tolerated Upper Intake (TUL) established for adults by the U.S. Food and Nutrition Board, 1999–2001.

Adapted with permission from Mason JB. Consequences of altered micronutrient status. In: Goldman L, Bennett J, eds. *Cecil Textbook of Medicine.* 21st ed. Philadelphia: WB Saunders Co.; 2000:1172–1174.

(continued)

TABLE 7.2

	Biochemistry and Physiology	Deficiency (RDA*)	Toxicity (TUL**)	Assessment of Status
Fat-Soluble Vitamins (CONTINUED)				
Vitamin E	A group of at least 8 naturally-occurring compounds, some of which are tocopherols and some of which are tocotrienols. At present, the only dietary form that is thought to be biologically active in humans is alpha-tocopherol. Acts as an anti-oxidant and free radical scavenger in lipophilic environments; most notably in cell membranes. Acts in conjunction with other anti-oxidants such as selenium.	Deficiency due to dietary inadequacy rare in developed countries. Usually seen in (1) premature infants, (2) individuals with fat malabsorption, and (3) individuals with abetalipoproteinemia. Red blood cell fragility occurs and can produce a hemolytic anemia. Neuronal degeneration produces peripheral neuropathies, ophthalmoplegia, and destruction of posterior columns of spinal cord. Neurologic disease frequently irreversible if deficiency is not corrected early enough. May contribute to hemolytic anemia and retrolental fibroplasia in premature infants. Has been reported to suppress cell-medicted immunity. (15 mg)	Depressed levels of vitamin K-dependent procoagulants and potentiation of oral anticoagulants has been reported, as has impaired leukocyte function. Doses of 800 mg/d have been reported to slightly increase the incidence of hemorrhagic stroke. (1000 mg)	Plasma or serum concentration of alpha-tocopherol is most commonly used. Additional accuracy is obtained by expressing this value per mg of total plasma lipid. Red blood cell peroxide hemolysis test is not entirely specific but is a useful functional measure of the anti-oxidant potential of cell membranes.
Vitamin K	A family of napthoquinone compounds with similar biologic activity. Phylloquinone (vitamin K_1) is derived from plants; a variety of menaquinones (vitamin K_2) are derived from bacterial sources. Serves as an essential co-factor in the post-translational gamma-carboxylation of glutamic acid residues in many proteins. These proteins include several circulating pro- and anti-coagulants as well as proteins in the bone matrix and renal epithelium.	Deficiency syndrome uncommon except in (1) breast-fed newborns, where it may cause "hemorrhagic disease of the newborn", (2) adults with fat malabsorption or who are taking drugs which interfere with vitamin K metabolism (eg: coumarin, phenytoin, broad-spectrum antibiotics), and (3) individuals taking large doses of vitamin E and anti-coagulant drugs. Excessive hemorrhage is the usual manifestation. (F: 90 µg; M: 120 µg)	Rapid intravenous infusion of K_1 has been associated with dyspnea, flushing and cardiovascular collapse; this is likely related to the dispersing agents in the solution. Supplementation may interfere with coumarin-based anticoagulation. Pregnant women taking large amounts of the pro-vitamin, menadione, may deliver infants with hemolytic anemia, hyperbilirubinemia, and kernicterus. (no TUL established)	The prothrombin time is typically used as a measure of functional K status; it is neither sensitive nor is it specific for vitamin K deficiency. Determination of undercarboxylated prothrombin in the plasma is more accurate but less widely available.
Water-Soluble Vitamins				
Thiamine (vitamin B_1)	A water-soluble compound containing substituted pyrimidine and thiazole rings and a hydroxyethyl side chain. The co-enzyme form is thiamin pyrophosphate. Serves as a co-enzyme in many alpha-keto acid decarboxylation and transketolation reactions. Inadequate thiamin availability leads to impairments of above reactions, resulting in inadequate ATP synthesis and abnormal carbohydrate metabolism, respectively. May have an additional role in neuronal conduction independent of above mentioned actions.	Classical deficiency syndrome ("beriberi") described in Asian populations consuming polished rice diet. Alcoholism and chronic renal dialysis are also common precipitants. High carbohydrate intake increases need for B_1. Mild deficiency commonly produces irritability, fatigue, and headaches. More pronounced deficiency produces various combinations of peripheral neuropathy, and cardiovascular and cerebral dysfunction. Cardiovascular involvement ("wet beriberi") includes congestive heart failure and low peripheral vascular resistance. Cerebral disease includes nystagmus, ophthalmoplegia, and ataxia (Wernicke's encephalopathy) as well as hallucinations, impaired short-term memory, and confabulation ("Korsakoff's psychosis"). Deficiency syndrome responds within 24 hours to parenteral thiamin but is partially or wholly irreversible after a certain stage. (F: 1.1 mg; M: 1.2)	Excess intake is largely excreted in the urine although parenteral doses of >400 mg/d are reported to cause lethargy, ataxia, and reduced tone of the gastrointestinal tract. (TUL not established)	The most effective measure of B_1 status is the erythrocyte transketolase activity coefficient, which measures enzyme activity before and after addition of exogenous TPP: red cells from a deficient individual express a substantial increase in enzyme activity with addition of TPP. Thiamin concentrations in the blood or urine are also used.

(continued)

TABLE 7.2

Water-Soluble Vitamins (CONTINUED)				
	Biochemistry and Physiology	Deficiency (RDA*)	Toxicity (TUL**)	Assessment of Status
Riboflavin (vitamin B_2)	A compound consisting of a substituted isoalloxazine ring with a ribitol side chain. The vitamin serves as a co-enzyme for a diverse array of biochemical reactions. The primary co-enzymatic forms are flavin mononucleotide (FMN) and flavin adenine dinucleotide (FAD). Riboflavin holoenzymes participate in oxidation-reduction reactions in a myriad of metabolic pathways.	Deficiency is usually seen in conjunction with deficiencies of other B vitamins. Isolated deficiency of riboflavin produces hyperemia and edema of nasopharyngeal mucosa, cheilosis, angular stomatitis, glossitis, seborrheic dermatitis, and a normochromic, normocytic anemia. (F: 1.1; M: 1.3)	Toxicity not reported in humans. (TUL not established)	The most common method of assessment is determining the activity coefficient of glutathione reductase in red blood cells (the test is invalid for individuals with glucose-6-phosphate dehydrogenase deficiency). Measurements of blood and urine concentrations are less desirable methods.
Niacin (vitamin B_3)	Refers to nicotinic acid and the corresponding amide, nicotinamide. The active co-enzymatic forms are composed of nicotinamide affixed to adenine dinucleotide, forming NAD or NADP. Over 200 apoenzymes use these compounds as electron acceptors or hydrogen donors, either as a co-enzyme or a co-substrate. The essential amino acid, tryptophan, is utilized as a precursor of niacin; 60 mg of dietary tryptophan yield approximately 1 mg of niacin. Dietary requirements are therefore partly dependent on tryptophan content of diet. Requirement is often determined on basis of caloric intake (ie: niacin equivalents/1000 kcal). Large doses of nicotinic acid (1.5–3.0 g/d) effectively lower LDL cholesterol and elevate HDL cholesterol.	*Pellagra* is the classical deficiency syndrome and is often seen in populations where corn is the major source of energy. Still endemic in parts of China, Africa, and India. Diarrhea, dementia (or associated symptoms of anxiety or insomnia), and a pigmented dermatitis that develops in sun-exposed areas are typical features. Glossitis, stomatitis, vaginitis, vertigo, and burning dysetheias are early signs. Reported to occasionally occur in carcinoid syndrome, because tryptophan is diverted to other synthetic pathways. (F: 14 mg; M: 16)	Human toxicity known largely through studies examining hypolipidemic effects. Includes vasomotor phenomenon (flushing), hyperglycemia, parenchymal liver damage, and hyperuricemia. (35 mg)	Assessment of status is problematic: blood levels of vitamin not reliable. Measurement of urinary excretion of the niacin metabolites, N-methylnicotinamide and 2-pyridone are thought to be the most effective means of assessment at present.
Vitamin B_6	Refers to several derivatives of pyridine, including pyridoxine (PN), pyridoxal (PL) and pyridoxamine (PM), which are interconvertible in the body. The co-enzymatic forms are pyridoxal-5-phosphate (PLP) and pyridoxamine-5-phosphate (PMP). As a co-enzyme, B_6 is involved in many transamination reactions (and thereby in gluconeogenesis), in the synthesis of niacin from tryptophan, in the synthesis of several neurotransmitters, and in the synthesis of delta-aminolevulinic acid (and therefore in heme synthesis). It also has functions that are not related to co-enzymatic activity: PL and PLP bind to hemoglobin and alter O_2 affinity; PLP also binds to steroid receptors, inhibiting receptor affinity to DNA and thereby modulates steroid activity.	Deficiency usually seen in conjunction with other water-soluble vitamin deficiencies. Stomatitis, angular cheilosis, glossitis, irritability, depression, and confusion occur in moderate to severe depletion; normochromic, normocytic anemia has been reported in severe deficiency. Abnormal EEGs and, in infants, convulsions have also been observed. Some sideroblastic anemias are responsive to B_6 administration. Isoniazid, cycloserine, penicillamine, ethanol, and theophylline are drugs which can inhibit B_6 metabolism. (ages 19–50: 1.3 mg; >50: 1.5 mg for women, 1.7 mg for men)	Chronic use with doses exceeding 200 mg per day (in adults) may cause peripheral neuropathies and photosensitivity. (100 mg)	Many useful laboratory methods of assessment exist. The plasma or erythrocyte PLP levels are most common. Urinary excretion of xanthurenic acid after an oral tryptophan load or activity indices of RBC alanine or aspartic acid transaminases (ALT and AST, respectively) are all functional measures of B_6-dependent enzyme activity.

(continued)

TABLE 7.2

Water-Soluble Vitamins (CONTINUED)				
	Biochemistry and Physiology	**Deficiency (RDA*)**	**Toxicity (TUL**)**	**Assessment of Status**
Folate	A group of related pterin compounds. Over 35 forms of the vitamin are found naturally. The fully oxidized form, folic acid, is not found in nature but is the pharmacologic form of the vitamin. All folate functions relate to its ability to transfer one-carbon groups. It is essential in the *de novo* synthesis of nucleotides, in the metabolism of several amino acids, and is an integral component for the regeneration of the "universal" methyl donor, S-adenosylmethionine. Inhibition of bacterial and cancer cell folate metabolism is the basis for the sulfonamide antibiotics and chemotherapeutic agents such as methotrexate and 5-fluorouracil, respectively.	Women of childbearing age are the most likely individuals to develop deficiency. The "classical" deficiency syndrome is megaloblastic anemia. The hemopoeitic cells in the bone marrow become enlarged and have immature nuclei, which is a reflection of ineffective DNA synthesis. The peripheral blood smear demonstrates macroovalocytes and polymorphnuclear leukocytes with an average of more than 3.5 nuclear lobes. Megaloblastic changes also occur in other epithelia that proliferate rapidly such as the oral mucosa and gastrointestinal tract, producing glossitis and diarrhea, respectively. Sulfasalazine and diphenytoin inhibit absorption and predispose to deficiency. (400 μg of dietary folate equivalents (DFE); 1 μg folic acid=1 μg DFE; 1 μg food folate=0.6 μg DFE)	Doses >1000 μg per day may partially correct the anemia of B_{12} deficiency and may therefore mask (and perhaps exacerbate) the associated neuropathy. Large doses also reported to lower seizure threshold in individuals prone to seizures. Parenteral administration rarely reported to cause allergic phenomena but is probably due to dispersion agents. (1000 μg)	Serum folate measures short-term folate balance whereas RBC folate is a better reflection of tissue status. Serum homocysteine rises early in deficiency but is non-specific since B_{12} or B_6 deficiency, renal insufficiency, and advanced age may also cause elevations.
Vitamin C (ascorbic and dehydro-ascorbic acid)	Ascorbic acid readily oxidizes to dehydroascorbic acid in aqueous solution. Since the latter can be reduced *in vivo*, it possesses vitamin C activity. Total vitamin C is therefore measured as the sum of ascorbic, and dehydroascorbic, acid concentrations. Due to its reductant properties, it serves primarily as a biological antioxidant in aqueous environments. The biosyntheses of collagen, carnitine, bile acids, and norepinephrine, as well as proper functioning of the hepatic mixed-function oxygenase system, are all dependent on this property. Vitamin C in foodstuffs increases the intestinal absorption of non-heme iron.	Overt deficiency uncommonly observed in developed countries. The classical deficiency syndrome is *scurvy*: characterized by fatigue, depression, and widespread abnormalities in connective tissues such as inflamed gingivae, petechiae, perifollicular hemorrhages, impaired wound healing, coiled hairs, hyperkeratosis, bleeding into body cavities. In infants, defects in ossification and bone growth may occur. Tobacco smoking lowers plasma and leukocyte vitamin C levels. (F: 75 mg; M: 90 mg; increased requirement for cigarette smokers by 35 mg/d)	Quantities exceeding 500 mg per day (in adults) sometimes cause nausea and diarrhea. Acidification of the urine with supplementation, and the potential for enhanced oxalate synthesis, have raised concerns regarding nephrolithiasis but this has yet to be demonstrated. Supplementation may interfere with laboratory tests based on redox potential (e.g., fecal occult blood testing, serum cholesterol, and glucose). Withdrawal from chronic ingestion of high doses of vitamin C supplements should occur gradually over a month since accommodation does seem to occur, raising a concern of "rebound scurvy." (2 g)	Plasma ascorbic acid concentration reflects recent dietary intake whereas leukocyte levels more closely reflect tissue stores. Women's plasma levels are approximately 20% higher than men for any given dietary intake.

(continued)

TABLE 7.2

Water-Soluble Vitamins (CONTINUED)				
	Biochemistry and Physiology	**Deficiency (RDA*)**	**Toxicity (TUL**)**	**Assessment of Status**
Vitamin B_{12}	A group of closely related cobalamin compounds composed of a corrin ring (with a cobalt atom in its center) connected to a ribonucleotide via an aminopropanol bridge. Microorganisms are the ultimate source of all naturally-occurring B_{12}. The two active co-enzyme forms are desoxyadenosylcobalamin and methylcobalamin. These co-enzymes are needed for the synthesis of succinyl CoA, which is essential in lipid and carbohydrate metabolism, and for the synthesis of methionine. The latter reaction is essential for amino acid metabolism, for purine and pyrimidine synthesis, for many methylation reactions, and for the intracellular retention of folates.	Dietary inadequacy is a rare cause of deficiency except in strict vegetarians. The vast majority of cases of deficiency arise from loss of intestinal absorption: this may be a result of pernicious anemia, pancreatic insufficiency, atrophic gastritis, small bowel bacterial overgrowth, or ileal disease. Megaloblastic anemia, and megaloblastic changes in other epithelia (see "folate") are the result of sustained depletion. Demyelination of peripheral nerves, the posterior and lateral columns of the spinal cord, as well as nerves within the brain may occur. Altered mentation, depression, and psychoses occur. Hematologic and neurologic complications may occur independently. Folate supplementation, in doses exceeding 1000 µg per day, may partly correct the anemia, thereby masking (or perhaps exacerbating) the neuropathic complications. (2.4 µg)	A few allergic reactions have been reported to crystalline B_{12} preparations, and are probably due to impurities, not the vitamin. (TUL not established)	Serum, or plasma, concentrations are generally accurate. Subtle deficiency with neurologic complications, as described in the "deficiency" column, can best be established by concurrently measuring the concentration of plasma B_{12} and serum methylmalonic acid, since the latter is a sensitive indicator of cellular deficiency.
Biotin	A bi-cyclic compound consisting of a ureido ring fused to a substituted tetrahydrothiophene ring. Endogenous synthesis by the intestinal flora may contribute significantly to biotin nurtriture. Most dietary biotin is linked to lysine, a compound called biotinyl lysine, or biocytin. The lysine must be hydrolyzed by an intestinal enzyme called biotinidase before intestinal absorption occurs. Acts primarily as a co-enzyme for several carboxylases; each holoenzyme catalyzes an ATP-dependent CO_2 tranfer. The carboxylases are critical enzymes in carbohydrate and lipid metabolism.	Isolated deficiency is rare. Deficiency in humans has been produced experimentally (by dietary inadequacy), by prolonged total parenteral nutrition lacking the vitamin, and by ingestion of large quantities of raw egg white, which contains avidin, a protein which binds biotin with such high affinity that it renders it bio-unavailable. Alterations in mental status, myalgias, hyperesthesias, and anorexia occur. Later, a seborrheic dermatitis and alopecia develop. Biotin deficiency is usually accompanied by lactic acidosis and organic aciduria. (30 µg)	Toxicity has not been reported in humans with doses as high as 60 mg per day in children. (TUL not established)	Plasma and urine concentrations of biotin are diminished in the deficient state. Elevated urine concentrations of methyl citrate, 3-methylcrotonylglycine and 3-hydroxyisovalerate are also observed in deficiency.
Pantothenic acid	Consists of pantoic acid linked to β-alanine through an amide bond. It serves as an essential component of coenzyme A (CoA) and phosphopantetheine, which are essential for the synthesis and β-oxidation of fatty acids, as well as the synthesis of cholesterol, steroid hormones, vitamins A and D, and other isoprenoid derivatives. CoA is also involved in the synthesis of several amino acids and delta-aminolevulinic acid, a precursor for the corrin ring of vitamin B_{12}, the porphyrin ring of heme and of cytochromes. CoA is also necessary for the acetylation and fatty acid acylation of a variety of proteins.	Deficiency rare: only reported as a result of feeding semisynthetic diets or an antagonist to the vitamin. Experimental, isolated deficiency in humans produces fatigue, abdominal pain and vomiting, insomnia, and parathesias of the extremities. (5 mg)	In doses exceeding 10 grams per day, diarrhea is reported to occur. (TUL not established)	Whole blood and urine concentrations of pantothenate are indicators of status; serum levels are not thought to be accurate.

TABLE 7.3

Trace Elements				
	Biochemistry and Physiology	**Deficiency (RDA*)**	**Toxicity (TUL**)**	**Assessment of Status**
Chromium	Dietary chromium consists of both inorganic and organic forms. Its primary function in humans is to potentiate insulin action. It accomplishes this function as a circulating complex called "Glucose Tolerance Factor." It thereby affects carbohydrate, fat, and protein metabolism.	Deficiency in humans only described in long-term TPN patients whose TPN contained insufficient chromium. Hyperglycemia, or impaired glucose intolerance, is uniformly observed. Elevated plasma-free fatty acid concentrations, neuropathy, encephalopathy, and abnormalities in nitrogen metabolism are also reported. Whether supplemental chromium may improve glucose tolerance in mildly glucose intolerant but otherwise healthy individuals remains controversial. (F: 25 μg; M: 35 μg)	Toxicity after oral ingestion is uncommon and seems confined to gastric irritation. Airborne exposure may cause contact dermatitis, eczema, skin ulcers, and bronchogenic carcinoma. (TUL not established)	Plasma or serum concentration of chromium is a crude indicator of chromium status; it appears to be meaningful when the value is markedly above or below the normal range.
Copper	Copper is absorbed by a specific intestinal transport mechanism. It is carried to the liver where it is bound to ceruloplasmin, which circulates systemically and delivers copper to target tissues in the body. Excretion of copper is largely through bile, and then into the feces. Absorptive and excretory processes vary with the levels of dietary copper, providing a means of copper homeostasis. Copper serves as a component of many enzymes, including amine oxidases, ferroxidases, cytochrome c oxidase, dopamine β-hydroxylase, superoxide dismutase, and tyrosinase.	Dietary deficiency is rare; it has been observed in premature and low birth weight infants fed exclusively a cow's milk diet and in individuals on long-term total parenteral nutrition without copper. The clinical manifestations include depigmentation of skin and hair, neurological disturbances, leukopenia and hypochromic, microcytic anemia, and skeletal abnormalities. The anemia arises from impaired utilization of iron, and is therefore a conditioned form of iron deficiency anemia. The deficiency syndrome, except the anemia and leukopenia, is also observed in Mencke's disease, a rare inherited condition associated with impaired copper utilization. (900 μg)	Acute copper toxicity has been described after excessive oral intake and with absorption of copper salts applied to burned skin. Milder manifestations include nausea, vomiting, epigastric pain, and diarrhea; coma and hepatic necrosis may ensue in severe cases. Toxicity may be seen with doses as low as 70 μg/kg/d. Chronic toxicity is also described. Wilson's disease is a rare, inherited disease associated with abnormally low ceruloplasmin levels and accumulation of copper in the liver and brain, eventually leading to damage to these two organs. (10 mg)	Practical methods for detecting marginal deficiency are not available. Marked deficiency is reliably detected by diminished serum copper and ceruloplasmin concentrations, as well as low erythrocyte superoxide dismutase activity.
Fluorine	Known more commonly by its ionic form, fluoride. It is incorporated into the crystalline structure of bone, thereby altering its physical characteristics.	Intake of <0.1 mg/d in infants and 0.5 in children is associated with an increased incidence of dental caries. Optimal intake in adults is between 1.5 and 4 mg/d. (F: 3 mg; M: 4 mg)	Acute ingestion of >30 mg/kg body weight fluoride is likely to cause death. Excessive chronic intake (0.1 mg/kg/d) leads to mottling of the teeth (dental fluorosis), calcification of tendons and ligaments, and exostoses and may increase the brittleness of bones. (10 mg)	Estimates of intake or clinical assessment are used because no good laboratory test exists.

*Recommended Daily Allowance (RDA) established for female (F) and male (M) adults by the U.S. Food and Nutrition Board, 1999-2001. In some instances insufficient data exist to establish an RDA, in which case the Adequate Intake (AI) established by the Board is listed.

**Tolerated Upper Intake (TUL) established for adults by the U.S. Food and Nutrition Board, 1999-2001.

Adapted with permission from Mason JB. Consequences of altered micronutrient status. In: Goldman L, Bennett J, eds. *Cecil Textbook of Medicine.* 21st ed. Philadelphia: WB Saunders Co.; 2000:1172-1174.

(continued)

TABLE 7.3

Trace Elements (CONTINUED)				
	Biochemistry and Physiology	Deficiency (RDA*)	Toxicity (TUL**)	Assessment of Status
Iodine	Readily absorbed from the diet, concentrated in the thyroid and integrated into the thyroid hormones, thyroxine (T_4), and tri-iodothyronine (T_3). These hormones circulate largely bound to thyroxine-binding globulin. They modulate resting energy expenditure and, in the developing human, growth and development.	In the absence of supplementation, populations relying primarily on food from soils with low iodine content have endemic iodine deficiency. Maternal iodine deficiency leads to fetal deficiency, which produces spontaneous abortions, stillbirths, hypothyroidism, cretinism, and dwarfism. Rapid brain development continues through the second year, and permanent cognitive deficits may be induced by iodine deficiency over that time period. In the adult, compensatory hypertrophy of the thyroid (goiter) occurs along with varying degrees of hypothyroidism. (150 µg)	Large doses (>2 mg/d in adults) may induce hypothyroidism by blocking thyroid hormone synthesis. Supplementation with >100 µg per day to an individual who was formerly deficient occasionally induces hyperthyroidism. (1.1 mg)	Iodine status of a population can be estimated by the prevalence of goiter. Urinary excretion of iodine is an effective laboratory means of assessment. The TSH (thyroid stimulating hormone) level in the blood is an indirect, and therefore not an entirely specific, means of assessment.
Iron	Conveys the capacity to participate in redox reactions to a number of metalloproteins such as hemoglobin, myoglobin, the cytochrome enzymes, and many oxidases and oxygenases. Primary storage form is ferritin and, to a lesser degree, hemosiderin. Intestinal absorption is 15%–20% for "heme" iron and 1%–8% for the iron contained in vegetables. Absorption of the latter form is enhanced by the ascorbic acid in foodstuffs, by poultry, fish, or beef and by an iron deficient state; it is decreased by phytate and tannins.	The most common micronutrient deficiency in the world. Women of child-bearing age constitute the highest risk group because of menstrual blood losses, pregnancy and lactation. The classical deficiency syndrome is hypochromic, microcytic anemia. Glossitis and koilonychias ("spoon" nails) are also observed. Easy fatiguability often develops as an early symptom, before the appearance of anemia. In children, mild deficiency of insufficient severity to cause anemia is associated with behavioral disturbances and poor school performance. (postmenopausal F and M: 8 mg; premenopausal F: 18 mg)	Iron overload typically occurs when habitual dietary intake is extremely high, when intestinal absorption is excessive, when repeated parenteral administration of iron occurs, or if a combination of these factors exist. Excessive iron stores usually accumulate in the reticuloendothelial tissues and cause little damage ("hemosiderosis"). If overload continues, iron will eventually begin to accumulate in tissues such as the hepatic parenchyma, pancreas, heart, and synovium, damaging these tissues ("hemochromatosis"). Hereditary hemochromatosis arises as a result of homozygousity of a common, recessive, trait. Excessive intestinal absorption of iron is observed in homozygotes. (45 mg)	Negative iron balance initially leads to depletion of iron stores in the bone marrow: a bone marrow biopsy or the concentration of serum ferritin are accurate and early indicators of such depletion. As the severity of deficiency proceeds, serum iron (SI) decreases and total iron binding capacity (TIBC) increases: an iron saturation (=SI/TIBC) of <16% suggests iron deficiency. Microcytosis, hypochromia, and anemia ensue as latter stages of the deficient state. Elevated levels of serum ferritin or an iron saturation over 60% raises the suspicion of iron overload, although systemic inflammation elevates serum ferritin irrespective of iron status.
Manganese	A component of several metalloenzymes. Most manganese is in mitochondria, where it is a component of manganese superoxide dismutase.	Manganese deficiency in the human has not been conclusively demonstrated. It is said to cause hypocholesterolemia, weight loss, hair and nail changes, dermatitis, and impaired synthesis of vitamin K-dependent proteins. (F: 1.8 mg; M: 2.3 mg)	Toxicity by oral ingestion unknown in humans. Toxic inhalation causes hallucinations, other alterations in mentation, and extrapyramidal movement disorders. (11 mg)	Until the deficiency syndrome is better defined, an appropriate measure of status will be difficult to develop.
Molybdenum	A cofactor in several enzymes, most prominently xanthine oxidase and sulfite oxidase.	A probable case of human deficiency is described as being secondary to parenteral administration of sulfite and resulted in hyperoxypurimenia, hypouricemia, and low sulfate excretion. (45 µg)	Toxicity is associated with nausea, diarrhea, alterations in mental status, peripheral neuropathy, and loss of hair and nails; such symptoms were observed in adults who inadvertently consumed between 27 and 2400 mg. (2 mg)	Erythrocyte glutathione peroxidase activity and plasma, or whole blood, selenium concentrations are moderately accurate indicators of status.

(continued)

TABLE 7.3

Trace Elements (CONTINUED)

	Biochemistry and Physiology	Deficiency (RDA*)	Toxicity (TUL**)	Assessment of Status
Selenium	Most dietary selenium is in the form of an amino-acid complex. Nearly complete absorption of such forms occurs. Homeostasis is largely performed by the kidney, which regulates urinary excretion as a function of selenium status. Selenium is a component of several enzymes, most notably glutathione peroxidase and superoxide dismutase. These enzymes appear to prevent oxidative and free radical damage of various cell structures. Evidence suggests that the anti-oxidant protection conveyed by selenium operates in conjunction with vitamin E, since deficiency of one seems to enhance damage induced by a deficiency of the other. Selenium also participates in the enzymatic conversion of thyroxine to its more active metabolite, tri-iodothyronine.	Deficiency is rare in North America but has been observed in individuals on long-term TPN lacking selenium. Such individuals have myalgias and/or cardiomyopathies. Populations in some regions of the world have marginal intake of selenium, most notably some parts of China. It is in these regions of China that *Keshan's disease* is endemic, a condition characterized by cardiomyopathy. Keshan's disease can be prevented (but not treated) by selenium supplementation. (55 μg)	Toxicity is associated with nausea, diarrhea, alterations in mental status, peripheral neuropathy, loss of hair, and nails: such symptoms were observed in adults who inadvertently consumed between 27 and 2400 mg. (400 μg)	Erythrocyte glutathione peroxidase activity and plasma, or whole blood, selenium concentrations are the most commonly used methods of assessment. They are moderately accurate indicators of status.
Zinc	Intestinal absorption occurs by a specific process that is enhanced by pregnancy and corticosteroids and diminished by co-ingestion of phytates, phosphates, iron, copper, lead, or calcium. Diminished intake of zinc leads to an increased efficiency of absorption and decreased fecal excretion, providing a means of zinc homeostasis. Zinc is a component of over 100 enzymes; among these are DNA polymerase, RNA polymerase and tRNA synthetase.	Deficiency of zinc has its most profound effect on rapidly proliferating tissues. Mild deficiency causes growth retardation in children. More severe deficiency is associated with growth arrest, teratogenecity, hypogonadism and infertility, dysgeusia, poor wound healing, diarrhea, a dermatitis on the extremities and around orifices, glossitis, alopecia, corneal clouding, loss of dark adaptation and behavioral changes. Impaired cellular immunity is observed. Excessive loss of gastrointestinal secretions through chronic diarrhea, fistulas, etc., may precipitate deficiency. *Acrodermatitis enteropathica* is a rare, recessively inherited disease in which intestinal absorption of zinc is impaired. (F: 8 mg; M: 11 mg)	Acute zinc toxicity can usually be induced by ingestion of >200 mg of zinc in a single day (in adults). It is manifested by epigastric pain, nausea, vomiting, and diarrhea. Hyperpnea, diaphoresis and weakness may follow inhalation of zinc fumes. Copper and zinc compete for intestinal absorption: chronic ingestion of >25 mg zinc/d may lead to copper deficiency. Chronic ingestion of >150 mg/d has been reported to cause gastric erosions, low HDL cholesterol levels and impaired cellular immunity. (40 mg)	There are no accurate indicators of zinc status available for routine clinical use. Plasma, erythrocyte, and hair zinc concentrations are frequently misleading. Acute illness, in particular, is known to diminish plasma zinc levels, in part by inducing a shift of zinc out of the plasma compartment and into the liver. Functional tests which determine dark adaptation, taste acuity, and rate of wound healing lack specificity.

TABLE 7.4A

1979 Guidelines for Daily Delivery of Parenteral Micronutrients in Adults[1]	
Vitamins	
A	1000 μg
D	5 μg
E	10 mg
K	2-4 mg once weekly
C	100 mg
folate	400 μg
niacin	40 mg
riboflavin	3.6 mg
thiamin	3 mg
B_6	4 mg
B_{12}	5 μg
pantothenic acid	15 mg
biotin	60 μg
Trace elements	
copper	0.5–1.5 mg
chromium	10–15 μg
manganese	0.15–0.8 mg
zinc	2.5–4.0 mg

TABLE 7.4B

1988 Guidelines for Daily Delivery of Parenteral Micronutrients in Children	
Vitamins	
A	700 μg
D	10 μg
E	7 mg
K	200 μg
C	80 mg
folate	140 μg
niacin	17 mg
riboflavin	1.4 mg
thiamin	1.2 mg
B_6	1.0 mg
B_{12}	1.0 μg
pantothenic acid	5 mg
biotin	20 μg
Trace elements (μg/kg/d)	
copper	20
chromium	0.2
manganese	1.0
zinc	50
molybdenum	0.25
iodide	1.0
selenium	2.0
iron	1-2 mg/d

Adapted with permission from Greene H, Hambidge KM, Schanler R, et al. Guidelines for the use of vitamins, trace elements, calcium, magnesium, and phosphorus in infants and children receiving TPN. *Am J Clin Nutr.* 1988;48:1324–1342; Erratum of reference 2. *Am J Clin Nutr.* 1989;49:1332; and Erratum of reference 2. *Am J Clin Nutr.* 1989;50:560.

teral nutrition (TPN) lacking the elements resulted in deficiency states.

The biochemical functions of trace elements have not been as well characterized as those for the vitamins but most of their functions appear to be as components of prosthetic groups or as co-factors for a number of enzymes. Determination of essential trace element status is quite problematic except for iron, selenium, and iodine. The vanishingly low concentrations of these elements in body fluids and tissues, the fact that blood levels frequently do not correlate well with levels in the target tissues, and the fact that functional tests cannot be devised until biochemical functions are better understood preclude an accurate and convenient laboratory method of assessment for most of the trace elements. Assessing trace element status is further obscured in the critically ill patient because factors associated with acute illness may alter the measurements that are typically used for assessment. The prototype example of this is plasma zinc, where systemic inflammation causes a shift of zinc out of the plasma compartment and into the liver.[6,7]

Is the Micronutrient Content of Standard Enteral and Parenteral Feeding Solutions Sufficient to Meet the Needs of the Critically Ill Patient?

In a critically ill adult patient who does not otherwise have extraordinary needs for particular micronutrients, the majority of standard enteral and parenteral formulas available in the United States contain suitable quantities of vitamins and microminerals. The issue is a rather straightforward one in TPN because parenteral solutions are individually compounded for each patient, and as long as the standardized quantities of multivitamin and trace element mixtures are included daily, the needs of most patients are met.

The issue becomes somewhat more complex in the patient being fed an enteral nutritional formula, because such formulas are received by the healthcare provider in a finished form. Nevertheless, manufacturers are quite aware of this concern and therefore they routinely formulate adult enteral solutions so that 100%–120% of the RDA for vitamins and microminerals is delivered in 2000 kcal. Complicating this matter, however, is the current trend to feed as little as 25 kcal/kg/d. This is thought to meet the needs of most mechanically ventilated, ill patients,[8] and therefore one might ask whether most tube feeding formulas will still provide sufficient micronutrients if a philosophy of conservative caloric delivery is subscribed to. The answer is yes: a review of 59 pre-formulated liquid nutritional supplements available in the United States revealed only two products that would deliver less than 85% of the RDA in a daily volume sufficient to provide 25 kcal/kg/d (Table 7.5). Given the margin of safety that is built into the RDAs, it is almost always adequate to meet only 85% of the RDA over a matter of weeks to a couple of months, although for patients on long-term support, one should strive to meet 100% of the RDA.

A concern over insufficient micronutrient delivery in enteral formulas may also arise in other circumstances where a relatively small number of calories is being provided per kg of body weight, although this concern is probably more theoretical than real in most cases. Examples include the very obese patient, where an "adjusted ideal body weight"[9] is often used to calculate macronutrient needs, thereby leading to a low micronutrient delivery per kilogram of actual weight or when intentional hypocaloric feeding regimens are used for obese patients,[10] as has become popular in some medical centers during the past decade. In practice, however, there is little evidence that the obese person has elevated micronutrient needs substantially above those of a non-obese person of similar height. A genuine concern should arise, however, in those instances where a critically ill patient has repeated interruptions in tube feeding, a phenomenon that occurs all too frequently.[11] This warrants supplementation with a liquid multivitamin and multimineral preparation.

Are There Situations Where Supraphysiologic Supplementation Is Indicated?

Certainly, there is little debate that supraphysiologic supplementation is indicated for a brief period when a frank deficiency of a micronutrient is identified. As a general guideline, the provision of 5 to 10 times the RDA on a daily basis for 5–7 days, either enterally or parenterally, will suffice as a means of repletion. On occasion, even larger doses are appropriate. Rapid reversal of iron deficiency, for instance, can be effected by calculating the estimated iron deficit[12] and administering intravenous iron dextran in doses of 100–500 mg/d until the deficit is corrected. Since it remains unclear as to whether the rare anaphylactoid

TABLE 7.5

A Survey of the Micronutrient Content of Common Liquid Nutritional Supplements

Formulas containing less than 100% of the RDAs in 1750 kcal* have the percentage indicated in bold.

Advera® §	Isosource HN® ‡	NutriVent® †	RenalCal® **(87.5%)**# †
AlitraQ® §	Isosource VHN® ‡	Optimental® §	Replete® †
Compleat® ‡	Isotein HN® **(83%)** ‡	Osmolite® **(87.5%)** §	Replete® with fiber †
Crucial® †	Jevity® §	Osmolite HN® §	Respalor® ††
Deliver® 2.0 **(88%)**††	Jevity Plus® §	Oxepa® §	Sandosource Peptide® ‡
Fibersource® ‡	Lipisorb® ††	Peptamen® †	Subdue® ††
Fibersource HN® ‡	Nepro® **(92%)** §	Peptamen 1.5® †	Subdue Plus® ††
Glucerna® §	Novasource® 2.0 **(92%)** ‡	Peptamen VHP® †	Suplena® **(92.4%)** §
Glytrol® †	Novasource Renal® **(87.5%)** ‡	Perative® §	Traumacal® **(58%)**@ §
Impact® ‡	Novasource Pulmonary® ‡	Probalance® †	TwoCal® HN **(92.4%)** §
Impact 1.5® **(93%)** ‡	Nutren 1.0® †	Promote® §	Ultracal® ††
Isocal® **(87%)**††	Nutren 1.0 with fiber® †	Protain XL® ††	Vital HN§
Isocal HN® ††	Nutren 1.5® †	Pulmocare® §	Vivonex Plus® **(97%)** ‡
Isosource® ‡	Nutren 2.0® †	Reabilan® **(87.5%)** †	Vivonex TEN® **(87.5%)** ‡
Isosource 1.5® ‡	NutriHep® †	Reabilan HN® **(87.5%)** †	

*Equivalent to providing 25 kcal/kg/d to a 70 kg person. All figures derived from published contents by manufacturer.
Contains only Zn and selenium as trace elements
@ No chromium added
§ Ross Laboratories, Columbus, Ohio
† Nestle, Deerfield, Illinois
‡ Novartis, Minneapolis, Minnesota
†† Mead Johnson, Evansville, Indiana

reactions to parenteral iron dextran are dose-related, it is my habit to not administer more than 100 mg of iron per day via this route. Repletion of vitamin B_{12} deficiency should also be accomplished with large doses of the vitamin. The neurologic complications of B_{12} deficiency become irreversible after a point, and since repletion with small doses can take weeks or months, the daily administration of 100–1000 μg parenterally for 5 days is the most prudent course to take for rapid repletion.

The remainder of this section contains discussions about other situations where the question of supraphysiologic supplementation often arises in critically ill patients. Each discussion examines whether there is sufficient scientific evidence to justify such supplementation.

Chromium and Hyperglycemia

Frank chromium deficiency induces glucose intolerance, and repletion corrects this deficit, apparently by potentiating the effect of insulin.[13] This property of chromium is thought to be mediated through its participation in a circulating "Glucose Tolerance Factor [GTF]," although the biochemical nature of GTF continues to elude characterization. Many studies have been performed to see whether chromium supplementation might improve glucose intolerance and/or hyperglycemia. The results of the studies are not entirely consistent and therefore the matter remains one of controversy. Nevertheless, the consensus of studies indicates that it is unlikely that chromium-replete individuals have anything to benefit from supplementation[14–16]; only when individuals are maintained on a low chromium diet (consuming about 4 μg/d: one-sixth of the mean daily intake in the United States) do subjects consistently display improved glucose tolerance with supplementation.[17] Consistent with this consensus is the FDA's interim rule, prohibiting foods from making the claim that chromium can improve glucose intolerance or prevent hyperglycemia.[18]

Routine supplementation of critically ill patients with hyperglycemia is therefore not indicated. Nevertheless, if there is a high index of suspicion that an individual might have had a sustained period of inadequate chromium intake due to a severely restrictive diet, etc., daily supplementation (200 μg/d orally as chromium-rich yeast or picolinate or 8 μg/d parenterally) over a period of a week would be a reasonable therapeutic trial.

Antioxidant Micronutrients and Critical Illness

Marked degrees of systemic inflammation are associated with increases in free radical generation, diminished concentrations of antioxidants such as vitamin E and selenium in the plasma,[19–21] and increases in several biomarkers of oxidation.[21,22] It is hypothesized that an excessive load of free radicals and oxidant stress might overwhelm endogenous antioxidants and contribute to the tissue damage seen in conditions such as adult respiratory distress syndrome and SIRS, and therefore clinical trials with antioxidant nutrients have been conducted. Although supplementation of these critically ill patients with vitamin E, C, carotenoids and selenium raises plasma levels of these nutrients and even attenuates rises in indicators of oxidant damage,[20,23] there is little or no evidence to date that such treatment has any impact on clinical endpoints.[21,23] Administering supplemental levels of these nutrients to such patients for the purposes of improving outcomes should therefore continue to be in the setting of clinical trials.

Zinc and Critical Illness

There are a few issues pertinent to zinc in critical illness. The first pertains to the fact that urinary zinc losses increase in response to systemic inflammation, increasing from a mean of approximately 0.6 mg/day in healthy individuals to as much as 7 mg/day in critically ill patients.[24] Interestingly, patients who are sedated with propofol, which contains the chelating agent, EDTA, have much higher excretion than patients receiving other sedating agents not containing EDTA.[24] This level of enhanced excretion is a clinically relevant one since total body losses usually only amount to about 2–4 mg/d[25] and many enteral and parenteral formulas are based on the excretion observed in the healthy situation. Flagrant zinc deficiency is only rarely diagnosed in the intensive care unit, and one could therefore argue that it should be of no concern. However, establishing a diagnosis of zinc deficiency is a difficult task because the clinical manifestations are non-specific: rash, impaired immunity, and poor wound healing. Furthermore, the difficulty of arriving at a diagnosis is exacerbated by the lack of an effective diagnostic test. In view of this, it may be prudent in the critically ill, parenterally fed patient to ensure that the daily intravenous delivery amounts to 10 mg: this exceeds the 1979 AMA recommendations (2.5–4 mg/d) as well as the amount typically found in the standard dose of trace element solution

(2 mg). The bioavailabilty of zinc from commercial tube feedings has not been investigated systematically, but if one assumes an average availability from dietary sources, zinc balance in a critically ill patient would be met with an enteral intake of about 25 mg/d. The increased amount of zinc delivery suggested here for critically ill patients does not exceed the TUL of 40 mg/d.[25]

Under normal circumstances, the gastrointestinal tract is the major source of zinc loss from the body. Sustained diarrhea and high-output fistulas from the GI tract may therefore lead to depletion and a frank deficiency of zinc, a consequence that has been reported on many occasions in chronic diarrhea arising from inflammatory bowel disease.[26] Fistulas arising high in the intestine rather than more distally have secretions higher in zinc because pancreatic secretions are a major source of zinc in the intestinal effluent. Balance studies indicate that zinc requirements may double or triple in the setting of uncontrolled diarrhea,[27] and this situation therefore warrants supplementation. The empiric delivery of 12–15 mg of parenteral zinc per day, or 40 mg of oral elemental zinc/d, to such a patient should suffice in this setting. Enterally, the zinc should be administered on a BID or TID schedule, and is available as a chelate or a variety of salts.

Evaluation of zinc status remains problematic, and this is particularly true in the critically ill patient since systemic inflammation induces shifts in zinc from the blood compartment to the liver,[6,7] so it is best to guide therapy based on the clinical scenario rather than plasma zinc levels.

Iron, B_{12} and Folate in Erythropoietin Therapy

Erythropoietin has proven to be a useful agent for enhancing bone marrow erythropoiesis in several settings, such as chronic renal failure, recovery from chemotherapy, and following bone marrow transplantation. It is well recognized that the response to erythropoietin is blunted if its use is superimposed on a deficiency of iron, folate or B_{12}.[28] A related question is whether utilization of these micronutrients is sufficiently increased during erythropoietin therapy to effectively increase the daily requirement and therefore warrant routine supplementation, even in patients who are considered replete by conventional standards. Several trials in patients with chronic renal failure have tested this question and the results are inconsistent. In regard to folate, most studies have found that no additional supplements are necessary if the patient has normal folate status at the onset of therapy,[29,30] although one small uncontrolled study suggested otherwise.[31] Intravenous iron supplementation, at a dose of 100 mg twice per week, enhanced the response to erythropoeitin in one trial even though the subjects started with serum ferritin levels >100 ng/mL.[32] The mean ferritin at the end of the latter study was 750 ng/mL, which is of some concern in regard to iron overload, and it is well worth remembering in ill patients receiving transfusions that each unit of packed red blood cells contains approximately 350 mgs of bioavailable iron.

It is difficult to draw a firm conclusion regarding this issue. Certainly, if there is a clinical suspicion of iron, folate or B_{12} deficiency or if a patient has a suboptimal response to erythropoeitin, then diagnostic testing for these micronutrients should be performed and corrected if necessary. It is presently not the practice of this author to routinely provide supplemental levels of B_{12}, folate and iron to acutely ill patients who are receiving erythropoietin and who can otherwise take in these three nutrients at levels approximating the RDA.

Is Iodide Supplementation Necessary for Patients on Total Parenteral Nutrition?

Iodide, the ionic form of iodine, is not a conventional additive to TPN, nor is it contained in conventional trace element additive solutions, but it is clearly essential for normal health. Nevertheless, there is a conspicuous lack of reports of goiter or hypothyroidism in the literature on long-term TPN. The issue has been examined in infants and children and there has been no evidence of impaired thyroid function in either short- or long-term TPN.[33,34] In one study, iodine contamination of commercial 2-in-1 parenteral solutions was shown to be approximately 10 μg/L and in IV lipid emulsions, about 4 μg/200 mL bottle of 20% emulsion.[34] This falls short of the estimated average parenteral requirement that would be needed by an adult (85 μg: extrapolated from reference 35), and it remains unclear what source the remainder of the iodine requirement comes from. Nevertheless, there is no evidence that iodine supplementation is necessary in TPN, even that which extends over several years.

Are There Situations Where Administering Less Than Conventional Amounts of Micronutrients Is Indicated?

VITAMIN A IN CHRONIC RENAL INSUFFICIENCY

The renal parenchyma normally degrades senscent retinol binding protein. In chronic, but NOT acute, renal insufficiency, removal of the senescent protein does not occur, and the concentrations of serum retinol-binding protein and retinol rise several-fold.[36,37] This is particularly true of individuals receiving long-term hemodialysis. Whether this leads to an enhanced risk of vitamin A toxicity is not entirely clear, but in some instances, such individuals have been noted to have significantly elevated concentrations of vitamin A in their tissues.[38,39] Furthermore, hypercalcemia and elevations in alkaline phosphatase (presumably from the osteolytic activity of vitamin A toxicity[40]) have been reported in chronic hemodialysis patients who have taken vitamin A supplements containing as little as 750 μg (2500 I.U.) of vitamin A, biochemical abnormalities which then disappeared when the vitamin A was discontinued.[41,42]

Most disturbing of all is the report of three chronic hemodialysis patients who developed elevated retinol levels, various biochemical indicators of vitamin A toxicity (e.g., hypertriglyceridemia, hypercalcemia, and elevated transaminases) as well as clinical signs and symptoms of toxicity (e.g., headaches, diplopia, hepatomegaly, skin scaliness) while receiving only 450 μg of retinol in their TPN, which is less than one-half of the recommended dose for parenteral nutrition.[43] The indicators of toxicity in these three patients normalized when the vitamin A was removed.

Although the latter report described toxicity that developed within 10 days after the institution of parenteral vitamin A, this concern is probably one that is most prone to occur with TPN that is administered over weeks or months. Until we understand this issue better, it is prudent to not administer any oral vitamin supplements containing pre-formed vitamin A to patients with substantial chronic renal insufficiency (creatinine clearance <25 mL/min), particularly those on hemodialysis, and to halve the amount of vitamin A parenterally in such patients who have long-term dependence on TPN. Reduction of vitamin A in TPN is problematic at this point because the vitamin A added to TPN is typically administered in a preformulated mix with the other vitamins. It also would behoove the clinician to develop an index of suspicion for vitamin A toxicity in the critically ill patient who is a chronic hemodialysis patient, who is receiving TPN, and who has developed some of the signs and symptoms of toxicity.

IS IRON UNSAFE IN THE TPN OF PATIENTS WHO ARE BACTEREMIC?

Many pathogenic bacteria have an absolute requirement for iron[44,45] and some serious infections, such as those caused by Yersinia enterocolitica and several species of Vibrio, are more prone to occur in iron-overloaded hosts.[46,47] Nevertheless, there is no evidence that the provision of conventional levels of iron dextran in TPN (1–2 mg/d) predisposes to, or enhances the severity of, such infections. The only modification in clinical practice that this author makes in deference to this issue is refraining from administering repletion doses of intravenous iron (~100 mg/d) to patients who are actively bacteremic.

VITAMIN K AND WARFARIN THERAPY

Warfarin sodium, which induces hypocoagulability by interrupting vitamin K-mediated protein carboxylation in the liver, is used extensively as an anticoagulant. Exogenously administered vitamin K, however, can overcome the warfarin inhibition of carboxylation through a warfarin-insensitive pathway.[48] Traditionally, clinicians use 1–10 mg of vitamin K to rapidly reverse warfarin-induced anticoagulation.[49] However, it has become clear that far less amounts of vitamin K are capable of partially or wholly reversing the warfarin effect, and therefore it is important to be aware that the vitamin K in either enteral or parenteral solutions may serve as a clinically significant warfarin antagonist. There is a marked degree of inter-individual variation in this regard, but enteral formulas delivering as little as 25–115 μg of vitamin K have been reported to cause clinically relevant degrees of warfarin resistance.[50,51] Partial reversal of warfarin anticoagulation has been reported to occur with 500 μg of intravenously administered vitamin K[52] and, in this regard, it is worth noting that the existing recommendations for vitamin K in TPN are approximately 400 μg/d or 3 mg per week.[1] Furthermore, intravenous lipid emulsions are an additional source of vitamin K, containing up to 150 μg of K in 250 mL of 20% lipid.[53] A single bottle of intravenous lipid emulsion is sufficient to partially reverse the subclinical anticoagulation produced by ingesting 1 mg of warfarin a day.[54] Clinically, this may be important since 1 mg of warfarin per day ("minidose warfarin") is commonly used as a prophylactic against the thrombosis of central venous catheters,[55] and is monitored without biochemical guidance since no rise in prothrombin time is induced by this low dose of the drug.

Although the complexity of anticoagulation therapy as well as the big inter-individual variation in response to vitamin K precludes having a convenient algorithm that applies to all patients on warfarin, the clinician needs to be aware of these principles so that inadvertent vitamin K administration in enteral and parenteral feeding solutions can be reduced if necessary.

Conclusions

Modern-day enteral and parenteral feeding solutions are formulated to ensure that they meet the needs of most critically ill individuals. However, given how complex the critically ill patient is, it is not surprising that there are many exceptions where a particular patient requires either more or less of certain micronutrients. In order to prevent micronutrient deficiencies or excesses from remaining uncorrected, the clinician taking care of critically ill patients needs to be familiar with clinical scenarios where deficiencies or excesses are likely to occur. The clinician should also be familiar with the situations that arise in the intensive care unit that demand custom delivery of micronutrients so that appropriate adjustments can be made.

References

1. AMA Nutrition Advisory Group. Multivitamin and trace element preparations for parenteral use: a statement by the Nutrition Advisory Group. *J Parenter Enteral Nutr.* 1979; 3:258–267.
2. Greene H, Hambidge KM, Schanler R, et al. Guidelines for the use of vitamins, trace elements, calcium, magnesium, and phosphorus in infants and children receiving TPN. *Am J Clin Nutr.* 1988;48:1324–1342.
3. Erratum of reference 2. *Am J Clin Nutr.* 1989;49:1332.
4. Erratum of reference 2. *Am J Clin Nutr.* 1989;50:560.
5. *Modern Nutrition in Health and Disease, 9th ed.* Shils M, Olson J, Shike M, Ross AC, eds. Baltimore: Williams and Wilkins; 1999.
6. McMillan D, Sattar N, Talwar D, et al. Changes in micronutrient concentrations following anti-inflammatory treatment in patients with gastrointestinal cancer. *Nutrition.* 2000;16:425–428.
7. Schroeder J, Cousins R. Interleukin 6 regulates metallothionein gene expression and zinc metabolism in heptocyte monolayer cultures. *Proceed Nat Acad Sci.* 1990; 87:3137–3141.
8. McClave SA, Lowen CC, Kleber MJ, et al. Are patients fed appropriately according to their caloric requirements? *J Parenter Enteral Nutr.* 1998;22:375–381.
9. Glynn C, Greene G, Winkler M, et al. Predictive versus measured energy expenditure using limits-of-agreement analysis in hospitalized, obese patients. *J Parenter Enteral Nutr.* 1999;23:147–154.
10. Dickerson R, Rosato E, Mullen J. Net protein anabolism with hypocaloric parenteral nutrition in obese stressed patients. *Am J Clin Nutr.* 1986;44:747–755.
11. Kemper M, Weissman C, Hyman A. Caloric requirements and supply in critically ill surgical patients. *Crit Care Med.* 1992;20:344–348.
12. Fairbanks V. Iron in medicine and nutrition. In: Shils M, Olson J, Shike M, eds. *Modern Nutrition in Health and Disease, 8th ed.* Philadelphia: Lea & Febiger; 1994:185–213.
13. Jeejeebhoy K, Chu R, Marliss E, et al. Chromium deficiency, glucose intolerance and neuropathy reversed by chromium supplementation in a patient receiving long-term total parenteral nutrition. *Am J Clin Nutr.* 1977;30: 531–538.
14. Trow L, Lewis J, Greenwood R, et al. Lack of effect of dietary chromium supplementation on glucose tolerance, plasma insulin and lipoprotein levels in patients with type 2 diabetes. *Int J Vit Nutr Res.* 2000;70:14–18.
15. Joseph L, Farrell P, Davey S, et al. Effect of resistance training with or without chromium picolinate supplementation on glucose metabolism in older men and women. *Metabolism.* 1999;48;546–553.
16. Uusitupa M, Mykkanen L, Siitonen O, et al. Chromium supplementation in impaired glucose tolerance of elderly: effects on blood glucose, plasma insulin, c-peptide and lipid levels. *Br J Nutr.* 1992;68:209–216.
17. Anderson R, Polansky M, Bryden N, et al. Supplemental chromium effects on glucose, insulin, glucagon, and urinary chromium losses in subjects consuming controlled low-chromium diets. *Am J Clin Nutr.* 1991;54:909–916.
18. Food labeling health claims; chromium and the risk in adults of hyperglycemia and the effects of glucose intolerance. *Fed Regist.* 1998;63:34104–34107.
19. Forceville X, Vioux D, Gauzit R, et al. Selenium, systemic immune response syndrome, sepsis and outcome in critically ill patients. *Crit Care Med.* 1998;26:1536–1544.
20. Parenteral selenium supplementation in critically ill patients—effects on antioxidant metabolism. *Z Ernahrungswiss.* 1998;37(suppl 1):106–109.
21. Rotstein O. Oxidants and antioxidant therapy. *Crit Care Clin.* 2001;17:239–247.
22. Dasgupta A, Malhotra D, Levy H, et al. Decreased total antioxidant capacity but normal lipid hydroperoxide concentrations in sera of critically ill patients. *Life Sci.* 1997; 60:335–340.

23. Preiser J, Van Gossum A, Berre J, et al. Enteral feeding with a solution enriched with antioxidant vitamins A, C, and E enhances the resistance to oxidative stress. *Crit Care Med.* 2000;28:3828–3832.
24. Higgins T, Murray M, Kett D, et al. Trace element homeostasis during continuous sedation with propofol containing EDTA versus other sedatives in critically ill patients. *Intensive Care Med.* 2000;S413–S421.
25. Dietary Reference Intakes for Vitamin A, vitamin K, arsenic, boron, chromium, copper, iodine, iron, manganese, molybdenum, nickel, silicon, vanadium, and zinc. *Food and Nutrition Board, Institute of Medicine*. Washington, DC: National Academy Press; 2001:351–398.
26. McClain C, Soutor C, Zieve L. Zinc deficiency: a complication of Crohn's Disease. *Gastroenterology.* 1980;78:272–279.
27. Wolman S, Anderson G, Marliss E, et al. Zinc in TPN: requirements and metabolic effects. *Gastroenterology.* 1979; 76:458–467.
28. Drueke T. Modulating factors in the hematopoietic response to erythropoietin. *Am J Kidney Dis.* 1991;18(suppl 1):87–92.
29. Klemm A, Sperschneider H, Lauterbach H, Stein G. Is folate and vitamin B12 supplementation necessary in chronic hemodialysis patients with EPO treatment? *Clin Nephrol.* 1994;42:343–345.
30. Ono K, Hisasue Y. Is folate supplementation necessary in hemodialysis patients on erythropoeitin therapy? *Clin Nephrol.* 1992;38:290–292.
31. Pronai W, Riegler-Keil M, Silberbauer K, et al. Folic acid supplementation improves erythropoeitin response. *Nephron.* 1995;71:395–400.
32. Fishbane S, Frei G, Maesaka J. Reduction in recombinant human erythropoeitin doses by the use of chronic intravenous iron supplementation. *Am J Kidney Dis.* 1995;26:41–46.
33. Gough D, Laing I, Astley P. Thyroid function on short-term total parenteral nutrition without iodine supplements. *J Parenter Enteral Nutr.* 1982;6:439–440.
34. Moukarzel A, Buchman A, Salas J, et al. Iodine supplementation in children receiving long-term parenteral nutrition. *J Pediatr.* 1992;121:252–254.
35. Dietary reference intakes for vitamin A, vitamin K, arsenic, boron, chromium, copper, iodine, iron, manganese, molybdenum, nickel, silicon, vanadium, and zinc. *Food and Nutrition Board, Institute of Medicine*. Washington, DC: National Academy Press; 2001:185–213.
36. Cano N, DiCostanzo-Dufetel J, Calaf R, et al. Prealbumin-retinol binding protein-retinol complex in hemodialysis patients. *Am J Clin Nutr.* 1988;47:664–667.
37. Stewart W, Fleming L. Plasma retinol and retinol binding protein concentrations in patients on maintenance haemodialysis with and without vitamin A supplements. *Nephron.* 1982;30:15–21.
38. Yatzidis H, Digenis P, Fountas P. Hypervitaminosis A accompanying advanced chronic renal failure. *Br Med J.* 1975;3:352–353.
39. Vahquist A, Berne B, Berne C. Skin content and plasma transport of vitamin A and beta-carotene in chronic renal failure. *Eur J Clin Invest.* 1982;12:63–67.
40. Binkley N, Krueger D. Hypervitaminosis A and bone. *Nutr Rev.* 2000;58:138–144.
41. Farrington K, Miller P, Vaghese Z, et al. Vitamin A toxicity and hypercalcemia in chronic renal failure. *Br Med J (Clin Res Ed).* 1981;282:1999–2002.
42. Fishbane S, Frei G, Finger M, et al. Hypervitaminosis A in two hemodialysis patients. *Am J Kidney Dis.* 1995;25: 346–349.
43. Gleghorn E, Eisenberg L, Hack S, et al. Observations of vitamin A toxicity in three patients with renal failure receiving parenteral alimentation. *Am J Clin Nutr.* 1986; 44:107–112.
44. Lindsay J, Riley T. Staphylococcal iron requirements siderophore production, and iron-regulated protein expression. *Infect Immun.* 1994;62:2309–2314.
45. Mengaud J, Horwitz M. The major iron-containing protein of Legionella pneumophilia is an aconitase homologous with the human iron-responsive element-binding protein. *J Bacteriol.* 1993;175:5666–5676.
46. Adamkiewicz T, Berkovitch M, Krishnan C, et al. Infection due to Y. enterocolitica in a series of patients with beta-thalassemia. *Clin Infect Dis.* 1998;27:1362–1366.
47. Hor L, Chang T, Wang S. Survival of Vibrio vulnificus in whole blood from patients with chronic liver diseases: association with phagocytosis by neutrophils and serum ferritin levels. *J Infect Dis.* 1999;179:275–278.
48. Sadowski J, Booth S, Mann K, et al. Structure and mechanism of activation of vitamin K antagonists. In: Poller L, Hirsh J, eds. *Oral Anticoagulants*. New York: Arnold; 1996: 19–29.
49. Litin S, Gastineau D. Current concepts in anticoagulant therapy. *Mayo Clin Proceed.* 1995;70:266–272.
50. Howard P, Hannaman K. Warfarin resistance linked to enteral nutritional products. *J Am Diet Assoc.* 1985;85:713–715.
51. Martin J, Lutomski D. Warfarin resistance and enteral feedings. *J Parent Enteral Nutr.* 1989;13:206–208.
52. Shetty H, Backhouse G, Bentley D, et al. Effective reversal of warfarin-induced excessive anticoagulation with low dose vitamin K1. *Thromb Haemost.* 1992;647:13–15.
53. Lennon C, Davidson K, Sadowski J, et al. The vitamin K content of intravenous lipid emulsions. *J Parent Enteral Nutr.* 1993;17:142–144.
54. Camilo M, Jatoi A, O'Brien M, et al. Bioavailability of phylloquinone from an intravenous lipid emulsion. *Am J Clin Nutr.* 1998;67:716–721.
55. Bern M, Lokich J, Wallach S, et al. Very low doses of warfarin can prevent thrombosis in central venous catheters: a randomized prospective trial. *Ann Int Med.* 1990;112:423–428.
56. Mason JB. Consequences of altered micronutrient status. In Goldman L, Bennett J, eds. *Cecil Textbook of Medicine*, 21st edition. Philadelphia: WB Saunders Co.; 2000:1170–1178.

CHAPTER 8

Assessment and Management of Fluid and Electrolyte Abnormalities

Vincent W. Vanek, M.D., F.A.C.S., C.N.S.P.

INTRODUCTION 79
FLUID ABNORMALITIES 79
ELECTROLYTE ABNORMALITIES 85
SODIUM (NA^+) 86
POTASSIUM (K^+) 89
CALCIUM (CA^{++}) 93
PHOSPHORUS 96
MAGNESIUM (MG^{++}) 98
CHLORIDE (CL^-) 100
CONCLUSIONS 100
REFERENCES 100

Introduction

For optimal physiological function, the human body must maintain fluids and electrolytes within fairly narrow limits. Extensive homeostatic mechanisms function to maintain these balances. However, critically ill patients frequently have fluid and electrolyte abnormalities that overcome these homeostatic mechanisms and require early recognition and treatment to avoid morbidity and mortality. This chapter reviews the principles of fluids and electrolytes and how to recognize and treat any abnormalities.

Fluid Abnormalities

Approximately 60% of the human body by weight consists of water.[1,2] This proportion of body water changes throughout the life cycle and also varies with sex and body habitus (Table 8.1). At birth, 80% of the body is composed of water. This percentage slowly decreases to about 60% for adults and then decreases further to about 50% once an individual is over 60 years of age. The proportion of body water is similar for both males and females until puberty, after which males in general have a greater proportion of their body weight composed of water.

Body water is divided into several compartments (Figure 8.1).[1,3] Approximately two-thirds of the body water, approximately 40% of the body weight, is located within the cells of the body, the intracellular fluid (ICF) compartment. The remaining one-third of the body water, approximately 20% of the body weight, is located outside of the cells of the body, the extracellular fluid (ECF) compartment. The ECF compartment can be further divided. One-quarter of the ECF resides in the intravascular compartment, blood plasma, and it accounts for 5% of the body weight. The remaining three-fourths of the ECF is in

TABLE 8.1

Total Body Water as a Percentage of Body Weight in Relation to Age, Sex, and Lean Body Mass

	Premature Infant	3 Months	6 Months	10–18 Years	Adults: Emaciated	Adults: Lean	Adults: Normal	Adults: Obese	Age >60 years
Male	80%	70%	60%	59%	70%–75%	70%	60%	50%	52%
Female	80%	70%	60%	57%	70%–75%	60%	50%	42%	46%

Adapted with permission from Whitmire SJ. Fluids and electrolytes. In: Matarese LE, Gottschlich MM, eds. Contemporary Nutrition Support Practice: A Clinical Guide, 1st ed. Philadelphia: WB Saunders; 1998:129.

the interstitial compartment and accounts for 15% of the body weight.[2]

Semi-permeable membranes separate these compartments. The ICF and the interstitial fluid compartment are separated by the cell membranes, while the interstitial fluid and intravascular compartments are separated by the capillary membranes. Epithelial membranes separate ECF compartment from the transcellular fluid, i.e. fluid within the bowel lumen, peritoneal cavity, pleural space, pericardial space, cerebrospinal fluid, etc. Very small molecules, such as water, pass easily through all membranes, while larger molecules, such as proteins, do not readily pass through membranes unless there is an active transport system or the membranes become altered and are "leaky."[1]

Body fluids contain electrolyte and non-electrolyte substances. Non-electrolyte substances do not dissociate in solution and consist of solutes such as glucose, urea, and creatinine. Electrolytes dissociate into positively charged ions (cations) and negatively charged ions (anions). Figure 8.1 shows the distribution of the major electrolytes among the three major fluid compartments. The concentration of electrolytes is significantly different between the ICF and ECF.

Sodium (Na^+) and Chloride (Cl^-) are the most common extracellular cation and anion, respectively, while intracellularly, they are potassium (K^+) and inorganic phosphate (PO_4^-). These concentration gradients are maintained by an active transport system (Na^+–K^+–ATPase pump). This requires a carrier substance in the cell wall membrane plus energy. However, electrical neutrality must be maintained at all times. So if a cation moves from the ECF to the ICF, it must be accompanied by an anion or it must be exchanged for another cation.[1]

The direction and extent of water movement between fluid compartments is determined by the osmolality. Osmolality is the number of osmotically active particles per kg of solvent and in clinical practice is expressed as milliosmoles per liter (mOsm/L). Water will diffuse among the body fluid compartments to equalize the osmolality such that the osmolality should be the same for both the ECF and ICF. Normal osmolality is 290 to 310 mOsm/L.[1,2] Serum osmolality can be measured or it can be calculated using the following equation:[1,4]

$$\text{Serum osmolality (mOsm/L)} = (2 \times ([Na^+] + [K^+])) + \text{BUN}/2.8 + [\text{serum glucose}]/18$$

BUN = Blood Urea Nitrogen

mEq/L Water

	Blood Plasma CATIONS (154 mEq/L)		Blood Plasma ANIONS (154 mEq/L)		Interstitial CATIONS (154 mEq/L)		Interstitial ANIONS (154 mEq/L)		Intracellular CATIONS (205 mEq/L)		Intracellular ANIONS (205 mEq/L)	
	Na^+	142	Cl^-	103	Na^+	145	Cl^-	103	K^+	160	HPO_4^-	140
			HCO_3^+	27			HCO_3^-	27	Mg^+	35	Proteins	55
			Proteins	16			Proteins	16	Na^+	10		
	Ca^+	5	Organic Acids	5	K^+	4	Organic Acids	5			HCO_3^-	8
	K^+	4	HPO_4^-	2	Ca^+	3	HPO_4^-	2			Cl^-	2
	Mg^+	3	SO_4^{-+}	1	Mg^+	2	SO_4^{-2}	1				

% BODY WT. VOLUME (70 kg man)	BLOOD PLASMA	INTERSTITIAL FLUID	INTRACELLULAR FLUID
	5%	15%	40%
	3,500 mL	10,500 mL	28,000 mL
	EXTRACELLULAR FLUID (ECF) 20% 14,000 mL		

Figure 8.1

Distribution of Body Fluids and Electrolyte Composition

Abbreviations: Na^+—Sodium; Ca^{++}—Calcium; K^+—Potassium; Mg^{++}—Magnesium; Cl^-—Chloride; HCO_3^-—bicarbonate; HPO_4^-—Inorganic phosphate; SO_4^{-2}—Inorganic sulfate

Adapted with permission from Whitmire SJ. Fluids and electrolytes. In: Matarese LE, Gottschlich MM, eds. Contemporary Nutrition Support Practice: A Clinical Guide, 1st ed. Philadelphia: WB Saunders; 1998:128; and Shires GT, Canizaro PC, Shires III GT, et al. Fluid, electrolyte and nutritional management of the surgical patients. In: Schwartz SI, ed. Principles of Surgery, 7th ed. New York: McGraw-Hill; 1999:54.

TABLE 8.2

Average Daily Fluid Gains and Losses in Adults			
Fluid Gains		**Fluid Losses**	
Sensible		Sensible	
Oral fluids	1100-1400 mL	Urine	1200-1500 mL
Solid foods	800-1000 mL	Intestinal	100-200 mL
Insensible		Insensible	
Oxidative metabolism	300 mL	Lungs	400 mL
		Skin	500-600 mL
Total	2200-2700 mL	**Total**	2200-2700 mL

Reprinted with permission from Whitmire SJ. Fluids and electrolytes. In: Matarese LE, Gottschlich MM, eds. Contemporary Nutrition Support Practice: A Clinical Guide, 1st ed. Philadelphia: WB Saunders; 1998:129.

Table 8.2 shows the sources and amounts of fluid gains and losses from the body. Normally, the majority of the fluid gains are from ingestion of oral fluids; however, a substantial amount of fluids are extracted from "solid food." Also some fluid is gained from the metabolism of carbohydrates, proteins, and fats, since the end product of metabolism is water, CO_2, and energy, in the form of adenosine triphosphate (ATP).

The urine accounts for the majority of the fluid losses from the body, with the kidneys being primarily responsible for regulation of fluid and electrolytes. Of the 180 L of fluid that is filtered through the renal glomerulus daily, all but about 1500 mL is reabsorbed back into the body. The kidneys' maximal concentrating capacity is about 1400 mOsm/L so at least 400 mL of urine is required to excrete the normal daily load of metabolic waste.[1]

Fluid is lost from the skin by two mechanisms. Evaporation of fluid from the skin surface is one mechanism, and these losses are increased in patients who have sustained second- or third-degree burns or who have fever. This fluid loss contains no electrolytes so it is free water loss. Fluid can also be lost from the skin in the form of sweat, which has a modest amount of electrolytes (15 to 60 mEq Na^+/L), but it is still hypotonic.[1] The amount of fluid loss from sweat varies with the ambient temperature and the individual's activity level. Normally about 500 to 600 mL of fluid is lost from the skin daily; however, under extreme conditions, up to 2 L/h can be lost from the skin.[5] Also, fans blowing directly on patients or patients on specialty beds that rely on constant air flow through the beds can also increase evaporative fluid losses.

Insensible fluid losses also occur from the lungs. These fluid losses vary with the humidity of the inspired gases and the minute ventilation, which is determined by the rate and depth of respiration. Normally, approximately 400 mL of fluid is lost from the lungs daily; however, hyperventilation and inhalation of unhumidified air through a tracheostomy can result in as much as 1.5 L/d.

The amount of fluid secreted and its electrolyte content vary throughout the GI tract (Table 8.3); but

TABLE 8.3

Volume and Electrolyte Concentrations of Fluids Throughout the GI Tract

Type of Secretion	Volume (mL/24 hrs.)	Sodium (mEq/L)	Potassium (mEq/L)	Chloride (mEq/L)	Bicarb (mEq/L)
Saliva	1500 (500-2000)	10 (2-10)	26 (20-30)	10 (8-18)	30
Stomach	1500 (100-4000)	60 (9-116)	10 (0-32)	130 (8-154)	0
Duodenum	Variable (100-2000)	140	5	80	0
Ileum	3000 (100-9000)	140 (80-150)	5 (2-8)	104 (43-137)	30
Colon	Variable	60	30	40	0
Pancreas	Variable (100-800)	140 (113-185)	5 (3-7)	75 (54-95)	115
Bile	Variable (50-800)	145 (131-164)	5 (3-12)	100 (89-180)	35

Reprinted with permission from Whitmire SJ. Fluids and electrolytes. In: Matarese LE, Gottschlich MM, eds. Contemporary Nutrition Support Practice: A Clinical Guide, 1st ed. Philadelphia: WB Saunders; 1998:130.

TABLE 8.4

Calculating Maintenance Fluid Requirements	
Age	**Daily Maintenance Fluid Needs**
Newborn to young adult	■ 100 mL/kg for first 10 kg ■ 50 mL/kg for second 10 kg ■ 20 mL/kg for every kg over 20 kg
25 years to 55 years	■ 35 mL/kg
56 years to 65 years	■ 30 mL/kg
Over 65 years	■ 25 mL/kg

Adapted with permission from Naitove A, Evans DB, Ihde JK. Fluid and electrolyte balance. In: Lawrence PF, Bilbao M, Bell RM, et al., eds. Essentials of General Surgery, 1st ed. Baltimore: Lippincott Williams & Wilkins; 1988:66.

generally, the GI fluids are isotonic to hypotonic. Large amounts of fluids pass through the gastrointestinal (GI) tract, about 6 to 8 L/d. However, the intestine, mainly the right side of the colon, normally reabsorbs all but about 100 to 200 mL of this fluid. However, large amounts of fluids can be lost from the GI tract in patients with vomiting, diarrhea, fistula drainage, large amount of nasogastric tube drainage, bowel resections (especially the right colon), etc., and if these losses are not replaced, significant fluid, electrolyte, and acid-base abnormalities can occur.[1]

Estimating an individual's daily fluid needs requires calculating his or her maintenance fluid needs, then assessing for any extraordinary fluid needs and/or the presence of conditions that would decrease fluid needs. Maintenance fluid needs slowly decrease with the age of the patient (Table 8.4) and are based on the patient's body weight.

Factors that increase fluid needs include fever (12.5% for each 1°C above normal), severe sweating (10% to 25%), hyperventilation (10% to 60%), hyperthyroidism (25% to 50%), hypovolemia, dehydration, or extraordinary urinary or GI (nasogastric tube drainage, fistula drainage, etc.) losses.[1] Fluid can also be lost into "third spaces," which are areas such as the peritoneal cavity, pleural space, lumen of the bowel, etc. This does not change the total body water but decreases the fluid available to the ECF compartment.[2]

Up to 10% depletion of the ECF, approximately 1500 mL in a 70 kg adult, can occur with minimal signs or symptoms (Table 8.5). Clinical signs or symptoms begin occurring at approximately 20% ECF deficit, approximately 3000 mL. The earliest signs of ECF deficit are tachycardia and orthostatic hypotension. Orthostatic hypotension is defined as an increase of heart rate by 20 or decrease of systolic blood pressure by 20 mm Hg when the patient goes from lying position to a standing position. Also, there is a moderate

TABLE 8.5

Signs and Symptoms of ECF Depletion According to the Degree of Depletion				
Degree of Depletion	**ECF Lost[1]**	**Signs and Symptoms**	**Urine Output**	**Laboratory**
Mild (10%)	1500 mL	■ 2% weight loss ■ Symptoms mild and may be overlooked ■ patient may be thirsty	Mild reduction (30–40 mL/h)	■ Mild elevation of Hct[2] ■ Mild elevation urine sp. gr.[3]
Moderate (20%)	3000 mL	■ 4% weight loss ■ Tachycardia and orthostatic hypotension[4] ■ Apathy, drowsiness, decreased skin turgor, dry mucous membranes and tongue	Moderate reduction (<30 mL/h)	■ Moderate elevation of Hct[2] ■ Urine sp. gr. >1.020, urine osmolarity >500, urine Na <10-15 mEq/L ■ Moderate increase in BUN with relatively normal creatinine (Cr) with BUN/Cr >10:1
Severe (30%)	4000 mL	■ 6% weight loss ■ Shock with hypotension and severe tachycardia (weak, thready pulse) ■ Skin cool, pale, cyanotic, and poor turgor ■ Eyes sunken ■ Stupor or coma	Severe reduction (<10-15 mL/h)	■ Severe elevation of Hct[2] ■ Urine changes same as above but more severe ■ Further increase in BUN with some increase in Cr with BUN/Cr >10:1[5]

[1]Based on 70 kg adult
[2]Hematocrit (Hct) increases 1% for every 500 mL decrease in ECF
[3]Urine sp. gr.—urine specific gravity (normal 1.003–1.015)
[4]Check BP and heart rate lying down then repeat while standing (or at least sitting with legs over side of bed) and orthostatic hypotension present if heart rate increases ≥20 or systolic BP decreases by ≤20
[5]Unless patient develops acute tubular necrosis; then see intrinsic renal causes of low urine output in next section

Adapted with permission from Naitove A, Evans DB, Ihde JK. Fluid and electrolyte balance. In: Lawrence PF, Bilbao M, Bell RM et al., eds. Essentials of General Surgery, 1st ed. Baltimore: Lippincott Williams & Wilkins; 1988:53.

reduction in urine output and elevation in hematocrit, urine specific gravity, and BUN. Once the ECF deficit reaches 30%, or approximately 4000 mL, the body's ability to compensate is surpassed and the patient develops the classic signs and symptoms of shock such as pale, cool, clammy skin; weak thready pulse; and hypotension. The patient also has severe reduction in urine output and severe elevation of hematocrit and BUN.

Low urine output (<30 mL/h for an adult or <0.5 mL/kg/h for children and infants) can be a sign of ECF deficit; however, it can be caused by multiple other conditions.[2] Causes for low urine output can be divided into three categories, pre-renal, intrinsic renal, and post-renal (Table 8.6). Post-renal causes require obstruction of both kidneys since obstruction of only one kidney will be compensated for by the other kidney. Since it is rare that one condition can obstruct both ureters, post-renal causes for low urine output usually occur at the level of the urethra or bladder neck. So a urethral urinary catheter can be inserted to evaluate this. If a urethral catheter is already in place, it should be irrigated to ensure that it is not obstructed. Also, an ultrasound of the kidneys can detect hydronephrosis indicating distal obstruction.

The most difficult categories of low urine output to differentiate are pre-renal and intrinsic renal problems. Urine and serum electrolytes, BUN, creatinine (Cr), and osmolality can be very helpful in this regard (Table 8.7). Probably the most accurate of these tests is the fractional excretion of sodium. This represents the percentage of the sodium that is filtered through the glomerulus that eventually ends up in the urine. With pre-renal situations, the kidneys are maximally reabsorbing sodium in order to also reabsorb water. So the fractional excretion of sodium should be less than 1%. In the setting of intrinsic renal failure, the kidneys lose some of their concentrating capacity and the fractional excretion of sodium is greater than 2%. If the result is between 1% and 2%, it is equivocal and either situation or both could be present. This test can also be affected by administering diuretics, especially loop diuretics, in which case the fractional excretion of sodium will be artificially elevated. However, if the patient has had diuretics and the fractional excretion of sodium is still less than 1%, a pre-renal cause is most likely present.

Some patients can have an abnormally high urine output. This could be a sign of volume overload or it could be pathological and could lead to an ECF deficit if not properly diagnosed and treated. Plasma osmolality and urine osmolality, sodium, and potassium can help differentiate between these different causes of polyuria (urine output >3000 mL/d) (Figure 8.2). If the cause is due to too much oral free water or intravenous (IV) saline or dextrose, the treatment is to decrease the fluid intake. If it is one of the other causes, the patient should be given adequate and appropriate

TABLE 8.6

Categories and Etiologies of Low Urine Output or Azotemia	
Categories	Etiologies
Pre-renal	■ Hypovolemia—hemorrhage, GI losses, burns, peritonitis, diuretics ■ Impaired cardiac function—congestive heart failure, myocardial infarction, pericardial tamponade, pulmonary embolus ■ Peripheral vasodilation—bacteremia, antihypertensive medications ■ Increased renal vascular resistance—anesthesia, surgery, hepatorenal syndrome ■ Renal vascular obstruction (must be bilateral)—renal artery embolism or thrombosis
Intrinsic renal (renal failure)	■ Ischemic disorders (acute tubular necrosis (ATN))—major trauma, massive hemorrhage, severe hypotension, severe dehydration, crush syndrome, septic shock, transfusion reactions, myoglobinuria ■ Nephrotoxins—IV contrast, antimicrobial agents (such as aminoglycosides, amphotericin B, etc.), heavy metals (mercury, arsenic, lead, etc.), ethylene glycol, carbon tetrachloride, organic solvents, pesticides, fungicides, etc. ■ Disease of the glomeruli and small blood vessels—glomerulonephritis from various etiologies such as lupus, subacute bacterial endocarditis, Goodpasture's Syndrome, malignant hypertension, drug-related vasculitis, etc. ■ Major blood vessel disease—renal artery thrombosis, embolism, or stenosis or bilateral renal vein thrombosis
Post-renal (obstruction)	■ Urethral obstruction—obstructed urethral catheter, etc. ■ Bladder neck obstruction—benign prostatic hypertrophy (BPH), bladder cancer, bladder infection, neuropathic bladder ■ Bilateral ureteral obstruction—tumors (cervix, prostate, uterine, etc.), retroperitoneal fibrosis, iatrogenic injury (ligation or division of the ureters), bilateral ureteral stones or blood clots, bilateral necrotizing papillitis

Adapted with permission from Yaqoob MM, Alkhunaizi AM, Edelstein CL et al. Acute renal failure: pathogensis, diagnosis, and management. In: Schrier RW, ed. Renal and Electrolyte Disorders, 5th ed, Philadelphia: Lippincott-Raven Publishers; 1997:450, 480, 481.

TABLE 8.7

Urine and Serum Laboratory Tests to Differentiate Pre-Renal from Intrinsic Renal Causes for Low Urine Output or Azotemia[5–7]

Laboratory Test	Pre-renal Azotemia	Acute Renal Failure
Serum BUN:Cr ratio	>20:1	<20:1
Urine osmolality (mOsm/L)	>500	<400
Urine osmolality: plasma osmolality ratio	>1.5:1	<1.1:1
Urine specific gravity	>1.020	Approximately 1.010
Urine Cr/plasma Cr	>40	<20
Urine sodium (mEq/L)	<20	>40
Fractional excretion of sodium*	<1%	>2%
Urine sediment	Normal or occasional granular casts	Brown granular casts, cellular debris

*Fractional excretion of sodium = (Urine (Na) × Plasma (Cr))/(Plasma (Na) × Urine (Cr)) × 100

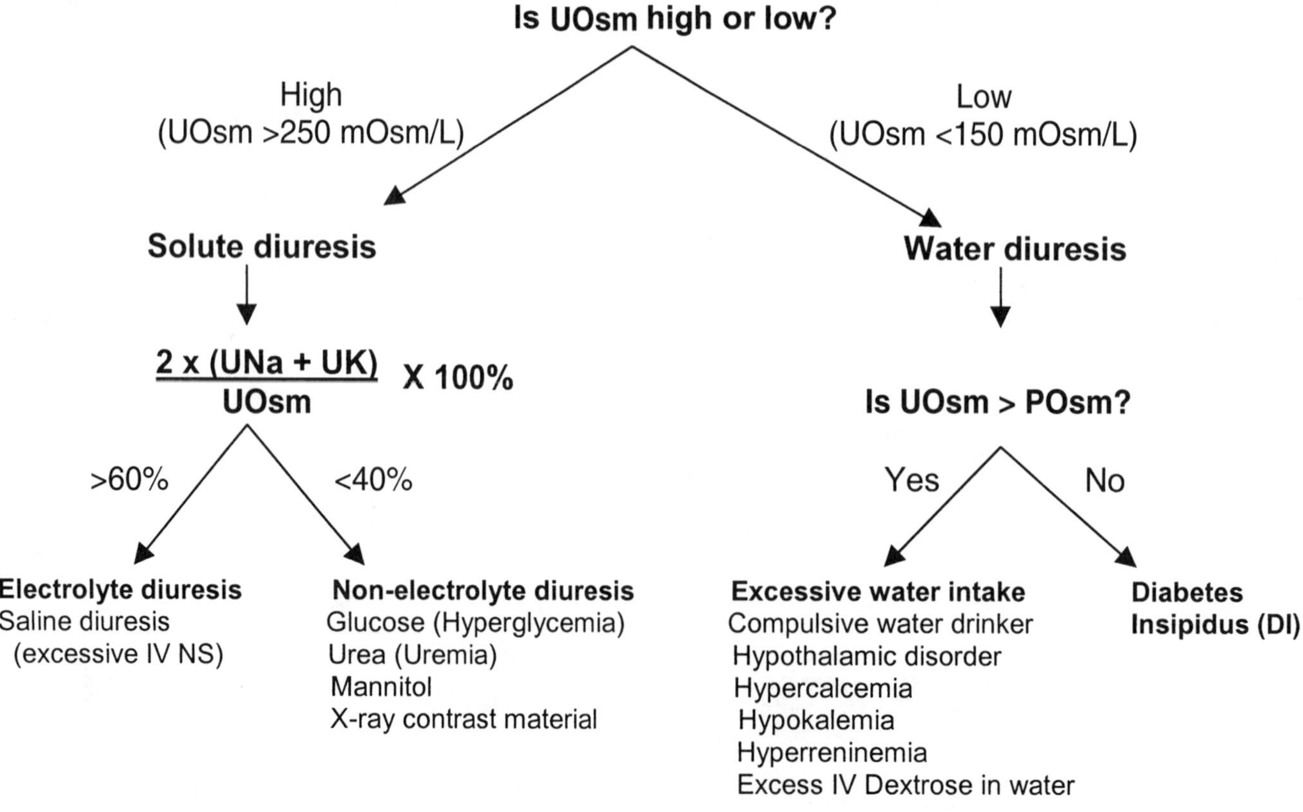

Figure 8.2

Evaluation of Patients with High Urine Output (polyuria; U.O. >3000 mL/d)

Adapted with permission from Gonzalez JM, Suki WN. Polyuria and nocturia. In: Massry SG, Glassock RJ, eds. Text Book of Nephrology, Vol 1, 3rd ed. Baltimore: Williams & Wilkins; 1995:551.

fluids to prevent ECF deficit while the underlying condition is treated.

Multiple different types of IV fluids are available for treatment of different clinical situations (Table 8.8). Dextrose in water is available in several concentrations, such as 5%, 10%, 50%, etc., with 5% dextrose in water (D_5W) being the most common concentration used for IV fluids. D_5W provides free water, which is distributed evenly throughout the ICF and ECF and is used in the treatment of total body water deficits.

Normal saline (NS) is 0.9% solution of saline. It approximates the serum concentration of Na^+; however, NS has 154 mEq/L of Na^+ so it is slightly hypertonic. NS expands the ECF only and it does not enter the ICF. It is used for abnormal fluid losses or as an expander of the intravascular volume.[1] There are also derivatives of NS such as one-half NS (77 mEq/L) and one-fourth NS (38.5 mEq/L), which contain increasing amount of free water similar to D_5W. Hypertonic saline (3%) is used on rare occasion in patients with severe hyponatremia, but it must be used with caution. Ringer's Lactate (RL) was designed to approximate the electrolyte composition of serum and includes Na^+, K^+, Cl^-, and Ca^{++}. It also includes 28 mEq/L of lactate, which is converted by the liver into bicarbonate. It functions similarly to NS and is frequently used to resuscitate trauma or critically ill surgical patients. D_5W is routinely combined with RL or any derivation of NS but should not be used if large volumes of IV fluid will be needed since it may result in hyperglycemia.

Maintenance IV fluids for a 70-kg man is D_5W one-fourth NS with 20 mEq KCl/L at 105 mL/h (Table 8.9). If the patient has mild to moderate ECF deficit then D_5W one-half NS with 20 mEq KCl/L (amount of KCl depends on serum K^+ level and K^+ requirements) at 125 to 150 mL/h (125%–150% of maintenance). In cases of a severe ECF deficit such as trauma, hemorrhage, peritonitis, intestinal obstruction, etc., RL at 150 to 200 mL/h (150% to 200% maintenance) may be most appropriate.[2]

Factors that may decrease fluid needs include fluid overload associated with congestive heart failure, renal failure, hepatic failure, and acute respiratory distress syndrome (ARDS). Signs and symptoms of hypervolemia or fluid overload include shortness of breath, orthopnea, peripheral edema, pulmonary edema, hypertension, weight gain, distended neck veins, tachycardia, moist skin, and rhonchi, rales, and wheezes on auscultation of the lungs. Treatment of fluid overload is to restrict sodium and water and possibly treatment with diuretics. If the patient is in oliguric renal failure, peritoneal or hemodialysis or continuous arteriovenous or veno-venous hemofiltration may be required.[1]

Electrolyte Abnormalities

Electrolytes are measured either in millimoles (mmol) or milliequivalents (mEq). Moles or mmol are an expression of the number of particles per unit volume. A mole of any substance is its gram (g) molecular weight. A mmol is the same value expressed in milligrams (mg). For example, the molecular weight for sodium is 23 and for chloride is 35. So a mmol of sodium is 23 g, a mmol of chloride is 35 g, and a mmol of sodium chloride is 58 mg (23 + 35). A solution con-

TABLE 8.8

Electrolytes Composition and Osmolality of Common IV Fluids

IV Solution	Sodium (mEq/L)	Chloride (mEq/L)	Potassium (mEq/L)	Lactate (mEq/L)	Calcium (mEq/L)	Glucose (g/L)	Osmolality (mOsm/L)
5% Dextrose (D_5W)	0	0	0	0	0	50	252
$D_{10}W$	0	0	0	0	0	100	505
$D_{50}W$	0	0	0	0	0	500	2520
Hypertonic saline, 3%	513	513	0	0	0	0	1027
0.9% Saline (Normal saline (NS))	154	154	0	0	0	0	308
1/2 NS	77	77	0	0	0	0	154
Ringer's lactate (RL)	130	109	4	28	2.7	0	273
D_5W NS	154	154	0	0	0	50	560
D_5W 1/2 NS	77	77	0	0	0	50	406
D_5W RL	130	109	4	28	2.7	50	525

TABLE 8.9

Calculating Maintenance IV Fluids for a 70 kg 20-Year Old Man[2]		
	Maintenance Daily Requirements	Maintenance IV Orders
Fluids	2500 mL (based on guidelines from Table 8.4)	105 mL/h
Glucose	>100 gm (for protein sparing effect)	D_5W (125 g/d)
Sodium	1-1.5 mEq/kg =>70-105 mEq/d =>28-42 mEq/L	1/4 NS (39 mEq/L)
Potassium	0.5-0.75 mEq/kg =>35-52.5 mEq/d =>14-21 mEq/L	20 mEq KCl/L

taining 58 mg of sodium chloride in 1 liter of water would have 1 mmol/L of sodium and 1 mmol/L of chloride.[1]

Another method of quantifying electrolytes is by their chemical combining activity or equivalents. This depends on the valence of the ion. For univalent ions, such as Na^+, Cl^-, K^+, $HCO3^-$, and acetate$^-$, 1 mmol/L equals 1 mEq/L. However, for divalent ions, such as Mag^{++} and Ca^{++}, 1 mmol/L equals 2 mEq/L.[1]

Normal electrolyte concentrations may vary slightly from lab to lab, so any electrolyte result should be evaluated in light of the normals for that lab. Electrolyte abnormalities can occur with or without fluid abnormalities. Electrolyte abnormalities should be prevented with proper fluid and electrolyte management when possible; however, when they do occur, failure to promptly diagnose and treat them can result in significant morbidity or even mortality.[1]

Sodium (Na^+)

Total body Na^+ is estimated to be 40 mEq/kg (approximately 280 mEq for a 70-kg man).[2] Sodium is the principal ECF cation and is the main determinant of serum osmolality.[2] Therefore, water shifts between the body compartments mainly in response to ECF Na^+ concentration. So changes in serum Na^+ can reflect either changes in total body Na^+, changes in body water, or both.[1] Normal serum Na^+ ranges from 135 to 145 mEq/L.[2] Na^+ enters the body via oral diet, medications, or IV fluids and is lost from the body through the urine, sweat, and GI secretions.

Under normal circumstances regulation of Na^+ and water balance is primarily performed in the kidney. Assuming normal renal perfusion and membrane function, Na^+ and water are both filtered at the glomerulus. In the proximal tubules large amounts of each are recovered. However, selective processes occurring in the distal tubules determine renal conservation or excretion of Na^+ and water.[2] The kidneys are normally very efficient at reabsorbing Na^+, especially when ECF deficits are present and reabsorption of water is important.[1]

Aldosterone, an adrenal cortical hormone, causes Na^+ to be reabsorbed in the distal tubules in exchange for either potassium or hydrogen ions. Aldosterone helps to maintain both ECF volume and osmolality. ECF deficit, particularly in the intravascular space, is a potent stimulus for aldosterone release. This response is triggered by a decrease in renal perfusion, which promotes the juxtaglomerular apparatus in the kidney to secrete renin. Renin then promotes secretion of angiotensin I and its conversion to angiotensin II, which causes increased aldosterone secretion. Volume receptors in the right atrium also stimulate aldosterone secretion when there is a decrease in intravascular volume.[2]

Decreased ECF Na^+ concentrations also stimulate aldosterone secretion. Aldosterone secretion is also increased by increased serum concentrations of potassium or adrenocorticotropic hormone (ACTH). Aldosterone secretion is suppressed by ECF volume expansion, increased serum Na^+ concentration, and/or decreased serum potassium concentration.[2]

Antidiuretic hormone (ADH) is produced and released from the posterior pituitary gland and has a potent direct effect on the kidney to increase tubular reabsorption of water. This effect and its modulation are important in the regulation of fluid volumes and osmolality in the body. Intracranial osmoreceptors serve as the sensors that initiate the events resulting in increased ADH secretion when the serum osmolality increases and inhibits ADH secretion when serum osmolality decreases. ADH production and release are also dependent upon volume receptors in the right and left atrium, with decreased ECF volume causing increased ADH secretion and vice versa. Volume dependent responses can and usually do override the influences of the osmoreceptor controlling system when the two are in conflict.[2]

Hyponatremia

Hyponatremia can be divided into hypotonic, isotonic, or hypertonic based on serum osmolality (Figure 8.3). Isotonic hyponatremia can then be divided into hypovolemic, isovolemic, and hypervolemic depending on the patient's fluid status. Urinary Na^+ concentration can also help further determine the underlying etiology.

In the surgical patient, dilutional hyponatremia commonly is caused by the infusion or ingestion of too much water, or the use of hypotonic fluids to replace isotonic gastrointestinal or third-space fluid losses. Accumulations of sodium-free water also can be generated metabolically by the catabolic breakdown of body tissues, as occurs with surgical stress and caloric deprivation (approximately 1 liter of water is generated for

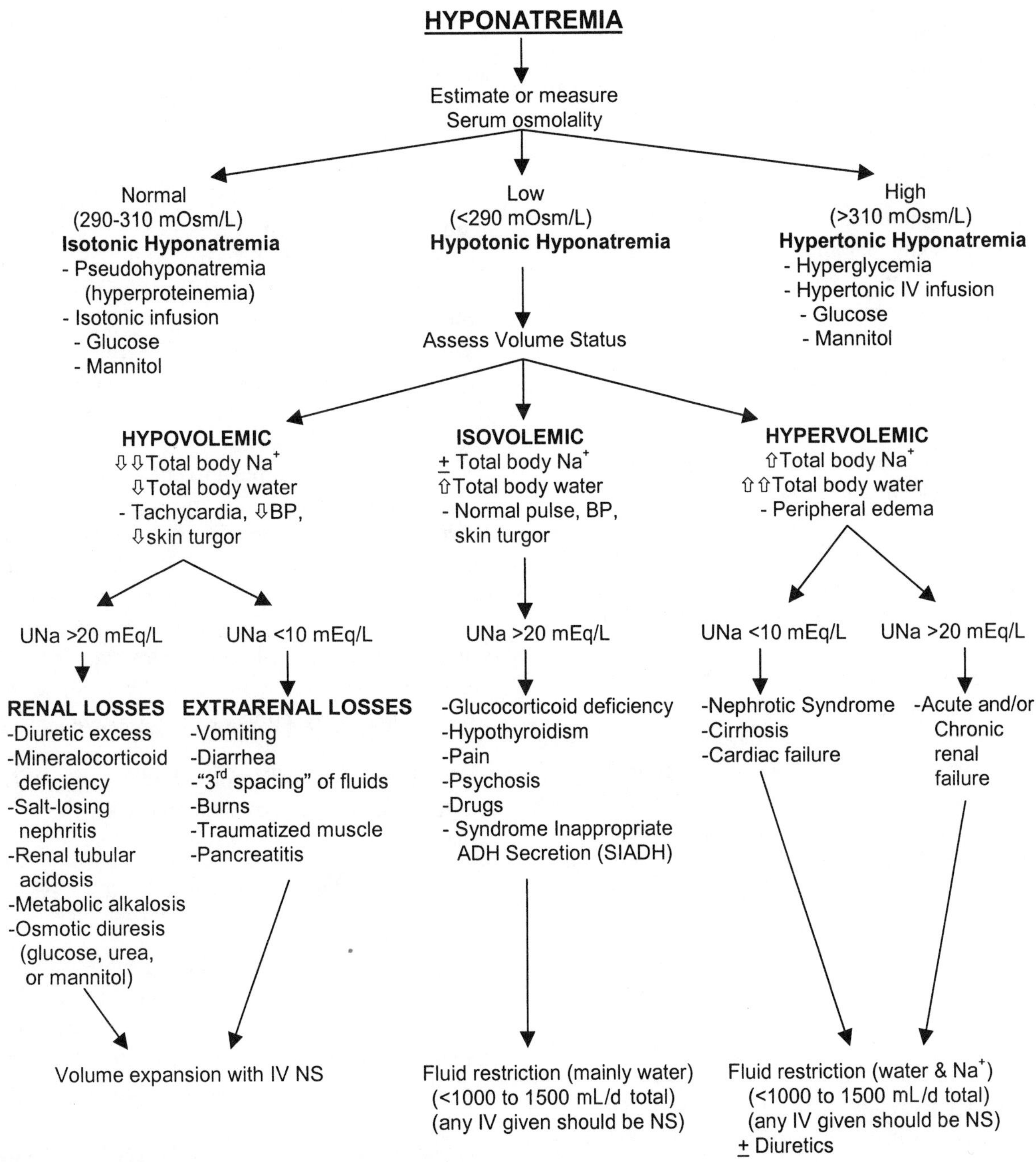

Figure 8.3

Evaluation, Etiology, and Treatment of Hyponatremia

Adapted with permission from Whitmire SJ. Fluids and electrolytes. In: Matarese LE, Gottschlich MM, eds. Contemporary Nutrition Support Practice: A Clinical Guide, 1st ed. Philadelphia: WB Saunders; 1998:134; and Berl T, Schrier RW. Disorders of water metabolism. In: Schrier RW, ed. Renal and Electrolyte Disorder, 5th ed. Philadelphia: Lippincott-Raven Publishers; 1997:41.

every 1 kg of body fat or muscle metabolized). Perioperatively or post-traumatically, the usual compensatory mechanisms leading to renal excretion of excess water and correction of the hypotonic state may not be functional. In these situations, secretion of high circulating levels of ADH induced by the number of stress-related stimuli is not subject to hyposmolar inhibition, so hypotonic fluid retention persists. Similarly, hyponatremia secondary to unremitting ADH-induced accumulation of water in excess of Na^+ is characteristic in patients with advanced diseases of the heart, kidney, or liver. Dilutional hyponatremia can be caused by the syndrome of inappropriate ADH secretion (SIADH). This can be due to tumors of the lung, pancreas, and duodenum; intracranial disease; trauma; surgery; or various medications.[2]

Signs and symptoms of hyponatremia are directly related to both the absolute value of the serum Na^+ as well as to the rapidity with which the hyponatremia develops. Hyponatremia is rarely symptomatic until the serum Na^+ goes below 130 mEq/L, in which case weakness, fatigue, hyperactive deep tendon reflexes, and muscle twitching can occur. This is particularly true when the serum Na^+ decreases rapidly, 10 to 15 mEq/L or more over 24 to 48 hours. Serum Na^+ below 120 mEq/L and progressing toward 110 mEq/L may be associated with confusion, convulsions, coma, areflexia, and even death. However, patients can have severe hyponatremia, serum Na^+ <120 mEq/L, and be relatively asymptomatic if it developed over a prolonged period of time.[2]

Treatment of hyponatremia consists of treating the underlying disorder as well as manipulation of the patient's fluid and electrolyte management (Figure 8.3). In the case of hypovolemic hyponatremia, IV NS should be given with the goal of volume expansion. In the case of isovolemic or hypervolemic hyponatremia, the patient's oral, enteral, and parenteral fluids should be restricted and any IV fluids given should be NS so as not to worsen the hyponatremia. In the case of hypervolemic hyponatremia, diuretics or even dialysis, if the patient is in renal failure, may be necessary.[1,2]

Rarely, in severe symptomatic hyponatremia, hypertonic saline (3% or 5% saline solution) may need to be used judiciously. This is usually when the patient has severe hyponatremia (serum Na^+ <120 mEq/L) and the patient is manifesting mental status changes (decreased mentation, confusion, convulsions, etc.). In this situation, the sodium deficit is calculated by the following equation:

$$Na^+ \text{ deficit (mEq)} = (140 \text{ mEq/L} - \text{Measured serum } Na^+) \times (0.6 \times \text{Weight in kg})$$

Replace half of this deficit with IV 3% or 5% saline solution over 12 to 18 hours then replace the other half over 24 to 48 hours. The serum Na^+ should be repeated frequently during this time period to ensure the serum Na^+ is not being corrected too fast (goal is to increase serum Na^+ approximately 1 mEq/L/h).[1,2]

Hypernatremia

Hypernatremia is always associated with a hypertonic state so measuring serum osmolality does not help differentiate the underlying cause. It also is always associated with movement of free water from the ICF to the ECF causing cellular dehydration.[1] It can be associated with hypovolemia, isovolemia, or hypervolemia. Assessment of the volume status and the urinary Na^+ can help determine the etiology (Figure 8.4). Signs and symptoms of hyponatremia can start to appear once the serum Na^+ is >150 mEq/L and may include restlessness, weakness, decreased salivation and lacrimation, dry mucous membranes, dry flushed skin, decreased skin turgor, oliguria, fever, tachycardia, and hypotension. Once the serum Na^+ exceeds 160 mEq/L, the patient is at risk for delirium, coma, convulsions, and even death.[1,2]

Treatment of hypernatremia should be aimed at treating the underlying etiology and adjusting the fluids and electrolytes (Figure 8.4). When the volume deficits are modest and the underlying condition can be controlled, simple oral ingestion of water or IV administration of D_5W can reduce sodium concentration to normal relatively easily. However, if the hypernatremia is more prolonged and severe, serum Na^+ ≥160 mEq/L, correcting the condition becomes more complicated.[2]

In patients with hypovolemic hypernatremia, the fluid deficit can be calculated with the following equation:

$$\text{Water deficit (L)} = 0.6 \times \text{Weight in kg} \times (1 - (140/\text{measured serum } Na^+))$$

Approximately half of the calculated fluid deficit should be replaced over the first 12–24 hours with hypotonic saline (1/2 NS). The rest of the deficit can be replaced over the subsequent 24 to 48 hours, frequently re-evaluating the patient's fluid and electrolyte status.[1,2]

Overly aggressive correction of hypernatremia can cause rapid fluid shifts from the ECF to the ICF compartment, resulting in cerebral edema and severe neurological consequences. The reason for this is that brain cells accommodate to slowly developing extracellular hypertonicity by accumulating extra intracellular

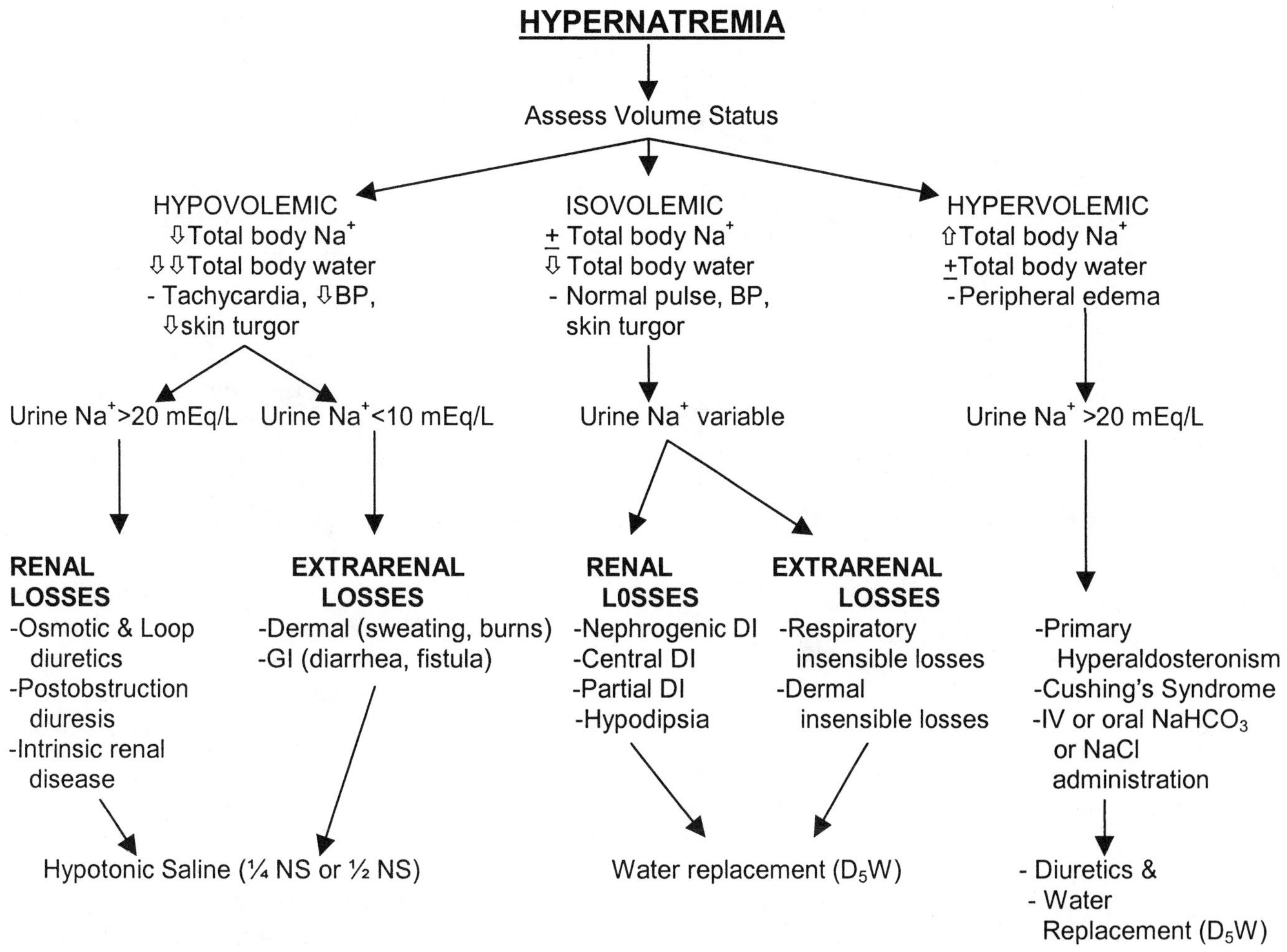

Figure 8.4

Evaluation, Etiology, and Treatment of Hypernatremia

Adapted with permission from Whitmire SJ. Fluids and electrolytes. In: Matarese LE, Gottschlich MM, eds. Contemporary Nutrition Support Practice: A Clinical Guide, 1st ed. Philadelphia: WB Saunders; 1998:135; and Berl T, Schrier RW. Disorders of water metabolism. In: Schrier RW, ed. Renal and Electrolyte Disorder, 5th ed. Philadelphia: Lippincott-Raven Publishers; 1997:21.

solute. A sudden decrease in ECF osmolality without time for elimination of these extra intracellular milliosmoles leads to rapid swelling of brain cells, which then causes serious neurologic dysfunction.[1,2] So if a hypernatremic patient has severe ECF deficit with hypotension, signs and symptoms of poor tissue perfusion, and shock, then NS may need to be infused until hemodynamic stability is restored, then the patient can be administered hypotonic solutions at a slower rate.[2]

Potassium (K^+)

Potassium is the main intracellular cation and it is the most abundant cation in the body with total body K^+ of approximately 50 to 55 mEq/kg or 3,500 mEq in a 70 kg man.[2,9] Normal serum K^+ is about 3.6 to 5.0 mEq/L.[2,9] Only about 2% of the total body K^+ is present in the ECF.[1,2] Therefore, the serum K^+ level is only the tip of the iceberg when evaluating potassium disorders and relatively small changes in serum K^+, with no change in the intracellular:extracellular K^+ concentration, can account for a large change in total body K^+. For example, if the serum K^+ decreases from a normal value of 4.2 mEq/L to 3.0 mEq/L, this accounts for approximately 13% total body deficit of K^+ (Figure 8.5), which is approximately 455 mEq in a 70 kg man. Conversely, if the serum K^+ increases from a normal of 4.2 mEq/L to 6.0 mEq/L, this accounts for about a 13% increase in total body K^+ (Figure 8.5) or an increase of approximately 455 mEq total body K^+.

Potassium is important in maintaining cell volume, hydrogen ion concentration (pH), enzyme function, protein synthesis, and cell growth.[1] Changes in the intracellular:extracellular ratio of K^+ can adversely af-

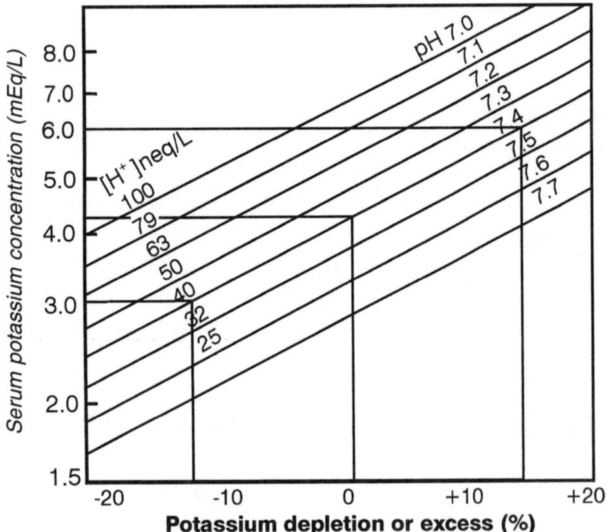

Figure 8.5

Relationship of Serum Potassium to Total Body Potassium

Adapted with permission from Gabow PA, Peterson LN. Disorders of potassium metabolism. In: Schrier RW, ed. Renal and Electrolyte Disorders, 2nd ed. Boston: Little, Brown and Company; 1980:207.

fect neuromuscular and cardiac function by altering nerve and muscle cell resting membrane potentials.[1] Factors that cause an intracellular shift of K^+ include alkalosis, rapid cellular growth, thyrotoxicosis, drugs (such as digitalis overdose and depolarizing muscle relaxants such as succinylcholine), and certain hormones (such as insulin, catecholamines, and aldosterone). Factors that cause an extracellular shift of K^+ include acidosis, exercise, necrosis or tissue injury, hyperosmolality, and drugs or toxins (such as barium intoxication).[9]

In order to maintain a normal serum pH, the body shifts H^+ ions into and out of the ICF as needed (Figure 8.6). In the presence of acidosis, H^+ ions are shifted into the cells. In order to maintain electrical neutrality, the H^+ ions are exchanged for K^+ ions leaving the cells. This results in an increase in the serum K^+ and hyperkalemia. The reverse happens with alkalosis, H^+ ions are shifted out of the cells and are exchanged for K^+ ions entering the cells, resulting in a decrease in the serum K^+ and a hypokalemia.[1] Figure 8.7 shows the relationship between serum pH and serum potassium levels. With no change in the total body potassium levels, a rise in serum pH from the normal pH of 7.4 to 7.7 would result in a decrease of serum pH from normal of 4.2 mEq/L to 2.8 mEq/L. Vice versa, a drop in the serum pH to 7.1 will cause the serum potassium to increase to 6.0 mEq/L.

Potassium enters the body through food, medications, and IV fluids. Losses occur through the kidneys, GI tract, and skin (generally negligible). The kidneys are the principle regulator of potassium homeostasis; however, they are not as efficient at preserving K^+ as they are Na^+.[1,9]

Hypokalemia

Hypokalemia can occur with or without a total body K^+ deficit and a K^+ deficit can occur without hypokalemia (Table 8.10). Clinical signs and symptoms of hypokalemia include muscle weakness, ileus (nausea, vomiting, or abdominal distention), EKG changes (flattened T waves, prominent U waves, prolongation of the P-R interval, and widening of the QRS complex), cardiac arrhythmias (premature ventricular con-

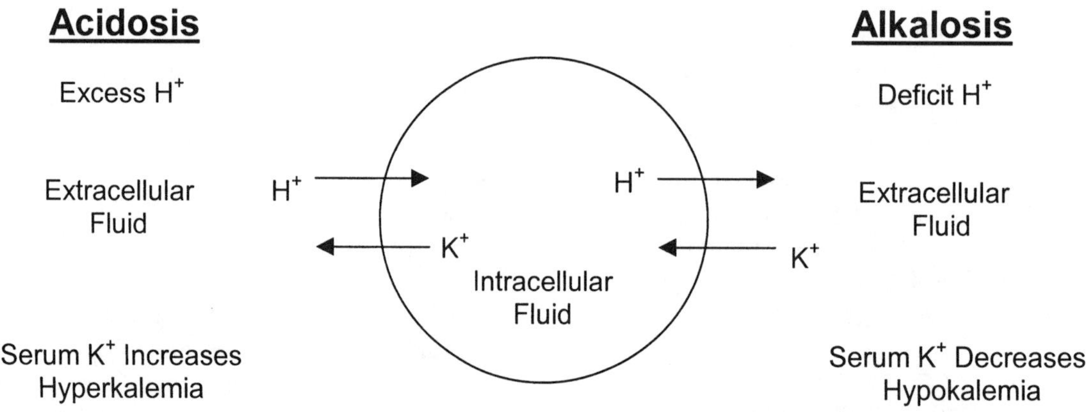

Figure 8.6

Effects of Acidosis and Alkalosis on Intracellular: Extracellular Ratio of Potassium

Adapted with permission from Whitmire SJ. Fluids and electrolytes. In: Matarese LE, Gottschlich MM, eds. Contemporary Nutrition Support Practice: A Clinical Guide, 1st ed. Philadelphia: WB Saunders; 1998:140.

tractions (PVC), ventricular tachycardia, and ventricular fibrillation), hyporeflexia, and paralysis (the latter two symptoms usually do not occur until the serum K^+ is <2.5 mEq/L).[2,9]

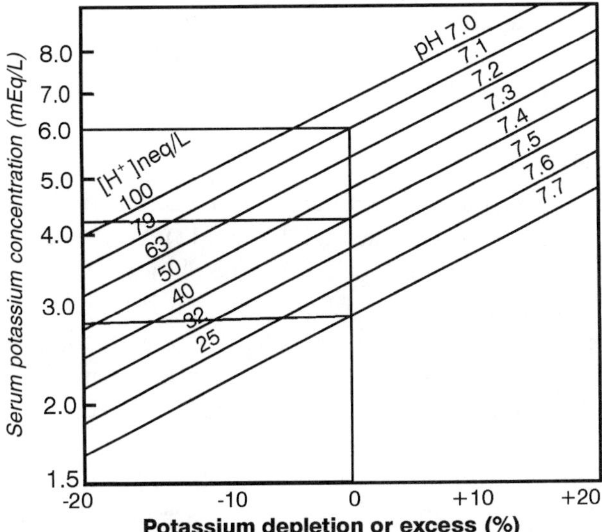

Figure 8.7

Relationship of Serum pH to Serum Potassium Levels

Adapted with permission from Gabow PA, Peterson LN. Disorders of potassium metabolism. In: Schrier RW, ed. Renal and Electrolyte Disorders, 2nd ed. Boston: Little, Brown and Company; 1980:207.

Treatment of hypokalemia is aimed at the underlying etiology, and GI and urinary K^+ losses can be differentiated by measuring a urine K^+ level (Table 8.10). Any existing alkalosis should be corrected. If hypokalemia still exists after correction of any acid-base abnormalities, potassium replacement should be initiated. If the patient has a functioning GI tract and the hypokalemia is mild to moderate, oral potassium supplements are preferred. Oral K^+ can be replaced at a rate of 30 to 60 mEq daily.[2,9]

If the GI tract is not functional and/or the hypokalemia is severe, then IV KCl should be given. If the hypokalemia is mild to moderate, the KCl can be added to the patient's maintenance IV, usually 20 to 40 mEq/L depending on the severity of the deficit. If the deficit is severe or symptomatic, IV KCl boluses can be given with doses ranging from 20 to 80 mEq depending on the degree of hypokalemia and the patient's renal function.[11,12] Potassium can be administered up to 10 mEq/h safely; however, the patient should be on a continuous cardiac monitor if given potassium at a rate faster than this, and it is mandatory for rates equal to or greater than 20 mEq/h.[2] The bolus should not exceed 20 mEq/h except in extreme emergency, in which case the K^+ can be given as fast as 40mEq/h.[11,12] Potassium should never be given as an IV push.[13] Potassium can be very irritating to peripheral veins, so IV KCl boluses may require central

TABLE 8.10

Etiologies of Hypokalemia[9,10]	
Categories	**Etiologies**
Hypokalemia without K^+ deficit	■ Respiratory alkalosis ■ Familial hypokalemic periodic paralysis ■ Athletes ■ Leukocytosis ■ Insulin and glucose administration ■ Drugs/toxins (beta agonists and barium intoxication)
Hypokalemia with K^+ deficit	■ Poor dietary intake—"tea and toast diet," alcoholism, anorexia nervosa, geophagia ■ Cellular incorporation—nutrition support in severally malnourished patient ("refeeding syndrome"), treatment of megaloblastic anemia ■ GI losses (urinary K^+ <20 mEq/L)—protracted vomiting, diarrhea, GI fistula, laxative abuse, ureterosigmoidostomy, obstructed or long ileal conduit, colonic villous adenoma ■ Urinary losses (urinary K^+ >20 mEq/L) □ Excessive mineralocorticoid effect—primary or secondary hyperaldosteronism, Bartter's syndrome, excessive glucocorticoid hormones (Cushing's syndrome), licorice abuse, excessive ACTH □ Renal tubular acidosis □ Endogenous or exogenous osmotic diuretic □ Diuretic therapy □ Carbenicillin or penicillin therapy □ Leukemias
K^+ deficit without hypokalemia	■ K^+ deficit along with acidosis ■ Uremia ■ Congestive heart failure

venous access since the recommended maximal concentration of K+ that should be given through a peripheral IV is 80 mEq/L. There is no specified maximum K concentration for central venous administration.[11]

However, recommendations for IV potassium replacement have been inconsistent with few recommendations based on clinical studies, so one study[13] retrospectively reviewed over a 5-month period of time all medical intensive care patients who received a KCl bolus. The hospital's standard KCl bolus was 20 mEq in 100 mL of NS IV over 1 hour. A total of 1462 infusions were administered during the review period, but 111 were excluded because post-infusion K+ was not obtained within 12 hours.

On average, the serum K+ level increased by 0.25 mEq/L for each 20 mEq KCl infused. A significant number of the study patients had impaired renal function and 21 patients had oliguric renal failure. Despite this, the serum creatinine level did not correlate with rise in serum K+ after the KCl bolus, and no patient with renal insufficiency developed hyperkalemia. However, these were selected patients with severe hypokalemia and ongoing extrarenal K+ losses. So KCl boluses can be safely administered to patients with renal impairment, but this must be done cautiously. The majority of KCl boluses reviewed in this study were infused into a central vein; however, 23% of the boluses were infused into a peripheral vein. Even though this far exceeded the previously stated recommended maximum concentration of K+ infusion through a peripheral vein (200 mEq/L compared to the recommended maximum of 80 mEq/L), only three patients, 2.6% of the peripheral K boluses, had documented pain necessitating discontinuance of the KCl bolus. However, some of these patients were sedated or had altered mental status such that their pain threshold or ability to report pain was altered.[13] So this concentration of KCl bolus, 20 mEq in 100 mL NS, can be infused through a peripheral venous catheter, but the patient should be monitored for pain or other signs of phlebitis. If this occurs, the bolus can be slowed down, but if the pain or other symptoms persist, the bolus may need to be discontinued and given through a central venous catheter.

Another study[14] prospectively analyzed the efficacy and safety of KCl boluses in critically ill patients. Depending on the patient's severity of hypokalemia, either 20 mEq, 30 mEq, or 40 mEq of KCl were placed in 100 mL of NS and infused over 1 hour. The mean increase in serum K+ 1 hour after the bolus was 0.5 ± 0.3 mEq/L, 0.9 ± 0.4 mEq/L, and 1.1 ± 0.4 mEq/L for the 3 different levels of KCl boluses, respectively. This is a significantly greater increase compared to the previous study.[13] The prospective study[14] included only a small number of patients with significant renal impairment, and only one patient was anuric. But these patients had similar responses to the KCl bolus compared to those patients with normal renal function, which was also seen in the above retrospective study.[13] All KCl boluses in the prospective study[14] were administered through central venous catheters.

Hyperkalemia

Hyperkalemia can be an artifact of a traumatic blood draw, pseudohyperkalemia (Table 8.11). So if a serum K+ level is not appropriate for the clinical setting or out of line with other recent values, it is best to perform a stat repeat level before aggressively treating the hyperkalemia. True hyperkalemia can be secondary to redistribution, decreased K+ excretion, or increased input (Table 8.11). Hyperkalemia is usually not clinically significant until the serum K+ is above 6.0 mEq/L.[2] The clinical signs of hyperkalemia are muscle weakness and cardiotoxicity. Muscle weakness can progress to paralysis if hyperkalemia is severe.[1,2] The appearance of adverse cardiac effects are accelerated by acute acidosis, hypocalcemia, hyponatremia, and rapid increase of the serum K+. In the absence of these factors, peaked T waves, most dramatic in the precordial leads, appear at serum K+ of 6.0 to 7.0 mEq/L. At serum K+ of 7.0 to 8.0, electrocardiographic (EKG) changes consist of diminished P waves, increased P-R intervals, heart block, decreased Q-T intervals, widening of the QRS complexes, and depressed S-T segments. Elevations of serum K+ over 8.0 mEq/L can result in loss of T waves, asystole, and death.[2,9]

Severe hyperkalemia, serum K+ >6.5 mEq/L, should be treated acutely with administration of IV insulin and glucose, IV sodium bicarbonate, and albuterol aerosol (Table 8.12). These treatments all cause an intracellular shift of the K+ and a lowering of the serum K+. If the serum K+ reaches 7.5 mEq/L, IV calcium gluconate should be given (Table 8.12). This does not affect the serum K+ level but rather stabilizes the myocardial cell membranes, making them less sensitive to the effects of the hyperkalemia. However, these are only temporary measures. Long-term correction of hyperkalemia requires treating the underlying cause. If the problem is excessive amounts of potassium in the body then the potassium must be removed (Table 8.12). It can be removed through the urine with loop diuretics if the kidneys are functioning.[15] However, frequently, when hyperkalemia occurs, the kid-

TABLE 8.11

Etiologies of Hyperkalemia	
Categories	**Etiologies**
Pseudohyperkalemia	■ Hemolysis from traumatic blood draw ■ Blood sample contaminated by infused potassium solution ■ Thrombocytosis ■ Leukocytosis ■ Mononucleosis
Increased intake or tissues release	■ Excessive IV or oral potassium administration ■ Hemolysis ■ Rhabdomyolysis ■ Tumor lysis ■ Massive transfusion with old stored blood
Redistribution	■ Acidosis ■ Diabetic ketoacidosis (insulin deficiency) ■ Periodic paralysis ■ Exercise ■ Tissue damage ■ Drugs (β-adrenergic blockade, arginine HCl, succinylcholine, digitalis overdose)
Renal origin	■ Glomerular filtration rate <20 mL/min □ Acute and/or chronic renal failure ■ Glomerular filtration rate >20 mL/min □ Aldosterone deficiency ➥ Addison's disease ➥ Hereditary adrenal enzyme defects ➥ Hyporeninemic hypoaldosteronism ➥ Drugs (heparin, non-steroidal anti-inflammatory drugs, angiotensin-converting enzyme inhibitors, cyclosporine) □ Tubular hyperkalemia without aldosterone deficiency ➥ Obstructive uropathy ➥ Post renal transplant ➥ Systemic lupus erythematosus (SLE) ➥ Amyloidosis ➥ Sickle cell nephropathy ➥ Interstitial nephritis ➥ AIDS ➥ Drugs (potassium-sparing diuretics, cyclosporine, pentamidine, trimethoprim) ➥ Pseudohypoaldosteronism

Adapted with permission from Peterson LN, Levi M. Disorders of potassium metabolism. In: Schrier RW, ed. Renal and Electrolyte Disorders, 5th ed. Philadelphia: Lippincott Williams & Wilkins; 1997:231–232.

neys are not functioning properly and may not respond to diuretics. Potassium can also be removed through the GI tract with cation exchange resins such as Kayexalate, which can be given orally or by retention enema. Lastly, potassium can be removed via hemodialysis, which may be necessary if the patient is in renal failure.[9,15]

Calcium (Ca^{++})

Calcium is one of the most abundant ions in the body and is an important regulator of many neuromuscular functions and enzymatic process. Almost all of the total body Ca^{++} is in the bones and teeth in the form of calcium carbonate or calcium phosphate, with less than 1% located in the ECF. Serum Ca^{++} levels are regulated by parathyroid hormone (PTH) and calcitonin. Low serum Ca^{++} levels stimulate release of PTH, which increases bone resorption, stimulates renal conservation of Ca^{++}, and activates vitamin D, which increases GI Ca^{++} absorption. Calcitonin is released by the thyroid gland in response to increased serum Ca^{++} levels and acts by inhibiting bone resorption.[1]

Serum Ca^{++} exists in three forms, bound, complexed, and ionized. Approximately 40% of serum Ca^{++} is bound to serum proteins and 80% to 90% of this is bound to serum albumin. About 15% are complexed to phosphate, citrate, sulfate, lactate, or bicarbonate. The majority of the serum Ca^{++}, about 45%, is ionized, which is the metabolically active form of serum Ca^{++}. The ratio of ionized to total serum Ca^{++} is altered by changes in serum pH and protein levels.[1,16]

TABLE 8.12

Treatment of Hyperkalemia[2,9,15]					
Medication	Mechanism of Action	Dosage	Onset	Peak Effects	Duration
Temporary Treatments					
For serum K^+ >6.5 mEq/L					
Insulin & Glucose	Shifts potassium into intracellular space	10 units regular insulin & 1 ampule of $D_{50}W$ IV	15–30 minutes	30–60 minutes	2–4 hours
Sodium bicarbonate	Shifts potassium into intracellular space	1 ampule Na bicarb IV over 5 minutes; can repeat within 30 minutes	15–30 minutes	30–60 minutes	1–2 hours
Albuterol	Beta 2-adrenergic agonist shifts potassium into intracellular space	20 mg in nebulized form	—	30–60 minutes	—
For serum K^+ >7.5 mEq/L					
Calcium gluconate	Antagonism of membrane actions	10 mL (1 ampule) 10% solution IV over 2–3 minutes	minutes	5 minutes	1 hour
Long-Term Treatments					
Loop diuretics	Increases excretion of potassium in the urine (if the kidneys are functioning)	? Furosemide 40 g to 80 mg IV	15–30 minutes	30–60 minutes	4 hours
Kayexalate	Binds with potassium in the GI tract and excretes it in the stool	20 g in 100 mL 20% Sorbitol given orally or as retention enema	60 minutes	2–4 hours	4 hours
Hemodialysis	Removes potassium from the body	—	minutes	minutes	variable

Most commonly the total serum Ca^{++} is what the laboratory reports, with the normal level being between 9.5 and 10.5 mg/dL. However, since the ionized serum Ca^{++} is the metabolically active component, the measured total serum Ca^{++} must be adjusted when there is an alteration in the acid-base status or hypoalbuminemia. Acidosis increases the ionized fraction, so total Ca^{++} should be increased by 2 mg/dL for every 0.1 decrease in serum pH. Conversely, alkalosis decreases the ionized fraction, so total Ca^{++} should be decreased by 2 mg/dL for every 0.1 increase in serum pH. With hypoalbuminemia, total serum Ca^{++} should be adjusted up 0.8 mg/dL for each 1 g/dL decrease in serum albumin below 4.0 g/dL. However, these are only approximations. The most accurate method of accessing for calcium abnormalities is to measure ionized Ca^{++} directly.[1,16]

Hypocalcemia

Hypocalcemia frequently occurs secondary to hypoalbuminemia; however, this is not significant as long as the ionized Ca^{++} remains normal. Causes of symptomatic hypocalcemia include decreased vitamin D activity (vitamin D deficiency, hyperphosphatemia, pseudohypoparathyroidism, acute and chronic renal failure), decreased PTH activity (acute pancreatitis, hypomagnesemia, hypoparathyroidism), "hungry bone" syndrome (can occur after parathyroidectomy for hyperparathyroidism or thyroidectomy), massive soft tissue damage or infection (crush injuries, rhabdomyolysis, necrotising fasciitis), and massive blood transfusions (secondary to the citrate preservative in the bank blood binding with the serum Ca^{++}).[1,2,16]

Hypocalcemia is usually not clinically significant until the corrected serum total Ca^{++} is less than 8 mg/dL.[2] Clinical signs and symptoms of hypocalcemia include neuromuscular excitability, circumoral paresthesias, numbness and tingling of the tips of the fingers, muscle and abdominal cramps, hyperactive deep tendon reflexes, positive Chvostek sign (twitching of the facial muscles with tapping over the facial nerve in front of the tragus of the ear), tetany with carpopedal spasms, EKG changes (prolonged QT interval), convulsions, stupor, coma, and death.[1,2] Severity of the signs and symptoms depend not only on the absolute serum Ca^{++} level, but also the rapidity with which the hypocalcemia developed.[1] Treatment consists of reversing the underlying cause if possible.[1,2] Oral calcium replacement (400 mg BID), with or without supplemental vitamin D, should be adequate if the symptoms are minimal or if long-term replacement is necessary.[12] If the hypocalcemia is acute and symptomatic, IV 10% calcium gluconate (10 mL ampule = 90 mg elemental calcium = 4.5 mEq Ca^{++}) or 10% calcium chloride (10 mL ampule = 270 mg elemental calcium = 13.5 mEq Ca^{++}) should be administered. Recommended dose is 4.5 to 18 mEq, depending on the severity of the hypocalcemia and the serum phosphorous concentration, in 250 ml of NS or D_5W. The preferred rate of administration is 1.5 mEq/h with the maximal rate for emergency use of 4.5 mEq/h. The recommended maximum daily dose is 36 mEq. If hyperphosphatemia is present, this should be treated as well. If the hyperphosphatemia is severe, calcium replacement may need to be delayed until the phosphorous is correct for fear of calcium phosphate precipitates.[12]

Hypercalcemia

Hyperparathyroidism and cancer with bone metastasis (breast cancer being most common) account for the majority of cases of hypercalcemia; however, there is a long list of other potential causes as well (Table 8.13). Hypercalcemia is usually not clinically significant until the total serum calcium level is over 11 to 12 mg/dL.[2] Clinical signs and symptoms of hypercalcemia include weakness, fatigue, anorexia, nausea, vomiting, headaches, muscle pain, polyuria, EKG changes (shortening of Q-T interval and widening of T waves), psychosis, somnolence, stupor, coma, and death. Life threatening complications usually do not occur until the serum Ca^{++} level is >15 mg/dL.[1,2] Chronic hypercalcemia can result in polydipsia, polyuria, and metastatic calcium deposits, which is most likely to occur when the product of the total serum Ca^{++} and phosphorus is >70 mg/dL.[1]

If the patient is hypercalcemic, then Ca^{++} intake, orally, enterally, and parenterally, should be limited or totally eliminated. The main initial treatment of hypercalcemia is aggressive (200 to 250 mL/h) IV hydration with NS. This results in an expansion of the

TABLE 8.13

Causes of Hypercalcemia
▪ Primary hyperparathyroidism
□ Parathyroid adenoma—most common
□ Parathyroid hyperplasia—more common in familial hyperparathyroidism
□ Parathyroid carcinoma—very infrequent cause
▪ Secondary hyperparathyroidism
□ Malabsorption and vitamin D deficiency
□ Chronic renal failure
□ Following kidney transplant
▪ Neoplastic diseases
□ Malignant tumor with lytic bone metastasis
□ Tumors secreting parathyroid hormone-like substances
□ Tumors secreting humoral non-parathyroid-like substances and various cytokines
□ Multiple myeloma and other lymphoproliferative disease—"osteoclast-activating factor"
▪ Familial hypocalciuric hypercalcemia
▪ Hyperabsorptive hypercalciuria
▪ Hypervitaminosis D
▪ Hypervitaminosis A
▪ Granulomatous diseases—sarcoidosis, tuberculosis, histoplasmosis, coccidioidomycosis, leprosy, foreign body granulomas
▪ Hyperthyroidism
▪ Adrenocortical insufficiency
▪ Infantile hypercalcemia
▪ Immobilization
▪ Hypophosphatemia
▪ Milk-Alkali Syndrome
▪ Parenteral nutrition
▪ Hypercalcemia associated with acute renal failure
▪ Medications—thiazides, lithium, theophylline, calcium-ion exchange resins

Adapted with permission from Popovtzer MM, Knochel JP, Kumar R. In: Schrier RW, ed. Renal and Electrolyte Disorders, 5th ed. Philadelphia: Lippincott Williams & Wilkins; 1997:270.

ECF causing an increase in the urine output and therefore increased urinary excretion of Ca^{++}. The additional sodium from the NS also increases Ca^{++} excretion in the urine by competing for tubular reabsorption.[1,2,16] Fluid status must be monitored closely for volume overload, especially in elderly patients and patients with cardiopulmonary compromise.[16]

IV NS hydration and correction of the underlying etiology usually is sufficient to treat hypercalcemia. However, if the serum Ca^{++} is still not decreasing, loop diuretics, such as furosemide, can be given to further increase urinary excretion of Ca^{++}. However, if loop diuretics are given without adequate hydration, volume contraction can occur, resulting in increased reabsorption of urinary Ca^{++}, actually worsening the hypercalcemia.[2,16]

Biphosphonates can also be used in the treatment of hypercalcemia. They bind tightly to calcified bone matrix and interfere with osteoclast function, with net effect of decreasing bone reabsorption. Didronel is a first-generation biphosphonate, and its effectiveness is limited because it not only reduces bone resorption but also inhibits bone mineralization. Clodronate and Pamidronate are second-generation biphosphonates. They are more successful in treating hypercalcemia because they inhibit bone resorption with minimal effects on bone mineralization. They are approved in the United States for treatment of malignancy-related hypercalcemia, with proven decrease in bone pain and pathologic fractures in these patients. Alendronate, risedronate, and tiludronate are third-generation biphosphonates and are more effective than the second generation in inhibiting bone resorption. But they are not yet approved for use in the U.S.[16]

Glucocorticoids are effective in lowering serum Ca with vitamin D intoxication, sarcoidosis, and malignancy (especially lymphoma, leukemia, and multiple myeloma). The exact mechanism is unknown, but they may suppress bone resorption and decrease intestinal absorption. The recommended dose is 3 to 4 mg/kg/d hydrocortisone IV or orally. This will usually cause decreases in serum Ca^{++} within 1 to 2 days.[16]

Calcitonin inhibits bone resorption and increases urinary Ca excretion. Its therapeutic action has a limited duration since osteoclast becomes resistant to its effects within several days of starting therapy. Mithramycin is a cytotoxic chemotherapeutic agent that suppresses bone resorption. The recommended dose is 25 μg/kg IV (which is lower than the treatment dose for cancer), and its effect starts 24 to 48 hours after administration and last for several days. Phosphates bind with Ca^{++} to lower serum Ca^{++}; however, CaPhos deposits can form in the tissues, especially the kidneys, causing renal failure. Phosphates are contraindicated in patients with hyperphosphatemia or renal insufficiency.[16]

Gallium nitrate can be used to inhibit bone resorption but it is nephrotoxic. Somatostatin can be used to inhibit PTH-like hormone secretion from pancreatic neoplasms that secrete this substance. Propranolol has been successful in hypercalcemia from thyrotoxicosis and theophylline toxicity. Chelating agent (Na-EDTA) can be given IV to complex with Ca, which is then excreted through the kidneys, but it is nephrotoxic. Hemodialysis and peritoneal dialysis can also be used in renal-failure patients to correct hypercalcemia.[16]

Phosphorus

Phosphorus is a vital component of all the body organs, structurally as well as by participating in many of the different metabolic pathways of the body. Phosphorus is one of the main structural components of bone and teeth along with calcium. It facilitates normal nerve and muscle function, and acts as an acid-base buffer in the urine. Phosphorus is the main intracellular anion. Approximately 85% of phosphorus is in the bones and about 14% is in the body's soft tissues. Only 1% of total body phosphorus is in the ECF, and the exchange between the ECF and the other forms of phosphorus is relatively slow. Therefore, serum phosphorus levels may not correlate with intracellular or total body phosphorus levels.[1,2]

The laboratory measurements are that of elemental phosphorus. However, almost all plasma phosphorus exists in either free or protein-bound phosphate. Free phosphate exists in univalent ($H_2PO_4^-$) and divalent (HPO_4^{-}) forms. At the normal levels of serum pH, the ratio of divalent to univalent ions is about 2:1. So in converting millimoles of phosphorus to milliequivalents, an average of 1.7 valence is used.[1]

Phosphate levels are affected by intake, intestinal absorption, renal excretion, and hormonal regulation associated with bone metabolism. Phosphorus can be shifted intracellularly by alkalosis, glucose and insulin administration, or catecholamines. Extracellular shift can be a result of acidosis.[1,16]

Hypophosphatemia

There are many causes for moderate hypophosphatemia (Table 8.14) and severe hypophosphatemia (Table 8.15). Hypophosphatemia was initially the hallmark of Refeeding Syndrome; however, the more

TABLE 8.14

Causes of Moderate Hypophosphatemia

- Pseudohypophosphatemia
  - Mannitol
  - Bilirubin
  - Acute leukemia
- Decreased dietary intake
- Decreased intestinal absorption
  - Vitamin D deficiency
  - Malabsorption
  - Steatorrhea
  - Vomiting
  - Phosphate binding antacids
- Shift from ECF to ICF
  - Respiratory alkalosis secondary to
    - Sepsis
    - Heat stroke
    - Neuroleptic malignant syndrome
    - Hepatic coma
    - Salicylate poisoning
    - Gout
    - Panic attacks
    - Psychiatric depression
  - Hormonal effects
    - Insulin
    - Glucagon
    - Epinephrine
    - Androgens
    - Cortisol
    - Anovulatory hormones
  - Nutrient effects
    - Glucose
    - Fructose
    - Glycerol
    - Lactate
    - Amino acids
    - Xylitol
- Cellular Uptake Syndromes
  - Recovery from hypothermia
  - Burkitt's lymphoma
  - Histiocytic lymphoma
  - Acute myelomonocytic leukemia
  - Acute myelogenous leukemia
  - Chronic myelogenous leukemia in blast crisis
  - Treatment of pernicious anemia
  - Erythropoietin therapy
  - Erythrodermic psoriasis
  - Hungry bone syndrome
    - After parathyroidectomy
    - Acute leukemia
- Increased excretion into the urine
  - Hyperparathyroidism
  - Renal tubular defects
    - Fanconi's syndrome
    - Hereditary hypophosphatemic rickets
    - Polyostotic fibrous dysplasia
    - Panostotic fibrous dysplasia
    - Neurofibromatosis
    - Kidney transplantation
    - Oncogenic osteomalacia
    - Recovery from hemolytic-uremic syndrome
  - Aldosteronism
  - Licorice ingestion
  - Volume expansion
  - Syndrome of inappropriate secretion of antidiuretic hormone (SIADH)
  - Mineralocorticoid and corticosteroid administration
  - Diuretics
  - Aminophylline therapy

Reprinted with permission from Popovtzer MM, Knochel JP, Kumar R. In: Schrier RW, ed. Renal and Electrolyte Disorders, 5th ed. Philadelphia: Lippincott Williams & Wilkins; 1997:296.

modern definition of Refeeding Syndrome encompasses multiple different fluid and electrolyte abnormalities, including hypophosphatemia, hypokalemia, and hypomagnesemia, as well as different organ system dysfunctions.[17,18]

Hypophosphatemia has several well documented clinical sequela and some proposed adverse effects (Table 8.16). Hypophosphatemia results in reduced levels of 2,3-diphosphoglycerate (2,3-DPG), which interacts with hemoglobin to promote release of oxygen, and adenosine triphosphate (ATP), which is how the body stores and transfers energy. This interferes with the ability of the erythrocyte to release oxygen at the cellular level and result in tissue anoxia. This and the deficiency of ATP are the probable causes of most the adverse clinical effects of hypophosphatemia. Hypophosphatemia can cause respiratory failure and require intubation or impair weaning if the patient is already on a ventilator.[2,16]

Treatment of hypophosphatemia is phosphorus replacement. If the GI tract is functioning, oral sodium or potassium phosphate can be given at a dose of 16 to 32 mmol BID to QID depending on renal function.[12] If the GI tract is not functional or the hypophosphatemia is severe, IV sodium or potassium phosphate should be given. Phosphate is the only electrolyte ordered in mmol; the others are usually ordered in mEq. The way that phosphate dissociates for every 3 mmol of phosphorous released, 4 mEq Na^+ is released from sodium phosphate and 4.4 mEq of K^+ is released from potassium phosphate.[12,16] If the serum K^+ is <4.0 mEq/L, the KPhos should be used for the bolus; otherwise, NaPhos should be used. The recommended bolus dose ranges from 15 to 60 mmol Phos

TABLE 8.15

Causes of Severe Hypophosphatemia
■ Nutrition repletion (Refeeding Syndrome) ■ Chronic alcoholism and alcohol withdrawal ■ Dietary deficiency and phosphate binding antacids ■ Respiratory alkalosis ■ Severe thermal burns ■ Following major surgery ■ Neuroleptic malignant syndrome ■ Recovery from diabetic ketoacidosis ■ Recovery from exhaustive exercise ■ Kidney transplant ■ Therapeutic hyperthermia ■ Reye's syndrome ■ Periodic paralysis ■ Acute malaria ■ Drug therapy □ Ifosfamide □ Cisplatin ■ Acetaminophen intoxication ■ Cytosine infusions □ Tumor necrosis factor (TNF) □ Interleukin-2

Adapted with permission from Popovtzer MM, Knochel JP, Kumar R. In: Schrier RW, ed. Renal and Electrolyte Disorders, 5th ed. Philadelphia: Lippincott Williams & Wilkins; 1997:297.

TABLE 8.16

Consequences of Severe Hypophosphatemia
■ Definite consequences □ Red cell dysfunction ➡ Impaired release of oxygen to the tissues ➡ Rigidity of RBC, which can cause hemolysis □ Leukocyte dysfunction—impaired chemotactic, phagocytic, and bactericidal activity of granulocytes, which can increase the risk of infection or impair the body's ability to respond to infection □ Platelet dysfunction—thrombocytopenia and impaired function of platelets □ Respiratory failure—secondary to diaphragm and intercostal muscle weakness □ Central nervous system dysfunction—irritability, apprehension, weakness, numbness, paresthesias, dysarthria, confusion, obtundation, convulsions, and coma □ Cardiomyopathy □ Metabolic acidosis—secondary to impaired excretion of metabolic acid in the urine □ Osteolysis—if chronic, can cause bone pain and osteomalacia □ Rhabdomyolysis ■ Possible consequences □ Hepatocellular dysfunction—hyperbilirubinemia and possible hepatic encephalopathy □ Renal dysfunction—renal bicarbonate wasting and renal glycosuria □ Ketoacidosis □ Peripheral neuropathy

Adapted with permission from Popovtzer MM, Knochel JP, Kumar R. In: Schrier RW, eds. Renal and Electrolyte Disorders, 5th ed. Philadelphia: Lippincott Williams & Wilkins; 1997:301.

depending on the severity of hypophosphatemia and the renal function. The Phos bolus should not run any faster than 7.5 mmol/h.[12] However, the phosphorous should not be replaced too rapidly because it can cause hyperphosphatemia. The phosphorous can then bind to calcium and cause hypocalcemia or metastatic calcium phosphate deposits, which can cause organ dysfunction in those tissues with calcium phosphate deposits.[2,16]

Hyperphosphatemia

The most common cause of hyperphosphatemia is renal insufficiency or failure, which results in decreased excretion of phosphorus.[1] Also, hyperphosphatemia can be caused by endogenous release of phosphorus into the ECF from severe cellular destruction, such as with massive trauma, cytotoxic agents (especially with treatment of lymphomas or leukemias), hypercatabolic states, hemolysis, rhabdomyolysis, and malignant hyperthermia. Finally, hyperphosphatemia can be caused by a shift of phosphorus from the ICF to the ECF, which can be a result of respiratory or lactic acidosis and early stages of diabetic ketoacidosis.[1,2,16]

Consequences of hyperphosphatemia include hypocalcemia, metastatic deposits of calcium phosphate (occurs when the Ca-Phos product is >70 mg/dL), osmotic diuresis, dehydration, hypernatremia, and renal dystrophy with renal failure.[1,16] Treatment should include decreasing or eliminating all exogenous phosphate intake. Secondly, volume repletion in conjunction with diuretics can increase phosphorus excretion in the urine. Phosphate-binding antacids (calcium carbonate and aluminum hydroxide) can be given orally to bind the phosphate in the GI tract and thereby increase phosphorus elimination through the stool. Lastly, the patient may need dialysis especially in the setting of acute or chronic renal failure.[1,2]

Magnesium (Mg^{++})

Magnesium is the fourth most common cation in the body[19] and the second most common intracellular cation.[1] It plays important roles in protein and carbohydrate metabolism and intracellular electrolyte homeostasis by activating enzymes involved in the Na^+-K^+, calcium, and proton pumps. Magnesium is also crucial for the transmission of neuromuscular activity, central nervous system activity, and myocardial function.[1,19] The majority of the total body magnesium, 50% to 60%, is incorporated into bone. Only 1% is distributed to the ECF space, with the remainder in the ICF space.[1,2,19] One-third of serum magnesium is protein bound with a small portion complexed to citrate, bicarbonate, and phosphate. The remainder is free or ionized, which is the metabolically active portion.[1] Similar to calcium, hypoalbuminemia causes decreased total serum magnesium; however, the amount of ionized magnesium remains unchanged.[1] Magnesium is absorbed in the GI tract and excreted mainly in the urine.[1,19] Only about one-third of magnesium in the diet is actually absorbed.[1,19] Renal excretion of magnesium decreases with decreased sodium and calcium excretion, increased levels of PTH, and decreased ECF volume.[1]

Hypomagnesemia

Causes of hypomagnesemia include inadequate intake or GI absorption of magnesium, renal magnesemia wasting, or other miscellaneous causes (Table 8.17). Hypomagnesemia can induce hypocalcemia.[19] Clinical signs and symptoms of hypomagnesemia are similar to those of hypocalcemia, including muscle weakness, hyperreflexia, tremor, positive Chvostek sign, tetany with carpopedal spasms, cardiac arrhythmias (prolonged Q-T interval and ventricular arrhythmias), hypotension, increased vascular resistance, and hypokalemia that is usually resistant to correction until the magnesium is replaced. With severe hypomagnesemia, delirium, convulsions, stupor, and coma can occur.[1,2,19] The treatment is magnesium replacement. If the GI tract is functioning and the deficit is mild and asymptomatic, oral magnesium gluconate (500 mg tablet = 27 mg elemental magnesium = 2.2 mEq Mg^{++} or 1000 mg/5 mL solution) or magnesium oxide (400 mg tablet = 241.3 mg elemental magnesium = 19.9 mEq Mg^{++}) can be given at a dose of 400 mg daily to QID depending on the renal function.[12] These preparations cause less diarrhea than magnesium sulfate or magnesium citrate.[1] If the GI tract is not functioning or the deficit is severe, IV boluses of magnesium sulfate (1 g = 8 mEq Mg^{++}) can be given in doses of 2 to 8 g depending on the severity of the hypomagnesemia and the renal function. The recommended rate of administration is 0.5 to 1 g/h, with a maximal rate of 5 gm/h in emergency situations.[12,19] While correcting hypomagnesemia, any concomitant hypokalemia and hypocalcemia should also be treated.[19] Care should be taken not to overcorrect the hypomagnesemia, especially in the setting of renal impairment, since complications of hypermagnesemia may occur.[1,19]

TABLE 8.17

Causes of Hypomagnesemia[1,2,19]

- Inadequate intake or GI absorption of magnesium
  - Inadequate intake, starvation, or protein-calorie malnutrition (kwashiorkor)
  - Malabsorption syndromes
  - Inflammatory bowel disease
  - Severe diarrhea
  - Familial magnesium malabsorption
- Renal magnesium wasting
  - Volume expansion
  - Diuretics
  - Sodium loads
  - Diabetic ketoacidosis
  - Medications—aminoglycosides, cis-platinum, cyclosporine, pentamidine
  - Hyperaldosteronism, primary or secondary
  - Syndrome of inappropriate secretion of antidiuretic hormone (SIADH)
  - Bartter's Syndrome
  - Familial or sporadic renal magnesium-wasting
  - Hypercalciuria
- Miscellaneous
  - Nutritional repletion (Refeeding Syndrome)
  - Alcoholism
  - Acute pancreatitis
  - Burns
  - Thyrotoxicosis

Hypermagnesemia

Hypermagnesemia occurs mainly with acute or chronic renal failure. It can also occur with adrenocortical insufficiency, early burn injury, severe trauma or surgical stress, rhabdomyolysis, severe dehydration, severe acidosis, and with administration of large amounts of oral or parenteral magnesium, such as ingestion of large amounts of magnesium containing laxatives, treatment of premature labor, or correction of hypomagnesemia.[1,19] Clinical signs of hypermagnesemia include lethargy, weakness, diaphoresis, dilated pupils, nausea, vomiting, diarrhea, depressed deep tendon reflexes, muscle paralysis, respiratory depression, hypotension, cardiac arrhythmia (bradycardia, heart block, asystole), and death.[1,2,19]

Treatment of hypermagnesemia includes minimizing or eliminating all oral or parenteral magnesium. Oral or IV rehydration with or without loop diuretics can increase magnesium excretion in the urine. Correcting any acidosis present will help correct hypermagnesemia. Administration of IV calcium chloride or calcium gluconate (5 to 10 mEq) can directly antagonize the effects of hypermagnesemia, reversing potentially lethal respiratory depression or cardiac arrhythmia, as well as increasing urinary magnesium excretion. If renal failure is present, hemodialysis may be required to correct the hypermagnesemia.[1,2,19]

Chloride (Cl^-)

Isolated abnormalities do not occur because they accompany other electrolyte or acid-base abnormalities. Causes of hypochloremia include GI losses, such as nasogastric suction, diarrhea, GI fistulas, etc., and renal losses, such as diuretics, non-oliguric acute or chronic renal failure, etc. The main adverse effect is the development of hypochloremic, hypokalemic metabolic alkalosis. The treatment is chloride replacement with NaCl or KCl, usually IV. Rarely, ammonium chloride or hydrochloric acid may be needed in severe or life-threatening situations.[2]

Hyperchloremia is associated with hypernatremia, excess chloride administration, renal tubular acidosis, and ileal conduit or ureterosigmoidostomy. There are no specific signs of hyperchloremia, but rather those of the other associated underlying causes. Treatment is to address the underlying causes.[2]

Conclusions

Fluid and electrolyte abnormalities are common in critically ill patients and can result in serious adverse outcomes. Appropriate administration of IV fluids and electrolytes can prevent many of these complications. Appropriate clinical assessment and laboratory monitoring can lead to early detection and prompt treatment, which are essential in decreasing the morbidity and mortality that can be associated with fluid and electrolyte abnormalities.

References

1. Whitmire SJ: Fluids and electrolytes. In: Matarese LE, Gottschlich MM, eds. *Contemporary Nutrition Support Practice: A Clinical Guide*. 1st ed. Philadelphia: WB Saunders Company; 1998:127–144.
2. Naitove A, Evans DB, Ihde JK. Fluid and Electrolyte Balance. In: Lawrence PF, Bilbao M, Bell RM, Dayton MT, eds. *Essentials of General Surgery*. 1st ed. Baltimore: Williams & Wilkins; 1988:48–68.
3. Shires III GT, Barber A, Shires GT, et al. Fluid and electrolyte management of the surgical patient. In: Schwartz SI, ed. *Principles of Surgery*. 7th ed. New York, McGraw-Hill;1999:54.
4. Berl T, Schrier RW. Disorders of water metabolism. In: Schrier RW, ed. *Renal and Electrolyte Disorders*. 5th ed. Philadelphia: Lippincott-Raven Publishers; 1997:1–71.
5. Yaqoob MM, Alkhunaizi AM, Edelstein CL, Conger JD, Schrier RW. Acute Renal Failure: Pathogensis, Diagnosis, and Management. In: Schrier RW, ed. *Renal and Electrolyte Disorders*. 5th ed. Philadelphia: Lippincott-Raven Publishers; 1997:449–506.
6. Lyerly HK. The renal system. In: Lyerly HK, ed. *The Handbook of Surgical Intensive Care*. 2nd ed. Philadelphia: Lippincott-Raven Publishers; 1989:165–202.
7. Danielson RA, McDougal WS. Renal dysfunction. In: Berk JL, Sampliner JE, Artz JS, Vinocur B, eds. *Handbook of Critical Care*. 1st ed. Boston: Little, Brown and Company; 1976:389–417.
8. Gonzalez JM, Suki WN. Polyuria and nocturia. In: Massry SG, Glassock RJ, eds. *Textbook of Nephrology*. 3rd ed. Baltimore: Williams & Wilkins; 1995:547–552.
9. Peterson LN, Levi M. Disorders of potassium metabolism. In: Schrier RW, ed. *Renal and Electrolyte Disorders*. 5th ed. Philadelphia: Lippincott-Raven Publishers; 1997:192–240.
10. Gabow PA, Peterson LN. Disorders of Potassium Metabolism. In: Schrier RW, ed. *Renal and Electrolyte Disorders*. 2nd ed. Boston: Little, Brown, and Company; 1980: 183–222.
11. Lacy CF, Armstrong LL, Goldman MP, Lance LL. *Drug Information Handbook 2000–2001*. Lexi-Comp Inc., 1100 Terex Road, Hudson, OH 44236. 2000:784.
12. MacLaren R, Ramsay KB, Liiva MT, et al. The development and implementation of evidence-based electrolyte replacement guidelines in the intensive care unit. *CJHP*. 1999;52:393–398.
13. Kruse JA, Carlson RW. Rapid correction of hypokalemia using concentrated intravenous potassium chloride infusions. *Arch Intern Med*. 1990;150:613–617.
14. Hamill RJ, Robinson LM, Wexler HR, Moote C. Efficacy and safety of potassium infusion therapy in hypokalemic critically ill patients. *Crit Care Med*. 1991; 19:694–699.
15. Tyler DS. Fluid and electrolytes. In: Lyerly HK, ed. *The Handbook of Surgical Intensive Care*. 2nd ed. Chicago: Year Book Medical Publishers, Inc.; 1989:223–250.
16. Popovtzer MM, Knochel JP, Kumar R. Disorders of calcium, phosphorus, vitamin D, and parathyroid hormone activity. In: Schrier RW, ed. *Renal and Electrolyte Disorders*, 5th ed. Philadelphia: Lippincott-Raven Publishers; 1997: 241–319.
17. Solomon SM, Kirby DF. The refeeding syndrome: a review. *J Parenter Enteral Nutr*. 1990;14:90–97.
18. Brooks MJ, Melnik G. The refeeding syndrome: an approach to understanding its complications and preventing its occurrence. *Pharmacotherapy*. 1995;15:713–726.
19. Alfrey AC. Normal and abnormal magnesium metabolism. In: Schrier RW, ed. *Renal and Electrolyte Disorders*. 5th ed. Philadelphia: Lippincott-Raven Publishers; 1997:320–348.

CHAPTER

Assessment and Management of Acid-Base Abnormalities

Vincent W. Vanek, M.D., F.A.C.S., C.N.S.P.

INTRODUCTION	101	METABOLIC ALKALOSIS	108
RESPIRATORY ACIDOSIS	104	CONCLUSIONS	109
RESPIRATORY ALKALOSIS	105	REFERENCES	109
METABOLIC ACIDOSIS	105		

Introduction

As with fluids and electrolytes, the human body must maintain the balance between acids and bases within fairly narrow limits for optimal physiological function. Critically ill patients frequently develop acid-base abnormalities that overcome the normal homeostatic mechanisms and require early recognition and treatment to avoid morbidity and mortality. This chapter reviews the principles of acid-base homeostasis and the recognition and treatment of these disorders.

An acid is a compound that donates a H^+, while a base is a compound that accepts a H^+. Every acid (HA) has a corresponding base (A^-), and it is the dissociation constant (K_{eq}) that determines if the compound is a strong acid or strong base according to the following relationship[1]:

$$[HA] = K_{eq} \times [H^+]\,[A^-]$$

Acidity is measured as pH, which is a representation of the concentration of H^+ ions as follows[2]:

$$pH = \log (1 / [H^+])$$

Normal serum pH is 7.35 to 7.45 and the body must maintain the pH within a fairly narrow range in order for all organ systems to function properly.[2,3] This is accomplished by the combination of three mechanisms: (1) buffering systems present in body fluids that immediately offset changes in hydrogen ion concentration, (2) pulmonary ventilation changes that can promptly adjust the excretion of carbon dioxide, and (3) renal tubular function that can increase or decrease the urinary excretion of acid or base.[3]

Buffers consist of a poorly dissociating acid (HA) and its anion base (A^-).[1] Figure 9.1 demonstrates how if an acid (H^+) is added to a buffered solution, the buffer will blunt the change in pH.[1] In the extracellular fluid (ECF) compartment, the bicarbonate buffer is the major buffer, while proteins and the inorganic phosphate buffer act as minor buffers. However, the inorganic phosphate buffer is the major intracellular fluid (ICF) compartment buffer and the bicarbonate buffer and proteins are the minor buffers.[1,2] The bicarbonate buffer functions as follows:

$$H^+ + HCO_3^- \overset{K_{eq}}{\longleftrightarrow} H_2CO_3 \longleftrightarrow S \times pCO_2$$

where H_2CO_3 is carbonic acid, S is a solubility coefficient, and pCO_2 is partial pressure of CO_2 in the serum.[1,4] By combining the two previous equations, the following equation demonstrates the relationship between pH and the metabolic component (HCO_3^-) and the respiratory component (pCO_2) of the acid-base system.[1,2]

$$pH = pK + \log \frac{[HCO_3^-]}{pCO_2}$$

If there is a primary abnormality of one component, the other component will try to compensate by changing in the opposite direction in order to attempt to normalize the pH. Respiratory compensation occurs rapidly, in minutes, compared to metabolic compensation, which depends on changes in the kidney that can

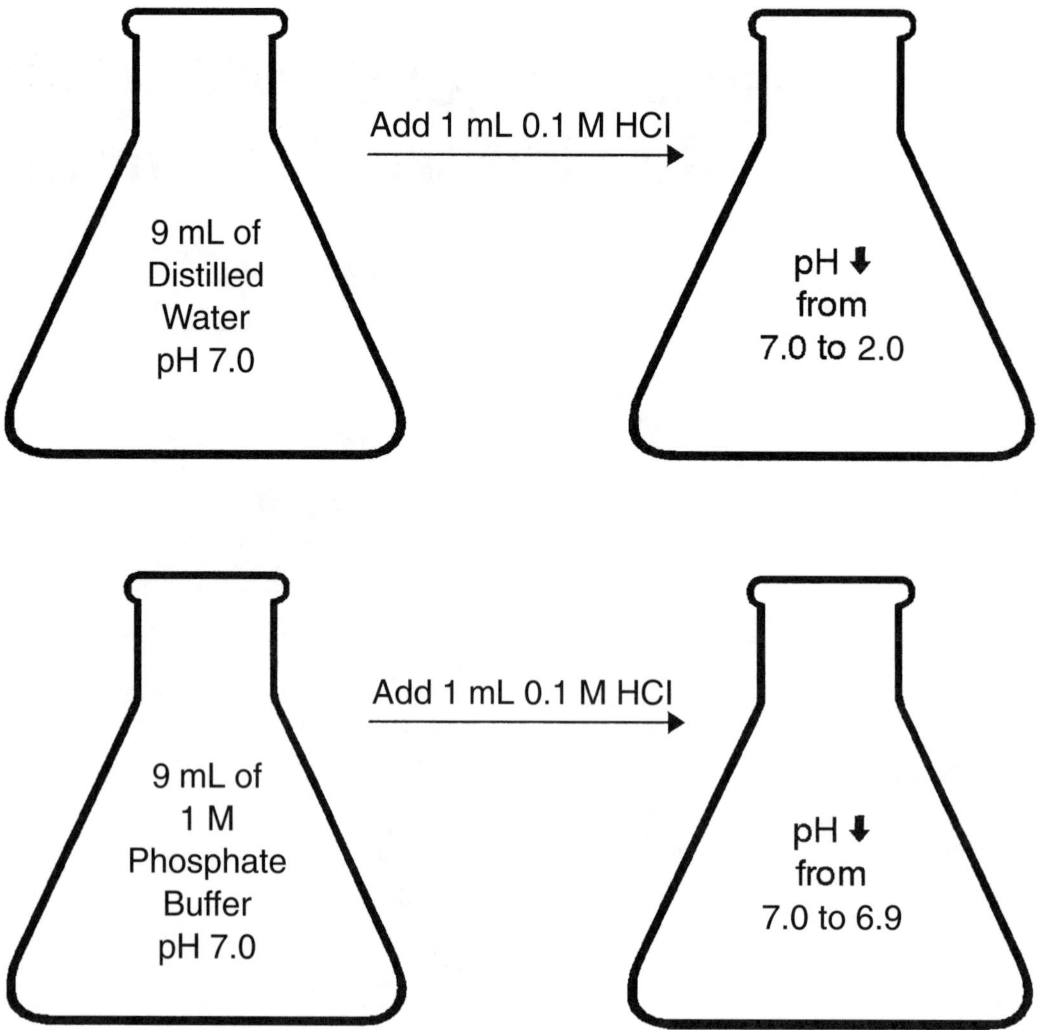

Figure 9.1

Effects of Adding an Acid to a Un-Buffered Solution Compared to a Buffered Solution

take hours or days.[2] However, compensation alone will never bring the pH completely back to normal and will not "overshoot" and cause the pH to be abnormal in the opposite direction from the primary abnormality.[1] Table 9.1 shows the expected changes in pH, pCO_2, and HCO_3^- for uncompensated and compensated primary respiratory and metabolic acid-base abnormalities.[5]

Mixed acid-base abnormalities can occur with primary problems of both the respiratory and metabolic components. This situation is easy to recognize if the abnormalities of both components are in the same direction, i.e. both acidosis or both alkalosis (Table 9.2). However, if the abnormalities are in opposite directions, one acidosis and one alkalosis, the pH can be quite variable (Table 9.2) and it can be difficult to differentiate compensatory changes from mixed acid-base abnormalities.

The best way to diagnosis acid-base abnormalities is to obtain an arterial blood gas (ABG). The partial pressure of oxygen in arterial blood (pO_2) is not helpful in determining the presence or absence of an acid-base abnormality but it should be assessed since hypoxemia can cause or be a result of acid-base abnormalities and may need to be treated with supplemental oxygen or even mechanical ventilator assistance.[2]

In diagnosing an acid-base abnormality, the pH should be assessed first (Table 9.3). If the pH is >7.45 then there is an alkalosis present, if the pH is <7.35 then there is an acidosis, and if the pH is normal then either no abnormality exists or there is a mixed acid-base abnormality. Next pCO_2 is assessed. If it is

TABLE 9.1

Expected Changes in pH, pCO_2, and HCO_3^- Associated with Primary Respiratory and Metabolic Acid-Base Abnormalities with and without Compensatory Changes

Type of Acid-Base Abnormality	ACUTE (uncompensated) pH	pCO$_2$	HCO$_3^-$	CHRONIC (partially compensated) pH	pCO$_2$	HCO$_3^-$
Respiratory acidosis	⇓⇓	⇑⇑	N	⇓	⇑⇑	⇑
Respiratory alkalosis	⇑⇑	⇓⇓	N	⇑	⇓⇓	⇓
Metabolic acidosis	⇓⇓	N	⇓⇓	⇓	⇓	⇓⇓
Metabolic alkalosis	⇑⇑	N	⇑⇑	⇑	⇑	⇑⇑

Abbreviations: N is normal; ⇓ or ⇓⇓ is mild or moderately to severely decreased; and ⇑ or ⇑⇑ is mild or moderately to severely increased

Adapted with permission from Shires III GT, Barber A, Shires GT. Fluid and electrolytes management of the surgical patient. In: Schwartz SI, Shires GT, Spencer FC, et al, eds. Principles of Surgery. 7th ed. New York: McGraw-Hill, 1999:60.

>45 mmHg then a respiratory acidosis (primary or compensatory) exists, if it is <35 mmHg then a respiratory alkalosis (primary or compensatory) exists, and if it is normal then either no respiratory abnormality or an uncompensated or mixed acid-base abnormality exists. Next the HCO_3^- is assessed. If it is <22 mEq/L then a metabolic acidosis (primary or compensatory) exists, if it is >26 mEq/L then a metabolic alkalosis (primary or compensatory) exists, and if it is normal then either no metabolic abnormality or an uncompensated or mixed acid-base abnormality exists.[1,2] The HCO_3^- obtained off of the arterial blood gas is not directly measured but rather is calculated from the measured pH and pCO_2. Alternatively, the serum total CO_2 obtained from the serum electrolytes can be used to assess the metabolic acid-base component. It includes both the serum HCO_3^- and the pCO_2 that is dissolved into the serum. The serum total CO_2 should be about 1 or 2 mEq/L greater than the arterial HCO_3^-. The normal values for HCO_3^- and pCO_2 vary from lab to lab, so one should check the normal values for their lab.[2]

The final step in assessing acid-base abnormalities is to determine which component, respiratory or metabolic, is the primary abnormality (usually the component that is in the same direction as the pH) and if the change in the other component is uncompensated or compensated, or a mixed abnormality exists. This can be done by one of two methods. The first is to calculate the expected compensation of the component opposite to the component with the primary abnormality (Table 9.4). If the observed changes are not consistent with the expected changes, there is a mixed acid-base abnormality.[2,6] The other method is to use a

TABLE 9.2

Expected Changes in pH, pCO_2, and HCO_3^- Associated with Mixed Respiratory and Metabolic Acid-Base Abnormalities

	pH	pCO$_2$	HCO$_3^-$
Respiratory acidosis & Metabolic alkalosis	⇓, N, or ⇑	⇑⇑	⇑⇑
Respiratory acidosis & Metabolic acidosis	⇓⇓⇓	⇑⇑	⇓⇓
Respiratory alkalosis & Metabolic alkalosis	⇑⇑⇑	⇓⇓	⇑⇑
Respiratory alkalosis & Metabolic acidosis	⇓, N, or ⇑	⇓⇓	⇓⇓

Abbreviations: N is normal; ⇓, ⇓⇓, or ⇓⇓⇓ is mild, moderately, or severely decreased; and ⇑, ⇑⇑, or ⇑⇑⇑ is mild, moderately, or severely increased.

Adapted with permission from Kaehny WE. Pathogenesis and management of respiratory and mix acid-base disorders. In: Schrier RW, ed. Renal and Electrolyte Disorders, 5th ed. Philadelphia: Lippincott Williams & Wilkins; 1997:183.

TABLE 9.3

Diagnosis of Acid-Base Abnormalities

	Acidosis	Normal	Alkalosis
Arterial pH	<7.35	7.35 to 7.45	>7.45
Arterial pCO$_2$, mmHg (Respiratory component)	>45	35 to 45	<35
Arterial HCO$_3^-$, mEq/L * Serum Total CO$_2$, mEq/L (Metabolic component)	<22 <23	22 to 26 23 to 30	>26 >30

Adapted with permission from Androgue HJ. Normal cshemistry and physiology of acid-base homestasis. In: Massry SG, Glassock RJ, eds. Textbook of Nephrology. 3rd ed. Baltimore: Williams & Wilkins; 1995:420.

TABLE 9.4

The "Rules of Thumb" Listed Below Predict the Compensatory Changes Anticipated by the Opposite Component with the Maximal Limits for Compensation		
Primary abnormality	Compensatory Response	Limits
Metabolic acidosis	⇓ $PaCO_2$ (mmHg) by 1.0–1.5 × ⇓ HCO_3^- (mEq/L)	$PaCO_2$ of 10 mmHg
Metabolic alkalosis	⇑ $PaCO_2$ (mmHg) by 0.25–1.0 × ⇑ HCO_3^- (mEq/L)	$PaCO_2$ of 55 mmHg
Respiratory acidosis—acute	⇑ HCO_3^- (mEq/L) by 0.1 × ⇑ $PaCO_2$ (mmHg)	HCO_3^- of 30 mEq/L
Respiratory acidosis—chronic	⇑ HCO_3^- (mEq/L) by 0.3–0.4 × ⇑ $PaCO_2$ (mmHg)	HCO_3^- of 45 mEq/L
Respiratory alkalosis—acute	⇓ HCO_3^- (mEq/L) by 0.1–0.3 × ⇓ $PaCO_2$ (mmHg)	HCO_3^- of 16–18 mEq/L
Respiratory alkalosis—chronic	⇓ HCO_3^- (mEq/L) by 0.2–0.5 × ⇓ $PaCO_2$ (mmHg)	HCO_3^- of 12–15 mEq/L

Adapted with permission from Shapiro JI, Kaehny WD. Pathogenesis and management of metabolic acidosis and alkalosis. In: Schrier RW, ed. Renal and Electrolyte Disorders. 5th ed. Philadelphia: Lippincott-Raven Publishers; 1997: 137 and from Androgue HJ. Normal chemistry and physiology of acid-base homeostasis. In: Massry SG, Glassock RJ, eds. Textbook of Nephrology. 3rd ed. Baltimore: Williams & Wilkins; 1995:423.

nomogram, as shown in Appendix Figure 9.2. It is possible to have three or all four primary acid-base abnormalities simultaneously; however, it is difficult to predict the changes in pH, pCO_2, and HCO_3^- in these situations.[6]

Respiratory Acidosis

The causes of respiratory acidosis can be divided into acute and chronic respiratory acidosis (Table 9.5). The main treatment of respiratory acidosis is to identify and treat the underlying cause.[2,6] Overfeeding can result in excess CO_2 generation and respiratory acidosis. So if the patient is on nutrition support, the patient should be assessed for overfeeding.[2] If this is the case, the nutrition support should be appropriately reduced. If the patient is not being overfeed, the fat calories can be increased and CHO calories reduced to take advantage of the lower respiratory quotient (RQ) for fats.[7,8]

Some general supportive measures may also be needed while the underlying cause is being diagnosed and treated. Supplemental oxygen should be given as needed to maintain adequate oxygenation.[3] If the underlying cause is not readily reversible and the pa-

TABLE 9.5

Causes of Respiratory Acidosis[2,6]		
	Acute	Chronic
Alveolar hypoventilation	Narcotic, sedative, tranquilizer, alcohol CNS lesions (head injury, CVA, infections, etc.) Spinal cord injury (high level) Guillain-Barré Syndrome Myasthenia Gravis Botulism/Tetanus/Poisonings Muscle abnormality (myositis, hypokalemia, hypophosphatemia)	Chronic narcotic or sedative ingestion Primary hypoventilation Obesity/Pickwickian syndrome Poliomyelitis Diaphragmatic paralysis Hypothyroidism CNS lesion, tumor, MS, etc. Muscular dystrophy/myositis/ALS
Ventilation-perfusion mismatch	Acute airway obstruction —Laryngospasm —Bronchospasm/asthma —Aspiration/foreign body —Sleep apnea Ventilatory restriction —Hemo- or pneumothorax —Severe pneumonia —Smoke inhalation —Severe pulmonary edema/ARDS —Massive pulmonary embolism	Obstructive disease —Chronic obstructive pulmonary disease (COPD) Restrictive disease —Kyphoscoliosis —End-stage interstitial pulmonary disease (sarcoid, silicosis, etc.) —Fibro- or hydrothorax —Chronic radiation pneumonitis —Ascites —Chronic peritoneal dialysis
Other	Nutrition support with overfeeding	

tient is deteriorating, such as but not limited to pH <7.2, pCO_2 >60 (unless baseline pCO_2 elevated), or decreased mentation, consider endotracheal intubation and mechanical ventilation. If the patient is already intubated and on a ventilator, the tidal volume and/or respiratory rate can be increased.[3,6] IV sodium bicarbonate is not indicated in the treatment of respiratory acidosis and can be harmful, as will be discussed later in conjunction with the treatment of metabolic acidosis.

Respiratory Alkalosis

The causes of respiratory alkalosis can be divided into those that cause central stimulation of respiration, those that cause peripheral stimulation of respiration, and miscellaneous causes (Table 9.6). The main treatment for respiratory alkalosis, again, is to identify and treat the underlying cause.[2,6] While doing this, adequate oxygenation must be maintained, which may occasionally require supplemental oxygen. In mechanically ventilated patients, the minute ventilation can be decreased by decreasing the rate and/or tidal volume or dead space can be added to the ventilator system. If manipulating the ventilator does not help, the patient may need to be sedated or pharmacologically paralyzed in order to take total control of the patient's ventilation. Patients who are not mechanically ventilated can be cautiously given narcotics or sedatives if they are in pain or anxiety; however, adequate oxygenation must be maintained. If the patient is awake and alert, he or she can breathe into a paper bag to increase the pCO_2 gas in the inspired air and reverse the respiratory alkalosis.[6]

Metabolic Acidosis

The serum anion gap (SAG) is the difference between the serum Na^+ and the combination of the serum Cl^- and total CO_2. The SAG represents the difference between the "unmeasured" cations (K^+, Ca^{++}, and Mg^{++}) and anions (SO_4^{-2}, $H_2PO_4^-$, HPO_4^{-2}, albumin, and organic anions). The normal SAG used to be reported as 12 mEq/L; however, with more sensitive laboratory techniques for measuring Cl^-, the normal SAG is 9 mEq/L with a range of 6 to 12 mEq/L. But each lab should report its own normal value for SAG depending on the technique used for measuring serum electrolytes. Since serum albumin is one of the "unmeasured" anions, hypoalbuminemia will decrease the SAG, approximately 3 mEq/L for every 1 g/dL decrease in serum albumin, even without any acid-base abnormality.[1,2]

The causes of metabolic acidosis can be divided into gap acidosis, those with an increased SAG; and non-gap acidosis, those with a normal SAG (Table 9.7). The non-gap metabolic acidosis is secondary to excess loss of HCO_3^- resulting in a hyperchloremic metabolic acidosis, which is also termed a mineral acidosis. The gap metabolic acidosis involves the ingestion, increased production, or decreased excretion of some type of organic acids, which is also termed an organic acidosis. While the SAG is helpful in differentiating gap from non-gap metabolic acidosis, it is not absolute. At times, an organic acidosis may have a normal SAG, especially early in the process and when the patient also has severe hypoalbuminemia, which will decrease the SAG. Likewise, occasionally a mineral acidosis will have a mildly elevated SAG. However, if the SAG is >26 mEq/L an organic acidosis exists.[1]

The main treatment for all types of metabolic acidosis is to identify and treat the underlying cause.[1,2] For example, lactic acidosis from shock can be corrected by restoring adequate tissue perfusion by reversing and treating the etiology of the shock. Diabetic ketoacidosis (DKA) is treated with insulin and once the glucose comes into acceptable range, if the DKA

TABLE 9.6

Causes of Respiratory Alkalosis[2,6]		
Central Stimulation of Respiration	Peripheral Stimulation of Respiration	Other
Anxiety/pain Head trauma CNS tumors/infection CVA/Stroke Salicylates/nicotine Fever Pregnancy	Pulmonary emboli Pulmonary edema/ARDS Interstitial lung diseases Pneumonia Asthma Hemodialysis Carbon monoxide poisoning Severe anemia High altitude	Hyperventilation —Mechanical (ventilator) —Voluntary Miscellaneous (pathophysiology uncertain) —Hepatic insufficiency/severe cirrhosis —Gram-negative septicemia

TABLE 9.7

Causes of Metabolic Acidosis[1,2]	
Non-Anion Gap (hyperchloremic)	Increased Anion Gap
Gastrointestinal loss of HCO_3^- —Diarrhea —Small bowel or pancreatic drainage or fistula —Ureterosigmoidoscopy —Long or obstructed ileal loop conduit —Anion exchange resins —Ingestion of $CaCl_2$, $MgCl_2$	Increased acid production —Diabetic ketoacidosis —Lactic acidosis —Starvation ketoacidosis —Alcoholic ketoacidosis —Inborn errors of metabolism
Renal loss of HCO_3^- —Carbonic anhydrase inhibitors —Renal tubular acidosis (RTA) —Hyperparathyroidism —Hypoaldosteronism	Ingestion of toxic substances —Salicylate overdose —Paraldehyde poisoning —Methanol ingestion —Ethylene glycol ingestion
Miscellaneous —Dilutional acidosis —Addition of HCl or its congeners —Parenteral nutrition acidosis —Sulfur ingestion	Failure of acid excretion —Acute renal failure —Chronic renal failure

persists, then a combination of glucose and insulin.[2] Alcoholic ketoacidosis is a combination of alcohol toxicity, starvation, and dehydration and it is treated with replacement of fluid volume, glucose, potassium, magnesium, phosphorus, and vitamins.[1,2]

Sodium bicarbonate ($NaHCO_3$) has been used to treat severe metabolic acidosis while the underlying etiology is being identified and treated. Previous indications for the use of IV $NaHCO_3$ were if the pH was <7.2 (because it was thought that at this pH cardiac output begins to decrease and pulmonary impairment begins to occur) or the acidosis was causing significant cardiovascular impairment.[9,10] In these situations, 1 to 2 amps of $NaHCO_3$ (44.5 mEq to 89 mEq HCO_3^-) have been given by slow IV push. In cases of severe and persistent gap metabolic acidosis, a bicarbonate IV drip has been administered by putting 1 to 2 amps of $NaHCO_3$ in 500 mL D_5W at about 40 to 60 mL/h and adjusted according to frequent follow-up ABG.[9] Patients with chronic renal failure may require chronic oral sodium bicarbonate therapy. However, hemodialysis may be required in patients with severe acidosis due to either acute or chronic renal failure.[5]

However, more recently, two extensive literature reviews have shown no benefit to $NaHCO_3$ therapy in humans and have demonstrated potential harm with this treatment.[11,12] One of these reviews[12] focused mainly on the use of $NaHCO_3$ in the treatment of lactic acidosis. Only two small prospective randomized controlled studies have been performed on humans assessing the hemodynamic effects of $NaHCO_3$ therapy in critically ill patients with lactic acidosis. The first study[13] involved 14 patients who were randomized to receive either $NaHCO_3$ therapy or equimolar sodium chloride infusion. Correction of acidemia with $NaHCO_3$ did not improve hemodynamics or the cardiovascular response to vasopressors but it did decrease serum ionized calcium levels and increase arterial pCO_2. The second study[14] randomized 10 patients again finding no improvement in the patients' hemodynamic status with $NaHCO_3$ therapy; however, there was also no worsening of tissue oxygenation.

Four studies analyzed patients with DKA treated with or without IV $NaHCO_3$. Two of these studies found no differences in the neurologic status, incidence of hypokalemia or hypoglycemia, or rate of correction of acidemia between the two groups.[15,16] However, the other two studies suggested a delay in clearance of ketones and lactate in DKA patients treated with IV $NaHCO_3$.[17,18] So there is no role for IV $NaHCO_3$ in the treatment of DKA.

The other literature review[11] evaluated the use of $NaHCO_3$ during cardiopulmonary resuscitation. Of the 11 prospective randomized controlled animal studies reviewed, four showed a survival benefit with the use of $NaHCO_3$ and the remainder revealed no difference. None of these studies showed a decreased survival with the use of $NaHCO_3$. Fourteen animal studies assessed myocardial performance. None of these studies showed any benefit with the use of $NaHCO_3$, 2 studies showed no effect, and 12 studies demonstrated a significant impairment of myocardial function with the administration of $NaHCO_3$.[11]

Twenty human studies were reviewed and none showed any beneficial effects associated with the use of $NaHCO_3$ during cardiopulmonary resuscitation.[11] Twelve studies showed no difference, while 8 studies actually showed deleterious effects associated with administering IV $NaHCO_3$ in this clinical setting. However, the majority of these human studies were prospective or retrospective cohort, case control, or case-series studies. There was only one published prospective randomized controlled human study.[19] It was conducted in Norway and included 502 out-of-hospital cardiopulmonary arrest patients who presented with asystole or ventricular fibrillation that did not respond to one initial defibrillation. The placebo group, which received 250 mL of normal saline IV, showed a slight but not statistically significant survival advantage over the treatment group, which received 250 mL of a sodium bicarbonate-trometamol-phosphate buffer solution (14% vs. 10% survival, p=0.18).

Factors that could explain the discrepancies between the findings of the animal and human studies include the difference in experimental conditions, timing and dosage of buffer agents, timing of blood sampling, use of vasopressors in the human studies, level of perfusion, and confusion of results by variable amounts of fluid administration. However, combining the findings of the articles included in the above literature review, several theoretical advantages and disadvantages of using $NaHCO_3$ during cardiopulmonary resuscitation were formulated.[11] Potential advantages include enhanced action of epinephrine, reversal of extracellular metabolic acidosis, and improved rate of defibrillation (demonstrated in only one dog study and not reproduced in other animal and human studies).[11,12] But these seem to be outnumbered by the potential disadvantages.

Overzealous administration of IV $NaHCO_3$ can cause an "overshoot" metabolic alkalosis.[10] This can cause a rapid shift of the oxyhemoglobin dissociation curve to the left, causing an increase in the affinity of hemoglobin for oxygen, resulting in a decrease in the release of oxygen from the hemoglobin in the peripheral tissues and impaired oxygen delivery.[10,11,12,20] Arterial alkalosis also causes intracellular shifts of calcium and potassium that can lead to fatal cardiac arrhythmias.[10,11] The sodium load from the IV $NaHCO_3$ can cause hypernatremia and a hyperosmolality state, especially in chronic renal failure patients.[10,11] In the presence of severely compromised circulation, as with cardiopulmonary arrest, the CO_2 produced by the buffering of hydrogen ion, especially with exogenously administered $NaHCO_3$ may result in increased tissue and venous hypercarbia.[11]

Although administration of $NaHCO_3$ can reliably increase arterial pH, its effect on intracellular pH is variable. In a review of 18 studies[12] involving this issue, only one study showed a rise in intracellular pH with administration of exogenous buffer solution, while six studies showed no change, and nine studies actually demonstrated a decrease in intracellular pH. The other two studies showed either an increase or a decrease in intracellular pH depending on which of the two different buffers was administered. Only one such study[21] has been conducted in humans and this involved five normal volunteers. Infusion of $NaHCO_3$ was found to increase pCO_2, increase cerebral blood flow, and decrease intracellular pH, which could cause impairment of the central nervous system as well as other organ systems.

Finally, one of the initial rationales for the administration of IV $NaHCO_3$ during the treatment of cardiopulmonary arrest was based on early studies that demonstrated the presence of metabolic acidosis during cardiac arrest and that cardiac muscle function was impaired by acidosis. However, subsequent studies have shown that myocardial contractility is more profoundly reduced by increased intracellular pCO_2 than by extracellular pH such that administration of IV $NaHCO_3$ actually impairs myocardial function rather than improving it.[11,12,20]

As a result of the preponderance of evidence in the medical literature regarding the potential adverse effects of IV $NaHCO_3$, the most recently revised Advanced Cardiac Life Support (ACLS) guidelines no longer recommend the routine administration of IV $NaHCO_3$ during cardiopulmonary resuscitation.[11,14,22] The ACLS guidelines further state that $NaHCO_3$ is only indicated for preexisting hyperkalemia, metabolic acidosis, or tricyclic or barbiturate overdose and possibly after prolonged cardiopulmonary arrest or persistent severe acidosis upon return of circulation.[22]

The causes of non-gap metabolic acidosis may not be readily reversible. Severe symptomatic acute non-gap metabolic acidosis can be temporarily corrected by giving IV $NaHCO_3$ based on the amount of deficit by the following equation:

$$HCO_3^- \text{ deficit} = (\text{normal serum } [HCO_3^-] - \text{measured serum } [HCO_3^-]) \times 0.5 \times BW$$

BW is body weight in kg. Half of this deficit is given over 12 to 24 hours and then the acid-base status is reevaluated, again being careful to avoid overshoot alkalosis.[2] Chronic acidosis due to uncorrectable causes can be treated with oral sodium and/or potassium bicarbonate.[1]

Parenteral amino acid solutions used in parenteral nutrition (PN) contain chloride. In addition to this, sodium and potassium are frequently added to PN as the chloride salt. Sodium bicarbonate is not used in PN because of the potential complications of precipitation. But acetate can be added to the PN as sodium or potassium acetate and the acetate is converted to HCO_3^- by the liver, assuming that the liver is functioning normally. However, if the acetate is not added in sufficient quantities or the liver is severely impaired, a hyperchloremic metabolic acidosis can occur.[8] Care must also be taken not to add too much acetate to the PN as it can cause or worsen an alkalosis.[2,8]

Metabolic Alkalosis

The causes of metabolic alkalosis can be divided into sodium chloride-responsive, sodium chloride-resistant, and other causes (Table 9.8). Like all other acid-base abnormalities, the main treatment of metabolic alkalosis is to treat the underlying cause.[1,2] However, some treatments are common to all types of metabolic alkalosis.

The initial treatment is hydration with sodium chloride and potassium chloride containing fluids, usually IV. This will allow the kidneys to excrete HCO_3^- and retain sodium and potassium chloride. The chloride deficit can be calculated as follows:[2]

$$Cl^- \text{ deficit (mEq)} = 0.2 \times BW \times (Cl^-_{normal} - Cl^-_{measured})$$

BW stands for body weight in kg. The initial dose should not exceed 4 mEq Cl^-/kg.[2]

Chloride replacement is helpful in most varieties of metabolic alkalosis and can completely correct the problem in sodium chloride-sensitive causes of metabolic alkalosis.[1,2] Sodium chloride-resistant metabolic alkalosis secondary to secretory tumors require removal or ablation of the tumor or blockade of the renal tubular effects of the mineralocorticoids with spironolactone.[1]

Acetazolamide is a carbonic anhydrase inhibitor that produces large increases in renal HCO_3^- and potassium secretion. It may be given by mouth or IV and it requires adequate potassium repletion to avoid hypokalemia. It is useful in situations where patients are already volume overloaded or intolerant to volume loads such as a patient with congestive heart failure.[1] Histamine (H_2) blockers or proton pump inhibitors may be useful to reduce gastric hydrochloric acid secretion and loss in causes involving gastrointestinal losses.[1] In renal failure patients on hemodialysis, using a dialysate with low HCO_3^- or acetate can help correct the alkalosis.[1]

Patients with severe alkalosis (pH >7.60) can develop life-threatening cardiac arrhythmias and seizures that can be prevented only by acutely lowering pH. This usually occurs in cases of mixed metabolic and respiratory alkalosis.[1,2]

Hydrochloric acid (HCl), arginine chloride, or ammonium chloride have been used when the metabolic alkalosis has been refractory to standard chloride replacement, volume or electrolyte constraints preclude adequate NaCl or KCl administration, or in rare cases of severe life-threatening alkalosis.[1,2] The amount of HCl needed to correct the metabolic alkalosis can be calculated as follows[2]:

$$\text{HCl (mEq)} = 0.3 \times \text{base deficit} \times BW$$

Using 0.1 N to 0.2 N HCl, the above calculated amount of HCl can be infused slowly over 6 to 24 hours with frequent, every 4 hours, ABG and electrolyte assessments to avoid too rapid of a correction or

TABLE 9.8

Causes of Metabolic Alkalosis[1,2]		
Sodium Chloride-Responsive (urine Cl <10 mEq/L)	Sodium Chloride-Resistant (urine Cl >20 mEq/L)	Unclassified
Gastrointestinal disorders —Vomiting —Gastric drainage —Villous adenoma of the colon —Chloride diarrhea Diuretic therapy Correction of chronic hypercapnia Cystic fibrosis Volume contraction or depletion	Excess mineralocorticoid activity —Hyperaldosteronism —Cushing's Syndrome —Bartter's Syndrome —Excessive licorice intake Severe potassium depletion Laxative abuse	Administration of bicarbonate or one of its precursors such as acetate Milk-alkali syndrome Massive blood transfusion Hypercalcemia Hypoparathyroidism Carbohydrate loading after starvation Large doses of carbenicillin or penicillin

over correction.[2] However, some authors[1] feel that use of these agents have potentially severe complications (such as hemolysis and tissue necrosis with HCl and ammonia toxicity with ammonium chloride) and do not work fast enough to prevent the above life threatening complications. Alternatively, the pH can be acutely decreased by controlling ventilation and elevating pCO_2. This requires pharmacological paralysis and sedation and mechanical hypoventilation; however, care should be taken to maintain adequate oxygenation.[1]

Conclusions

Acid-base disorders are frequently seen in critically ill patients and require an arterial blood gas for diagnosis. If the arterial pH is low (<7.35) then an acidemia is present; if it is high (>7.45), an alkalemia is present; and if it is normal, either there is a mixed acid-base disorder or no disorder present. Assessment of the pCO_2 will give an indication if there is a respiratory acidosis (<35 mmHg) or respiratory alkalosis (>45 mmHg), while examining the HCO_3^- level will give an indication if there is a metabolic acidosis (<22 mmHg) or metabolic alkalosis (>26 mmHg). Serum electrolytes and calculation of the serum anion gap can also be helpful especially in the assessment of metabolic acidosis. Utilizing either an acid-base nomogram or established guidelines for appropriate changes in pCO_2 and HCO_3^- with primary acid-base disorders, the acid-base disorder can be categorized as primary with or without compensation or a mixed acid-base disorder. Treatment is aimed at the underlying cause of the acid-base abnormality along with appropriate supportive care.

References

1. Shapiro JI, Kaehny WD. Pathogenesis and management of metabolic acidosis and alkalosis. In: Schrier RW, ed. *Renal and Electrolyte Disorders*. 5th ed. Philadelphia: Lippincott-Raven Publishers; 1997:130–171.
2. Whitmire SJ. Fluids and electrolytes. In: Matarese LE, Gottschlich MM, eds. *Contemporary Nutrition Support Practice: A Clinical Guide*. 1st ed. Philadelphia: WB Saunders Company; 1998:127–144.
3. Naitove A, Evans DB, Ihde JK. Fluid and Electrolyte Balance. In: Lawrence PF, Bilbao M, Bell RM, Dayton MT, eds. *Essentials of General Surgery*. 1st ed. Baltimore: Williams & Wilkins, 1988:48–68.
4. Androgue HJ. Normal chemistry and physiology of acid-base homeostasis. In: Massry SG, Glassock RJ, eds. *Textbook of Nephrology*. 3rd ed. Baltimore: Williams & Wilkins, 1995:413–424.
5. Shires III GT, Barber A, Shires GT. Fluid and electrolytes management of the surgical patient. In: Schwartz SI, Shires GT, Spencer FC, et al., eds. *Principles of Surgery*. 7th ed. New York: McGraw-Hill, 1999:53–75.
6. Kaehny WD. Pathogenesis and management of respiratory and mixed acid-base disorders. In Schrier RW, ed. *Renal and Electrolyte Disorders*. 5th ed. Philadelphia: Lippincott-Raven Publishers, 1997:172–191.
7. Cerra FB. Complications and their management. In: Cerra FB, ed. *Pocket Manual of Surgical Nutrition*. 1st ed. St. Louis: The C.V. Mosby Company, 1984:156–175.
8. Krzywda EA, Schulte WJ. Surgical nutrition. In: Condon RE, Nyhus LM, eds. *Manual of Surgical Therapeutics*. 9th ed. Boston: Little, Brown and Company, 1993:203–211.
9. Gump FE. Acid-base disturbances. In: Berk JL, Sampliner JE, Artz JS, Vinocur B, eds. *Handbook of Critical Care*. 1st ed. Boston: Little, Brown and Company, 1976:255–272.
10. Berlauk J. Acid-base balance. In: Cerra FB, ed. *Manual of Critical Care*. 1st ed. St. Louis: The C.V. Mosby Company, 1987:146–175.
11. Levy MM. An evidence-based evaluation of the use of sodium bicarbonate during cardiopulmonary resuscitation. *Critical Care Clinics*. 1998;14:457–483.
12. Forsythe SM, Schmidt GA. Sodium bicarbonate for the treatment of lactic acidosis. *Chest*. 2000;117:260–267.
13. Cooper DJ, Walley KR, Wiggs BR, et al. Bicarbonate does not improve hemodynamics in critically ill patients who have lactic acidosis: a prospective, controlled clinical study. *Ann Intern Med*. 1990;112:492–498.
14. Mathieu D, Neviere R, Billard V, et al. Effects of bicarbonate therapy on hemodynamics and tissue oxygenation in patients with lactic acidosis: a prospective, controlled clinical study. *Crit Care Med*. 1991;19:1352–1356.
15. Lever E, Jaspan JB. Sodium bicarbonate therapy in severe diabetic ketoacidosis. *Am J Med*. 1983;75:263–268.
16. Morris LR, Murphy MB, Kitabchi AE. Bicarbonate therapy in severe diabetic ketoacidosis. *Ann Intern Med*. 1986;105:836–840.
17. Hale PJ, Crase J, Nattrass M. Metabolic effects of bicarbonate in the treatment of diabetic ketoacidosis. *Br Med J (Clin Res Ed)*. 1984;289(6451):1035–1038.
18. Okuda Y, Adrogue HJ, Field JB, et al. Counterproductive effects of sodium bicarbonate in diabetic ketoacidosis. *J Clin Endocrinol Metab*. 1996;81:314–320.
19. Dybvik T, Strand T, Steen PA. Buffer therapy during out-of-hospital cardiopulmonary resuscitation. *Resuscitation*. 1995;2992:89–95.
20. Arieff AI. Efficacy of buffers in the management of cardiac arrest. *Crit Care Med*. 1998;26:1311–1313.
21. Nakashima K, Yamashita T, Kashiwagi S, et al. The effect of sodium bicarbonate on CBF and intracellular pH in man: stable Xe-CT and 31P-MRS. *Acta Neurol Scand Suppl*. 1996;166:96–98.
22. Bar-Joseph G. Is sodium bicarbonate therapy during cardiopulmonary resuscitation really detrimental? *Crit Care Med*. 2000;28:1693–1694.

CHAPTER

10 Hazards of Overfeeding

Gordon L. Jensen, M.D., Ph.D., Jeff Binkley, Pharm.D., B.C.N.S.P.

INTRODUCTION	111	RECOMMENDED APPROACH	114
MACRONUTRIENTS	111	CASE STUDY	115
REFEEDING SYNDROME	113	REFERENCES	117

Introduction

Appropriate feeding of the critically ill patient often involves more clinical judgment than adherence to a textbook assessment of the patient's needs. Practitioners should avoid the dictum that "more is better," and should instead heed the rule of "minimize harm." In the early days of parenteral nutrition practitioners often intentionally provided more macronutrients than patients required (hyperalimentation); thus, many patients developed complications that resulted not from the substrates themselves, but from the provision of excess energy (Table 10.1). Unrealistic expectations of what nutrition support can accomplish for the critically ill patient are a major concern. In highly stressed patients, desired goals of attaining positive nitrogen balance, meaningful weight gain, and increased visceral proteins are not often achievable outcomes. More realistic goals for providing nutrition to the critically ill patient should be to provide nutrients to support vital organ system functions and promote necessary immune and wound healing responses. Appropriate manifestations of inflammatory response, which include decline in visceral proteins, must not be misinterpreted as evidence that increased protein or other macronutrients are required. Hazards of overfeeding can include metabolic complications and organ system dysfunction.[1] Interventions to avoid overfeeding include appropriate initial patient assessment, scrutiny in follow-up, and utilization of a multidisciplinary team approach to patient management. Indeed, some authors have advocated modest underfeeding for selected acutely ill patients.[2–4] Nutrition support may be deferred altogether during acute resuscitation from shock.

Response to injury or inflammation is mediated by the cytokines interleukin-1, interleukin-6, and tumor necrosis factor, as well as the counter-regulatory hormones glucagon, epinephrine, cortisol, and growth hormone.[5–7] Increased hepatic glucose production and hyperglycemia often result.[8,9] The patient's resting energy expenditure may be elevated.[10] Erosion of body cell mass can result from muscle catabolism to provide amino acids for gluconeogenesis.[11,12] Over the short run (3 to 7 days), this catabolism is an appropriate and likely beneficial adaptation of inflammatory response. It is with the advent of modern critical care that patients may survive for protracted periods in highly pro-inflammatory states and suffer decline and adverse outcomes. It is telling that many survivors of prolonged critical illness suffer dramatic declines in body cell mass even with state-of-the-art nutrition support.

Macronutrients

Overfeeding with macronutrient substrates may further complicate metabolic response to injury or inflammatory condition.[1,13,14] The development of

TABLE 10.1

Impact of Overfeeding
Hyperglycemia
Phagocyte dysfunction
Osmotic diuresis
Increased risk of infection
Intracellular shifts of electrolytes
Excessive CO_2 Production
Respiratory failure
Prolonged mechanical ventilation requirements
Organ System Dysfunction
Hepatic dysfunction (steatosis)
Cardiac dysfunction (refeeding syndrome)
Respiratory dysfunction (refeeding syndrome)
Neurologic dysfunction (refeeding syndrome)

hepatic steatosis, or fatty liver, was more commonly encountered in the early days of parenteral nutrition.[15] The provision of large doses of carbohydrates promotes lipogenesis, ultimately resulting in accumulation of fat in the liver.[16,17] Hepatic steatosis can be recognized by increased liver function tests and hyperbilirubinemia. Complications associated with fatty liver can include intrahepatic cholestasis, hepatocyte dysfunction, and changes in immune competence from Kupffer cell dysfunction. Hepatic steatosis may be reversible when energy provision is appropriately reduced.[18]

Overfeeding with carbohydrates can also lead to hyperglycemia and, theoretically, increased carbon dioxide production. Hyperglycemia can cause a milieu of problems that include impaired immune function with phagocyte dysfunction, osmotic diuresis, and stimulation of insulin secretion.[9,19] Intracellular shifts of potassium and phosphorus may result. Patients with underlying diabetes or those receiving steroid therapy are at particularly increased risk of developing hyperglycemia when they are stressed. Rosmarin et al.[20] performed a retrospective study to evaluate whether there was an increased incidence of hyperglycemia occurred in patients who received total parenteral nutrition (TPN) but were not predisposed to hyperglycemia (n=102). All patients whose dextrose load was maintained at or below 4 mg/kg/min (n=19) were devoid of hyperglycemia. Eighteen of the 37 patients who received dextrose at a dose greater than 5 mg/kg/min exhibited hyperglycemia.

The end products of carbohydrate metabolism are energy, in the form of adenosine triphosphate (ATP), as well as carbon dioxide (CO_2) and water. Overfeeding with carbohydrates can therefore lead to increased CO_2 retention and ultimately may contribute to respiratory failure in patients with limited pulmonary capacity.[21–23] This can translate to prolonged requirements for mechanical ventilation or even precipitate respiratory failure in the marginally compensated patient.[24] A variety of enteral formulations have been marketed with reduced carbohydrate and increased lipid contents for patients with respiratory compromise. Such an approach is rarely indicated as long as overfeeding is not implemented.

Energy requirements of critically ill patients may be reasonably estimated at 25–35 kcal/kg/d.[25] The use of Harris-Benedict equations with empiric stress factors can also be utilized to determine energy goals.[25,26] Estimation of energy needs may be enhanced through the use of indirect calorimetry.[24,27] Measurement of oxygen consumption and carbon dioxide production using a metabolic cart for a short period of time, usually 30 minutes to an hour, allows the practitioner to measure resting energy expenditure (REE). Total energy expenditure can be estimated as 10% to 20% above the measured REE to cover fluctuations throughout the day. The subjective nature of this estimation requires clinical acumen to account for metabolic changes, body composition changes, and concurrent disease processes that impact total energy expenditure. Limitations of indirect calorimetry include inability to accommodate high FIO_2 (>0.70), difficulty in achieving steady state measurements, and perturbation by gas leaks or analyzer errors.[25] Gas exchange measurements with a metabolic cart study allows for calculation of the respiratory quotient (RQ), which is carbon dioxide production divided by oxygen consumption. The RQ reflects the utilization of substrates oxidized as energy sources and can aid the practitioner in determining if the patient is overfed, underfed, or appropriately fed. Given the limitations, personnel time, and cost of metabolic cart studies, these measurements may be best reserved for those patients who are otherwise difficult to assess and/or those who will require protracted nutrition support. Frail older persons may be particularly susceptible to overfeeding in view of their reduced lean mass.[29,30]

Overfeeding with fats can lead to hypertriglyceridemia.[27] Overzealous administration of fat emulsion can even lead to severe reactions described as fat overload syndrome, which is characterized by respiratory distress, coagulopathies, and abnormal liver function tests.[1,31–33] Hansen et al.[34] described lipid infusion in children and reported severe reactions in 2.5% of the 159 children observed. These severe reactions were allergic reactions that were associated with doses greater than 4 grams per kilogram of body weight. In reports of children who received home TPN, symptoms developed after 6 weeks of administration of 3.2 g/kg of body weight over 14 hours, after 2 months of a dose of 5.4 g/kg over 12 hours daily, and after 24 hours of a dose of 3.4 g/kg over 10 hours. In adults, fat overload syndrome has been reported after 100 grams or more of lipids per day were infused for 2 to 29 days.[35–37] A report of lipid dosing of 2.5 grams or less per kilogram of body weight per day over 4 hours for up to 2 weeks showed no evidence of intolerance.[34]

Immune compromise is theorized as a possible outcome from overfeeding with fats.[38–40] The reticuloendothial system (RES) normally utilizes phagocytosis and cytokine secretion for immune defense. RES dysfunction has been described in animals and humans receiving intravenous fat emulsion, with impairment of Kupffer cell activity as the proposed primary mechanism.[41] One study[38] found a dose response relationship between intravenous fat emulsion (IVFE) and RES dysfunction; another study[42] suggested that a continuous infusion of IVFE as a part of a total nutrient admixture (TNA) had no adverse impact upon RES system function. Therefore, IVFEs are most likely best tolerated in moderate doses provided as a continuous infusion. Pro-inflammatory pathways have the potential to be fueled with n6 fats found in conventional lipid emulsions. Alternative lipid substrates like n3 fats are being actively studied. In order to avoid immune dysfunction associated with standard lipid emulsion infusion, it is recommended that fat be administered continuously at a dose that approximates one-third of the total energy prescription (typical dosing 30–70 g of fat).

Amino acids are deaminated in the liver to produce urea, which circulates in the bloodstream and is excreted by the kidneys.[43] When the rate of production exceeds the rate of excretion, there is a build up of urea nitrogen in the blood, known as azotemia. During stress, cytokine-mediated catabolism of skeletal muscle occurs. Adrenal hormones and catecholamines also promote muscle catabolism. Acutely ill patients with an increase in proteolysis combined with large amounts of amino acid intake from aggressive feeding may be predisposed to azotemia.[44] Additionally, practitioners should moderate amino acid load for patients with acute renal failure who are not being dialyzed and for patients with severe hepatic failure or hepatic encephalopathy.

Refeeding Syndrome

Patients with severe weight loss or poor nutrient intake can experience the syndrome of "refeeding." Refeeding syndrome has been defined as both the metabolic and physiologic consequences associated with the depletion, repletion, and compartmental shifts of phosphorus, potassium, and magnesium as well as alterations in glucose metabolism and fluid status[45] (see Table 10.2). Vitamin deficiencies may also occur. Accompanying clinical sequellae can be significant if the intracellular shifts of electrolytes are severe; indeed, death may result from overzealous refeeding.[46] Although phosphorus depletion has been the focus of studies in the past, Brooks and Melnik[47] suggest that the refeeding syndrome should be more broadly characterized as a syndrome of generalized fluid and electrolyte imbalance.

TABLE 10.2

Effects of Refeeding Syndrome
Hypophosphatemia
Altered cardiac function
Altered hematologic effects
Hepatic dysfunction
Neuromuscular effects
Respiratory effects
Hypokalemia
Cardiac
Gastrointestinal effects
Metabolic effects
Neuromuscular effects
Renal effects
Hypomagnesemia
Cardiac effects
Gastrointestinal effects
Neuromuscular effects
Glucose and Fluid Intolerance

First observed after World War II, the refeeding syndrome has been reported for over 50 years. In the 1940s, when starvation victims in Leningrad, the Netherlands, and Japan were liberated, malnourished subjects developed hypertension, cardiac insufficiency, peripheral edema, coma, and convulsions that were temporally related to the restoration of normal food and fluid intake.[48–49] The Minnesota Experiment in the 1940s studied previously healthy conscientious objectors who underwent semi-starvation for six months.[50] During the subsequent refeeding phase, some volunteers experienced cardiac failure. When parenteral nutrition solutions were fed to chronically ill patients in the 1970s and 1980s, the severe cardiopulmonary and neurologic complications associated with refeeding were "rediscovered."

Paresthesias, convulsions, and coma were reported in three patients who had experienced significant weight loss and were hypophosphatemic.[51] Within a week after the initiation of hypercaloric infusions, two of the patients experienced paresthesias and convulsions, while the third died after becoming comatose. In another report two cases of chronically malnourished patients whose baseline phosphorus levels were normal became severely hypophosphatemic (1.1 mg/dL and 0.7 mg/dL, respectively) within 24 hours after parenteral nutrition was initiated, and developed sudden cardiopulmonary decompensation resulting in death within 48 hours.[46]

Although serum laboratory values may be within normal range, total body stores of electrolytes may be depleted from starvation. Therefore, it is important to identify malnourished patients who may be at risk for refeeding syndrome even when serum laboratory profiles at first appear normal. In a retrospective review by Thompson and Hodges[52] examining 61 patients who received 68 courses of parenteral nutrition, 12% of patients had low serum phosphorus levels prior to feeding; however, 42% of patients developed hypophosphatemia during the initiation of parenteral nutrition. Additionally, malnourished patients who are refed orally or enterally may also be at risk for developing hypophosphatemia. Severe hypophosphatemia was observed in 25 postoperative surgical intensive care unit patients after they were orally fed.[53] The levels corrected after oral repletion of phosphates. Warning signs for risk for refeeding syndrome include a history of weight loss, disease states associated with weight loss, and behaviors associated with poor nutrient intake.

Patients with a history of semi-starvation will exhibit signs of marasmus, including loss of body mass that is readily detected by weight measurements and anthropometry. Critically ill patients will also generally have low visceral proteins, such as albumin or prealbumin, in response to acute inflammatory stress or injury. Fluid retention and edema are often associated with reduced visceral protein status, rendering body weight and anthropometrics of limited utility. Patients with weight loss of greater than 10% of usual body weight should, however, signal the practitioner to approach nutrition repletion cautiously. Conditions associated with weight loss would include malabsorption from intestinal disease or chemotherapy, excessive diarrhea, short bowel syndrome, enteroenteric fistulae, and recent gastrointestinal surgery. Behaviors associated with poor nutrient intake may include anorexia nervosa, substance abuse, and fad diets.

During pure chronic starvation, a number of metabolic changes occur. Endogenous fat oxidation becomes the primary source of energy, with the stimulation of ketone body production. Energy expenditure declines. As refeeding is initiated, glucose rapidly shifts to become the primary fuel source. This results in a shift from a hypoinsulinemic state to one of hyperinsulinemia. As glycolysis occurs, the demand for phosphorus increases as a necessary component in the production of phosphorylated intermediates such as adenosine triphosphate (ATP), 2,3-Diphosphoglycerate (2-3DPG), and glycerol-3-phosphate dehydrogenase (G-3-PD).[53] Increased demand for phosphorus and intracellular shifts induced by insulin promote a decrease in extracellular phosphorus. In addition, potassium and magnesium are shifted intracellularly. Fluid retention is common. Cardiac decompensation and neuromuscular dysfunction may be complications of these electrolyte and fluid imbalances.[48] Patients with severe malnutrition may suffer nutritional cardiomyopathy with loss of myocardium and limited cardiac reserve to compensate for increased fluid challenge. Congestive heart failure and arrhythmias may result.

Thiamine deficiency may play a role in the refeeding syndrome, but its exact contribution has not been elucidated. Malnourished individuals are often deficient in thiamine stores. Patients with alcohol abuse are often considered at risk for Wernicke's encephalopathy because of their decreased thiamine stores, but any malnourished patient can be at risk.[54] The cardiomyopathies of thiamine deficiency and alcohol abuse can contribute to hemodynamic compromise. Thiamine is an important cofactor in carbohydrate metabolism; thus, the risk of acute deficiency can be increased in malnourished patients who are administered carbohydrates or dextrose.

Recommended Approach

Precautions used to prevent the refeeding syndrome include knowledge of the phenomenon and identifying patients at risk.[45] Severely malnourished patients should receive empiric thiamine administration acutely. Abnormalities of potassium, phosphorus, or magnesium should be addressed prior to the initiation of nutrition support, whether parenteral or enteral. Strict recordings of fluid intake and output, daily weights, and daily electrolytes should be monitored in patients at risk. Excessive weight gain due to fluid retention may promote fluid overload and may precipitate heart failure. Additional intravenous fluids and sodium should be minimized to the degree feasible. Invasive procedures and instrumentation should be avoided if possible. Electrocardiogram changes with low voltage and prolonged Q-T interval may indicate nutritional cardiomyopathy. Nutrition support should be initiated slowly and advanced over several days as the patient exhibits tolerance to the regimen. Declines in levels of potassium, magnesium, and phosphorus should be restored prior to any further advance toward protein and calorie goals.

Interventions to prevent overfeeding include appropriate patient assessment, careful selection of the nutrition regimen, sensible monitoring, and a multidisciplinary team approach to nutrition management. Appropriate assessment in critical care uses a combination of objective parameters such as body weight and visceral proteins but also requires the subjective clinical acumen of the practitioner. Regimen selection includes route of administration, as well as prescription of total daily doses of macronutrients and micronutrients. Recognition of all potential sources of dextrose calories, including intravenous fluids used for volume maintenance and occasionally dialysate solutions for peritoneal dialysis or continuous veno-venous hemodialysis, must be taken into account. Sedative and antifungal drugs that are administered in lipid emulsions should also be considered. The nutrition regimen, whether parenteral or enteral, should be designed carefully to approximate the patient's energy needs. Several days of cautious underfeeding are often required while fluid, electrolyte, and other concerns are resolved.

Practitioners should anticipate adverse refeeding sequellae. For example, with the severely malnourished patient who is started on a nutrition regimen, the practitioner can anticipate a shift of electrolytes and can empirically give additional amounts of potassium, phosphorus, and magnesium even when the patient's baseline serum levels are normal. Empiric supplementation of thiamine, folate, and vitamin B_{12} is often appropriate.

A multidisciplinary team approach to nutrition management may help to minimize complications as well as overall healthcare costs.[55,56] Severe undernutrition does not happen overnight but usually over weeks and months. Accordingly it often takes weeks or months to fully resuscitate the undernourished patient. There are few nutrition "emergencies"; however, the practitioner should recognize that the patient at risk for severe refeeding difficulties warrants cautious management by skilled nutrition consultants.

Case Study

The following hypothetical case demonstrates the multiple hazards of overfeeding a critically ill patient. JT is a 23-year-old male brought to the Emergency Department after he sustained a gasoline burn to his face, upper chest, and left upper and lower extremities. He was intubated in the field and fluid resuscitated. JT was evaluated and found to have second- and third-degree burns on 25% total body surface area. After 2 days of hemodynamic instability, the patient resuscitated. Questioning his family members, revealed that JT had a history of active Crohn's disease with a recent exacerbation and a 15-pound weight loss. He was on steroid therapy and received stress steroid coverage in the setting of his burn injury. Physical findings on hospital day 3 were as follows:

Patient Height 175 cm (69 inches)
Weight (admission) 42 kg
Weight (current) 58 kg

Physical Exam:

General: Intubated, sedated, with facial burns, singed eyelashes and eyebrows

Vitals:

Temperature 38.7

Pulse 120

Blood Pressure 105/56

Respirations 20

Oropharynx: Lips swollen, mucus membranes moist, pink, without lesions

Neck: Supple with second degree burns, dressing intact, no lymphadenopathy

Respiratory: Ventilated, lung sounds coarse, ronchi scattered throughout

Skin: Second and third degree burns

Gastrointestinal: Abdomen soft, nontender, bowel sounds hypoactive

Neurologic: Sedated

Extremities: Second and third degree burns

Laboratory Values:

WBC Count 15.3×10^3 cells/mm^3
(normal 4.8–10.8 $\times 10^3$ cells/mm^3)

Hemoglobin 6.5 mmol/L
(normal 8.7–11.2 mmol/L)

Hematocrit 0.26
(normal 0.42–0.52)

RBC Count 3.5×10^{12} cells/L
(normal 4.6–6.2 $\times 10^{12}$ cells/L)

Sodium 135 mEq/L
(normal 135–145 mEq/L)

Potassium 3.1 mEq/L
(normal 3.5–4.5 mEq/L)

Chloride 110 mEq/L
(normal 95–110 mEq/L)

CO_2 15 mmol/L
(normal 20–30 mmol/L)

BUN 14 mg/dL
(normal 8–15 mg/dL)

Creatinine 1.0 mg/dL
(normal 0.5–1.0 mg/dL)

Glucose 188 mg/dL
(normal 85–120 mg/dL)

Magnesium 1.6 mEq/L
(normal 1.8–2.5 mEq/L)

Phosphorus 2.1 mmol/L
(normal 2.5–4.5 mmol/L)

Calcium (ionized) 3.89 mEq/L
(normal 4–4.5 mEq/L)

Albumin 2.1 mg/dL
(normal 3.5–4.5 mg/dL)

The house officer suspected that the patient's degree of catabolism was great, and thus he wanted to provide a large amount of energy to the patient. Because of the nature of his facial burns, a nasoenteric feeding tube could not be readily placed at the onset. Instead, the resident ordered TPN and started the following regimen: amino acids 120 grams (480 kcal), dextrose 353 grams (1200 kcal), lipids 80 grams (720 kcal) for a total of 2400 kcal, which represented 2.8 g/kg protein and 57 kcal/kg of body weight (42 kg). He selected the standard electrolyte concentrations for TPN for the first bag. On the morning after the first TPN bag was administered, the following labs were observed:

Laboratory Values:

WBC Count 19.3×10^3 cells/mm^3
(normal 4.8–10.8 $\times 10^3$ cells/mm^3)

Hemoglobin 6.8 mmol/L
(normal 8.7–11.2 mmol/L)

Hematocrit 0.28
(normal 0.42–0.52)

RBC Count 3.9×10^{12} cells/L
(normal 4.6–6.2 $\times 10^{12}$ cells/L)

Sodium 130 mEq/L
(normal 135–145 mEq/L)

Potassium 2.8 mEq/L
(normal 3.5–4.5 mEq/L)

Chloride 110 mEq/L
(normal 95–110 mEq/L)

CO_2 16 mmol/L
(normal 20–30 mmol/L)

BUN 14 mg/dL
(normal 8–15 mg/dL)

Creatinine 1.0 mg/dL
(normal 0.5–1.0 mg/dL)

Glucose 454 mg/dL
(normal 85–120 mg/dL)

Magnesium 1.4 mEq/L
(normal 1.8–2.5 mEq/L)

Phosphorus 1.3 mmol/L
(normal 2.5–4.5 mmol/L)

Calcium (ionized) 3.89 mEq/L
(normal 4–4.5 mEq/L)

Albumin 2.1 mg/dL
(normal 3.5–4.5 mg/dL)

JT exhibited at least two signs of overfeeding related to his initial TPN: hyperglycemia and the refeeding syndrome. He demonstrates hyperglycemia due to an aggressive nutrition regimen in a severely stressed individual receiving steroid therapy. Additionally, the intracellular shifts of potassium, phosphorus, and magnesium are classic findings of a patient with refeeding issues. In light of his confounding history of Crohn's disease, a more appropriate approach to prescribe an initial TPN for JT would include the following:

1. Select more moderate initial goals for his nutrition intervention (for example, 1.8 g protein/kg and 25–30 kcal/kg adjusted weight as a target).
2. Start the parenteral nutrition below his goals and monitor the patient's glucose and electrolyte tolerance.
3. Anticipate electrolyte shifts with the provision of energy. The concentrations of potassium, phosphorus, and magnesium should have been empirically increased in the parenteral nutrition.
4. Expect hyperglycemia since he already demonstrated elevated blood sugar levels prior to the initiation of TPN. A reasonable amount of insulin could have been safely administered in the TPN with additional sliding scale insulin coverage to manage his sugars.

JT remained on the house officer's formulation for 2 days. His serum blood concentration range was 256–452 mg/dL, with sliding scale insulin coverage provided every 4 hours. He was started on an insulin drip for better control. The multidisciplinary Nutrition Support Team (NST) evaluated JT on the morning after the second TPN had been administered. The consult service recommended that the nutrition regimen be adjusted to provide fewer calories while the patient demonstrated the signs of stress and intolerance to the current regimen. The NST suggested that a metabolic cart study might aid in determining the patient's energy requirements. The test was performed, and the following results were evaluated: Measured Energy Expenditure (MEE) 1800 kcal, Respiratory Quotient (RQ) 1.09. Because the ordered nutrition regimen delivered 600 kcal more energy than his measured needs and because the respiratory quotient was also consistent with overfeeding, the house staff agreed to reduce the macronutrient content of his regimen.

References

1. Klein, CJ, Stanek GS, Wiles CE. Overfeeding macronutrients to critically ill adults: metabolic complications. *J Am Dietetic Assoc.* 1998;98:795–805.
2. Choban PS, Burge JC, Scales D, Flancbaum L. Hypoenergetic nutrition support in hospitalized obese patients: a simplified method for clinical application. *Am J Clin Nutr.* 1997;66:546–550.
3. Shikora SA, Jensen GL. Hypoenergetic nutrition support in hospitalized obese patients. *Am J Clin Nutr.* 1997;66: 679–680.
4. Patino JF, de Pimiento SE, Vergara A, et al. Hypocaloric support in the critically ill. *World J Surg.* 1999;23:553–559.
5. Kushner I. Regulation of the acute phase response by cytokines. *Perspect Biol Med.* 1993;36:611–622.
6. Michie HR. Metabolism of sepsis and multiple organ failure. *World J Surg.* 1996;20:460–464.
7. Roubenoff R. Inflammatory and hormonal mediators of cachexia. *J Nutr.* 1997;127 (supplement):1014S–1016S.
8. Chiolero R, Revelly JP, Tappy L. Energy metabolism in sepsis and injury. *Nutrition.* 1997;13:45S–51S.
9. McMahon MM, Rizza RA. Nutrition support in hospitalized patients with diabetes mellitus. *Mayo Clin Proc.* 1996; 71:587–594.
10. Vrees MD, Albina JE. Metabolic Response to Illness and Its Mediators. In: Rombeau JL, Caldwell MD, eds. *Clinical Nutrition: Parenteral Nutrition.* 3rd ed. Philadelphia: WB Saunders; 2001:21–34.
11. Roubenoff R, Roubenoff RA, Cannon JG, et al. Rheumatoid cachexia: cytokine driven hypermetabolism and loss of lean mass in chronic inflammation. *J Clin Invest.* 1994;93: 2379–2386.
12. Roubenoff R, Roubenoff RA, Ward LM, et al. Rheumatoid cachexia: depletion of lean body mass in rheumatoid arthritis. Possible associations with tumor necrosis factor. *J Rheumatol.* 1992;19:1505–10.
13. Chan S, McCowen KC, Blackburn GL. Nutrition management in the ICU. *Chest.* 1999;115:145S–148S.
14. Jebb SA, Prentice AM, Goldberg GR, et al. Changes in macronutrient tolerance balance during over- and underfeeding assessed by 12-d continuous whole-body calorimetry. *Am J Clin Nutr.* 1996;64:259–266.
15. Sax HC, Bower RH. Hepatic complications of total parenteral nutrition. *J Parenter Enteral Nutr.* 1988;12:615–618.
16. Li S, Nussbaum MS, Teague D, et al. Increasing dextrose concentrations in total parenteral nutrition (TPN) causes alterations in hepatic morphology and plasma levels of insulin and glucagon in rats. *J Surg Res.* 1988;4:639–648.
17. Hall RI, Grant JP, Ross LH, et al. Pathogenesis of hepatic steatosis in the parenterally fed rat. *J Clin Invest.* 1984;74: 1658–1668.
18. Nussbaum MS, Li S, Bower RH, et al. Addition of lipid to total parenteral nutrition prevents hepatic steatosis in rats by lowering the portal venous insulin/glucagon ratio. *J Parenter Enteral Nutr.* 1992;16:106–109.
19. Yamamoto T. Metabolic response to glucose overload in surgical stress: energy disposal in brown adipose tissue. *Surg Today Jpn J Surg.* 1996;26:151–157.
20. Rosmarin DK, Wordlaw GM, Mirtallo J. Hyperglycemia associated with high, continuous infusion rates of total parenteral nutrition dextrose. *Nutr Clin Pract.* 1996;11: 151–156.
21. Sullivan DJ, Marty TL, Barton RG. A case of overfeeding complicating the management of adult respiratory distress syndrome. *Nutrition.* 1995;11:375–378.
22. Askanazi J, Elwyn DH, Silverberg BS, et al. Respiratory distress secondary to a high carbohydrate load: a case report. *Surgery.* 1980;87:596.
23. Askanazi J, Rosenbaum SH. Respiratory changes induced by the large glucose loads of total parenteral nutrition. *JAMA.* 1990;234:1444.
24. Liposky JM, Nelson LD. Ventilatory response to high caloric loads in critically ill patients. *Crit Care Med.* 1994;22: 796–802.
25. Frankenfield D. Energy and Macrosubstrate Requirements. In: Gottschlich, MM, ed. *The Science and Practice of Nutrition Support: A Core-Based Curriculum.* Dubuque: Kendall/Hunt Publishing Company; 2001:31–52.
26. Harris JA, Benedict FG. *A Biometric Study of Basal Metabolism in Man.* Publication No. 279. Washington, DC: Carnegie Institute; 1919.
27. Long CL, Schaffel N, Geiger JW, et al. Metabolic response to injury and illness: Estimation of energy and protein needs from indirect calorimetry and nitrogen balance. *J Parenter Enteral Nutr.* 1979;18:398–403.
28. Trujillo EB, Chertow GM, Jacobs DO. Metabolic Assessment. In: Rombeau JL, Caldwell MD, eds. *Clinical Nutrition: Parenteral Nutrition.* 3rd ed., Philadelphia: WB Saunders; 2001:80–108.
29. Sullivan DH, Sun S, Walls RC. Protein energy undernutrition among elderly hospitalized patients. A prospective study. *JAMA.* 1999;281:2013–2019.
30. Anderson CF, Moxness K, Meister J, et al. The sensitivity and specificity of nutrition-related variables in relationship to the duration of hospital stay and rate of complications. *Mayo Clin Proc.* 1984;59:477–483.
31. Belin RP, Bivins BA, Jona JZ, et al. Fat overload with a 10% soybean emulsion. *Arch Surg.* 1976;111:1391–1393.
32. Haber LM, Hawkins EP, Seilheimer DK, et al. Fat overload syndrome: an autopsy study with evaluation of the coagulopathy. *Am J Clin Pathol.* 1988;89:223–227.
33. Meng HC, Kuyama T, Thompson SW, et al. Toxicity testing of fat emulsions, I: tolerance study of long-term intravenous administration of intralipid in rats. *Am J Clin Nutr.* 1965;16:29–36.

34. Hansen LM, Hardie WR, Hildago J. Fat emulsion for intravenous administration: clinical experience with Intralipid 10%. *Ann Surg.* 1976;184:80–88.

35. Roth B, Nilsson-Ehle P, Eliasson I. Possible role of short-term nutrition with fat emulsions for development of haemophagocytosis with multiple organ failure in a patient with traumatic brain injury. *Intensive Care Med.* 1993;19: 111–114.

36. Freund U, Krausz Y, Levij IS, et al. Iatrogenic lipidosis following prolonged intravenous hyperalimentation. *Am J Clin Nutr.* 1975;28:1156–1160.

37. Taylor RF, Buckner CD. Fat overload from 10 percent soybean oil emulsion in a marrow transplant recipient. *West J Med.* 1982;136:345–349.

38. Seidner DL, Mascioli EA, Istfan NW, et al. Effects of long-chain triglyceride emulsions on reticuloendothelial system function in humans. *J Parenter Enteral Nutr.* 1989; 13:614.

39. Klein S, Miles JM. Metabolic effects of long-chain and medium-chain triglycerides in humans. *J Parenter Enteral Nutr.* 1994;18:396–397.

40. Battistella FD, Widergren JT, Anderson JT, et al. A prospective, randomized trial of intravenous fat emulsion administration in trauma victims requiring parenteral nutrition. *J Trauma: Injury, Infection, and Critical Care.* 1997;43: 52–58.

41. Driscoll DF, Adolph M, Bistrian BR. Lipid Emulsions in Parenteral Nutrition. In: Rombeau JL, Caldwell MD, eds. *Clinical Nutrition: Parenteral Nutrition.* 3rd ed., Philadelphia: WB Saunders; 2001:35–59.

42. Jensen GL, Mascioli EA, Seidner DL, et al. Parenteral infusion of long and medium-chain triglycerides and reticuloendothelial system function in man. *J Parenter Enteral Nutr.* 1990;14:467–471.

43. Fan ST, Poon RTP. Liver Disease and Parenteral Nutrition. In: Rombeau JL, Caldwell MD, eds. *Clinical Nutrition: Parenteral Nutrition.* 3rd ed., Philadelphia:WB Saunders; 2001:392–406.

44. Matarese LE. Metabolic Complications of Parenteral Nutrition Therapy. In: Gottschlich, MM, ed. *The Science and Practice of Nutrition Support: A Core-Based Curriculum.* Dubuque: Kendall/Hunt Publishing Company; 2001:269–286.

45. Solomon SM, Kirby DF. The refeeding syndrome: a review. *J Parenter Enteral Nutr.* 1990;14:90–97.

46. Weinsier RL, Krundieck CL. Death resulting from overzealous total parenteral nutrition: the refeeding syndrome revisited. *Am J Clin Nutr.* 1981;34:393–399.

47. Brooks MJ, and Melnik G. The refeeding syndrome: an approach to understanding its complications and preventing its occurrence. *Pharmacotherapy.* 1995;15:713–726.

48. Brozek J, Chapman CB, Keys A. Drastic food restriction: Effect on cardiovascular dynamics in normotensive and hypertensive conditions. *JAMA.* 1948;137:1569–1574.

49. Schnitker MA, Mattman PE, Bliss TL. A clinical study of malnutrition in Japanese prisoners of war. *Ann Intern Med.* 1951;35:69–96.

50. Keys A, Brozek J, Henschel A, et al. *The Biology of Human Starvation*, Vols 1,2. Minneapolis: University of Minnesota Press, 1950.

51. Silvas SE, Paragas Jr, PD. Paresthesias, weakness, seizures, and hypophosphatemia in patients receiving hyperalimentation. *Gastroenterology.* 1972;62:513–520.

52. Thompson JS, Hodges RE. Preventing hypophosphatemia during total parenteral nutrition. *J Parenter Enteral Nutr.* 1984;8:137–139.

53. Hyek ME, Eisenberg PG. Severe hypophosphatemia following the institution of enteral feedings. *Arch Surg.* 1989; 124:1325–1328.

54. Reuler JB, Girard DE, Cooney TG: Wernicke's encephalopathy. *N Engl J Med.* 1985;312:1035–1039.

55. ChrisAnderson D, Heimburger DC, Morgan SL, et al. Metabolic complications of total parenteral nutrition: effects of a nutrition support service. *J Parenter Enteral Nutr.* 1996;20:206–210.

56. Trujillo EB, Young LS, Chertow GM, et al. Metabolic and monetary costs of avoidable parenteral nutrition use. *J Parenter Enteral Nutr.* 1999;23:109–113.

CHAPTER

11 Parenteral vs. Enteral Nutrition

Kenneth A. Kudsk, M.D.

INTRODUCTION 119

ENTERAL VS. PARENTERAL FEEDING: IMPACT ON CLINICAL OUTCOME 119

STUDIES OF ENTERAL VS. PARENTERAL FEEDING IN TRAUMA PATIENTS 120

Blunt and Penetrating Torso Trauma 120

Head Injury 122

Summary of Trauma Studies 122

STUDIES OF ENTERAL VS. PARENTERAL FEEDING IN NONTRAUMA PATIENTS 122

General Surgical Patients 122

Inflammatory Bowel Disease 123

Pancreatitis 123

Transplantation 124

Pediatric Studies 124

HYPOTHESES FOR REDUCED SEPTIC COMPLICATIONS WITH ENTERAL DELIVERY OF NUTRIENTS 124

Hyperglycemia and Increased Incidence of Infectious Complications with TPN 124

Mucosal Alterations with Increases in Gut Permeability and Bacterial Translocation 125

Alterations in Small Intestinal Microcirculation and Alterations in the Response to Inflammation 126

Mucosal Immunity 127

CONCLUSIONS 128

REFERENCES 128

Introduction

Prior to the late 1960s, there was no safe and practical way to deliver adequate amounts of macro- and micronutrients to a patient with a nonfunctional gastrointestinal tract due to fistula, ileus, or loss of absorptive surface. Central vein infusion of concentrated nutrients provided an effective solution to this problem, preventing progressive starvation-induced malnutrition and loss of lean tissue that further depressed the ability to heal wounds and fight infection.[1] In the 1980s, the first clinical[2,3] and laboratory evidence[4,5] surfaced, suggesting that additional benefits are gained when nutrients are delivered enterally that are not gained when similar nutrients are provided parenterally. While reduction in cost with enteral feeding is generally accepted, more compelling reasons to provide enteral nutrition would be improved host defenses, reduced infectious complications, and maintenance of a more "physiologic" state of the GI tract. Certainly, enteral feeding allows more diverse and complex nutrients that can be provided parenterally; for example, in the United States, parenteral supplemental fat is limited to omega-6 fatty acids while varying combinations of saturated, unsaturated, and polyunsaturated fatty acids containing both omega-3 and omega-6 fatty acids can be provided enterally. Experimentally and clinically, these compounds are capable of exerting profound biochemical effects.[6] However, enteral provision of nutrients and the ability to advance to a desirable nutrient rate requires significant time and effort.

Enteral vs. Parenteral Feeding: Impact on Clinical Outcome

Nutrition support—whether parenteral or enteral—is a highly technical therapy capable of inducing both benefits and injury. Interpretation of results from randomized clinical studies of either parenteral or enteral feeding requires consideration of the risk-benefit ratio of patients entered into the study. For example, if patients with little likelihood of developing nutrition-related complications are randomized into clinical trials, results will only demonstrate the risk of therapy with little likelihood of showing benefit. However, if patient selection is limited to groups with increased risk of (mal)nutrition-related complications, the actual advantage (and risk) of the therapy may be established in patients who might benefit from therapy. The Veterans Administration (VA) study of 395 patients requiring laparotomy or noncardiac thoracotomy demonstrates this effect.[7] Patients were randomized to 7 to 15 days of preoperative nutrition or no specialized nutrition support and evaluated for postoperative complications. Rates of major noninfectious complications, such as wound or anastomotic dehiscence, were similar between unfed and parenterally fed patients with *mild to moderate malnutrition*, but parenterally fed patients sustained significantly more infectious complications. However, patients with preexisting *severe* malnutrition sustained a significant reduction in the same major noninfectious complications with a trend toward a reduction in infectious complications. Thus, parenteral nutrition increased the rate of complications in patients at low risk of nutrition-related complications but improved outcome in a select high-risk group. Similarly, Brennan et al.[8] randomized 117 mildly malnourished patients to either postoperative parenteral nutrition or to IV fluids alone. In this relatively low nutritionally at-risk patient population, infectious complications were significantly greater in parenterally fed patients due to a higher rate of intra-abdominal abscess formation. Therefore, interpretation of clinical studies warrants an examination of both the clinical outcome as well as the patient population entered into the clinical trials to assess the clinical effectiveness of one therapy versus another.

Studies of Enteral vs. Parenteral Feeding in Trauma Patients

Blunt and Penetrating Torso Trauma

Most studies comparing routes of feeding that show a reduction in septic morbidity have been in patients sustaining blunt and penetrating trauma. Moore et al.[3] first randomized moderately severely injured trauma patients using the Abdominal Trauma Index (ATI). The ATI (Table 11.1) allows calculation of the risk of post-injury sepsis at the time of surgery by quantifying the number of organs injured within the peritoneal cavity and their likelihood of causing subsequent septic complications.[9] Organs at high risk of septic complications include major vascular injuries and injuries to the colon, pancreas, liver, or duodenum. By multiplying the risk factor of that organ by magnitude of injury to that organ and summing the individual scores, risk for sepsis can be predicted. With an ATI of 15 or greater, the incidence of sepsis is approximately 16%; if the ATI is ≥25, 25%; if the ATI is ≥35, 43%; or if the ATI is ≥45, a sepsis rate of 60% is expected. The ability to successfully advance tube feedings to goal rate is more difficult in patients with an ATI >40, blood loss >25 units in 2 hours, or with severe pelvic fractures.[10] In this study, only patients with an ATI between 15 and 40 were recruited so that the feeding rate could be advanced to 80% of goal within 3 days. Patients received either early enteral feeding with a defined formula diet or IV fluids alone. TPN was provided to 26% of unfed patients who did not tolerate a diet by the fifth postoperative day. Early enteral feeding significantly reduced the incidence of infectious complications (primarily intra-abdominal abscess) compared with the unfed controls. In a follow-up study,[11] the Denver group randomized moderately severely injured patients with similar ATI values to either early enteral or early parenteral feeding. Septic complications, primarily pneumonia, were significantly reduced in patients receiving enteral feedings, but the incidence of intra-abdominal abscess also was lower.

In a larger study which included a more severely injured group, Kudsk[12] randomized patients to either enteral feeding with a chemically defined diet or an isonitrogenous, isocaloric parenteral solution and documented significant reductions in pneumonia, intra-abdominal abscess, and line sepsis with early enteral feeding. Patients were classified both by ATI and the Injury Severity Score (ISS), a scoring system which calculates the magnitude of injury to the three most severely injured body systems, including head, face and neck, chest, abdomen, soft tissues, and lower extremities.[13] In general, an ISS >19–20 is considered severely injured. In this study, benefits of enteral feeding were primarily found in the most severely injured patients, i.e., those with an ATI ≥25 or an ISS >20. Patients with lesser injuries had no significant differences in outcome because of the low incidence of infectious complications.

Two studies demonstrated no significant reduction in infectious complications with early enteral feeding after trauma. Adams et al.[14] randomized patients to jejunal or parenteral feeding after trauma. Both the enteral formula and the rate of administration were changed approximately one-third of the way through this study. Although there were no differences in infectious complications, patients receiving the enteral diet had three times as many severe chest injuries, three times as many severe pelvic fractures, nearly twice as many severe head injuries, and six times as many severe soft tissue injuries. Fever, leukocytosis, infiltrates, and significant growth on sputum cultures were used to diagnose pneumonia, but these criteria over diagnose the incidence of pneumonia, particularly with underlying lung injury.[15] With the chest injuries, increased severity of injury, and the inaccuracy of the diagnosis of pneumonia after chest trauma, the comparability of the patient populations is questionable.

TABLE 11.1

Calculated Risk of Sepsis by the Abdominal Trauma Index (ATI)

Organ Injured	Risk Factor	Scoring	Organ Injured	Risk Factor	Scoring
High Risk			**Low Risk**		
Pancreas	(5)	1. Tangential 2. Through-and-through (duct intact) 3. Major debridement or distal duct injury 4. Proximal duct injury 5. Pancreaticoduodenectomy	Kidney	(2)	1. Nonbleeding 2. Minor debridement or suturing 3. Major debridement 4. Pedicle or major calyceal 5. Nephrectomy
Large intestine	(5)	1. Serosal 2. Single wall 3. <25% wall 4. >25% wall 5. Colon wall and blood supply	Ureter	(2)	1. Contusion 2. Laceration 3. Minor debridement 4. Segmental resection 5. Reconstruction
Major vascular	(5)	1. <25% wall 2. >25% wall 3. Complete transection 4. Interposition grafting or bypass 5. Ligation	Bladder	(1)	1. Single wall 2. Through-and-through 3. Debridement 4. Wedge resection 5. Reconstruction
Moderately High Risk					
Duodenum	(4)	1. Single wall 2. <25% wall 3. >25% wall 4. Duodenal wall and blood supply 5. Pancreaticoduodenectomy	Extrahepatic Biliary	(1)	1. Contusion 2. Cholecystectomy 3. <25% wall 4. >25% wall 5. Biliary enteric reconstruction
Liver	(4)	1. Nonbleeding peripheral 2. Bleeding, central, or minor debridement 3. Major debridement or hepatic artery ligation 4. Lobectomy 5. Lobectomy with caval repair or extensive bilobar debridement	Bone	(1)	1. Periosteum 2. Cortex 3. Through-and-through 4. Intra-articular 5. Major bone loss
Moderate Risk					
Stomach	(3)	1. Single wall 2. Through-and-through 3. Minor debridement 4. Wedge resection 5. >35% resection	Small bowel	(1)	1. Single Wall 2. Through-and-through 3. <25% wall 4. >25% wall 5. Wall and blood supply or >5 injuries
Spleen	(3)	1. Nonbleeding 2. Cautery or hemostatic agent 3. Minor debridement or suturing 4. Partial resection 5. Splenectomy	Minor vascular	(1)	1. Nonbleeding small hematoma 2. Nonbleeding large hematoma 3. Suturing 4. Ligation of isolated vessels 5. Ligation of named vessels

Adapted from Borlase BC, Moore EE, Moore FA. The Abdominal Trauma Index—a critical reassessment and validation. *J Trauma.* 1990;30:1341. With permission of the McGraw-Hill Companies.

Despite a greater severity of injury, the patients fed via the jejunum sustained complications at rates similar to less severely injured patients receiving parenteral feeding.

Eyer et al.[16] randomized blunt trauma patients to either early enteral feeding using a nasojejunal tube or to delayed enteral feeding and showed no benefit with the early enteral feeding. The infectious complication rate was higher in the early fed group, but this was due to eye, sinus, or urinary infections, which are unlikely to be protected by enteral feeding. The type and magnitude of injuries were not provided in the article, but the incidence of severe lung injury with a P_aO_2/F_iO_2 <150 (comparable to a 20% shunt) was three times as common in patients receiving the early enteral formula. Thus, the patient populations did not appear compatible at the outset which may have precluded accurate assessment of nutrition. The inaccuracy in diagnosing pneumonia with such severe lung injury applies to interpretation of these data as well.

Head Injury

The outcome effects of nutrition after blunt and penetrating torso trauma may not be applicable to patients sustaining severe closed-head injury for several reasons. First, patients with low Glasgow Coma Scale (GCS) scores often remain paralyzed, intubated, and mechanically ventilated for a week or longer to control intracranial pressure. Pulmonary toilet is limited and hypostatic pneumonia frequently complicates the outcome of this severely injured patient population. Patients with severely altered GCS scores often develop a severe, but temporary, gastroparesis which limits the ability to successfully feed intragastrically. As a result, few studies of patients sustaining severe head injury have shown any benefit with enteral feeding.

Rapp et al.[17] randomized 38 patients with severe head injuries to either parenteral feeding or to intragastric feeding within 48 hours of admission. Intragastric feeding was delayed until bowel sounds were present and gastric drainage dropped below 300 cc/d. Over the first week, delayed intragastric feeding resulted in a caloric intake of less than 600 kcal/d compared with 2,000 kcal/d in the TPN group. No enterally fed patient received more than 1,000 kcal/d over the first 10 days. Mortality was reduced and neurologic outcome improved at three months in the parenterally fed patients, although this difference disappeared at follow-up. However, these promising benefits in neurologic outcome could not be duplicated by the same authors.[18] In a follow-up study, patients were randomized to parenteral feeding or intragastric feeding using the same criteria for instituting intragastric feedings. Enteral patients received significantly less nutrition than parenterally fed patients over the first 7 days because of "gastroparesis," but infectious complications were approximately 30% in both groups with no significant neurologic improvement in patients receiving parenteral feeding. Borzotta[19] found similar results in head injury patients with a GCS ≤8 randomized to TPN or to surgical jejunostomy. Even with feedings started within 72 hours, outcome was similar with no differences in infectious complications. In a recent study,[20] patients randomized to early nasojejunal feeding with an immune-enhancing diet or to intragastric feeding started on the second or third day as gastroparesis resolved showed no significant differences in infectious complications between the early and "very early" fed group.

Only one study noted improvement with early enteral feeding. Patients with a GCS ≤10 were randomized to either nasojejunal feeding started within 36 hours of admission or intragastric feeding on day 3 as gastroparesis resolved. Grahm[21] noted a significantly lower rate of respiratory bacterial infections, but the majority was tracheobronchitis, which was poorly defined in the article.

Summary of Trauma Studies

Both parenteral and enteral nutrition can meet nutrient goals. In patients sustaining severe blunt or penetrating trauma of the torso, the preponderance of data shows that enteral feeding significantly improves outcome by reducing infectious complications compared with parenteral feeding. The results are less dramatic in injured patient populations with a low ATI or ISS. Studies that detect no differences between routes of feeding do not appear to have comparable patient populations. There is little convincing evidence that enteral feeding influences infectious morbidity or neurologic outcome after severe head injury. This discrepancy between the blunt and penetrating torso in the closed-head injury patient population may reflect the prolonged intubation, paralysis, immobilization, and other neurologic maneuvers used to reduce intracranial pressure. Under these conditions, pneumonia may develop despite adequate nutrition support. Early intragastric feeding can be instituted within 2 to 3 days of head injury since gastroparesis resolves much quicker than suggested by early studies. There is no convincing evidence that the expense and trouble in placing a nasojejunal tube for earlier jejunal feedings will provide a significant benefit following head injury.

Studies of Enteral vs. Parenteral Feeding in Nontrauma Patients

General Surgical Patients

Administration of either enteral or parenteral feeding to well-nourished or mildly malnourished patients will not improve clinical outcome because the rate of complications under these conditions is low. The studies by the VA cooperative group[7] and by Brennan et al.[8] noted above support this concept. In addition, Heslin et al.[22] followed 195 patients without malnutrition undergoing esophageal, pancreatic, or gastric surgery comparing early enteral feeding with IV fluids alone and noted no significant difference in hospital mortality, length of stay, or in the number of major, minor, or infectious complications. Protein-sparing therapy administered to 678 patients with relatively normal nutritional status also showed no significant benefit in patients undergoing major, elective abdominal surgery.[23]

Several studies that include malnourished general surgical patients have shown a benefit of early enteral feeding. Shirabe et al.[24] randomized 26 patients undergoing major hepatic resection to either early enteral feeding or parenteral nutrition. The study was small with only 13 patients in a group. Infectious complications were higher in the parenterally fed group (31%) compared with the enterally fed group (8%), but this failed to reach statistical significance. Several immunologic parameters, such as PHA response, NK cell reactivity, and lymphocyte number, were improved in the enteral-fed group. Gianotti[25] undertook a multi-institutional study, randomizing patients requiring pancreatectomy, pancreatoduodenectomy, or gastrectomy for malignancy to either a standard enteral diet, parenteral nutrition, or a diet supplemented with arginine, omega-3 fatty acids, and RNA. The infectious complications were highest in the parenterally fed group (a 28% incidence) compared with patients receiving the supplemented diet, and length of stay was also significantly increased in the parenterally fed group. Patients receiving the standard diet had an infection rate midway between those receiving parenteral feeding and those receiving the supplemental diet, suggesting effects of both type and route of nutrition. Sand et al.[26] found fewer infectious complications (23%) in patients fed enterally after a curative total gastrectomy for gastric malignancy compared with parenterally fed patients (31% infectious complications), but this failed to reach statistical significance. The acute-phase protein response was significantly lower in the enterally fed group by day 6.

In summary, enteral delivery of nutrition in patient populations undergoing elective general surgical procedures who are at risk of developing septic complications appears to be associated with an improved clinical outcome that reaches statistical significance in a few studies. In certain circumstances, a specialty diet may significantly shorten hospital stay. There is no apparent benefit, however, in patients who are well nourished or have only mild malnutrition.

Inflammatory Bowel Disease

Patients with inflammatory bowel disease often suffer from an inadequate absorptive surface, chronic and acute inflammation, poor appetite and poor oral intake, and catabolic effects from steroid therapy. Disease remission does not appear to be different in enterally and parenterally fed patients sustaining ulcerative colitis.[27] In 42 patients receiving a polymeric enteral diet or isonitrogenous, isocaloric parenteral solution, there were few adverse outcomes, few postoperative infections, and an improvement in serum albumin in the group receiving the early enteral feeding in patients with ulcerative colitis.[28] In patients with Crohn's disease, there are no randomized, prospective studies of enteral and parenteral feeding, although several studies suggest that an elemental enteral diet is equivalent to steroid therapy in inducing disease remission. It is unknown, however, whether there is any additional benefit of the enteral feeding compared with the administration of parenteral nutrition under these conditions.

Pancreatitis

Intragastric feeding is considered contraindicated in patients sustaining severe pancreatitis because hormonal stimulation of pancreatic secretions aggravates the pancreatitis and gastroparesis limits absorption. Under these conditions, gastric decompression is usually necessary, and intravenous nutrition is an important part of the management of these patients unless surgery is indicated and access is obtained distal to the ligament of Treitz. Mild pancreatitis, however, may permit access beyond the ligament of Treitz without surgery. In a group of 30 patients admitted with mild acute pancreatitis,[29] clinical outcome parameters measured by the Ranson criteria improved significantly in the group randomized to nasojejunal feeding compared with patients receiving an isocaloric, isonitrogenous parenteral formula. Cost of nutrition care and stress-induced hyperglycemia were also reduced in the enterally fed group. In a study by Windsor et al.,[30] patients were stratified according to the degree of acute pancreatitis and randomized to either enteral feeding for 1 week or parenteral nutrition. The enteral-fed group had significant improvement in the incidence of sepsis, organ failure, ICU stay, and other markers of the systemic inflammatory response syndrome. In addition, there were improvements in the acute-phase protein response and disease severity score that remained unchanged in patients administered parenteral feeding.

In summary, the majority of patients sustaining pancreatitis do not require nutrition support since they will recover uneventfully. Because of gastroparesis and the potential stimulation of pancreatic and duodenal secretions, intragastric feeding is contraindicated in patients with severe pancreatitis. If access is obtained beyond the ligament of Treitz, nutrition can be provided into the small intestine with minimal hormonal stimulation.[31] In case of mild but prolonged pancreatitis, access beyond the ligament of Treitz is technically easier and is useful in the occasional patient.

TRANSPLANTATION

There has been only one small study of patients randomized to jejunal feeding of parenteral nutrition in the transplant population, and no difference in outcome was noted between the two groups.[32] Hasse,[33] however, randomized 50 patients receiving transplant to either IV fluids alone or jejunal feedings and noted a significant reduction in viral infections in patients fed via the gastrointestinal tract with a trend toward a reduction in bacterial infections (29% vs. 14%). There were no differences, however, in hospital costs, length of stay, ventilator days, or organ rejection. Mehta et al.[34] started enteral feeding via jejunostomy tube and parenteral nutrition in 21 transplant patients and noted an increased incidence of diarrhea (73% vs. 25%) in the enteral-fed patients but also noted a reduction in the incidence of postoperative ileus and a more rapid resumption of enteral intake.

PEDIATRIC STUDIES

There are relatively few studies of enteral and parenteral feeding in the pediatric population. In a study of 29 patients requiring extracorporal membrane oxygenation,[35] patients receiving parenteral and enteral nutrition achieved caloric goals at approximately the same time. There were no complications associated with enteral feeding. Although it did not reach statistical significance, survival was increased in the enteral-fed group (100% vs. 79%). The only clear benefit of enteral feeding was a reduction in cost of the nutrition.

Hypotheses for Reduced Septic Complications with Enteral Delivery of Nutrients

Several themes have emerged to explain the increased incidence of infectious complications in parenterally fed patients. These include: (1) an increase in hyperglycemia, (2) increased permeability of the GI mucosa to bacteria and enteral toxins, (3) augmented inflammatory response through intestinal priming of neutrophils, and (4) a generalized reduction in mucosal immunity.

HYPERGLYCEMIA AND INCREASED INCIDENCE OF INFECTIOUS COMPLICATIONS WITH TPN

Until recently, clinical studies had a propensity to overfeed patients with parenteral feeding which led to hyperglycemia. Over the last decade, particularly with information derived through metabolic cart measurements, recommendations for the provision of nutrients in critically ill patients have gradually decreased from approximately 40 total kcal/d or more to 30 kcal/d. Recently, Bistrian et al.[36] noted a significant increase in infectious complications of diabetic patients in the postoperative period if blood glucose values exceeded 220 mg/dL during the first 2 days of hospitalization, and speculated that hyperglycemia might explain outcome differences in prior clinical studies. They pointed out that TPN patients in the VA Cooperative study[7] were overfed by contemporary standards, and episodes of hyperglycemia (glucoses >300 mg/dL) occurred frequently. Also, in the meta analysis of enteral feeding studies by Moore et al.,[37] blood glucose values were significantly higher in parenterally fed patients at all points during the study but were especially elevated near the end, with differences approaching 100 mg/dL. However, in both of these publications, the relationship between the timing of the hyperglycemic episodes and the infectious complications was unclear.

Since infectious processes induce a stress response that increases catecholamines, cortisol, and hyperglycemia, hyperglycemia could be preceded or coincided with the episodes of sepsis. We examined[38] this in patients in our two clinical trials of enteral nutrition that compared enteral versus parenteral feeding,[12] or a specialty diet enhanced with arginine, omega-3 fatty acids, glutamine, and nucleotides with a standard isonitrogenous, isocaloric enteral diet.[39] In the latter study, a group of patients who met eligibility criteria by injury but who had no enteral access and, thus, could not receive enteral feeding, were also followed prospectively. The majority of the latter group received no nutrition support prior to the development of infectious complications. In the enteral versus parenteral study, there were no significant differences in serum glucose values between the two groups until the fourth or fifth day when glucose values became significantly higher in the TPN group as complications developed, suggesting that hyperglycemia was a response to infectious complications rather than a cause of the infectious complications. Although blood sugars tended to be higher—15 mg/dL—in the parenterally fed patients compared with the enterally fed group, the overall average glucose values were far below the 220 mg/dL suggested as an important etiologic factor in the development of infections (Table 11.2). In most cases, the hyperglycemic incidents were isolated, sporadic events, and the majority of infections in parenterally fed patients occurred without a single episode of hyperglycemia. In the second trial, patients randomized to a specialty immune-enhancing diet or an isonitrogenous, isocaloric control diet sustained very few episodes of hyperglycemia at all. The unfed patients had almost identical serum glucose values to the fed groups despite a rate of infectious complications, which was much higher. Thus, unless one postulates that the mechanism for development of infectious complications in trauma patients in the first study was totally different than the second, it is difficult to implicate hyperglycemia as *the* important etiologic factor in infectious complications with parenteral feeding.

It is possible that diabetic patients are different and that maintenance of reasonable glucose levels is more important in this chronic disease state. Unfortunately, intensive management with antihyperglycemic therapy in diabetic patients was unable to reduce the rate of infectious complications.[40]

Mucosal Alterations with Increases in Gut Permeability and Bacterial Translocation

The gut mucosa is a metabolically active organ that responds to the presence or absence of enteral stimulation. Several classic experimental studies in rats provided insights into mucosal changes associated with enteral feeding. Rats starved 6 days lose small bowel weight and intestinal and mucosal protein out of proportion to total body losses.[41] Particularly within the proximal half of the small intestine, parenteral feeding results in significant reductions in mucosal weight, mucosal DNA, and mucosal protein, characteristic of both atrophy and hypoplasia within the tissues.[42] Reinstitution of enteral feeding to protein-depleted rats results in retention of a high proportion of enterally administered protein within the mucosa until the mucosal mass recovers.[43] These changes occur primarily in the small intestine since colonic mucosa is less responsive to the lack of enteral nutrition. Histologic changes within the colonic mucosa are minimal although epithelial proliferation diminishes. Proliferation recovers with the administration of soluble fiber, such as pectins and gums, which are fermented by bacterial flora to short-chain fatty acids, primarily butyrate, which serves as the primary respiratory fuel of the colonocyte.[44]

TABLE 11.2

Maximal Serum Glucose Values in Enteral vs. Parenteral Study of Trauma Patients

Hospital Day	Enteral (g/dL)	TPN	
1	159 ± 41	157 ± 32	NS
2	142 ± 24	154 ± 34	NS
3	141 ± 34	155 ± 31	NS
4	146 ± 42	164 ± 38	p <0.05
5	145 ± 56	179 ± 63	p <0.02

The response of the mucosa to an insult, such as ischemia/perfusion, is influenced by its nutrition state. Ischemia/reperfusion results in significant disruption in the small intestine mucosa with microvilli alterations within 3 to 5 minutes of circulatory arrest.[45] The upper two-thirds of the villi become completely denuded within 30 minutes of ischemia, but recovery occurs very quickly unless ischemia is prolonged enough to cause total mucosal necrosis. Lactic acidosis, release of acid hydrolases, and liposomal breakdown have been implicated as etiologic factors in this mucosal breakdown. Surprisingly, several authors have noted that a previously fasted intestine appears to be more resistant to an ischemic insult,[46] although intraluminal glucose is protective.

Human histologic changes in the unfed gut are much more attenuated compared to rodent species. In humans, investigators have found only a 10% reduction in mucosal thickness after one to two weeks of parenteral nutrition[47] with most of the changes occurring within the villi; mucosal ulceration is uncommon. Although there are no clinical studies of histologic changes of the intestine in patients after moderate ischemic insults, changes in gut permeability have been noted after insults, such as burns,[48] sepsis,[49] or blunt and penetrating trauma,[50] using two inert markers of intestinal permeability, mannitol and lactulose, which are excreted unchanged into the urine. Approximately 40% of mannitol is absorbed under normal conditions compared with 0.4% of lactulose; therefore, the lactulose to mannitol ratio is low. As permeability increases, absorption of lactulose increases out of proportion to increases in mannitol, and the calculated lactulose-to-mannitol ratio rises. Deitch[48] demonstrated that the lactulose-mannitol (L:M) ratio tripled within 24 hours of an acute burn, and Ziegler[49] noted a proportional increase in intestinal permeability in relation to a calculated sepsis score that reflected the metabolic response to active infection. After blunt and penetrating trauma,[50] the L:M ratio increased in approximately one-third of patients. This rise in the L:M ratio correlated closely with systemic Interleukin IL-6 levels.[51] IL-6 is produced by the GI tract and other sites and is an important mediator in the inflammatory response and in the acute-phase hepatic protein response to injury.[52,53] IL-6 levels also are predictive of infectious complications following trauma, and the proportionate increase in IL-6 and L:M ratio suggests a relationship between gut permeability and infectious complications.

It has been postulated that increases in gut permeability increase levels of both bacteria and bacterial products that aggravate the development of multiple organ dysfunction.[54] Experimentally, this association was shown through translocation of intraluminal bacteria to mesenteric lymph nodes, the liver, and spleen.[55,56] Normally, lymph nodes and other organs are sterile, but bacteria can translocate from the lumen to the mesenteric lymph nodes and, under extreme circumstances, to the liver and spleen after shock, injury, and inflammation. Starvation by itself maintains the gut barrier and prevents translocation in animal models, but the addition of a stress or extraintestinal inflammatory site produces dramatic increases in bacterial translocation after starvation. Certain clinical conditions,[56] such as small bowel obstruction and inflammatory bowel disease, result in bacterial translocation in mesenteric lymph nodes.

There is no convincing evidence that this process results in an untoward outcome. Moore et al.[57] cannulated the portal vein of severely injured patients at the time of trauma celiotomy and sequentially cultured the portal circulation. Positive cultures from mesenteric lymph nodes correlated poorly with the development of multiple organ failure, and portal blood samples remain sterile almost uniformly. Evidence for bacterial translocation was found in 21 organ donors.[58] Cultures were positive in 14 of 21 donors, most of whom had been starved, were on multiple antibiotics, or had been administered vasoactive drugs. Endotoxin levels were elevated in the abdominal fluid of most of these patients. Despite this circumstantial evidence, however, the concept of bacterial translocation as a driving force in the development of extraintestinal infections or multiple organ dysfunction has fallen out of favor in the clinical and experimental literature.

Alterations in Small Intestinal Microcirculation and Alterations in the Response to Inflammation

Since the 1970s, advances in ICU management have increased the survival of critically ill and critically injured patients, and multiple organ dysfunction syndrome (MODS) has emerged as a major clinical problem. Although sepsis—recognized or unrecognized —was considered to be the primary factor in the development of MODS, it is clear that the gut can alter organ responses to sepsis and injury.

Shock, tissue injury, and other insults increase the inflammatory response, which is followed by an immunodepression,[59] resulting in infectious complications and late multiple organ dysfunction. Recently it became recognized that the early proinflammatory phase can also result in multiple organ dysfunction occurring within 3 to 5 days of injury. While bacterial translocation was initially considered a driving force in this process, the neutrophil (PMN) became suspect in the organ damage. The gastrointestinal tract can prime circulating PMNs soon after injury.[60–62] This gut priming occurs after upregulation of adhesion molecules in the small intestine microcirculation, which attracts PMNs and primes them through the local production of cytosolic phospolypase-A_2, platelet-activating factor, and other chemoattractants.[63] The newly primed PMNs are distributed throughout the body during reperfusion, and if a second inflammatory insult occurs, these previously primed PMNs produce an augmented cytolytic response that induces significant tissue injury leading to organ dysfunction.[51,62]

Route and type of feeding influence this response in both clinical and experimental studies. Clinically, patients administered an enteral diet enriched in arginine, omega-3 fatty acids, and nucleotides have a significant reduction in MODS compared with patients receiving standard enteral diet, suggesting that delivery of specific nutrients can influence this post-injury vulnerability.[64] Experimentally, lack of enteral feeding significantly changes the intestinal cytokines[65] and alters mRNA for cytokine production within the gut-associated lymphoid tissue (GALT).[66] As a result of these changes, IL-4 and IL-10 levels drop within the small intestine GALT with parenteral feeding. These two cytokines are important in at least two functions. IL-4 and IL-10 are important stimulants for IgA production for mucosal antibody protection by the GALT. This will be discussed in the subsequent section. Second, IL-4 and IL-10 suppress expression of intracellular adhesion molecule-1 (ICAM-1) on the vascular endothelium.[67] ICAM-1, together with other chemoattractants and adhesion molecules, attracts PMNs to the small intestine. Experimentally, when parenterally fed mice with high levels of gut neutrophils are exposed to a gut ischemia insult, lung and liver permeability increases, and there is an increase in mortality to that ischemic event.[68] Although the absolute number of PMNs within the lung are not increased after gut ischemia in parenterally fed mice, pulmonary PMNs express increased levels of the activation marker CD18, implicating the lack of enteral stimulation as a proinflammatory stimulus to a subsequent ischemic response.[69]

In summary, the intestine plays a key role in affecting the inflammatory response of the body to injury. Clinical evidence suggests that delivery of nutrients via the gastrointestinal tract can influence this inflammatory response, particularly when specialty nutrients are provided in the enteral formula. Experimentally, lack of enteral feeding leads to an upregulation of adhesion molecules within the small intestine. These primed neutrophils lead to an augmented inflammatory response at extraintestinal sites if subsequent insults are suffered by the animals.

Mucosal Immunity

The GALT provides immunologic protection against both infections and resident microflora. Approximately 60% to 70% of the body's total immunity is located beneath the single epithelial layer that lines the upper respiratory tract, trachea, stomach, intestine, and colon.[70] T and B cells within the lamina propria at these sites work in concert to produce IgA, which is immediately transported by the overlying epithelial cells onto their mucosal surfaces via secretory component. IgA binds to bacterial antigens and inhibits their ability to attach to the mucosa. If attachment is avoided, infection is prevented.[70] IgA does not stimulate an inflammatory response, an important characteristic for mucosal defenses.

Naive B and T cells are produced by the bone marrow, the peritoneum, the thymus, and possibly other sites. They circulate in the blood stream and gain entry into the mucosal-associated lymphoid tissue (MALT) through high endothelial venules (HEV) located in the Peyer's patches.[71] Mucosal addressin cellular adhesion molecule-1 (MAdCAM-1) on the HEV is an attractant for the L-selectin molecule on the naïve T and B cells, which are destined to produce cytokines and IgA, respectively, in the lamina propria of the MALT.[72] Cells that migrate into the Peyer's patches are sensitized to intraluminal antigens that have been absorbed by specialized M cells overlying the luminal surfaces of the Peyer's patches and processed by specialized dendritic cells. The sensitized T and B cells migrate to the mesenteric lymph nodes to proliferate and/or mature and then are released into the thoracic duct and vascular tree for distribution to both intestinal and extraintestinal sites where they function cooperatively in IgA production. In these sites, the T cells produce Th 2 IgA-stimulating cytokines (IL-4, IL-5, IL-6, IL-10, and IL-13), which are counterbalanced by the Th1 IgA-inhibiting cytokines (IFNγ and TNFβ). After production, IgA is immediately transported across the mucosa via secretory component located on the basal membranes of the mucosal cells.[71]

This mucosal immune system is exquisitely sensitive to the route and type of nutrition. MAdCAM-1 expression drops within hours of the institution of parenteral feeding, and Peyer's patches atrophy within 2 days as fewer T and B cells enter the MALT.[72] With 3 to 4 days of no enteral feeding, Peyer's patches shrink by approximately 50% with proportionate decreases in T and B cells within the lamina propria. As the lamina propria T cells decrease, a shift in the CD4:CD8 ratio occurs from 2:1 to 1:1.[73] This shift decreases the cytokines IL-4 and IL-10[65] within the homogenates of the small intestine and decreases the mRNA for these cytokines within isolated GALT lamina propria cells.[66] No changes occur in the Th1 IgA cytokines, which are known to inhibit IgA production. The effect of the change reduces IgA levels within the intestine. Respiratory tract IgA levels also drop, presumably because of reduced delivery of GALT cells to extraintestinal sites of mucosa.[74] With reinstitution of enteral feeding, MAdCAM-1 is upregulated within 24 hours with rapid repopulation of Peyer's patches and lamina propria cell numbers within 36 to 48 hours.

These cell changes induce functional effects. Animals who had previously been immunized against the influenza virus[75] or with *Pseudomonas* antigen[76] rapidly clear the virus or kill the bacteria after rechallenge with those organisms. Parenteral feeding significantly impairs established immunity against the virus[77] and totally destroys defenses against the *Pseudomonas* within 5 days so that all immune protection generated by the immunization is lost.[78] Memory of the antigen is still present since reinstitution of enteral feeding[79]—in association with recovery of GALT cell populations—regenerates an effective defense to the viral challenge. Thus, lack of enteral feeding significantly impairs IgA-mediated immunity against intraluminal bacteria, rendering the host susceptible to these challenges.

As host mucosal immunity decreases, bacteria respond with increased virulence. There is a normal symbiosis between intraluminal bacteria and the human intestinal environment. A generous food supply and warm, moist environment in a healthy host provide a nonhostile environment for bacteria to thrive. The predictable environment is mutually beneficial in health, but the environment becomes hostile to the bacteria through challenges, such as antibiotics, vasoactive drugs, and opiates, that reduce motility and starvation.[80] While a nonhostile environment keeps virulence genes downregulated in the bacteria, new stressors, such as starvation, elemental diets, and decreased blood flow, upregulate bacterial virulence genes in bacteria to increase adherence appendages on their surface.[80] Therefore, under conditions that decrease intestinal IgA and reduce human defenses, bacterial virulence and adherence are increased. Experimentally, this increased adherence results in decreases in cellular transepithelial resistance.[81,82] Bacteria harvested from fasted animals are more virulent when injected into other animals, and animals with nutritionally upregulated bacterial virulence are much less resistant to a surgical stress.

Conclusions

Both clinical and laboratory evidence suggest that route of nutrition alter the interactions between the intraluminal environment, mucosal defenses, and the systemic metabolic response to injury. Clinically, the enteral delivery of nutrients appears to improve host defenses and reduce the incidence of septic complications in some patient populations compared with parenteral feeding, but existing clinical literature must be interpreted with consideration of the patients entered into specific clinical protocols. Nutrition support—whether enteral or parenteral—is a highly technical therapy capable of both risks and benefits. When administered to patients who are unlikely to benefit, results are likely to demonstrate only the risk of therapy. However, when selectively administered to patients who are at risk of nutrition-related complications, nutrition support has been shown in multiple studies to improve clinical outcome. Under most circumstances, enteral feeding has been associated with an improved clinical outcome usually through reductions in septic complications compared with parenterally fed patients.

References

1. Dudrick SJ, Wilmore DW, Vars HM, et al. Long-term total parenteral nutrition with growth, development, and positive nitrogen balance. *Surgery.* 1968;64:134–136.
2. Alexander JW, Macmillan BG, Stinnett JD, et al. Beneficial effects of aggressive protein feeding in severely burned children. *Ann Surg.* 1980;192:505–517.
3. Moore EE, Jones TN. Benefits of immediate jejunostomy feeding after major abdominal trauma—a prospective, randomized study. *J Trauma.* 1986;26:874–879.
4. Kudsk KA, Carpenter G, Petersen S, Sheldon GF. Effect of enteral and parenteral feeding in malnourished rats with *E. coli*-hemoglobin adjuvant peritonitis. *J Surg Res.* 1981; 31:105–110.
5. Kudsk KA, Stone JM, Carpenter G, et al. Enteral and parenteral feeding influences mortality after hemoglobin-*E. coli* peritonitis in normal rats. *J Trauma.* 1983;23:605–609.
6. Kenler AS, Swails WS, Driscoll DF, et al. Early enteral feeding in postsurgical cancer patients: fish oil structured lipid-based polymeric formula versus a standard polymeric formula. *Ann Surg.* 1996;223:316–333.
7. The Veteran Affairs Total Parenteral Nutrition Cooperative Study Group. Perioperative total parenteral nutrition in surgical patients. *N Engl J Med.* 1991;325:525–532.
8. Brennan MF, Pisters PWT, Posner M, et al. A prospective, randomized trial of total parenteral nutrition after major pancreatic resection for malignancy. *Ann Surg.* 1994;220: 436–444.
9. Borlase BC, Moore EE, Moore FA. The Abdominal Trauma Index—a critical reassessment and validation. *J Trauma.* 1990;30(11):1340–1344.
10. Jones TN, Moore FA, Moore EE, et al. Gastrointestinal symptoms attributed to jejunostomy feedings after major abdominal trauma: a critical analysis. *Crit Care Med.* 1989; 17(11):1146–1150.
11. Moore FA, Moore EE, Jones TN, et al. TEN versus TPN following major abdominal trauma—reduced septic morbidity. *J Trauma.* 1989;29:916–923.
12. Kudsk KA, Croce MA, Fabian TC, et al. Enteral versus parenteral feeding: effects on septic morbidity after blunt and penetrating abdominal trauma. *Ann Surg.* 1992;215(5): 165–173.
13. Baker SP, O'Neill B, Haddon W, et al. The Injury Severity Score: a method for describing patients with multiple injuries and evaluating emergency care. *J Trauma.* 1974; 14:187–196.
14. Adams S, Dellinger EP, Wertz MJ, et al. Enteral versus parenteral nutritional support following laparotomy for trauma: a randomized prospective trial. *J Trauma.* 1986;26: 882–891.
15. Fagon JY, Chastre J, Hance AJ, et al. Detection of nosocomial lung infection in ventilated patients. Use of a protected specimen brush and quantitative culture techniques in 147 patients. *Am Rev Respir Dis.* 1988;138(1):110–116.
16. Eyer SD, Micon LT, Konstantinides FN. Early enteral feeding does not attenuate metabolic response after blunt trauma. *J Trauma.* 1993;34:639–644.

17. Rapp RP, Young B, Twymand D, et al. The favorable effect of early parenteral feeding on survival in head injured patients. *J Neurosurg.* 1983;58:906–911.

18. Young B, Ott L, Haack D, et al. Effect of total parenteral nutrition upon intracranial pressure in severe head injury. *J Neurosurg.* 1987;67:668–676.

19. Borzotta AP, Penning S, Papasadero B, et al. Enteral vs parenteral nutrition after severe closed head injury. *J Trauma.* 1994;37:459–468.

20. Minard G, Kudsk KA, Melton S, et al. Early versus delayed feeding with an immune-enhancing diet in patients with severe head injuries. *J Parenter Enteral Nutr.* 2000; 24(3):145–149.

21. Grahm TW, Zadrozny DB, Harrington T. The benefits of early jejunal hyperalimentation in the head-injured patient. *Neurosurgery.* 1989;25:729–735.

22. Heslin MJ, Latkany L, Leung D, et al. A prospective, randomized trial of early enteral feeding after resection of upper gastrointestinal malignancy. *Ann Surg.* 1997;226: 567–577.

23. Doglietto GB, Gallitelli L, Pacelli F, et al. Protein-sparing therapy after major abdominal surgery: lack of clinical effects. *Ann Surg.* 1996;223:357–362.

24. Shirabe K, Matsumata T, Shimada M, et al. A comparison of parenteral hyperalimentation and early enteral feeding regarding systemic immunity after major hepatic resection—the results of a randomized prospective study. *Hepatogastroenterology.* 1997;44:205–209.

25. Gianotti L, Braga M, Vignali A, et al. Effect of route of delivery and formulation of postoperative nutritional support in patients undergoing major operations for malignant neoplasms. *Arch Surg.* 1997;132:1222–1229.

26. Sand J, Luostarinen M, Matikainen M. Enteral or parenteral feeding after total gastrectomy: prospective randomized pilot study. *Eur J Surg.* 1997;163:761–766.

27. Dickinson RJ, Ashton MG, Axon AT, et al. Controlled trial of intravenous hyperalimentation and total bowel rest as an adjunct to routine therapy of acute colitis. *Gastroenterology.* 1980;79:1199–1205.

28. Gonzalez-Huix F, Fernandez-Banares F, Esteve-Comas M, et al. Enteral versus parenteral nutrition as adjunct therapy in acute ulcerative colitis. *Am J Gastroenterol.* 1993;88:227–232.

29. McClave SA, Greene LM, Snider HL, et al. Comparison of the safety of early enteral vs parenteral nutrition in mild acute pancreatitis. *J Parenter Enteral Nutr.* 1997;21:14–20.

30. Windsor AC, Kanwar S, Li AG, et al. Compared with parenteral nutrition, enteral feeding attenuates the acute phase response and improves disease severity in acute pancreatitis. *Gut.* 1998;42:431–435.

31. Bodoky G, Harsanyi L, Pap A, et al. Effect of enteral nutrition on exocrine pancreatic function. *Am J Surg.* 1991; 161:144–148.

32. Wicks C, Somasundaram S, Bjarnason I, et al. Comparison of enteral feeding and total parenteral nutrition after liver transplantation. *Lancet.* 1994;344:837–840.

33. Hasse JM, Blue LS, Liepa GU, et al. Early enteral nutrition support in patients undergoing liver transplantation. *J Parenter Enteral Nutr.* 1995;19:437–443.

34. Mehta TL, Alaka KJ, Filo RS, et al. Nutrition support following liver transplantation: comparison of jejunal versus parenteral routes. *Clin Transplant (Denmark).* 1995;9:364–369.

35. Pettignano R, Heard M, Davis R, et al. Total enteral nutrition versus total parenteral nutrition during pediatric extracorporeal membrane oxygenation. *Crit Care Med.* 1998;26:358–363.

36. Pomposelli JJ, Baxter JK, Babineau TJ, et al. Early postoperative glucose control predicts nosocomial infection rate in diabetic patients. *J Parenter Enteral Nutr.* 1998;22(2): 77–81.

37. Moore FA, Feliciano DV, Andrassy RJ, et al. Early enteral feeding, compared with parenteral, reduces postoperative septic complications: the results of a meta-analysis. *Ann Surg.* 1992;216(2):172–183.

38. Kudsk KA, Laulederkind A, Hanna MK. Most infectious complications in parenterally fed trauma patients are not due to elevated blood glucose levels. *J Parenter Enteral Nutr.* 2001;25:174–179.

39. Kudsk KA, Minard G, Croce MA, et al. A randomized trial of isonitrogenous enteral diets after severe trauma. An immune-enhancing diet reduces septic complications. *Ann Surg.* 1996; 224:531–540.

40. McCowen KC, Friel C, Sternberg J, et al. Hypocaloric total parenteral nutrition: effectiveness in prevention of hyperglycemia and infectious complications—a randomized clinical trial. *Crit Care Med.* 2000;28:3606–3611.

41. Steiner M, Bouges HR, Freeman LS, et al. Effect of starvation on tissue composition of the small intestine in the rat. *Am J Physiol.* 1968;215:75–77.

42. Johnson LR, Copeland EM, Dudrick SJ, et al. Structural and hormonal alterations in the gastrointestinal tract of parenterally fed rats. *Gastroenterology.* 1975;68:1177–1183.

43. Hirschfield JS, Kern F. Protein starvation and the small intestine. *J Clin Invest.* 1969;48:1224–1229.

44. Kripke SA, Fox AD, Berman JM, et al. Stimulation of intestinal mucosal growth with intracolonic infusion of short chain fatty acids. *J Parenter Enteral Nutr.* 1989;13:109–116.

45. Robinson JWL, Mirkovitch V, Winistorfer B, et al. Response of the intestinal mucosa to ischemia. *Gut.* 1981;22: 512–527.

46. Langkamp-Henken B, Kudsk KA, Proctor KG. Fasting-induced reduction of intestinal reperfusion injury. *J Parenter Enteral Nutr.* 1995;19:127–132.

47. Guedon C, Schmitz J, Lerebours E, et al. Decreased brush border hydrolase activities without gross morphologic changes in human intestinal mucosa after prolonged total parenteral nutrition of adults. *Gastroenterology.* 1986;90: 373–378.

48. Deitch EA. Intestinal permeability is increased in burn patients shortly after injury. *Surgery.* 1990;107:411–416.

49. Ziegler TR, Smith RJ, O'Dwyer ST, et al. Increased intestinal permeability associated with infection in burn patients. *Arch Surg.* 1988;123:1313–1319.

50. Langkamp-Henken B, Donovan TB, Pate LM, et al. Increased intestinal permeability following blunt and penetrating trauma. *Crit Care Med.* 1995;23:660–664.

51. Janu P, Li J, Minard G, et al. Systemic interleukin-6 (IL-6) correlates with intestinal permeability. *Surg Forum.* 1996;47:7.
52. Ohzato H, Yoshizaki K, Nishimoto N, et al. Interleukin-6 as a new indicator of inflammatory status: detection of serum levels of interleukin-6 and C-reactive protein after surgery. *Surgery.* 1992;111:201–209.
53. Mainous MR, Ertel W, Chaudry IH, et al. The gut: a cytokine-generating organ in systemic inflammation? *Shock.* 1995;4:193–199.
54. Deitch EA. Multiple organ failure: Pathophysiology and potential future therapy. *Ann Surg.* 1992;216:117–134.
55. Deitch EA, Winterton J, Ma L, et al. The gut as a portal of entry for bacteremia: role of protein malnutrition. *Ann Surg.* 1987;205:681–692.
56. Deitch EA. Does the gut protect or injure patients in the ICU? *Perspect Crit Care.* 1988;1:1–31.
57. Moore FA, Moore EE, Poggetti R, et al. Gut bacterial translocation via the portal vein: a clinical perspective with major torso trauma. *J Trauma.* 1991;31:629–638.
58. van Goor H, Rosman C, Grond J, et al. Translocation of bacteria and endotoxin in organ donors. *Arch Surg.* 1994; 129:1063–1066.
59. Moore FA, Moore EE, Sauaia A. Postinjury multiple-organ failure. In: Mattox KL, Feliciano DV, Moore EE, eds. *Trauma.* 4th ed. New York: McGraw-Hill; 2000:1427–1460.
60. Moore EE, Moore FA, Franciose RJ, et al. The postischemic gut serves as a priming bed for circulating neutrophils that provoke multiple organ failure. *J Trauma.* 1994; 37:881–887.
61. Moore FA, Moore EE. Evolving concepts in the pathogenesis of postinjury multiple organ failure. *Surg Clin North Am.* 1995;75:257–277.
62. Botha AJ, Moore FA, Moore EE, et al. Early neutrophil sequestration after injury: a pathogenic mechanism for multiple organ failure. *J Trauma.* 1995;39:411–417.
63. Patrick DA, Moore EE, Moore FA, et al. Reduced PAF-acetyl-hydrolase activity is associated with postinjury multiple organ failure. *Shock.* 1997;7:170–174.
64. Moore FA, Moore EE, Kudsk KA, et al. Clinical benefits of an immune-enhancing diet for early postinjury enteral feeding. *J Trauma.* 1994;37:607–615.
65. Wu Y, Kudsk KA, DeWitt RC, et al. Route and type of nutrition influence IgA-mediated intestinal cytokines. *Ann Surg.* 1999;229:662–668.
66. Fukatsu K, Kudsk KA, Wu Y, et al. TPN decreases IL-4 and IL-10 mRNA expression in lamina propria cells but glutamine supplementation preserves the expression. *Shock.* 2001;15:318–322.
67. Fukatsu K, Lundberg AH, Hanna MK, et al. Route of nutrition influences intercellular adhesion molecule-1 expression and neutrophil accumulation in intestine. *Arch Surg.* 1999;134:1055–1060.
68. Fukatsu K, Zarzaur BL, Johnson CD, et al. Enteral nutrition prevents remote organ injury and mortality following a gut ischemic insult. *Ann Surg.* 2001;233:660–668.
69. Fukatsu K, Kudsk KA, Zarzaur BL, et al. Increased ICAM-1 and β2 integrin expression in parenterally fed mice after a gut ischemic insult. *Shock.* (In Press)
70. Mestecky J, Abraham R, Ogra PL. Common mucosal immune system and strategies for the development of vaccines effective at the mucosal surfaces. In: Ogra PL, Lamm ME, McGhee JR, et al., eds. *Handbook of Mucosal Immunology.* New York: Academic Press, Inc; 1994:357–372.
71. Zarzaur BL, Kudsk KA. The mucosa-associated lymphoid tissue structure, function, and derangements. *Shock.* 2001: 15:411–420.
72. Fukatsu K, Zarzaur B, Johnson C, et al. MAdCAM-1 expression in Peyer's patches: a mechanism controlling the gut-associated lymphoid tissue (GALT). *Surgical Forum.* 2000;51:211–214.
73. Li J, Kudsk KA, Gocinski B, et al. Effects of parenteral and enteral nutrition on gut-associated lymphoid tissue. *J Trauma.* 1995;39:44–52.
74. King BK, Li J, Kudsk KA. A temporal study of TPN-induced changes in gut-associated lymphoid tissue and mucosal immunity. *Arch Surg.* 1997;132:1303–1309.
75. Renegar KB, Small PA. Immunoglobulin A mediation of murine nasal anti-influenza virus immunity. *J Virol.* 1991; 65:2146–2148.
76. Abraham E. Intranasal immunization with bacterial polysaccharide containing liposomes enhances antigen-specific pulmonary secretory antibody response. *Vaccine.* 1992;10: 461–468.
77. Kudsk KA, Li J, Renegar KB. Loss of upper respiratory tract immunity with parenteral feeding. *Ann Surg.* 1996; 223:629–638.
78. King BK, Kudsk KA, Li J, et al. Route and type of nutrition influence mucosal immunity to bacterial pneumonia. *Ann Surg.* 1999;229:272–278.
79. Janu P, Li J, Renegar KB, et al. Recovery of gut-associated lymphoid tissue (GALT) and upper respiratory tract (URT) immunity following parenteral nutrition (TPN). *Ann Surg.* 1997;225:707–717.
80. Kudsk KA, Alverdy JL. Host defenses and bacterial assaults: a delicate balance. In: Kudsk KA, Pichard C, eds. *From Nutritional Support to Pharmacologic Nutrition in the ICU.* Berlin: Springer-Verlag; 2000:15–25.
81. Laughlin RS, Musch MW, Hollbrook CJ, et al. The key role of Pseudomonas aeruginosa PA-1 lectin on experimental gut-derived sepsis. *Ann Surg.* 2000;232:133–142.
82. Alverdy J, Holbrook C, Rocha F, et al. Gut-derived sepsis occurs when the right pathogen with the right virulence genes meets the right host: evidence for in vivo virulence expression in Pseudomonas aeruginosa. *Ann Surg.* 2000; 232:480–489.

CHAPTER

12 Intravenous Access for Parenteral Nutrition in the Intensive Care Unit

Dion L. Franga, M.D.

INTRODUCTION 131
History 131
Anatomy 131
BASIC TENANTS OF CENTRAL VENOUS ACCESS 131
TECHNIQUES OF VENOUS CANNULATION 133
Percutaneous Infraclavicular Subclavian Catheterization 133
Percutaneous Supraclavicular Subclavian Catheterization 133
Percutaneous Internal Jugular Catheterization 133
Percutaneous External Jugular Venous Catheterization 133
Peripherally Inserted Central Catheter (PICC) 134
Femoral Venous Catheters 134
Long-term vs. Short-term Venous Catheters 134
COMPLICATIONS OF PARENTERAL ACCESS 134
Infectious Complications 134
Noninfectious Complications 135
CONCLUSIONS 136
REFERENCES 136

Introduction

Parenteral nutrition has evolved over the years as a useful adjunct to nutritional support when enteral nutrition is not an option. Infusion of nutrients is generally 3 to 4 times serum osmolarity and thus peripheral infusion is not possible without rapid onset of complications such as pain, peripheral vein thrombosis, and superficial thrombophlebitis. Goals of access should thus allow infusion into a high flow system, not limit mobility, and provide access for more than short-term duration when necessary.

HISTORY

Central venous access has long been described for hemodynamic monitoring. Aubaniac first described a percutaneous approach to the subclavian vein in patients with military battle injuries for resuscitation.[1] Techniques in percutaneous central venous access have improved over the years thanks to work by Dudrick, Yoffa, and Duffy.[2,3,4] Seldinger developed his technique utilizing a flexible guide wire, which is virtually universal as the current standard when central venous catheters are placed.[5]

ANATOMY

Peripheral and central venous anatomy of the upper extremity and torso are the main routes for administration of parenteral nutrition. The superficial veins of the arm important for parenteral access include the basilic, cephalic, and median antebrachial veins. These veins ultimately drain centrally by way of the subclavian vein. The subclavian and internal jugular veins join on each side of the chest to form brachiocephalic trunks that eventually form the superior vena cava. The superior vena cava is approximately 2–3 cm in diameter, roughly 6–7 cm long, and has flow rates of approximately 2 L/min. Thus, infusion of high-concentration parenteral nutrition is best performed into the superior vena cava.

Basic Tenants of Central Venous Access

Patient preparation for central venous access is crucial for successful outcome. In-depth discussion regarding the risk, benefits, and potential complication of central venous catheterization should be undertaken. Simply describing the procedure and offering reassurance while performing catheterization are beneficial. Often the assistance of support personnel familiar to the patient lowers anxiety levels. Rarely, sedation is necessary for temporary venous access but is almost mandatory for tunneled, more permanent access.

Positioning of the patient is incredibly important prior to initiation of the procedure. Individual physician preference and patient body habitus dictate the use of linens beneath the shoulder or longitudinally along the spine to assist in exposure of the upper body landmarks for access. If the upper venous system is to be accessed, Trendelenburg positioning can be helpful to distend the upper venous system to assist in venous cannulation and reduce the risk of air embolization. If the lower venous system is utilized, flat or reverse Trendelenburg position may be helpful. Access is named based on site of catheter insertion and location of the catheter tip.

Antiseptic skin preparation is vitally important. The skin must be thoroughly cleansed and free of exogenous materials such as adhesive or other dressings. A defatting solution should be used followed by a povidone-iodine skin preparation. Chlorhexidine or alcohol should be utilized in allergic patients. Patients with allergies to iodine often will tolerate small areas of skin preparation but skin testing should be performed.

Radiographic techniques have been found to be helpful in the placement of central venous catheters. Fluoroscopy helps to identify catheter position as well as direct catheter manipulation in the case of catheter malposition. The use of ultrasound guidance in the placement of central venous catheters has been reported and portable ultrasound devices are currently on the market. Ultrasound conveys benefit in identifying venous anatomy in difficult-to-place catheters, in obesity, and in coagulopathic states where multiple attempts at venous cannulation should be avoided.[6]

In stable patients in need of long-term access without current infection and those for whom home parenteral nutrition is possible, tunneled catheters designed for long-term access are preferred. Surgeons generally place these in an operative setting under strict sterile technique with sedation for patient comfort. For short-term access, temporary catheters are generally used and are not tunneled. Venous cutdown to any of these vessels can be safely accomplished but should be performed in a formal operative setting. Regardless of the type of catheter used, the basic technique is the same with some modifications for long-term catheters. Table 12.1 depicts various techniques with pros and cons for each.

TABLE 12.1

Site for Temporary Vascular Access

Technique	Pros	Cons
Subclavian	Low infection risk Patient comfort Exchangeable	Risk of pneumothorax higher Noncompressible vessel
Internal jugular	Lower risk of pneumothorax Infection risk low Exchangeable	Patient discomfort Injury
External jugular	Peripheral vein Exchangeable	Can be technically difficult
Femoral	Ease of placement Exchangeable	Higher infection rate Risk of deep venous thrombosis
Tunneled catheters	Lower infection rate	Operative placement More difficult to remove
Implantable ports	Lower infection rate Cosmetics	Not recommended for ICU setting More difficult to remove Frequent venipuncture/infiltration Operative placement
PICC	Bedside insertion Non-thoracic approach	Thrombophlebitis Infection Blood draw not always feasible

Techniques of Venous Cannulation

Percutaneous Infraclavicular Subclavian Catheterization

Patient preparation entails the Trendelenburg position. The right or left side is selected and the neck *and* chest wall are prepped and draped under sterile conditions. Local anesthetic is infiltrated from the junction of the middle and outer thirds of the clavicle down to the periosteum of the clavicle. Adequate anesthesia is a must because of the dense tissue of the clavicular fascia beneath the clavicle. An 18 gauge, 3-1/2 inch introducer needle is inserted 2–3 cm below and at the outer third of the clavicle in the anesthetized area. The needle is inserted to the clavicle directed to the sternal notch. Pressure is applied anteriorly to assist needle insertion below the clavicle. Syringe aspiration is performed as the needle is slid under the clavicle parallel to the coronal plane until the subclavian vein is entered. If no flash of blood is encountered, slowly withdraw the needle while aspirating as the subclavian vein may have been compressed on the initial pass. If the vessel is not entered, redirection more cephalad may be necessary. Once cannulation is completed, a flexible J-wire is passed through the needle. This should go easily and any difficulty usually means the wire is out of the vein, is abutting the internal jugular-subclavian junction, or has been passed into an accessory vein. The needle is removed from the end of the wire, a small incision made at the insertion site, and the tract to the subclavian vein is serially dilated depending on catheter size. It is crucially important that positive control of the wire is maintained at all times and that it remains still while passing the dilator through the subclavian puncture site. Keeping the catheter immobilized prevents the dilator from kinking the guidewire and causing a profound venous injury within the chest. The purpose of the dilator is to dilate a tract to the subclavian vein. Perforation of the subclavian vein, brachiocephalic vein, superior vena cava, and the right atrium have been described. After dilation is complete, the dilator is withdrawn and the catheter passed over the wire to its proper position at the atriocaval junction.

The purpose of prepping the neck and chest on the same side is to allow for a supraclavicular or internal jugular approach should the infraclavicular approach fail. Attempts to cannulate the contralateral side should ***never*** be undertaken until a chest roentogram has been performed to evaluate for a pneumothorax or other complications.

Percutaneous Supraclavicular Subclavian Catheterization

The same principles in patient preparation hold true for this approach as detailed above for the infraclavicular approach to the subclavian vein. The clavicular head of the sternocleidomastoid muscle (SCM) is identified and an area of skin and soft tissue is anesthetized with 1% lidocaine down to the periosteum of the clavicle. The introducer needle is inserted just deep to the clavicle, oriented to 45 degrees from the sagittal plane or roughly aimed at the contralateral nipple. Aspiration is performed until the vein is entered. The needle is lowered toward the shoulder and a wire is passed. The remainder of the procedure is similar to that outlined above.

Percutaneous Internal Jugular Catheterization

The borders of the internal jugular approach include the junction of the two heads of the sternocleidomastoid muscle and the ipsilateral nipple. An area of skin over the junction of the two heads of the SCM is infiltrated with 1% lidocaine. The carotid artery is palpated and should be medial to the junction of the two heads. An introducer needle is inserted and advanced at 45 degrees to the sagittal plane towards the ipsilateral nipple. The vein is entered and a flexible J-wire is used to guide the remainder of the procedure.

Percutaneous External Jugular Venous Catheterization

The external jugular vein may be utilized as the entry point for central venous catheters. The technique is essentially the same for the above-described approaches. Deep Trendelenburg positioning is important for this technique to raise the upper venous system pressures and facilitate venous filling.

The external jugular vein is entered in much the same way as for central access. Site of insertion should be as low as possible on the neck in a straight segment of vein to facilitate wire passage. Once cannulated the guide wire may be passed into the central venous system. Difficulty in passing the guidewire is often due to venous valves and the sharp angulation of the vessel. An alternative technique that can also be utilized with the external jugular approach is with a 16G angiocatheter. Once the vein is entered, the sheath can be advanced over the needle and then used for wire guidance and theoretically decrease the risk of vessel injury compared to introducer needles.

PERIPHERALLY INSERTED CENTRAL CATHETER (PICC)

These catheters are easily inserted and in most hospitals are done so by specialized nursing staff or phlebotomist. The antecubital fossa is most often the site of insertion. Prominent cephalic veins are easily cannulated as well. Ultrasound guidance is a useful adjunct in identification and placement of these catheters. A Seldinger technique is utilized after the vein is entered and a long guide wire is used to enter the central circulation. A 4 French 60 cm catheter is typically used to access the circulation, and post-placement chest film is obtained simply to confirm placement of catheter. These catheters are associated with a higher incidence of infection and are cumbersome at times to the patient and less suitable for long-term nutrition. Thus, these catheters should be avoided for long-term use.

FEMORAL VENOUS CATHETERS

Femoral catheters are alternatives to the above listed procedures. They are inserted in the same fashion as the above using the NAVEL (nerve, artery, vein, empty space, lymphatics from lateral to medial in the groin) mnemonic for identification of the femoral vein. These catheters are associated with a higher incidence of infection as well as deep venous thrombosis.[7] One author has described several patients in which this was the final option and maintained these patients on low dose anticoagulants for DVT prevention.[8] Ideal position of the catheter tip is above the renal arteries (T12–L1) given the higher flow rate in this region of the inferior vena cava. Fluoroscopy will aid in positioning of catheters or estimation with follow-up KUB roentogram can be performed to ensure appropriate positioning.

LONG-TERM VS. SHORT-TERM VENOUS CATHETERS

The techniques for long-term catheter insertion are only slightly different than for short-term access procedures. The mainstay of long-term catheters is tunneling through the subcutaneous tissues and the addition of a cuff to the outside of the catheter. Tunneling of these catheters aids in the prevention of infection, although this has been debated recently.[9,10,11] Tunneling generally places the catheter along the chest wall; therefore, the internal jugular, external jugular or subclavian approach can be utilized with suitable patient comfort. In addition, percutaneous inserted implantable catheters are available but are seldom used in the ICU setting. There is some evidence that these catheters convey some protection against catheter related infection but their use is limited in parenteral nutrition therapy because of frequent transcutaneous puncture.[12]

Complications of Parenteral Access

INFECTIOUS COMPLICATIONS

Nosocomial blood-related infections exceed 200,000 per year. Catheter related infections account for a majority of these cases. According to the CDC National Nosocomial Infections Surveillance Report, catheter infections are the third most common nosocomial infection in the intensive care unit.[13] The most common associated pathogens are listed in Table 12.2.

Central venous catheters come in varying sizes and are composed of a host of different materials (polyethylene, polyurethane, polyvinylchloride, silicone, and Teflon). Selection of catheter composition has implications on catheter-related infections. Silicone catheters have been recognized to reduce sensitivity of *Staphylococcus aureus* to antibiotics such as tetracycline, vancomycin, and penicillin.[14] Determination of the type, size, and number of lumens should guide your decision. Controversial evidence exists regarding increased infection rates for single vs. multi-lumen catheters. Early et al. compared single-lumen vs. dual-lumen Hickman catheters and found the infection rate for dual-lumen catheters to be greater than for single-lumen catheters with approximately 496 infection-free days vs. 1210 infection-free days, respectively.[15,16] Ideally, the smallest catheter necessary to provide therapy should be selected. In hospitalized patients and critically ill patients, this generally is in the form of .032 cm internal diameter, 20 cm triple-lumen catheter. These catheters provide access for parenteral nutrition as well as for other concomitant medical treatment and/or monitoring such as central venous pressure monitoring, and delivery of medication and blood products. Argument exists that central venous catheters used for parenteral

TABLE 12.2

Organisms Most Associated with Catheter-Related Infections
Staphylococcus epidermidis—30%
Staphylococcus aureus—13%
Enterococcus—13%
Candida sp.—6%

nutrition should be dedicated only for parenteral nutrition and not for other therapies or monitoring.

Catheter-related infection is the most common associated problem encountered in central parenteral access. Controversy exists regarding the practice of catheter site rotation in critically ill patients. The practice of guidewire directed catheter exchange and mandatory site rotation have met with mixed results. It is generally recognized that catheters should remain in place unless evidence of catheter-related sepsis or tunnel/insertion site infection occurs.[17] Centers for Disease Control recommendations advise placement of indwelling catheters in the subclavian position unless medically contraindicated to help prevent infection (see Table 12.3).[10]

New central venous catheters impregnated with antibiotics show promise in reducing the incidence of catheter-related infections. Hanley et al. reviewed catheter-related bloodstream infections in critically ill patients and found a 47% reduction in catheter-related infection with the use of silver sulfadiazine and chlorhexidine impregnated triple-lumen catheters. Patients receiving parenteral nutrition showed significantly decreased catheter-related infection in antibiotic-impregnated catheters compared to standard triple-lumen catheters.[18] However, in a similar randomized prospective study, Pemberton et al. failed to show any significant decrease in catheter-related infections between silver sulfadiazine/chlorhexidine impregnated catheters and standard non-impregnated catheters.[19] Darouiche et al. evaluated catheters impregnated with minocycline and rifampin vs. chlorhexidine and silver sulfadiazine. Minocycline/rifampin catheters are coated intraluminally as well as externally compared to the external surfaces only for chlorhexidine/silver sulfadiazine. Minocycline/rifampin catheters were less likely to become colonized and were associated with a significantly decreased number of catheter-related infections.[20] Therefore, these catheters should be selected for use when they are available.

TABLE 12.3

CDC Recommendations Regarding Techniques to Reduce Catheter-Related Infections
Head cover
Mask
Sterile gown
Sterile drape to cover field
Subclavian approach

Noninfectious Complications

The incidence of catheter insertion related complications is reported to be as high as 11% and is directly related to operator experience.[21] Possible complications include pneumothorax (0%–3%), arterial puncture or cannulation, catheter malposition, hemothorax and hemomediastinum, air embolus, nerve injury (brachial plexus/phrenic nerve), thoracic duct injury, puncture site bleeding, catheter dysfunction, and thrombosis of the vessel cannulated. Coagulation abnormalities should be corrected prior to attempting central catheter insertion. Location of catheter insertion helps define an acceptable level of coagulopathy and hence compressibility of the blood vessel. For example, the subclavian approach should not be performed unless the coagulopathy is corrected and platelet counts are normal in the event of an arterial puncture, since this vessel cannot be adequately compressed. An INR of less than 1.5 and platelet count of greater than 100,000 is recommended.

Kincaid recently reported a series of patients in which long-term indwelling catheters were placed in an outpatient clinic setting without the aid of real-time imaging modalities such as fluoroscopy. They reported a technical success rate of 92%. Only small-bore catheters, both percutaneous inserted or implantable, were used. Patients with significant comorbid illnesses were not selected. Their incidence of complications did not differ significantly from previously reported complications. A few patients (2.9%) required repositioning of their catheter tips. All patients received post-operative chest films. An average cost-savings of 57% to 63% was estimated compared to operating or radiology suite placed catheters.[22]

Guth also assessed the need for post-operative chest roentography following intraoperative placement of central venous catheters using fluoroscopy. He defined the need for post-operative x-ray as unilateral chest pain, air aspiration at time of placement, decreased breath sounds, and difficult catheter insertion. There were no missed pneumothoraces if these criteria were followed.[23]

Catheter placement in the internal jugular position has a lower overall incidence of insertion complications. Embolic cerebrovascular accidents have been reported after cannulation of carotid arteries. Femoral vein cannulation has a significantly higher incidence of complications, primarily catheter-related infection, given its proximity to the perineal region and is associated with higher incidence of vein thrombosis.[7] The femoral vein catheter should be for short-term access

TABLE 12.4

Complications of Central Venous Access
Catheter dysfunction/occlusion
Pneumothorax
Hemothorax/hemomediastinum
Arterial injury
Air embolus
Catheter pinch-off
Catheter malposition
Thoracic duct injury (left IJ/supraclavicular approach)
Vein thrombosis

only or when all upper extremity venous access has been eliminated.

Catheter occlusion is well recognized as a complication of central venous catheters. Diligent care of the catheter, "packing" unused ports with heparinized saline (1:1000), and flushing the catheter with heparinized saline prior to insertion can help in preventing catheter occlusion. Should this complication occur, use of tPA to the affected port may open the lumen. If this fails or if the catheter has been in place for an extended period of time, a fibrin sheath may have formed around the catheter. One of the first signs of this may be a catheter that flushes but aspiration meets resistance.

Wire exchange of the catheter should be performed but may prove to be unsuccessful. Prepping the catheter with antiseptic solution, passing a guidewire through the distal port, and then removing the catheter over the guidewire accomplishes this. A new catheter is then placed over the guidewire to the appropriate position. It is not always necessary to obtain a chest roentogram following this procedure.[24]

Conclusions

Parenteral access for nutritional support is best accomplished via the central venous system. Selection criteria for access location and catheter type should be thoroughly considered. When available, antibiotic-impregnated catheters should be used and if long-term access is needed, a tunneled catheter should be utilized. Long-term central venous catheters can be inserted outside of the operative setting in select patients. Knowledge of and early recognition of catheter-related complications is necessary to prevent patient morbidity and preserve patency of central venous catheters.

References

1. Aubaniac R. Une nouvelle voie d'injection ou de ponction veinuse: La voie sous-claviculaire. *Semin Hop Paris.* 1952; 28:3445–3447.
2. Dudrick SJ. Can intravenous feeding as the sole means of nutrition support growth in the child and restore weight loss in adults? An affirmative answer. *Ann Surg.* 1969;169: 974–984.
3. Yoffa D. Supraclavicular subclavian venipuncture and catheterization. *Lancet.* 1965;2:614–617.
4. Duffy BJ Jr. The clinical use of polyethylene tubing for intravenous therapy: a report of seventy-two cases. *Ann Surg.* 1949;130:929–936.
5. Seldinger SI. Catheter replacement of the needle in percutaneous arteriography. *Acta Radiol.* 1953;39:368–376.
6. Mallory DL. Ultrasound guidance improves the success rates of internal jugular vein canulation. A prospective, randomized trial. *Chest.* 1990;98:157–160.
7. Joynt GM. Deep venous thrombosis caused by femoral venous catheters in critically ill adult patients. *Chest.* 2000; 117:178–183.
8. Grant JP. Parenteral access. In: Rombeau JL, Caldwell MD, eds. *Clinical Nutrition: Parenteral Nutrition.* 3rd ed. Philadelphia: WB Saunders; 2001:109–117.
9. Raad I. Low infection rate and long durability of non-tunneled silastic catheters: a safe and cost-effective alternative for long-term use of venous access devices in patients with cancer. *Ann Intern Med.* 1993;28:851–858.
10. Pearson, ML. Guideline for prevention of intravascular device-related infections: Part 1. Intravascular device-related infections: An Overview. The Hospital Infection Control Practices Advisory Committee. *Am J Infect Control.* 1996;24:262–277.
11. Keohane PP. Effect of catheter tunneling and a nutrition nurse on catheter sepsis during parenteral nutrition: a controlled trial. *Lancet.* 1983;2:1388–1390.
12. Hollyoak MA. Critical appraisal of surgical venous access in children. *Pediatr Surg Int.* 1997;12:177–182.
13. CDC NNIS System. National Nosocomial Infections Surveillance (NNIS) Report, Data Summary from October 1986–April 1997, issued May 1997. *Am J Infect Control.* 1997;25:477–487.
14. Williams I. The effects of adherence to silicone surfaces on antibiotic susceptibility in Staphylococcus aureua. *Microbiology.* 1997;143:2407–2413.
15. Kemp L. The effect of catheter type and site on infection rates in total parenteral infection rates. *J Parenter Enteral Nutr.* 1994;18:71–74.
16. Early TF. Increased infection rate in double-lumen versus single-lumen Hickman catheters in cancer patients. *Southern Med J.* 1990;83:34–36.
17. Badley AD. Mayo Clinic Proceedings. Infectious rates of central venous pressure catheters: comparison between newly placed catheters and those that have been changed. 1996;71(9):838–846.

18. Hanley EM. Evaluation of an antiseptic triple lumen catheter in an intensive care unit. *Crit Care Med.* 2000;28:366–370.
19. Pemberton LB. No difference in catheter sepsis between standard and antiseptic central venous catheters. A prospective randomized trial. *Arch Surg.* 1996;131:986–989.
20. Darouiche RO. A comparison of two antimicrobial-impregnated central venous catheters. Catheter Study Group. *N Engl J Med.* 1999;340:1–8.
21. Padburg FT. Central venous catheterization for parenteral nutrition. *Ann Surg.* 1981;193:264–272.
22. Kincaid EH. "Blind" placement of long-term central venous access devices: report of 589 consecutive procedures. *Am Surgeon.* 1999;65:520–524.
23. Guth AA. Routine chest-x-rays after insertion of implantable long-term venous catheters: necessary or not? *Am Surgeon.* 2001;67:26–29.
24. Amshel CE. Are chest X-rays mandatory following central venous recatheterization over a wire? *Am Surgeon.* 1998; 64:499–501.

CHAPTER 13

Enteral Access—The Foundation of Feeding

William A. Arnold, M.D., Mark H. DeLegge, M.D., F.A.C.G., C.N.S.P., Steven D. Schwaitzberg, M.D., F.A.C.S.

INTRODUCTION 139
NASOENTERIC NUTRITIONAL ACCESS 139
Alternate Feeding Tube Technology 143
PERCUTANEOUS ENDOSCOPIC ENTERAL ACCESS 143
Small Bowel Access 144
Percutaneous Endoscopic Enteral Access 144
SURGICAL ACCESS 146
Methods of Surgically Placed Enteral Access 146
Complications of Surgically Placed Enteral Access 148
CONCLUSIONS 149
REFERENCES 149

Introduction

Nutritional support of the hospitalized patient has been important in improving patient outcomes. Over the past 40 years we have seen tremendous advances in our ability to deliver nutrition to at-risk patients. The use of parenteral nutrition was introduced in the 1960s and has continued to be an important tool for the nutritional support of patients with gastrointestinal impairment. However, in patients with a functioning GI tract the use of enteral nutrition is the preferred route of feeding, especially with the advances in the development of disease-specific enteral nutritional feeding products.[1] Enteral nutrition is less costly than parenteral nutrition, and has the advantages of reduced infectious and metabolic complications.[2] In addition, enteral nutrition maintains gut integrity and is fundamental is supporting gut immunity, an important defense system for the at-risk patient.[3]

In a patient who can eat and drink, the provision of enteral nutrition support is focused on the use of nutritional supplements, dietary counseling, and appetite stimulation. However, in those patients who will not or cannot eat, an enteral route can be established to provide feedings as necessary. As such, obtaining enteral access becomes the foundation of any attempt at providing enteral nutrition. The science of enteral access, and nutrition support in general, has evolved dramatically over the recent years. Even though the benefits of enteral nutrition are well accepted, the best method for delivery of enteral nutrition remains controversial. Options include short-term nasoenteric tubes placed either into the stomach, past the pylorus, or distal to the ligament of Treitz. Other options include surgically placed gastrostomy or jejunostomy tubes or percutaneous, endoscopically guided gastrostomy tubes or jejunostomy (PEG, PEG-J, or DPEJ, respectively).

Nasoenteric Nutritional Access

Tube feeds are usually considered in patients who are unable to sustain adequate nutritional intake and have a functioning gastrointestinal tract. Contraindications to tube feeding include mechanical bowel obstruction, ischemic bowel, high output fistulas, GI hemorrhage, and severe malabsorption states. Other mitigating factors in the decision to feed the gut are the patient's ability to protect the airway, potential for aspiration, and the degree of gastrointestinal dysmotility caused by various circumstances such as surgery, trauma, sepsis, use of sympathetic agonists, and concomitant use of narcotics.

Nasoenteric tubes (NET) are usually placed at the bedside. One of the simplest methods is the placement of a large-bore nasogastric tube into the stomach for administration of tube feeds. This method is appreciated for its relative ease of placement, although any blind passage of nasoenteric tubes carries a small risk of complications. Perforation of the esophagus and inadvertent passage into the trachea or bronchial tree are rare, but noted complications. In order to avoid placing the NGT through the cribriform plate and into the brain, the presence of complex facial or basilar skull fractures is a contraindication to the blind passage of nasoenteric tubes, thus avoiding a potentially lethal complication.[4] All nasoenteric tubes can cause local irritation, epistaxis, and/or sinusitis. Nasogastric tubes are relatively stiff and large bore compared to their softer, smaller caliber nasojejunal counterparts. The larger nasogastric tubes allow for decompression of the stomach. In fact a specialized tube that allows for naso-gastric decompression and post-pyloric feeding has been created. Nasogastric tubes do not clog as easily as the nasojejunal tubes and are better for the administration of medications. Intragastric feeds can be delivered as a bolus, whereas jejunal feeds must be given continuously. Given their larger diameter, there is some concern that the nasogastric tubes may stent open the lower esophageal sphincter and increase gastroesophageal reflux, although the clinical significance of this is controversial. Nasoduodenal or nasojejunal feeding tubes can also be placed at the bedside. Although there are many tubes available, they are commonly referred to as Dobbhoff tubes, the name being derived from the inventors Dobbie and Hoffmeister in 1976.[5] Nasojejunal tubes are softer, more pliable tubes that come with tungsten-weighted or non-weighted tips. The smaller-diameter tubes cause less discomfort but are more likely to become clogged or inadvertently dislodged.

Concern that altered GI motility, particularly gastroparesis, may increase gastric residual volume, gastroesophageal reflux, and aspiration rates has led many to advocate post-pyloric delivery of enteral nutrition, and many ICUs have adopted the policy of initiating tube feeds only after post-pyloric access has been secured. In certain subpopulations of critically ill patients, especially patients undergoing celiotomy, gastroparesis or postoperative gastric ileus is often the limiting factor for the initiation of intragastric feeds. The small intestine regains motility and absorptive capacity before the stomach or the colon. It takes approximately one to two days for the stomach and three to five days for the colon post-operatively to regain motility.[6] The implication is that tube feeds delivered to the small intestine can be safely started almost immediately postoperatively. Several animal studies have demonstrated the importance of early (<72 hours) versus late (>72 hours) enteral nutrition in terms of improved wound healing, reduced catabolic phase, and lower rate of bacterial translocation.[7–9] In humans with major abdominal trauma, it was demonstrated that those receiving enteral feedings within 12 to 18 hours of injury had a lower infection rate than control patients.[10] Despite the best intentions to initiate early enteral feeds, gaining access to the duodenum or jejunum often proves difficult and contributes significantly to the delay in starting tube feeds. Difficulty obtaining post-pyloric access has prompted numerous adjuvant measures and techniques to facilitate small bowel intubation. Difficulty with small bowel intubation has also led many institutions to rethink their policies regarding intragastric feeds—even in patients that are traditionally considered high risk.

Several techniques have been described to facilitate transpyloric placement of nasoenteric tubes. The method of spontaneous passage of nasoenteric tubes from the stomach to the small bowel rarely meets with success. In the clinically stable patient, less than half will achieve spontaneous transpyloric passage.[11] In the critically ill population the number of spontaneous passages drops to 5% at 48 hours.[12] Concomitant use of the prokinetic agent metoclopramide increased the rate to 14.7% spontaneous migration at 72 hours.[12] A combination of patient positioning, air insufflation with auscultation, bending the stylet 30 degrees, and using a corkscrew motion has met with better success. Thurlow reports success in 28 of 31 consecutive patients using this technique,[13] and Zolaga succeeded in 92% of 231 attempts. The average time of placement for Zolaga was 40 ± 14 minutes,[14] suggesting that blind identification of the pylorus requires not only a high level of experience but also a high degree of motivation.

With few exceptions, it has been our practice to utilize nasoduodenal or nasojejunal tube feeds rather than intragastric feeds for the short-term delivery of enteral nutrition for critically ill surgical patients. Our own surgical intensive care unit (authors WAA, SDS) favors the blind bedside insertion technique as described by Zaloga along with the use of adjuvant prokinetic agents. Metoclopramide is a cholinergic agonist and a dopamine receptor antagonist that is thought to promote contraction of the stomach and small bowel by its cholinergic properties and by blocking dopamine's inhibition of GI smooth muscle. Erythromycin mimics the effects of the GI hormone motilin. Cisapride has also been used in the past as a promotility agent. Its use has been limited by the FDA because of its association with cardiac arrhythmias particularly Toursade de Pointes in patients with prolonged Q-T intervals.[15]

Our protocol for blind bedside insertion of nasoenteric tubes begins with the intravenous administration of metoclopramide and erythromycin 10 minutes prior to the planned insertion. The stylet of the Dobbhoff tube is then bent to 30 degrees approximately 6.5 cm from the tip, forming a kink at the distal end of the tube. The tube is inserted with the patient in the right lateral decubitus position. Gastric intubation is confirmed by auscultation as approximately 200 cc of air are insufflated into the stomach. The tube is then advanced slowly with a clockwise twisting motion in an attempt to "hook" the pylorus. An experienced person can often sense when the tube loops back into the stomach by a sudden loss of resistance. The position of the Dobbhoff tube is then confirmed with a bedside plain abdominal radiograph (KUB) to ensure successful post-pyloric placement prior to the initiation of tube feeds.

In order to critically examine our use and insertion efficiency of nasoenteric feeding tubes, we performed a retrospective review of all patients in our surgical ICU receiving enteral nutrition over an 8-month period (authors WAA, SDS). The surgical ICU is utilized by the general, vascular, transplant, orthopedic, and neurosurgical services. Over an 8-month period, 58 patients received Dobbhoff nasoduodenal or nasojejunal tubes. Five of these patients had nasojejunal tubes placed at the time of laparotomy, 39 patients had Dobbhoff tubes placed at the bedside, and 14 patients failed bedside insertion and had nasojejunal tubes placed with the aid of fluoroscopy. The cumulative number of bedside attempts at small bowel intubation over an eight-month period was 120 separate attempts. Forty-three attempts utilized prokinetic agents; 77 attempts did not. The overall success rate for blind bedside insertion was 48% (58 of 120 attempts). In our experience, the use of prokinetic agents did not contribute significantly to the success of small bowel intubation. In cases where blind nasoduodenal or nasojejunal insertion failed, we found that insertion with fluoroscopic guidance had a 100% success rate. Fluoroscopic guidance is successful but can be impractical if critically ill patients have to be transported to a GI radiology suite. It can also be difficult for an already busy radiology department to accommodate requests for fluoroscopically guided feeding tubes.

To illustrate the difficulty of obtaining and maintaining post-pyloric access, consider that in our experience, it required an average of 3.1 separate Dobbhoff insertion attempts for each successful bedside post-pyloric access. An average of 3.5 plain abdominal x-rays were required per successful placement to confirm position; and despite our standing goal to deliver early enteral nutrition, a retrospective review found that an average of 3.5 days elapsed post-operatively before post-pyloric access was even attempted. Once post-pyloric feeds were started, it required an average of 5.3 days to reach tube feed goal rates. Thus, even in an institution that places great emphasis on post-operative nutrition, delivering adequate enteral nutrition can be a challenging endeavor.

There are several factors that contribute to the difficulty of obtaining and maintaining access. The first is the patient population. The irritation of indwelling nasal tubes in a drowsy or delirious patient often leads to the frustrating complication of self-decannulation; a complication that could be decreased by more liberal use of a nasal bridle to secure nasoenteric tubes. Another barrier to delivery of tube feeds is that critically ill patients often require adjuvant studies such as endoscopy or swallowing studies that mandate removal of nasoenteric tubes. Tube feeds are also commonly stopped for bedside maneuvers such as patient repositioning, which contributes to a delay in reaching goal rate of tube feeds. Tube feeds are often stopped or slowed significantly when aspiration of tube feeds is suspected or the patient develops signs or symptoms of gastrointestinal distress such as bloating, cramping, regurgitation, or diarrhea.

The difficulty with bedside insertion has spurred interest in several different adjuvant measures to assist bedside insertion of post-pyloric feeding tubes. Other than fluoroscopy, most of these measures have not been routinely adopted. These adjuvant measures include ultrasound-assisted placement, endoscopic placement, magnet-assisted placement, and pH assisted placement. Hernandez-Socorro compared blind bedside insertion to ultrasound assisted post-pyloric placement and found that only 25.7% of blind placements were successful compared to 84.6% of sonographically guided placements. Average time for ultrasound-assisted placement was 18 minutes.[16] Gabriel utilized a hand-held external magnet to negotiate a weighted nasoenteric tube through the pylorus with an 88% success rate on first attempt,[17] although others using the same method have had less success.[11] Endoscopically guided nasojejunal tube placement allows positioning beyond the ligament of Treitz under direct vision, but requires the expertise of a trained endoscopist. Brandt reported a success rate of 90.9% and a mean placement time of 15.2 minutes for 56 patients.[18] Finally, several groups have experimented with pH sensitive enteral feeding tubes. By use of continuous pH monitoring, an abrupt rise in the pH can suggest passage from the stomach to the duodenum. Success rates for pH assisted placement range from 53% to 97%.[19–21] As one might expect, this adjuvant measure is limited by the oft-employed acid suppression regimens used for critically ill patients to prevent stress gastritis.

Finally, there is always the option to place a nasoenteric feeding tube at the conclusion of celiotomy. Working in concert with the anesthesiologist, the surgeon can manually guide the tip of the feeding tube through the pylorus and into the duodenum or jejunum. Intraoperative placement should be considered in all patients that would benefit from early post-operative administration of enteral nutrition, as it is much easier to remove an unneeded feeding tube than to place one post-operatively at the bedside.

Frustration with the difficulty of obtaining post-pyloric feeding tube placement has led many institutions to liberalize their guidelines for feeding the stomach. As previously mentioned, nasogastric intubation is relatively easier and faster than post-pyloric intubation. Nasogastric tube placement generally requires less exposure to radiation, as there are fewer radiographs taken to confirm position. Gastric tube feeds should be avoided in patients with known or suspected gastroesophageal reflux, atonic stomach, or gastric outlet obstruction. For advocates of post-pyloric tube feeding, the most frequently sited reason to avoid nasogastric feeds is the risk of tube feed aspiration, particularly in patients with bowel dysmotility, altered sensorium, and impaired ability to protect the airway, conditions that describe many critically ill, post-surgical, or neurologically debilitated patients. Several studies and retrospective reviews have examined this issue of tube feed aspiration for nasoenteric and nasogastric tube feeds in particular. There are, however, several problems interpreting the results of these studies. First, there are few prospective, randomized, controlled studies and most studies lack the power to arrive at significant conclusions. Second, the patient populations of these studies demonstrate significant heterogeneity in terms of severity of illness and method of tube feed administration. Third, there is lack of consensus as to what defines tube feed aspiration or even enteral feeding complications in general.

Aspiration rates have been reported in the literature to be anywhere from 0.8% to 92% depending on the study design and patient population.[22,23] Klodell et al. reported a 4% aspiration rate in a series of 118 patients with traumatic brain injury (most had GCS <8) who received intragastric tube feeds exclusively.[24] Spain et al. compared gastric feeds to nasoenteric feeds in 74 patients with head injuries. They found that there was no difference in the tube feed aspiration rate between the two groups (7% and 6% respectively) and that there was no difference in the pneumonia rate between the two groups (69% vs. 81% respectively).[25] The large discrepancy in the reported tube feed aspiration rate and the pneumonia rate highlights the difficulty in interpreting the results of tube feeding studies. In the Spain et al. study, aspiration was defined as any gross recovery of tube feeds from the tracheobronchial tree. It should be kept in mind that patients can aspirate not only from reflux of stomach contents, but also from oropharyngeal secretions, which can cause pneumonia irrespective of the route of enteral feeding. Huxley et al. used a radiolabeled tracer (Indium-111) to document pulmonary aspiration of pharyngeal secretions in 45% of normal control subjects during sleep and in 70% of subjects who had impaired consciousness.[26]

In contrast to several studies that suggest it is safe to administer intragastric tube feeds, an almost equal number of studies suggest it is safer to administer tube feeds past the pylorus. Theoretically, by placing the tip of the feeding tube past the pylorus, the sphincter action of the pylorus will reduce the chance of reflux and pulmonary aspiration of tube feeds. Montecalvo et al. reported a 10.5% incidence of pneumonia in a group of ICU patients randomized to nasogastric tube feeds compared to 0% incidence of pneumonia in the group randomized to endoscopically placed nasojejunal feeds. They also report that the jejunal group also obtained a significantly higher percentage of their daily caloric goal and had significantly greater increases in prealbumin levels compared to the gastric group.[27] This study was limited by its small sample size of 38 patients.

The issue of gastric versus post-pyloric feeds has yet to be settled. Based on our own experience with critically ill surgical patients, we have adopted a policy of post-pyloric tube feeding for patients who are likely to have bowel (especially gastric) dysmotility or high-grade gastroesophageal reflux, or for patients who have an impaired ability to protect their airway via normal oropharyngeal and laryngeal reflexes. For such patients we feel the increased time and expense associated with obtaining post-pyloric access outweighs the consequences of serious aspiration pneumonia. For selected patients who have no significant gastroparesis or gastric outlet obstruction and are able to protect their airway, we have often elected to administer nasogastric tube feeds with few complications. Careful patient assessment and good clinical judgment usually are enough to predict the patients at greatest risk for tube feed related complications.

Alternate Feeding Tube Technology

An alternative to the conventional feeding tube was designed by Dr. S. Bengmark and is in use in Europe. A coil replaces the balloon or weight, usually found at the tip of the tube. The coil is designed to facilitate its transportation down to the region of the ligament of Treitz.[28] Increasing the adherence of the coil to the mucosa, using thin flexible fins at the out- and inside, and/or making the exterior surface frosty or hairy can further increase the motility of this tube. The tube is placed with the aid of a guide wire and the coil allowed to deploy into the lower part of the stomach. The gastro-duodenal motility is stimulated through a small meal (sandwich, pizza, spaghetti, fruit, preferably vegetable juice) and the tip of the tube (the coil), along with the food, is usually transported to its final and optimal position around the ligament of Treitz. The tube is not only made to be self-propelling/auto-positioning, but also self-anchoring. Dr. Bengmark's experience has demonstrated a low dislodgement rate. He feels that it is not necessary to verify the position of the tip before nutrition supply begins. If desired, this can easily be done by simple and repeat pH measurements. It has increasingly become the developer's practice to start feeding immediately after the tube has been placed in the stomach without further waiting for the coil to move to its final position. No attempts are made to control the position of the coil, as it almost always is found within minutes in the region of the ligament of Treitz. The tube is available on the European market (Bengmark Flo-Care tube, Royal Numico-Nutricia group, Zoetermeer, The Netherlands), but not yet in North America.

The tube is especially designed for patients with normal motility, and the tip of the tube is most often and without pharmacological stimulation positioned in its optimal position within a few minutes, and always within 4 hours. Although the tube was intended as a tool only for patients with intact motility, e.g., introduced before surgery and used in connection with elective surgery, it has increasingly been tried in patients with reduced motility, introduced both with and without pharmacological stimulation of motility. Mangiante et al. also report successful intubations in very sick ICU patients, including in 10/10 patients with pancreatitis and in 6/6 patients with abdominal sepsis. Although all these patients demonstrated significantly reduced motility, the tip of the tube did reach its optimal position within an average of 5.2 hours, and always within 24 hours.[29]

Percutaneous Endoscopic Enteral Access

Patients who require enteral feeding for greater than 4 weeks need reliable access. Endoscopic percutaneous procedures are often the preferred means of achieving this (Table 13.1). These procedures include percutaneous gastrostomy (PEG), percutaneous gastrojejunostomy (PEG-J) and direct percutaneous jejunostomy (DPEJ). All of these procedures require the use of an endoscope and usually conscious sedation. In comparison to nasogastric access, PEG has been shown to be a more reliable enteral access tube, allowing patients to receive more calories per day because of the reduction in tube dysfunction.[30]

Ponsky and Gauderer developed percutaneous endoscopic gastrostomy in the early 1980s (see Appendix Figure 13.1a).[31] This procedure involves the placement of a percutaneous gastrostomy tube after endoscopic transillumination of the stomach for an appropriate PEG access position. After appropriate patient selection and consent the patient receives standard upper endoscopy. These patients are often at risk of aspiration by the nature of their underlying disease, requiring PEG placement and the presence of other co-morbid disease states. The patient should be maintained at 30 degrees during PEG placement with aggressive pharyngeal suctioning in an attempt to reduce the occurrence of aspiration. A point of appropriate PEG access is determined by a combination of abdominal wall transillumination with the endoscope and abdominal wall palpation that can be visualized during endoscopy. Failure to achieve appropriate transillumination is a contraindication to the procedure and may result in large or small bowel injury if the procedure is not aborted. Optimally the PEG is brought out through

TABLE 13.1

PEG Related Complications
Aspiration pneumonia (during PEG placement or with tube feeding)
Colocutaneous fistula (PEG placed through colon during placement)
Gastric or esophageal perforation
Gastric hemorrhage
Leakage around PEG tube
Liver hemorrhage (PEG placed through liver)
Necrotizing fasciitis (slough of abdominal wall secondary to infection)
Pain at PEG site
Peritonitis
Pneumoperitoneum (symptomatic)
Tube displacement (by patient or health care personnel)
Tube obstruction (tube feeding or medications)
Wound infection (at PEG tube site)

the anterior gastric wall in the region of the greater curve (see Appendix Figure 13.1b). An intradermal skin wheal is raised at the proposed insertion site. After Betadine cleansing of the abdominal wall, a 7mm–1 cm incision is made. This incision site will allow the PEG tube to exit the gastric cavity through the abdominal wall by the use of an attached PEG tube dilator. The use of prophylactic antibiotics prior to the procedure is important in the prevention of post-procedure infections.[32]

Placement of the PEG tube may be by either the Sachs-Vine (push) or Ponsky (pull) techniques. In the push techniques, a cannula is passed through the abdominal wall incision site into the gastric lumen under direct endoscopic visualization. A guidewire is passed through this cannula into the gastric lumen. The guidewire is snared and pulled out through the oral cavity with the endoscope. In the push technique, a PEG tube is pushed over the guidewire, into the gastric lumen and out the abdominal incision until the internal PEG tube bolster rests against the gastric mucosa. In the pull technique, the PEG tube is tied to the end of the guidewire and the PEG tube is pulled down into the gastric lumen and out the abdominal incision. A decision to use either technique is simply a matter of physician preference.[33] Prospective outcomes evaluations of PEG placement have found this procedure to be associated with few procedure-related complications (Table 13.2).[34] These are usually uncommon but may be devastating or even fatal in the case of intra peritoneal leakage, especially considering the population at risk requiring the PEG placement in the first place.

Once the PEG tube is in proper position, the skin bolster is pushed down over the PEG towards the exterior abdominal wall. Excessive tightening of the bolster can cause tissue ischemia, wound leakage, and potentially necrotizing fasciitis.[35] Nursing care is extremely important in preventing post PEG procedure complications of wound infection and tube obstruction. Tube feedings may begin within 3 to 6 hours of PEG tube placement.[36] Maintaining the head of the bed at 30 degrees will reduce the risk of tube feeding aspiration.

Small Bowel Access

Small bowel access placement techniques have been developed for the bedside, for use with endoscopy, for use with fluoroscopy, or to be placed during surgery. These techniques all have their indications, benefits, and risks. The final position of an enteral access tube is the jejunum. A patient who is intolerant of gastric feedings, such as a patient with gastroparesis, a patient who has had his or her stomach surgically removed, or a patient with acute pancreatitis will receive small bowel feedings. The use of small bowel feedings to prevent tube feeding aspiration events is a much more complicated and contentious issue. Some studies have shown a decrease in aspiration episodes in patients fed into the small bowel as compared to the stomach.[37,38] A recent, prospective trial by Neumann et al. directly compared the use of gastric feedings versus small bowel feedings in the intensive care unit. There was no difference in aspiration episodes between gastric or small bowel feedings. However, it took longer to initiate small bowel feedings because of the difficulty in obtaining adequate tube position.[39] This debate certainly will continue as further aspiration studies are performed. For patients who have known gastroparesis, patients who are intolerant to gastric feedings or patients who have had a witnessed tube feeding aspiration event with gastric feedings, small bowel access and feedings should be initiated.

TABLE 13.2

Enteral Access Methods

Type of Access	Used for	Length of Need
Nasal/Oral Access		
Gastric Tube	Gastric Feeding Gastric Decompression	<1 month
Gastrojejunal Tube	Gastric Feeding Jejunal Feeding Gastric Decompression	<1 month
Jejunal Tube	Jejunal Feeding	<1 month
Percutaneous Access		
Gastrostomy	Gastric Feeding Gastric Decompression	>1 month
Gastrojejunostomy	Gastric Feeding Jejunal Feeding Gastric Decompression	>1 month but <6 months
Jejunostomy	Jejunal Feeding	>1 month

Percutaneous Endoscopic Enteral Access

In those patients for whom small bowel feedings are desired, endoscopic, percutaneous small bowel access may be obtained by two methods. The first method, PEG-J, places a jejunal feeding tube through an existing PEG into the small bowel using a variety of over-the-guidewire methods. Early literature described poor outcomes with use of the PEG-J systems.[40] Previous J-tube placement techniques often required dragging a J-tube, using a grasping forceps, into the small intestine via an attached string. Attempts at removing the endoscope from the small bowel or the grasping forceps from the attached string often resulted in displacement of the J-tube back into the stomach. Jejunal tube failures were often secondary to migration or clogging. Improper positioning of the J-tube through the PEG into the small bowel will result in J-tube migration back into the stomach. Any loop of J-tube left in the stomach after placement will ultimately result in J-tube migration. The J-tube needs to be seen exiting the PEG and be seen directly passing through the pylorus into the small bowel with no evidence of gastric J-tube looping (see Appendix Figure 13.2). Proper jejunal tube placement through a PEG requires a modification of earlier techniques and commercial PEG/J kits. Success can be often obtained using an over-the-guide wire method. After the PEG is placed, the patient is re-endoscoped and an alligator or grasping forceps is passed through the PEG to the outside of the patient (see Appendix Figure 13.3). A guidewire is grasped by the forceps and pulled into the stomach. An air plug device is passed over the guidewire and secured into position on the external end of the PEG allowing insufflation of the stomach and adequate visualization. The endoscope, forceps and guide wire are pushed down to the third or fourth portion of the duodenum (see Appendix Figure 13.4). The grasping forceps are pushed 8–10 cm beyond the endoscope under direct visualization. The air plug is removed and tension is applied on the guidewire that still remains in the grasping forceps. The J-tube is lubricated and passed over the guidewire into position and locked into the distal end of the PEG. The endoscope is pulled back into the stomach while exchanging the grasping forceps forward. Once the endoscope is back in the stomach, the guide wire is released and removed. The grasping forceps is removed and the endoscope confirms proper passage of the J-tube through the PEG without looping.

DeLegge et al. reported a 100% success rate using this technique for PEG-J placement with a procedure time of approximately 26 minutes (see Appendix Figure 13.5).[41] There were no major complications. This PEG-J system allowed for both gastric decompression and small bowel feeding concurrently. The average longevity of this tube system was approximately 120 days when patients who died were excluded from the analysis of tube system longevity.

A newer PEG-J system includes a stiffening catheter in the J-tube to allow easier passage over the guide wire. The catheter is removed after proper J-tube positioning. More recently, Parasher et al. modified this technique by passing a stiffening catheter over the endoscopically placed guide wire under endoscopic visualization. The endoscope is pulled back into the stomach and the stiffening catheter is removed. The J-tube is passed over the guide wire into proper position under direct endoscopic visualization.[42]

With the development of smaller 5 mm endoscopes and 3.6 mm pediatric bronchoscopes, alternative PEG-J placement techniques have been developed. The mini-endoscopes are passed directly through the lumen of the PEG into the small bowel. A guide wire is passed through the biopsy channel of the endoscope into the small bowel. The endoscope is removed and a J-tube is passed over the guide wire into position or under fluoroscopic visualization.[43]

An alternative method of small bowel access, DPEJ, directly places a J-tube into the small bowel using an endoscope. This procedure requires the use of an enteroscope or a pediatric colonoscope to reach a puncture position beyond the ligament of Treitz. Once the abdominal wall site is appropriately transilluminated with the endoscope, a standard pull PEG technique is used to place the DPEJ (see Appendix Figure 13.6). It is often necessary to use intravenous glucagon during the procedure to paralyze the small bowel such that appropriate transillumination can be obtained. Mellert and Shike have reported good success with this procedure.[44,45] A standard 20 or 24 French PEG tube may be placed and used as the J-tube (see Appendix Figure 13.7). There were some reported minor complications, including local site infection, but no reported cases of peritonitis or bowel infarction.

The decision to use a J-tube for feeding also should warrant some very specific instructions regarding its care. The lumen of these J-tubes is much smaller than a gastric tube and therefore more prone to clogging. Jejunal feeding tubes should never be used to check for residual content, as they are a poor indicator of residual content of the small bowel. In addition, checking residuals through these small-bore tubes increases their probability of clogging. These tubes should be flushed after every tube feeding and medication instillation. Only liquid medications, or completely dissolved medications, should be placed through a J-tube in order to reduce the chances of tube occlusion. Care should be taken to stop tube feedings during infusion of medication such as theophylline or potassium chloride, products that are known to coagulate tube feedings or obstruct the J-tube. Since fastidious nursing care is required to maintain tube patency, some physicians do not allow any medication to be placed via the J-tube. Collier et al. has shown that the use of a fiber-containing formula is quite safe, even through a 5 French needle catheter jejunostomy.[46] However, the use of supplemental protein powder in tube feedings or an immune enhancing formula may promote obstruction of smaller (<8 French) J-tubes.

Percutaneous endoscopic procedures are reliable methods for obtaining small bowel enteral access. Percutaneous endoscopic gastrojejunostomy allows both gastric decompression and jejunal feeding and should be used in patients who will require jejunal feedings for greater than 1 month, but less than 6 months. The J-tube component of this system may fail secondary to tube occlusion or tube displacement if left in place long-term. Direct percutaneous or surgically placed jejunostomy should be performed in those patients who will require long-term jejunal feedings.

Surgical Access

Endoscopic enteral access is often the preferred route in the majority of patients who cannot eat despite a functioning GI tract or who require long-term enteral access. However, surgically placed enteral access is indicated in a variety of situations. The most obvious indication occurs when a patient is already in the operating room, particularly during the conduct of an abdominal procedure. Surgeons should consider surgically placed enteral access during the performance of major upper intestinal procedures that involve anastomoses of the esophagus, stomach, duodenum, or pancreas or during the performance of any abdominal procedure where it is likely that the patient will be critically ill postoperatively, such as surgery for major sepsis or major trauma. This definition of critical illness should be broad enough in the surgeon's mind to include patients who are malnourished going into the operating room even if the procedure itself is not so catastrophic. The obvious benefits of postoperative enteral access have been demonstrated by Moore as well as others.[47] Realistically these benefits have to be weighed against the complications of surgically placed enteral access (see below), which are small but potentially devastating.[48–50] Patients who undergo major transthoracic or head and neck procedures are also candidates for potential concomitant surgically placed enteral access. While it has been shown that PEG is less expensive to perform than a surgically placed G-tube in a variety of settings,[51,52] this is not true when the patient is already under anesthesia where the G-tube/J-tube can be placed simultaneously with a major head and neck cancer procedure or while the primary team is waiting for frozen section diagnosis, etc.

Intensive care unit patients who need enteral access need a thoughtful approach to meeting their needs. One critical care team managing a patient who needs a tracheostomy and feeding access might choose to accomplish this by performing a bedside percutaneous tracheostomy and a PEG/PEG-J/DPEJ. Another team may opt to have a surgically placed tracheostomy and J-tube. Which approach is best? The answer depends on a lot of local factors such as comfort level and skill of the treating physicians, operating room accessibility, local costs, nursing factors, and previous experience. This last factor, often based on anecdotal experience, frequently drives the process. For instance, feeding access in a patient who is at risk for aspiration is arguably best placed in the jejunum.[25,53] In skilled hands, as noted above, PEG-J or direct percutaneous puncture can accomplish this. Such expertise is not always readily available.[54] Furthermore, in some patients, maintaining the transgastric jejunostomy tube in the jejunum has been problematic, and obtaining sufficient transillumination for direct percutaneous jejunostomy is not always achievable. In settings such as these, surgically placed enteral access would seem preferable. Finally, there are subsets of patients in whom endoscopic access would seem preferable but cannot be accomplished, such as in patients with a malignant stricture of the esophagus, a gastric cancer where the stomach cannot be juxtaposed to the abdominal wall, or simply when body habitus prevents successful transillumination for PEG placement.

Methods of Surgically Placed Enteral Access

Considering first the patient who is already on the operating table, we find that some patients may require both a G-tube and a J-tube, as in the event of major pancreatico-duodenal trauma or cancer surgery, but most patients will require only one or the other. G-tubes might be preferred when there is specific concern about placing a nasogastric tube (NGT), as in facial trauma, and a low concern about aspiration, allowing for subsequent gastric gavage feeding. From a surgeon's standpoint, G-tubes are placed for decompression more commonly than as the preferred route of feeding. Jejunostomies have been popular as a feeding route because the downstream location seems safer, a fact that has not always been corroborated.[25] Postoperative ileus recovery time is shorter in the jejunum, accounting in part for some of the popularity of this route.[6] Surgeons who have use for short-term needle catheter access routinely use the jejunum.

Preoperative surgical consultation for surgically placed enteral access poses some unique challenges. First and foremost is determining why the access is needed. This has several implications. Is the anticipated length of feeding greater than a month? If not, surgical intervention seems unwarranted in term of risk and benefit. Second, why has a *surgical* consultation been made? Would a PEG be sufficient? Third, what is the intended use of the access? Enteral access for placement in an extended care facility would probably be best served through a gastrostomy so that bolus feeding could be delivered instead of pump feeding through a jejunostomy tube. The care of a G-tube in this setting is a little more straightforward.[55] Fourth, what type of tube is being asked for? Has the patient been worked up for aspiration risk? In many cases where a jejunostomy has been requested, a gastrostomy would serve more than adequately. Fifth, what are the surgical considerations? Has the patient had previous surgery? What is the disease state? Is the patient obese? How will these factors affect the planned procedure? A patient who has had a gastric resection or who has a gastric malignancy may not have enough stomach free to reach the abdominal wall surgically, not to mention endoscopically. Multiple previous abdominal incisions may turn what is normally a relatively small surgical procedure into an ordeal for the surgeon and the patient. Finally, what are the anesthetic issues? Can this procedure be done under local anesthesia with some sedation or is a general anesthetic needed based on the nature of the patient, his or her disease, and previous surgical factors? A surgeon should be careful before committing to an abdominal procedure under local anesthesia.

A gastrostomy tube can be placed for permanent or temporary access. The creation of a surgical stoma using the Janeway gastric tube technique provides permanent gastric feeding access. An external tube is not necessary in between feedings; since the mucosa of the stomach is sewn to the skin, the tract will not close. This technique is accomplished by applying a linear stapler to a portion of the greater curvature of the stomach, creating a tube of stomach that is brought out to the skin level and secured.[56] Once healed, this can be accessed intermittently as needed.

For temporary, intermediate, or even long-term gastric access, the tube gastrostomy is the most common method by far. The Stamm gastrostomy is made by placing a purse string in a convenient location on the anterior portion of the stomach, usually near the greater curve. A gastrotomy is made and the tube is placed into the stomach. The purse string is then secured. A second purse string is placed around this to invert the entry site and minimize leakage. The tube is then brought out through the abdominal wall. The stomach should be secured to the underside of the abdominal wall, sealing the G-tube exit site to the peritoneum. Failure to do this will increase the intraabdominal leak rate of gastric secretions into the abdominal cavity.[50] The tube itself should be secured to the skin in such a way that prevents accidental dislodgement particularly in the early postoperative period.

There are three main tube choices for the initial G-tube placement. They are the Foley, Pezzer, and Malecot catheters (see Appendix Figure 13.8). The Foley catheter is commonly available, but is a poor choice for the initial tube placement. This is because tube retention is highly dependent on the security of the balloon at the end of the catheter. This can fail for a number of reasons in the early postoperative period, resulting in intraabdominal gastric leakage or the G-tube pulling away from the abdominal wall. After the initial tube is exchanged sometime after the first 30 days postoperatively, the Foley catheter can be used with excellent results. The Malecot catheter does not depend on a balloon and retains its shape in the stomach; unfortunately, a minimal traction force on the tube will result in dislodgement, making this a less than optimal choice as well. The Pezzer catheter is basically a disk at the end of a tube. The tip may be cut off or not prior to placement into the stomach. This creates a very secure gastrotomy tube that may be exchanged 1 month postoperatively. A 22 French catheter or larger is recommended for insertion. This will allow for a variety of food sources and minimize tube occlusion. Laparoscopic approaches have also been employed for G-tube placement.[57] This can be accomplished with a 5 or 10 mm umbilical incision for a camera port and a small incision for the tube itself (see Appendix Figure 13.9). This minimally invasive approach requires gastric insufflation via an NGT. The stomach is then sutured to the abdominal wall. A Seldinger technique is used to cannulate the stomach. The tract is then dilated until it is large enough for the G-tube.

Jejunostomy tubes are generally placed at least 20 centimeters distal to the ligament of Treitz. The caliber of the jejunum mandates a smaller tube than what is placed in the stomach, usually in the 16F range or smaller. The smallest jejunostomy is created with the needle catheter technique. This has been used very successfully for relatively short-term feeding.[58] Most people feel that elemental formulations work best with this size access in order to avoid tube obstruction. The most common technique for placing a J-tube is a Witzel jejunostomy. A standard red rubber or similar catheter is passed through an anti-mesenteric enterotomy and secured initially with a purse string suture. One to 2 inches of tube is then inverted into the anti-mesenteric bowel by sewing the bowel over the tube. This will create a "Witzel" tunnel of bowel that should seal down when the tube is removed or lost, minimizing intra-abdominal leakage of enteric contents. The jejunum is sewn to the underside of the abdominal wall, then the end of the tube is brought out through the abdominal wall and secured to the skin. The problem with this technique is that it is totally dependent on the sutures to hold the tube in the jejunum; they can become loose and allow the tube to simply slide out. As such, biliary T-tubes have been utilized as jejunostomies as well. The idea is that the "T" will help hold the tube in place with greater success.

The transverse Witzel T-tube jejunostomy has been described.[59] A near mesenteric enterotomy is made and the T-tube is inserted (see Appendix Figure 13.10a). The transverse Witzel suture line is created and the jejunum is secured as above (see Appendix Figure 13.10b). Laparoscopic approaches to feeding jejunostomy have been worked out. This approach is technically more difficult than laparoscopic gastrostomy, requiring more ports to provide instrumention to manipulate the omentum and bowel in order to locate the ligament of Treitz and avoid misplacement of the feeding tube.[61]

The management of these tubes requires attention to detail to avoid tube obstruction, dislodgement, or skin excoriation. The smaller the caliber of the tube, the more likely it is that medications placed through the tube or a failure to flush the tube after use will result in tube obstruction. Once this occurs a variety of "cocktails" involving pancreatic enzymes or popular colas have been proposed to digest the obstruction in the tube.[62–64] Finally, sutures that were placed during the surgical procedure to hold the tube in place will cut through the patient's skin or loosen along the tube over time. Replacing the sutures or using an adequate taping system is required periodically to avoid dislodgement.

Complications of Surgically Placed Enteral Access

The corollary to the old saying "nature abhors a vacuum" equivalent to "the human body abhors a foreign body." Regardless of the method of insertion, feeding tubes are subject to a variety of complications. In fact the mortality of these procedures can be surprisingly high considering the simplicity of the concept of the surgery. This is in part due to the nature of the population requiring feeding access. Mortality rates as high as 11.4% have been reported.[48] Some complications are technique related. Shellito showed that failure to suture gastrostomy tube to the underside of the abdominal wall resulted in a 7% intraabdominal leak rate if the tube became dislodged or removed.[50] Erosion of the tube along the intestinal mucosa can cause gastrointestinal hemorrhage. While endoscopic techniques might control the bleeding, tube removal or even laparotomy is often required to control the hemorrhage.

Bowel obstruction can occur as a complication of either G-tubes or J-tubes when a loop of small bowel passes between the tube exit site and the abdominal wall, creating an internal hernia. The patient is subject to this even after the tube is removed since the symphysis between the tube exit site and the abdominal wall remains permanently. Laparotomy is required to correct this situation. Another mechanism of small bowel obstruction can occur when balloon catheters are used in the jejunum. If the balloon is over inflated, proximal small bowel obstruction occurs when the lumen is occluded.[65] (Bowel perforation may also result from over inflation of the balloon.) In this scenario, feedings are generally tolerated since the tip of the catheter is distal to the balloon. Vomiting is prominent but the abdomen is not distended because the obstruction is generally very proximal. Often the balloon is increasingly inflated because gastrointestinal contents are seen to exude around the J-tube skin exit site. This often exacerbates the problem because the balloon is already partially obstructing the lumen forcing the material out around the tube in the first place. This complication is avoided by using the minimal occlusion volume in the balloon, making sure that the balloon has not traveled downstream from the bowel exit site.

The most devastating complication of surgically placed enteral access is gastrointestinal leakage, perforation, or volvulus leading to necrosis, usually from a freshly placed tube. This has been observed 4% of the time in a recent large series.[66] Any patient who develops fever, tachycardia, abdominal tenderness, or a rising white blood cell count in any combination should be evaluated for a leaking tube site. The simplest way to evaluate this is with a contrast tube study. Alternatively, a computerized tomography study with contrast via the gastrointestinal tract and the tube in question is effective as well. Or if a surgical drain happens to be in the vicinity and functioning, methylene blue can be injected into the J-tube/G-tube and the drain is then observed for the appearance of the dye indicating leakage. Once diagnosed, laparotomy is indicated to repair the intestinal defect. Often a new tube may be placed safely at a new site downstream from the injury in the case of a J-tube or elsewhere in the stomach when repairing a leaking G-tube/PEG.

Conclusions

We have demonstrated a wide variety of techniques for providing enteral access. The choice for any one patient will depend on the myriad of factors illustrated above, carefully balancing nutritional need, surgical risk, and expected benefit.

References

1. Daly JM, Lieberman MD, Goldfine J, et al. Enteral nutrition with supplemental arginine, RNA, and omega-3 fatty acids in patients after operation: immunologic, metabolic, and clinical outcome. *Surgery.* 1992;112:56–67.
2. Kudsk KA, Croce MA, Fabian TC, et al. Enteral versus parenteral feeding. Effects on septic morbidity after blunt and penetrating abdominal trauma. *Ann Surg.* 1992;215: 503–511; discussion 511–513.
3. DeWitt RC, Kudsk KA. The gut's role in metabolism, mucosal barrier function, and gut immunology. *Infect Dis Clin North Am.* 1999;13:465–481.
4. Ferreras J, Junquera LM, Garcia-Consuegra L. Intracranial placement of a nasogastric tube after severe craniofacial trauma. *Oral Surg Oral Med Oral Pathol Oral Radiol Endod.* 2000;90:564–566.
5. Boyes RJ, Kruse JA. Nasogastric and nasoenteric intubation. *Crit Care Clin.* 1992;8:865–878.
6. Hiyama, DT, Zinner, MJ. Surgical complication: In: Schwartz SI, Shires GT, Spencer FC, eds. *Principles of Surgery.* New York: McGraw Hill Inc., 1994:476.
7. Heyland D, Cook DJ, Winder B, et al. Enteral nutrition in the critically ill patient: a prospective survey. *Crit Care Med.* 1995;23:1055–1060.
8. Inoue S, Epstein MD, Alexander JW, et al. Prevention of yeast translocation across the gut by a single enteral feeding after burn injury. *J Parenter Enteral Nutr.* 1989;13:565–571.
9. Zaloga GP, Bortenschlager L, Black KW, et al. Immediate postoperative enteral feeding decreases weight loss and improves wound healing after abdominal surgery in rats. *Crit Care Med.* 1992;20:115–118.
10. Moore EE, Jones TN. Benefits of immediate jejunostomy feeding after major abdominal trauma—a prospective, randomized study. *J Trauma.* 1986;26:874–881.
11. Levy H. Nasogastric and nasoenteric feeding tubes. *Gastrointest Endosc Clin N Am.* 1998;8:529–549.
12. Marian M, Rappaport W, Cunningham D, et al. The failure of conventional methods to promote spontaneous transpyloric feeding tube passage and the safety of intragastric feeding in the critically ill ventilated patient. *Surg Gynecol Obstet.* 1993;176:475–479.
13. Thurlow PM. Bedside enteral feeding tube placement into duodenum and jejunum. *J Parenter Enteral Nutr.* 1986;10: 104–105.
14. Zaloga GP. Bedside method for placing small bowel feeding tubes in critically ill patients. A prospective study. *Chest.* 1991;100:1643–1646.
15. Wysowski DK, Corken A, Gallo-Torres H, et al. Postmarketing reports of QT prolongation and ventricular arrhythmia in association with cisapride and Food and Drug Administration regulatory actions. *Am J Gastroenterol.* 2001;96:1698–1703.
16. Hernandez-Socorro CR, Marin J, Ruiz-Santana S, et al. Bedside sonographic-guided versus blind nasoenteric feeding tube placement in critically ill patients. *Crit Care Med.* 1996;24:1690–1694.
17. Gabriel SA, Ackermann RJ, Castresana MR. A new technique for placement of nasoenteral feeding tubes using external magnetic guidance. *Crit Care Med.* 1997;25:641–645.
18. Brandt CP, Mittendorf EA. Endoscopic placement of nasojejunal feeding tubes in ICU patients. *Surg Endosc.* 1999;13:1211–1214.
19. Krafte-Jacobs B, Persinger M, Carver J, et al. Rapid placement of transpyloric feeding tubes: a comparison of pH-assisted and standard insertion techniques in children. *Pediatrics.* 1996;98:242–248.
20. Botoman VA, Kirtland SH, Moss RL. A randomized study of a pH sensor feeding tube vs a standard feeding tube in patients requiring enteral nutrition. *J Parenter Enteral Nutr.* 1994;18:154–158.
21. Berry S, Orr M, Schoettker P, et al. Intestinal placement of pH-sensing nasointestinal feeding tubes. *J Parenter Enteral Nutr.* 1994;18:67–70.
22. Cataldi-Betcher EL, Seltzer MH, Slocum BA, et al. Complications occurring during enteral nutrition support: a prospective study. *J Parenter Enteral Nutr.* 1983;7:546–552.
23. Jacobs S, Chang RW, Lee B, et al. Continuous enteral feeding: a major cause of pneumonia among ventilated intensive care unit patients. *J Parenter Enteral Nutr.* 1990;14: 353–356.
24. Klodell CT, Carroll M, Carrillo EH, et al. Routine intragastric feeding following traumatic brain injury is safe and well tolerated. *Am J Surg.* 2000;179:168–171.
25. Spain DA, DeWeese RC, Reynolds MA, Richardson JD. Transpyloric passage of feeding tubes in patients with head injuries does not decrease complications. *J Trauma.* 1995; 39:1100–1102.

26. Huxley EJ, Viroslav J, Gray WR, et al. Pharyngeal aspiration in normal adults and patients with depressed consciousness. *Am J Med.* 1978;64:564–568.
27. Montecalvo MA, Steger KA, Farber HW, et al. Nutritional outcome and pneumonia in critical care patients randomized to gastric versus jejunal tube feedings. The Critical Care Research Team. *Crit Care Med.* 1992;20: 1377–1387.
28. Jeppsson B, Tranberg K, Bengmark S. Technical developments. A new self-propelling nasoenteric feeding tube. *Clin Nutr.* 1992;11:373–375.
29. Mangiante G, Marini P, Fratucello GB, et al. The Bengmark tube in surgical practice and in the critically ill patient. *Chir Ital.* 2000;52:573–578.
30. Park RH, Allison MC, Lang J, et al. Randomised comparison of percutaneous endoscopic gastrostomy and nasogastric tube feeding in patients with persisting neurological dysphagia. *BMJ.* 1992;304:1406–1409.
29. Gauderer MW, Ponsky JL, Izant RJ, Jr. Gastrostomy without laparotomy: a percutaneous endoscopic technique. *Nutrition.* 1980;14:736–738.
30. Jain NK, Larson DE, Schroeder KW, et al. Antibiotic prophylaxis for percutaneous endoscopic gastrostomy. A prospective, randomized, double-blind clinical trial. *Ann Intern Med.* 1987;107:824–828.
31. Hogan RB, DeMarco DC, Hamilton JK, et al. Percutaneous endoscopic gastrostomy—to push or pull. A prospective randomized trial. *Gastrointest Endosc.* 1986;32:253–258.
32. Larson DE, Burton DD, Schroeder KW, et al. Percutaneous endoscopic gastrostomy. Indications, success, complications, and mortality in 314 consecutive patients. *Gastroenterology.* 1987;93:48–52.
33. DeLegge M, Lantz G, Kazacos E et al. Effect of external bolster tension on PEG tube tract formation. *Gastrointest Endosc.* 1996;43:349.
34. Choudhry U, Barde CJ, Markert R, et al. Percutaneous endoscopic gastrostomy: a randomized prospective comparison of early and delayed feeding. *Gastrointest Endosc.* 1996;44:164–167.
35. Burtch GD, Shatney CH. Feeding jejunostomy (versus gastrostomy) passes the test of time. *Am Surg.* 1987;53:54–57.
36. Ho CS, Yee AC, McPherson R. Complications of surgical and percutaneous nonendoscopic gastrostomy: review of 233 patients. *Gastroenterology.* 1988;95:1206–1210.
37. Neumann D, DeLegge M. Gastric versus small bowel feeding in the ICU: a prospective comparison of efficacy. *Gastroenterology.* 2000;118:A774.
38. DiSario JA, Foutch PG, Sanowski RA. Poor results with percutaneous endoscopic jejunostomy. *Gastrointest Endosc.* 1990;36:257–260.
39. DeLegge MH, Patrick P, Gibbs R. Percutaneous endoscopic gastrojejunostomy with a tapered tip, nonweighted jejunal feeding tube: improved placement success. *Am J Gastroenterol.* 1996;91:1130–1134.
40. Parasher VK, Abramowicz CJ, Bell C, et al. Successful placement of percutaneous gastrojejunostomy using steerable glidewire—a modified controlled push technique. *Gastrointest Endosc.* 1995;41:52–55.
41. Baskin W, Johnson JF. Trans-PEG endoscopy for rapid PEJ placement. *Am J Gastroenterol.* 1994;89:1701–1704.
42. Mellert J, Naruhn MB, Grund KE, et al. Direct endoscopic percutaneous jejunostomy (EPJ). Clinical results. *Surg Endosc.* 1994;8:867–9; discussion 869–870.
43. Shike M, Berner YN, Gerdes H, et al. Percutaneous endoscopic gastrostomy and jejunostomy for long-term feeding in patients with cancer of the head and neck. *Otolaryngol Head Neck Surg.* 1989;101:549–554.
44. Collier P, Kudsk KA, Glezer J, et al. Fiber-containing formula and needle catheter jejunostomies: a clinical evaluation. *Nutr Clin Pract.* 1994;9:101–103.
45. Moore FA, Moore EE, Jones TN, et al. TEN versus TPN following major abdominal trauma—reduced septic morbidity. *J Trauma.* 1989;29:916–922; discussion 922–923.
46. Ephgrave KS, Buchmiller C, Jones MP, Cullen JJ. The cup is half full. *Am J Surg.* 1999;178:406–410.
47. Sonawane RN, Thombare MM, Kumar A, et al. Technical complications of feeding jejunostomy: a critical analysis. *Trop Gastroenterol.* 1997;18:127–128.
48. Shellito PC, Malt RA. Tube gastrostomy. Techniques and complications. *Ann Surg.* 1985;201:180–185.
49. Sartori S, Trevisani L, Tassinari D, et al. Cost analysis of long-term feeding by percutaneous endoscopic gastrostomy in cancer patients in an Italian health district. *Support Care Cancer.* 1996;4:21–26.
50. Harbrecht BG, Moraca RJ, Saul M, et al. Percutaneous endoscopic gastrostomy reduces total hospital costs in head-injured patients. *Am J Surg.* 1998;176:311–314.
51. Weltz CR, Morris JB, Mullen JL. Surgical jejunostomy in aspiration risk patients. *Ann Surg.* 1992;215:140–145.
52. DiSario JA, Foutch PG, Sanowski RA. Poor results with percutaneous endoscopic jejunostomy. *Gastrointest Endosc.* 1990;36:257–260.
55. Cogen R, Weinryb J, Pomerantz C, Fenstemacher P. Complications of jejunostomy tube feeding in nursing facility patients. *Am J Gastroenterol.* 1991;86:1610–1613.
56. Remine WH. Carcinoma of the stomach. In: Maingot R. and American Contributors. Maingot's Abdominal Operations. New York: Appleton-Century-Crofts; 1980:545–546.
57. Peitgen K, von Ostau C, Walz MK. Laparoscopic gastrostomy: results of 121 patients over 7 years. *Surg Laparosc Endosc Percutan Tech.* 2001;11:76–82.
58. Myers JG, Page CP, Stewart RM, et al. Complications of needle catheter jejunostomy in 2,022 consecutive applications. *Am J Surg.* 1995;170:547–550; discussion 550–551.
59. Schwaitzberg SD, Sable DB. Transverse Witzel-T-tube feeding jejunostomy. *J Parenter Enteral Nutr.* 1995;19:326–327.
60. Duh QY, Way LW. Laparoscopic jejunostomy using T-fasteners as retractors and anchors. *Arch Surg.* 1993; 128: 105–108.

61. Gama-Rodrigues J, Seid VE, Santos VR, et al. Unintentional ileostomy: a complication of the videolaparoscopic method? Report of the first case. *Surg Laparosc Endosc Percutan Tech.* 2000;10:253–257.

62. Marcuard SP, Stegall KL, Trogdon S. Clearing obstructed feeding tubes. *J Parenter Enteral Nutr.* 1989;13:81–83.

63. Marcuard SP, Stegall KS. Unclogging feeding tubes with pancreatic enzyme. *J Parenter Enteral Nutr.* 1990;14:198–200.

64. Mateo MA. Nursing management of enteral tube feedings. *Heart Lung.* 1996; 25:318–323.

65. Chester JF, Turnbull AR. Intestinal obstruction by overdistension of a jejunostomy catheter balloon: a salutary lesson. *J Parenter Enteral Nutr.* 1988;12:410–411.

66. Holmes JHt, Brundage SI, Yuen P, et al. Complications of surgical feeding jejunostomy in trauma patients. *J Trauma.* 1999;47:1009–1012.

CHAPTER

14 Drug-Nutrient Interactions

Mary S. McCarthy, R.N., M.N., C.N.S.N.,
Janet C. Fabling, R.D., C.N.S.D., David E. Bell, R.Ph.

INTRODUCTION 153
POPULATIONS AT RISK 154
EX VIVO BIOPHARMACEUTICAL INACTIVATIONS (PHYSICAL INCOMPATIBILITY WITH DELIVERY SYSTEM) 154
PARENTERAL NUTRITION 154
Cautions 154
Prevention of TPN Incompatibilities 155
ENTERAL NUTRITION 156
INCOMPATIBILITIES OF PHARMACEUTICAL PREPARATIONS AND ENTERAL NUTRITION FORMULAS 156
PREVENTION OF ENTERAL NUTRITION INCOMPATIBILITIES 156
ABSORPTION INTERACTIONS 160
EXAMPLES OF ABSORPTION INTERACTIONS 161
Presystemic Metabolism 161
Presystemic Transport 162
Presystemic Binding/Complexation 166
PREVENTING ABSORPTION INCOMPATIBILITIES WITH ENTERAL NUTRITION 166
FED VERSUS FASTED STATE 168
Interactions Affecting Systemic or Physiologic Dispositions 168
DRUG-NUTRIENT INTERACTION PAIRS 168
Warfarin and Vitamin K 168
Vitamin E and Vitamin K 168
Corticosteroids 168
VALPROIC ACID (VPA) 168
Sinemet (anti-Parkinson's) 168
Theophylline (bronchodilator) 169
Levodopa (Dopar) 169
Isoniazid (histaminase inhibitor) 169
Phenytoin (Dilantin, anticonvulsant), Fosphenytoin (Cerebyx, anticonvulsant) and Carbamazepine (Tegretol, anticonvulsant) 169
Methotrexate (antineoplastic, antipsoriatic, antirheumatic) 169
DRUG-NUTRIENT INTERACTIONS INVOLVING ALTERATION OF ELIMINATION OR CLEARANCE 169
MANAGEMENT OF DRUG-NUTRIENT INTERACTIONS INVOLVING ALTERED RENAL CLEARANCE 170
CONCLUSIONS 170
CASE STUDY 170
REFERENCES 171

Introduction

In today's intensive care unit (ICU) environment there is great risk for interactions between medications (prescription and non-prescription) and nutrients (foods, beverages, vitamin supplements). While some of these interactions are not clinically significant, others may be fatal.[1] Food-drug interactions vary according to the dosage, age, sex, and overall health of the patient.[2] Monitoring the medication regimen and educating patients about drug-nutrient interactions are part of our professional practice standards. This is further supported by the standards set by the Joint Commission on Accreditation of Healthcare Organizations (JCAHO) to ensure that practitioners monitor for potential drug-nutrient interactions.[3]

The following definitions will be used when describing the various drug-drug and drug-nutrient interactions: (1) Any inappropriate or undesirable effect of the interaction of two or more substances represents incompatibility between them,[4] and (2) an alteration of pharmacokinetics or pharmacodynamics of a drug or nutritional element, or a compromise in a nutritional status as a result of the addition of a drug.[5]

Populations at Risk

Any patient may have a drug-nutrient interaction but certain patient populations and clinical circumstances contribute to a greater potential for a reaction. Patient populations include the critically ill, who receive multiple potent medications for an extended period of time, and the elderly, because they often take multiple medications with an increased risk for interaction. Patients with impaired renal function are at an increased risk because the rate of renal clearance and/or excretion of drugs may be affected and dialysis will significantly alter drug bioavailability. Malnourished patients in whom metabolism of drugs by the liver is known to be depressed by starvation[6] may experience further depletion of vitamins and minerals that could reach critical values with administration of certain drugs.

Clinical circumstances that may contribute to drug-nutrient interactions include the use of enteral nutrition (EN) where the size of the tube, site of delivery, and medication formulation all must be taken into consideration, and total parenteral nutrition (TPN) where new additives present new opportunities for precipitation and incompatibility.[4]

In order to promote a standardized classification system based on mechanism of interaction, this chapter will incorporate the recently published classification system of drug-nutrient interactions described by Chan[5] and published by ASPEN. This system is based on our current understanding of drug and nutrient metabolism and drug-drug interactions. Drug-nutrient interactions will be categorized into four types: (1) ex vivo biopharmaceutical inactivations (physical incompatibility in the delivery system), (2) interactions affecting absorption phase, (3) interactions affecting systemic/physiologic dispositions, and (4) interactions affecting elimination/clearance.[5] Each category will be defined and described using examples. Management of the pharmacological issues will also be included. (A case study is presented at the end of the chapter.)

Ex Vivo Biopharmaceutical Inactivations (Physical Incompatibility with Delivery System)

The definition selected is the interaction between the drug and the nutritional element or formulation through biochemical or physical reactions.[5] The change is frequently evident on visual inspection. Precipitation is the most common physical incompatibility associated with parenteral nutrition; curdling is more often associated with enteral nutrition.

Examples of physical changes include flocculation, phase separation, and altered consistency or viscosity (thinning, thickening, coagulation, gelling). Variables that affect physical incompatibility include pH, cation-anion interaction, concentration and chemical complexity of individual components, temperature, time, and order of mixing.[4]

Parenteral Nutrition

Physical incompatibility is a major concern with TPN formulas. Drug-nutrient interactions may not be totally predictable by standard chemical solubility rules, and minor changes in the formula's content or temperature can alter the interaction. Each new additive must be monitored for resulting precipitation or potential adverse effects with other common components such as amino acids, electrolytes, acetate, insulin, vitamins, or lipids. A product may be acceptable for co-infusion with the parenteral nutrition solution, but not for direct mixing into the formula because of differences in dilution, contact time, and completeness of mixing.[4] Intravenous infusion of components that are physically incompatible may have grave consequences such as pulmonary deposition of crystals, occluded blood flow, respiratory distress, or even death.[7] The most problematic parenteral nutrition components in terms of compatibility with medications are trace elements, calcium, phosphorus, magnesium, and heparin.[4]

Cautions

Generally, antibiotics and TPN solutions should be administered through separate lines. In certain clinical situations, it would seem advantageous to mix the antibiotics with the TPN solution or to administer them at a Y-site with the TPN solution. However, a study by Zaccardelli et al.[8] examined the stability of imipenem-cilastatin sodium (Primaxin®), an antibiotic commonly used for the septic critically ill patient, in two different TPN solutions. The drug was found to be stable for only 15 minutes in the TPN solutions studied. The resulting recommendation is to administer the antibiotic through a separate line or Y-site while the TPN infusion is interrupted.[8]

Total nutrient admixtures, or "three-in-one solutions" (3:1) containing lipid emulsions, may obscure calcium-phosphate precipitation and cause destabilization of the solution.

PREVENTION OF TPN INCOMPATIBILITIES

1. Ensure adequate venous access to allow administration of parenteral nutrition separate from all other intravenous medications.
2. With limited venous access, consult with pharmacist prior to Y-site administration and refer to only updated compatibility charts in the institution (Table 14.1).

TABLE 14.1

Medication "Y-site" Administration with TPN		
Compatible with TPN	**Incompatible with TPN**	**Unknown or Limited Compatibility Data**
Anti-infectives	*Anti-infectives*	*Azole Anti-fungals*
Cephalosporins	Acyclovir	Fluconazole, Itraconazole
Chloramphenicol	Amphotericin B (steroid & liposomal)	Ciprofloxacin (may interact with Ca and Mg)
Clindamycin	Imipenem-cilastatin (Primaxin®)	Ganiclovir
Erythromycin Lactobionate	Metronidazole	Tetracyclines (may interact with Ca & Mg)
Gentamicin	Trimethoprim-Sulfamethoxazole (Bactrim®, Septra®)	*Other Medications*
Kanamycin	*Other Medications*	Ca and phosphate salts
Penicillins	Diazepam	Cyclosporin A (compatible with IV lipids, limited empiric evidence for TPN)
Azlocillin, Carbenicillin	Phenytoin	Gammaglobulin (IVIG)
Mezlocillin, Nafcillin	Sodium bicarbonate	Granisetron
Oxacillin, Penicillin G		Lorazepam (limited empiric evidence for TPN)
Piperacillin, Ticarcillin		Octreotide
(NOT Ampicillin)		Ondansetron
Tobramycin		Prochlorperazine
Vancomycin		Promethazine
Narcotic Analgesics		
Hydromorphone		
Meperidine		
Morphine		
Fentanyl		
Other Medications		
Digoxin		
Diphenhydramine		
Dopamine		
Droperidol		
Furosemide		
H_2 blockers		
Hydrocortisone		
Insulin, regular		
Lidocaine		
Metoclopramide		
Phytonadione		

*Use Y-site infusion with TPN only when other access cannot be obtained.

Compatibility is for Y-site administration only and assumes no other medications are in the TPN or given via the TPN line at the same time. Compatibility for IV lipids alone may differ. The recommended procedure for Y-site administration without documented compatibility is to stop the TPN, flush the line with 0.9% NaCl or D5W before and after administering the medication, then restart the TPN.

3. Filters: 1.2 micron air-eliminating for 3:1 solution; use 0.22 micron air-eliminating for non-lipid admixtures (bacterial retentive) to filter out precipitated salts resulting from pH, temperature, various unbalanced salt concentrations/amino acid concentrations, and prolonged infusion time. A filter will also protect against infusing large lipid particles resulting from emulsion destabilization.
4. Bedside clinicians should match contents on TPN label with MD order, observe formula periodically for signs of instability, and never allow the formula to hang beyond its intended time period, usually 24 hours.

Enteral Nutrition

The enteral route has many advantages for medication delivery including availability of a wider selection of oral medications, lower cost, and avoidance of the higher risk associated with IV administration.[9] Medications are sometimes added to enteral formulas for convenience of administration. However, there is much difficulty predicting the effect of some medications on the physical characteristics of the resulting formulations and the stability of the drugs in the formulations.[10] There may be clumping, thickening, or poor dispersion/dissolution of medication resulting in bolus administration. The osmolality of medications and electrolyte solutions has been implicated as a principal factor in physiologic incompatibility with enteral formulas. The main consequence of physical incompatibility with enteral formulas is clogged feeding tubes. This leads to decreased nutrient intake and discomfort and inconvenience for the patient, as well as valuable time spent unclogging or replacing the tube by the nurse or physician. Mixing medications with enteral nutrition also has the potential to contaminate feedings.[3,10]

Incompatibilities of Pharmaceutical Preparations and Enteral Nutrition Formulas

The form of protein (intact, hydrolyzed, or free amino acid) is the most critical property of enteral formulas. Acidic pharmaceutical preparations, especially syrups, caused the greatest problem during incompatibility testing with three intact protein formulas.[11] The same results were reported when high-nitrogen versions of the same formulas were tested. Better results have been achieved when testing acidic pharmaceutical preparations and oil-based products with hydrolyzed protein formulas.[12] Similarly, none of 39 medications tested were incompatible with the free amino acid formula Vivonex TEN®.[13]

Physical compatibility data on enteral feeding and drug administration are inadequate. One reason for the lack of conclusive data is the belief that the physical incompatibility in the GI tract does not result in life-threatening conditions such as precipitation or crystallization in the bloodstream. Therapeutic failure or lack of nutritional improvement may be the result of physical incompatibilities between enteral feeding formulas and drugs. Physical incompatibility commonly results from the hydrolytic process involving the direct mixing of enteral feeding formula and the vehicles used in oral liquid medications, such as syrups.[5]

Commonly used liquid formulations in the ICU setting include potassium chloride elixir, guaifenesin, metoclopramide hydrochloride, and ranitidine. In addition, sucralfate has been reported to bind with the protein in the food being administered and warfarin may be sequestered in the macromolecular fraction of the formula.[10] Another drug commonly implicated in drug-nutrient interactions is phenytoin. Splinter et al.[14] concluded from their experiments that the phenytoin oral suspension-enteral feeding formula interaction is pH dependent. Lower pH levels, as found in the stomach, account for the greatest difference in recovered phenytoin when it is combined with enteral formula.

Aluminum salts such as Amphojel and Maalox, and magnesium salts such as Mylanta and Milk of Magnesia, are well-known to bind calcium and phosphate in the gastrointestinal tract, but most likely exert this same effect on the calcium and phosphate in the enteral feeding formula in the bag or administration set. Such binding in the bag or tube could easily interrupt flow and result in a clogged feeding tube.

Table 14.2 summarizes available information regarding incompatibility of pharmaceutical preparations with enteral nutrition formulas.

Prevention of Enteral Nutrition Incompatibilities

To avoid administration of tablets by feeding tube, the recommended alternative is a different dosage form of the medication or a therapeutically similar medication, with changes in dosage and time intervals as necessary. Gora et al.[9] suggest several alternatives to crushed tablets, including granule formulations, effervescent tablets, and parenteral formulations. Different formulations of a particular tablet may exhibit different

TABLE 14.2

Pharmaceutical Preparations Physically Incompatible with Selected Enteral Formulas	
Drug	**Comments**
Aluminum hydroxide (Amphogel)	Thickens on contact
Al-mag hydroxide, double strength (Mylanta II)	Thickens on contact
Cibalith-S syrup (Lithium carbonate)	Clumping
Cimetadine HCL	Thickens on contact
Dicyclomine (Bentyl liquid)	Thickens on contact
Dimetane/Dimetapp Elixir	Gelatinous formation/enteral product breaks down
Ferrous sulfate (Feosol Elixir)	Complete gel formation
Fleet phospho-soda	Instant coagulation
Guaifenesin (Robitussin Syrup)	Flocculate precipitate
Magaldrate (Riopan)	Thickens on contact
Mandelamine suspension	Gelatinous tacky formulation
MCT oil	Adhesive gelatinous mass formation
Metoclopramide syrup (Reglan)	Compatible w/Two-Cal and Vivonex
Neo-calglucon syrup	Adhesive gelatinous mass formation
Paregoric elixir (opium, 45% alcohol)	Instant coagulation
Potassium chloride (some liquid forms; KCL liquid 10% & 20%, Klorvess syrup)	Interface incompatibility
Pseudophedrine syrup (Sudafed)	Viscous gelatinous formulation
Sucralfate suspension	Binds to protein in food
Thioridazine solution (Mellaril)	Granular formation
Thorazine concentrate	Granulation and particle formation
Triaminic syrup	Incompatible only with Two-Cal
Zinc sulfate capsules	Incompatible only with Two-Cal

*Enteral products tested included Ensure, Ensure HN, Ensure Plus HN, Enrich, Osmolite, Osmolite HN, and Two-Cal HN

tolerances for crushing (e.g., Erythromycin).[4] Gelatin capsules can be opened and the contents diluted in 10–15 mL of water, or the capsule can be dissolved in warm water. Other common medications such as K-Dur readily dissolve in warm water and have the added advantage of avoiding the gastrointestinal distress associated with potassium elixirs. When more than one medication is to be administered, 5–10 mL of water should be flushed through the tubing between medications. Ideally, medications should never be mixed together in a syringe.[10] Data to support co-mixing of medications are lacking. Intravenous form of a medication represents another alternative but most intravenous dosage forms are not designed to withstand conditions in the GI tract, specifically gastric acidity and digestive enzymes. Solutions for intravenous administration may form insoluble precipitates in an acid environment or may be rapidly degraded so that very little active medication reaches the blood[4] (Tables 14.3 and 14.4).

Irrigation both before and after administration of crushed or liquid medications is recommended, and volumes of 10 to 50 mL of irrigant are suggested. Most authors recommend irrigation with room-temperature or warm water.[15] Sterile water is often recommended for irrigation in the hospital setting, for immune-compromised patients in particular, to minimize the potential for bacterial contamination from tap water.[3] Studies indicate that water is as effective as cola and superior to cranberry juice in maintaining tube patency.[16] In fact, when soft drinks and juices are used as irrigants, their dried residues can further diminish the effective lumen of the tube and can actually contribute to clogging. Water is the most effective and available irrigant and leaves no residue.[16] The tendency for enteral feeding tube obstruction occurs in a

TABLE 14.3

Selected Oral Dosage Forms That Should Not Be Crushed			
Drug Product	**Manufacturer**	**Dosage Form**	**Comments**
ASA Enseals	Lilly	Tablet	Enteric coated
Atrohist Plus or Sprinkle	Adams	Tablet/Capsule	Slow release
Azulfidine Entabs	Pharmacia Labs	Tablet	Enteric coated
Bayer Aspirin, regular strength 325 mg	Sterling Health	Tablet	Enteric coated
Betachron E-R	Inwood	Capsule	Slow release
Biohist-LA	Wakefield	Tablet	Slow release
Bisacodyl	(various)	Tablet	Enteric coated
Bromfed	Muro	Capsule	Slow release
Calan SR	Searle	Tablet	Slow release
Cama Arthritis Pain Reliever	Sandoz Consumer	Tablet	Multiple compressed tablet
Cardizem	Marion-Merrell Dow	Tablet	Slow release
Cardizem CD	Marion-Merell Dow	Capsule	Slow release
Ciprofloxacin	Miles	Tablet	Taste; administration via NGT okay
Claritin-D	Schering Plough	Tablet	Slow release
Colace	Mead Johnson	Capsule	Taste; administration via NGT okay
Cotazym S	Organon	Capsule	Enteric coated
Depakote	Abbott	Capsule	Enteric coated
Diamox Sequels	Lederle	Capsule	Slow release
Dulcolax	Boehringer Ingelheim	Tablet	Enteric coated
E.E.S. 400	(various)	Tablet	Enteric coated
E-Mycin	Boots	Tablet	Enteric coated
Ergostat	Parke-Davis	Tablet	Sublingual form
Erythromycin base	(various)	Tablet	Enteric coated
Eskalith CR	Smith Kline Beecham	Tablet	Slow release
Feosol	Smith Kline Beecham	Tablet	Enteric coated
Fumatinic	Laser	Capsule	Slow release
Glucotrol XL	Pratt	Tablet	Slow release
Guaifenex PSE	Ethex	Tablet	Slow release
Humabid Sprinkle	Adams	Capsule	Slow release
Iberet 500	Abbott	Tablet	Slow release
Inderal LA	Wyeth-Ayerst	Capsule	Slow release
Indocin SR	MSD	Capsule	Slow release
Isoptin SR	Knoll	Tablet	Slow release
Isosorbide Dinitrate SR	(various)	Tablet	Sublingual form
Klorvess	Sandoz	Tablet	Effervescent tablet
K-Lyte/Cl/DS	Bristol Myers	Tablet	Effervescent tablet
K-Tab	Abbott	Tablet	Slow release
Mestinon	ICN Pharmaceutical	Tablet	Slow release
Motrin	Upjohn	Tablet	Taste; administration via NGT okay

(continued)

TABLE 14.3

Selected Oral Dosage Forms That Should Not Be Crushed (CONTINUED)			
Drug Product	Manufacturer	Dosage Form	Comments
MS Contin	Purdue Frederick	Tablet	Slow release
Naldecon	Bristol	Tablet	Slow release
Nitrostat	Parke-Davis	Tablet	Sublingual route
Nolamine	Carnick	Tablet	Slow release
Norpace CR	Searle	Capsule	Slow release form within a special capsule
Oramorph SR	Roxane	Tablet	Slow release
Oxycontin	Purdue Pharma	Tablet	Slow release
Pancrease	Ortho McNeil	Capsule	Enteric coated
Perdiem	Rhone-Poulenc Rorer	Granules	Wax coated
Phenergan	Wyeth-Ayerst	Tablet	Taste
Plendil	Astra Merck	Tablet	Slow release
Posicor	Roche	Tablet	Mucous membrane irritant
Prevacid	TAP Pharmaceutical	Capsule	Slow release
Prilosec	Astra Merck	Capsule	Slow release
Pro-Banthine	Schiapparelli Searle	Tablet	Taste
Procan SR	Parke-Davis	Tablet	Slow release
Procardia	Pfizer	Capsule	Delays absorption
Prozac	Dista	Capsule	Slow release
Quibron-T SR	Bristol-Myers Squibb	Tablet	Slow release
Ritalin SR	Ciba	Tablet	Slow release
Roxanol SR	Roxane	Tablet	Slow release
Sinemet CR	DuPont Pharm	Tablet	Slow release
Slo-Bid Gyrocaps	Rhone-Poulenc Rorer	Capsule	Slow release
Sorbitrate SA	Zeneca	Tablet	Slow release
Sorbitrate Sublingual	Zeneca	Tablet	Sublingual route
Tegretol-XR	Ciba Geigy	Tablet	Slow release
Theo-Dur	Key	Tablet	Slow release
Toprol XL	Astra	Tablet	Slow release
Trental	Hoechst-Marion Roussel	Tablet	Slow release
Volmax	Muro	Tablet	Slow release
Wellbutrin	Burroughs-Wellcome	Tablet	Anesthetizes mucous membranes
Wygesic	Wyeth-Ayerst	Tablet	Taste
Zyban	Glaxo Wellcome	Tablet	Slow release
Zymase	Organon	Capsule	Enteric coated

Alternatives to crushing:

- For some medications a liquid preparation may be available. The pharmacist should be consulted in the event that a dosage adjustment must be made for a liquid substitution.
- It may be possible to use the injectable form of a medication in a liquid, such as water or juice.
- Another alternative is to use a chemically different but clinically similar medication that is available in a liquid formulation.

TABLE 14.4

Dosage Form Selection and Administration Methods
1. Consider administration of medication orally, intravenously, or rectally, if possible. 2. Be aware of tube size and tube tip location. If the tube tip is in the small bowel be aware of the osmotic sensitivity in this area and dilute medications accordingly. Administer medication through feeding tube using the following procedure: a. Review and assess drug incompatibilities/interactions; initiate medication consultation with pharmacy. b. Flush feeding tube with 30 mL sterile water. c. Select medication dosage form (listed in order of preference): ■ Oral liquid: dilute with 10–30 mL water. ■ Oral immediate-release tablet: Crush to fine powder and mix with water to form slurry.* ■ Oral immediate-release capsule: Crush capsule contents to fine powder and mix with water to form slurry. ■ Oral soft gelatin capsule: Aspirate liquid contents. ■ IV liquid preparation *approved for oral use.* d. Administer medication via feeding tube. e. Flush feeding tube with 15–30 mL sterile water to clear residual medication and in between multiple medications to prevent drug-drug interactions. 3. Avoid mixing medications with formula to prevent clogging or drug-nutrient interactions. 4. Never add medications to the formula bag. (This may result in drug-nutrient interactions, clogging, or incomplete delivery of the medication.) 5. Consider the timing of the medication; should it be given on a full or empty stomach? Absorption of some medications (Warfarin, Ciprofloxacin, Dilantin) is enhanced if formula is held for 1 to 2 hours before and after medication administration. However, with multiple interruptions patient may not receive full nutritional support, so notify Registered Dietitian for possible rate adjustment, after pharmacy consult.

*The HandiCrush medication syringe (Welcon, Providence, RI) is one device available for the crushing and administration of medications while minimizing infection control risks and drug-drug interactions that occur with mortar & pestle crushing.

Special situations

Cardizem CD, Cardizem SR, Fergon, Prozac, Respbid oral capsules: Open capsule and pour intact pellets down feeding tube. Flush feeding tube with 30-mL water before and after administration.

Gastrocrom oral capsules: Open capsule, dissolve contents in water, pour down feeding tube. Flush feeding tube with 30-mL water before and after administration.

Lansoprazole (Prevacid) or Omeprazole (Prilosec) delayed-release capsules:

- Gastric feeding tube: Open capsule and pour intact pellets down feeding tube. Flush feeding tube with acidic fruit juice after administration. May use apple, cranberry, grape, grapefruit, orange, pineapple, prune, tomato, or V-8 juice.
- Intestinal feeding tube: Open capsule and pour intact pellets down feeding tube. Flush feeding tube with an alkaline liquid, such as water, milk, or saline.

variety of circumstances, including administration of both crushed and liquid medications, incompatibility of feeding formulas and gastric juices, drug-drug incompatibility, and drug-formula incompatibility.

The addition of medications to feeding formulas is discouraged altogether or recommended only on a limited basis.[8,17,18] Aggregation of formula and obstruction of feeding tubes can occur when liquid formulations that are acidic or buffered to a low pH come in contact with caseinate-based formulas. Marcuard and Stegall[19] and Powell et al.[20] recommend restricting liquid medications to elixirs and suspensions compatible with feeding formulas. Several charts of drug-formula compatibility are available[21] (see Table 14.2).

With known or suspected incompatibilities or potential loss of therapeutic effect of the drug, it is advised to interrupt the feeding 1 hour before and 1 to 2 hours after drug administration.[10] Holding enteral nutrition with a frequency of more than twice a day in order to administer medications may lead to inadequate caloric intake with difficulty achieving nutritional goals. Continuous feeding rates may have to be recalculated for less than 24-hour infusion time or drug dosages adjusted to account for decreased bioavailability if administered with the enteral feeding formula.

If the detrimental drug-formula interaction is pH-dependent, an alternate site for the tip of the feeding tube, and thus drug delivery, may solve the problem. For example, if the tip of the feeding tube is advanced from the stomach (pH 1–3) to the duodenum or jejunum (pH 7–7.5), the effects of the phenytoin suspension-enteral feeding interaction may be decreased.[14]

Absorption Interactions

The definition selected is that this type of interaction affects drugs and nutrients delivered only by mouth or via enteral delivery systems. The oral bioavailability of the drug or nutritional element is either increased or

TABLE 14.5

Management of Clogged Feeding Tubes
1. Withdraw any enteral solution remaining in tube.
2. Attempt to clear occlusion using the following methods in the order given:
Air method: Inject small volumes of air in rapid succession using a syringe ≥30 mL (to prevent tube rupture).
Warm water method: Inject 10–30 mL warm water into tube and clamp for 5 minutes. Flush with water until clear, and smooth flow is restored.
Alkalinized enzyme method:
1) Mix small amount of Papain (meat tenderizer/enzyme) with 5-10 mL warm water and inject into feeding tube. Clamp for 5 minutes. Flush with water until clear and smooth flow is restored.
2) Mix one crushed sodium bicarbonate (324 mg) tablet and the contents of either one Viokase capsule or other pancreatic-lipase enzyme (available from pharmacy) in 5 mL water. Inject into tube and clamp for 5 minutes. Attempt to flush with water until clear and flow is restored. Mixture may need to sit as long as 30 minutes in the tube to fully dissolve clog.
3) Use Clog-Zapper Kit (Corpak MedSystems, Wheeling, IL). Directions are with the kit. This kit contains an enzymatic mixture that is most effective if used immediately after the tube clogs. Use selectively, each kit costs $25.
Mechanical method:
The most recent report of a mechanical maneuver to clear obstructed feeding tubes involves the novel use of a catheter with minimal risks. A group of investigators demonstrated that clogged feeding tubes could be safely and reliably cleared using a Glo-tip 5-4-3 translucent TFE endoscopic retrograde cholangiopancreatography (ERCP) catheter (Wilson Cook, Winston Salem, NC). This bedside technique may avoid costly re-insertions and the inconvenience of transporting a critically ill patient to the procedure suite.[22] (Golioto, M. et al. *NCP* 16:284-285, Oct 2001)
3. Replace feeding tube—only if above suggestions have been unsuccessful in restoring patency of the feeding tube.

*Use only water (sterile water while hospitalized) to flush feeding tubes and not cola or cranberry juice, which may promote tube occlusion.[4]

decreased due to this interaction. The precipitant agent may affect the function of an enzyme (e.g., grapefruit juice and carbamazepine), a cofactor (phenytoin and folic acid), or a transporter (such as vitamin E liquid and cyclosporine) that is responsible for the transport of the drug or nutritional element. Chan[5] further divides absorption interactions into three subtypes: (1) presystemic metabolism, (2) presystemic transport, and (3) presystemic binding/complexation.

Examples of Absorption Interactions

Presystemic Metabolism

Presystemic metabolism usually involves the inhibition or induction of enzymes present in the gut or liver.

The mechanism by which grapefruit juice interacts with other medications is by selective downregulation of the intestinal cytochrome P450 (CYP) 3A4 isoenzyme. Some studies indicate that CYP3A4 in the liver is unaffected,[23] while others suggest that grapefruit juice not only inhibits the metabolism of cytochrome P450 isoenzyme 3A4 but also 1A2 and 2A6 in the liver.[24] It is thought that certain flavonoid compounds found in grapefruit juice are responsible for inhibiting the normal hepatic P450 metabolism of calcium-channel blockers, nifedipine, nicardepine, and felodipine.[2] Other drugs that have decreased metabolism when taken with grapefruit juice include cyclosporine, carbamazepine, dihydropyridine, midazolam, triazolam, lovastatin, and caffeine. This decrease in metabolism can lead to increased serum concentrations of these medications.[25] Both CYP2A6 and CYP3A4 metabolize warfarin (Coumadin®). Coumarin is metabolized by CYP2A6, and concomitant administration with grapefruit juice inhibits coumarin's metabolism. This would suggest that warfarin metabolism may also be affected by grapefruit juice, but when evaluated it was determined that there is no change in the prothrombin time.[23] Lilja et al.[24] confirmed that buspirone administration with grapefruit juice results in a 4.3-fold increase in maximum concentration and an increase in half-life from 1.8 to 2.7 hours. It is recommended that buspirone not be taken with large quantities of grapefruit juice due to its extensive first-pass metabolism.[23] It is noteworthy that the bioavailability of cyclosporine, tacrolimus, and itraconazole may be affected if the tip of the feeding tube is advanced from the stomach into the small bowel. The positioning of the feeding tube changes the exposure of the drugs to gut wall metabolism and transport by CYP3A4 and intestinal P-glycoprotein, therefore potentially altering absorption. However, Chan excludes this type of interaction from his classification of drug-nutrient interactions because the problem is caused by the tube placement, not a drug or nutrient.[5]

Orlistat decreases the absorption of dietary fat through inhibition of lipase in the GI tract. The unabsorbed fat acts as a vehicle to trap fat-soluble vitamins in the intestinal lumen and therefore reduces the bioavailability of these vitamins.[26]

Proton pump inhibitors work by inhibiting the hydrogen/potassium ATPase enzyme system in the gastric parietal cell; this in turn decreases vitamin B_{12} absorption from the GI tract.[27]

Presystemic Transport

Presystemic transport involves an alteration in the function of transporters, the transit time, or the dissolution of the drug or nutritional compound leading to a reduction in the bioavailability of the drug or nutritional element.

Phenytoin, with its numerous challenges for successful administration, may be classified in this subtype as well because one hypothesis holds that it decreases folate concentrations by inducing a metabolic process in the body that uses folate as a cofactor. It is also theorized that it may lead to malabsorption of dietary folate secondary to an increase in intraluminal pH.[28]

The amount and composition of food can affect drug absorption. Foods with a high fat content and/or meals served hot can delay gastric emptying. By keeping the drug in the stomach longer, the presentation of the drug to the absorptive surface of the small intestine where most medications are absorbed is delayed. Absorption of digoxin and the acid-labile penicillins is reduced when gastric emptying is delayed.[4] Lipid-soluble drugs, such as griseofulvin and theophylline products, have an increased bioavailability in the presence of a high-fat meal.[29] Atovaquone suspension is another such drug that has demonstrated significantly greater bioavailability when administered after food or a nutrition supplement with a moderate fat content.[30]

Large amounts of fluid stimulate intestinal motility and may decrease absorption secondary to decreased transit time. Conversely, a large amount of fluid may enhance a medication's dissolution, increasing the efficiency of absorption.[1] Laxatives are an example of medications that intentionally increase intestinal motility but may adversely affect fluid and electrolyte balance. Depletion of calcium, sodium, potassium, and vitamin D are the result of excessive laxative use. Mineral oil laxatives may additionally impair absorption of fat-soluble vitamins (A, D, E, and K) and their derivatives.[31] Cholestyramine and colestipol are agents that lower cholesterol by binding bile acids, but they also bind fat-soluble vitamins, which may lead to clinically significant deficiencies. Sorbitol is a hyperosmotic laxative commonly used to flavor distasteful medicines. Published data on the sorbitol content of liquid dosage forms demonstrate that the sorbitol content of a given medication varies by manufacturer. Sorbitol doses of 20 grams are reported to cause severe cramping and diarrhea in the majority of people, and doses of 5 to 10 grams cause bloating and flatulence in a substantial portion of people. Sorbitol is considered an inert excipient and thus, is not required to be listed as an ingredient on medication labels.[4] For this reason it is not listed as a drug-nutrient interaction, but an adverse effect. However, it has great potential to contribute to fluid and electrolyte losses due to excessive diarrhea. (see Tables 14.6 and 14.7). Dyes, such as the blue food coloring used to tint enteral feeding formulas or pediatric antibiotic suspensions, are also excipients that may result in adverse effects. Again, dye content is proprietary information and need not be listed on medication labels.

Some foods may affect drug absorption by stimulating gastric secretion of hydrochloric acid and digestive enzymes, damaging acid-labile drugs, such as proton pump inhibitors (omeprazole, lansoprazole, pantoprazole), penicillins, and erythromycin. The enteric coating of the preparations of proton pump inhibitors is designed to dissolve in the more alkalotic environment of the intestine where the drug is absorbed. Crushing the granules or dissolving them in an alkalotic liquid (e.g., milk) will impair the integrity of the enteric coating and result in drug degradation in the stomach acid.[1] Erythromycin formulations are especially susceptible to inactivation by gastric acid and decreased absorption if administered following a meal. The dissolution of basic drugs, such as amphetamines and tricyclic antidepressants, is enhanced in an acidic environment thus increasing absorption. By the same mechanism, the dissolution of acidic drugs, such as phenytoin, phenobarbital, and aspirin, is reduced.[32] Ketoconazole is expected to have poorer absorption when delivered into the small bowel than when delivered into the stomach, since it requires an acidic environment for dissolution and conversion to the hydrochloride salt that can be absorbed.[4]

Monoamine oxidase is an enzyme in the body that catalyzes the breakdown of serotonin, epinephrine, norepinephrine, and dopamine. It is also in the GI tract and metabolizes tyramine in food before it reaches the systemic circulation. The inhibition of monoamine oxidase via monamine oxidase inhibitors results in the accumulation of ingested tyramine in adrenergic neurons releasing large amounts of norepinephrine. The

TABLE 14.6

Osmolality of Selected Commercially Available Liquid Medications		
Product	**Manufacturer**	**Average Osmolality mOsm/Kg**
Acetaminophen elixir 65 mg/mL	Roxane	5400
Acetaminophen/codeine elixir	Wyeth	4700
Aminophylline liquid 21 mg/mL	Fisons	450
Amoxicillin suspension 50 mg/mL	Squibb	2250
Belladonna alkaloids elixir	Robins	1050
Cascara Sagrada Aromatic Extract	Roxane	1000
Cephalexin suspension 50 mg/mL	Dista	1950
Chloral Hydrate syrup 50 mg/mL	Pharmaceutical Associates	4400
Cimetadine solution 60 mg/mL	Smith, Kline & French	5550
Co-trimoxazole suspension (Bactrim®)	Burroughs Wellcome	2200
Dexamethasone elixir 0.1 mg/mL	Organon	3350
Dexamethasone elixir 1 mg/mL	Roxane	3100
Digoxin elixir 50 µg/mL	Burroughs Wellcome	1350
Diphenhydramine HCl elixir 2.5 mg/mL	Roxane	850
Diphenoxlate/atropine suspension	Roxane	8800
Docusate sodium syrup 3.3 mg/mL	Roxane	3900
Erythromycin ethylsuccinate susp 40 mg/mL	Abbott	1750
Ferrous sulfate liquid, 60 mg/mL	Roxane	4700
Furosemide solution 10 mg/mL	Hoiechst-Roussel	2050
Kaolin-pectin solution	Roxane	900
Haloperidol concentrate 2 mg/mL	McNeal	500
Hydroxyzine HCl syrup 2 mg/mL	Roerig	4450
Lactulose syrup 0.67 g/mL	Roerig	3600
Lithium citrate syrup 1.6 mEq/mL	Roxane	6850
Magnesium citrate solution	Medalist	1000
Metoclopramide HCl syrup 1 mg/mL	Robins	8350
Milk of Magnesia suspension	Pharmaceutical Associates	1250
Multivitamin liquid	Upjohn	5700
Nystatin suspension 100,000 U/mL	Squibb	3300
Phenytoin sodium suspension 20 mg/mL	Parke-Davis	2500
Phenytoin sodium suspension 25 mg/mL	Parke-Davis	1500
Potassium Chloride liquid 10%	Roxane	3550
Potassium Iodide saturated solution 1 g/mL	Upsher Smith	10950
Primidone suspension 50 mg/mL	Ayerst	450
Prochlorperazine syrup 1 mg/mL	Smith Kline French	3250
Promethazine HCl syrup 1.25 mg/mL	Wyeth	3500
Pyridostigmine bromide syrup 12 mg/mL	Roche	3800
Sodium Citrate liquid	Willen	2050
Sodium Phosphate liquid 0.5 g/mL	Fleet	7250
Theophylline solution 5.33 mg/mL	Berlex	800

Dilution of a hyperosmolar medication to approximately 300 mOsm/kg reduces the risk of medication-induced diarrhea. The volume of water required to achieve the desired osmolality can be calculated from the following: ((medication osmolality/desired osmolality) × medication volume in mL) – medication in mL = volume of sterile water.

Reprinted with permission from Dickerson RN, Melnick G. Osmolality of oral drug solutions and suspensions. *Am J Hosp Pharm.* 1988;45:832 © American Society of Health-System Pharmacists, Inc.

TABLE 14.7

Sorbitol Content of Selected Liquid Medications			
Generic	Trade Name	Manufacturer	% Sorbitol (w/v)
Acetaminophen Elixir	Tylenol	McNeil	<20
Acetaminophen Elixir		Roxane	35.0
Acetaminophen/Codeine	Generic	Capital	6.2
Aluminum Hydroxide Gel	Generic	Roxane	10.5
Aluminum Hydroxide/magnesium carbonate	Gaviscon	Marion-Merrell Dow	7.3
Aluminum/magnesium	Maalox	Rhône-Poulenc Rorer	4.5
Aluminum/magnesium	Maalox TC	Rhône-Poulenc Rorer	15.0
Aluminum/magnesium	Extra Strength Maalox Plus	Rhône-Poulenc Rorer	10.0
Aluminum/magnesium with simethicone	Generic	Roxane	10.6
Amantadine	Symmetrel	Du Pont	72.0
Aminophylline	Generic	Roxane	14.0
Brompheniramine/phenylephrine	Dimetane	A.H. Robins	42.2
Brompheniramine DM, pseudoephredrine	Dimetane DX	Wyeth-Ayerst	35.0
Calcium carbonate	Generic	Roxane	28.0
Carbamazepine	Tegretol	Geigy	17.0
Chloral Hydrate	Generic	UDL	3.5
Chlorpromazine	Chlorpromazine HCl intensol	Roxane	3.5
Cimetadine	Tagamet	SmithKline Beecham	46.1
Codeine	Generic	Roxane	28.0
Co-trimoxazole	Generic/ Bactrim	Biocraft Roche	10.0 7.0
Dexamethasone	Dexamethasone oral solution	Roxane	24.6
Diazepam	Generic	Roxane	21.0
Digoxin	Generic	Roxane	21.0
Diphenoxylate HCl/atropine	Lomotil/ Generic	Searle Roxane	21.0 45.0
Docusate	Colace/ Generic/ Generic/	Mead Johnson Roxane UDL	0.0 0.0 32.0
Doxepin	Generic	Warner Chilcott	25.7
Doxycycline	Vibramycin	Pfizer	70.0
Ferrous Sulfate	Fer-in-sol/ Generic	Mead Johnson Roxane	30.9 0.0
Furosemide	Lasix/ Generic	Hoechst-Roussel Roxane	35.0 49.0
Guaifenesin	Robitussin/ Generic	A.H. Robins Roxane	0.0 10.5
Guaifenesin/codeine	Robitussin AC	Wyeth-Ayerst	35.0
Guaifenesin/dextromethorphan	Generic	UDL	64.0
Haloperidol	Haldol/ Generic	McNeil Xactdose	0.0 0.0
Hydrocodone/homatropine	Hycodan	Du Pont	6.0
Hydrocodone/acetaminophen	Lortab	Russ	<1.0
Hydrocodone/guaifensin	Hycotuss/ Codiclear DH/ Kwelcoff	Du Pont Central Ascher	6.0 28.8

TABLE 14.7

Sorbitol Content of Selected Liquid Medications (CONTINUED)			
Generic	**Trade Name**	**Manufacturer**	**% Sorbitol (w/v)**
Hydrocodone/pseudoephedrine guaifenesin	Entuss D Jr.	Roberts	10.5
Hydrocodone/pseudoephedrine	Entuss D	Hauck	52.5
Hydroxyzine	Vistaril	Pfizer	116.0
Hydromorphone	Dilaudid	Knoll	13.0
Hyoscyamine	Levsin drops Levsin elixir Gastrosed	Schwarz Pharma Schwarz Pharma Hauck	18.2 2.9 43.4
Ibuprofen	Pedia-Profen/ Generic	McNeil Whitehall	0.0 10.0
Indomethacin	Indocin	Merck & Co	35.0
Isoniazid	Generic	Carolina Medical	70.0
Lithium Citrate	Cibatin-S/ Generic	Ciba Roxane	77.2 54.0
Loperamide	Imodium A-D	McNeil	0.0
Meperidine	Generic	Roxane	28.0
Mesoridazine	Serentil	Boehinger Ingelheim	2.8
Metaproterenol	Alupent Generic	Boehinger Ingelheim Roxane	21.5 28.0
Methadone HCl	Generic	Roxane	14.0
Metoclopramide	Reglan/ Generic/ Generic	Wyeth-Ayerst Roxane Biocraft	35.0 28.0 42.0
Minocycline	Minocin	Lederle	10.3
Morphine Sulfate	Generic	Roxane	8.4
Naproxen	Naprosyn	Syntex	9.0
Nortriptyline	Aventyl	Lilly	64.0
Oxybutynin	Ditropan	Hoechst Marion Roussel	26.0
Oxycodone	Roxicodone	Roxane	14.0
Phenylephrine chlorpheniramine	Novahistine	Hoechst Marion Roussel	34.0
Phenobarbital	Generic	Rugby	12.8
Potassium chloride	Generic	Roxane	0.0
Potassium chloride/potassium gluconate	Kolyum Liquid	Fisons	12.0
Potassium gluconate	Kaon	Adria	21.0
Prednisolone	Pediapred	Fisons	36.0
Promethazine/codeine	Promethazine VC	Warner Chilcott	0.05
Pseudoephredrine/triprolidine	Actifed	Burroughs Wellcome	49.0
Ranitidine	Zantac	Glaxo	10.0
Tetracycline	Sumycin	Bristol-Meyers Squibb	23.0
Theophylline	Generic	Roxane	21.0
Thioridazine	Thioridazine HCl	Roxane	21.0
Valproate sodium	Depakene	Abbott	15.0
Vitamin E	Aquasol	Astra	20.0

The sorbitol content of medications may change over time. Contact manufacturer for current information.

TABLE 14.8

Foods and Beverages Containing Pressor Agents (Tyramine, Dopamine, Phenylethylamine) to Avoid while Taking Monamine Oxidase Inhibitors
Cheese (especially aged)
Casseroles made with cheese, including pizza
Sour cream
Wine (especially red)
Tap beer
Coffee
Liver
Fermented meats (salami, pepperoni, summer sausage)
Herring (pickled or dry)
Soy sauce
Soya bean/paste
Fermented bean curd
Miso soup
Sauerkraut, kim chee
Fava, snowpea or broad bean pods
Overripe bananas
Concentrated yeast extracts

increased levels of norepinephrine may lead to severe headache, hypertensive crisis and cardiac dysrhythmias[1] (see Table 14.8).

PRESYSTEMIC BINDING/COMPLEXATION

Presystemic binding/complexation implies that the drug-drug or drug-nutrient substances are bound or complexed together resulting in a reduction in oral bioavailability. This interaction takes place inside the GI tract, rather than in the delivery set like ex vivo pharmaceutical inactivations. This usually doesn't involve enzymes or transporters but coadministration of drugs and enteral formulas. Bile acid binding resins and sucralfate bind with warfarin, phenprocoumon, and possibly other anticoagulants in the GI tract, reducing the anticoagulant response. Since warfarin and phenprocoumon undergo enterohepatic circulation, the binding cannot be completely avoided by spacing doses of the drugs.

Food may have a significant effect on drug absorption; the rate or extent of absorption of a medication may be altered by the presence of food through a variety of mechanisms. Most commonly, the presence of food in the GI tract can lead to a decrease in the amount of drug absorbed, leading to therapeutic failures. Food can also decrease the rate of absorption of a drug without having a significant effect on the total amount of drug absorbed. This usually does not alter the efficacy or toxicity of the medication.[1]

Fluoroquinolones, such as ciprofloxacin, ofloxacin, lomefloxacin, and enoxacin undergo a process called chelation with divalent cations (aluminum, calcium, magnesium, zinc) forming an inactive complex.[31] Ciprofloxacin normally is about 60% to 80% absorbed in the GI tract; however, concomitant administration with divalent cations reduces the bioavailability to 14% to 50%. Antacids, which may contain some or all of these troublesome cations, may decrease bioavailability of ciprofloxacin by as much as 90%.[33] Sucralfate contains aluminum and may decrease absorption of ciprofloxacin by as much as 30%.[34] Of interest is that a new fluoroquinolone, trovafloxacin, was administered via nasogastric tube to the stomach after being crushed, with and without concomitant enteral feeding, and was found to achieve absorption and tolerability comparable to orally administered trovafloxacin tablets.[35]

Enteral nutrition formulas and supplements are another source of divalent cations. Both Ensure® and Resource® were found to significantly decrease absorption of ciprofloxacin via the chelation mechanism. Numerous other medications are affected by the presence of food/enteral feeding formula. Antimicrobials such as tetracycline and doxycycline, as well as penicillins, isoniazid, ketoconazole and rifampin, all undergo reduced absorption in the presence of food.[25] Tetracycline specifically may form complexes with calcium and iron in the GI tract and prevent absorption of adequate amounts of these elements.[27] Another class of drug affected by the presence of food is the angiotensin converting enzyme (ACE) inhibitors. Food may decrease the absorption of captopril by 25% to 40%, which may have serious consequences for blood pressure control.[1]

The concomitant administration of phenytoin suspension and enteral formulas can result in significantly decreased serum concentrations secondary to decreased bioavailability. This is one drug in which a small change in the absorption can cause a significant change in the serum concentration.[1]

Preventing Absorption Incompatibilities with Enteral Nutrition

In order to prevent presystemic metabolism irregularities, most serious interactions will be avoided if grapefruit juice is not co-administered with the known target drugs (Table 14.9).

To preclude incompatibilities with presystemic transport, transit time or dissolution of the drug or nutritional compound, attention must be given to the mechanism of transport, the actual delivery site of the

TABLE 14.9

Potential Grapefruit Juice Interactions	
Drug	**Clinical Effect**
Alprazolam	Inhibits intestinal CYP 3A4 thereby ↑ levels of drugs
Astemizole*	Inhibits intestinal CYP 3A4 thereby ↑ levels of drugs
Cisapride*	Metabolized by intestinal CYP 3A4
Cyclosporine	↑ AUC & serum concentrations
Dihydropyridine	↑ AUC & serum concentrations
Calcium Channel Blockers Felodipine Nifedipine Nimodipine Amlodipine Nisoldipine Verapamil Diltiazem	↑ AUC & serum concentrations ↑ Serum concentrations from one study No significant effect
Triazolam	↑ Plasma concentration
Midazolam	↑ AUC & peak serum conc. No effect with IV form
Carbamazepine	↑ AUC & peak/trough plasma concentrations
Lovastatin	↑ AUC & C_{max}
Buspirone	↑ AUC & C_{max}
Caffeine	↑ AUC, ↑ $t_{1/2}$

Adapted from Hansten PD, Horn JR. *The Top 100 Drug Interactions. A Guide to Patient Management.* Edmonds, WA: H & H Publications; 2001, hanstenandhorn.com.
**removed from market*
CYP 3A4 = cytochrome enzyme 3A4; AUC = area under the curve

Several components such as flavonoids, nauringenin, or psoralen derivatives in grapefruit juice have been implicated. Since the content of these varies between different grapefruit juices it is not possible to determine if one is safer than another.

For drugs significantly affected by this interaction a single glass of grapefruit juice is sufficient to cause the interaction, and following regular ingestion the effect can last for up to 3 days. If the patient is receiving medication on a regular basis it appears prudent to avoid grapefruit juice altogether.

medication, and the fluid and electrolyte status of the patient.

Crushing an enteric-coated tablet for administration via a gastric feeding tube delivers the medication to an inappropriate site. An acid-labile medication will not be protected from stomach acid, resulting in destruction of the medication, or the stomach will not be protected from an irritating medication, and the risk of nausea, vomiting, or gastric erosion will increase. Likewise, crushing or dissolving a sustained-release product results in delivery of all doses of the medication intended for release over 12 to 24 hours. This could lead to a potential overdose or toxic situation.

Special forms of drugs must be evaluated individually by a pharmacist to determine if the medication can safely be altered. Minor alteration of the dosage form of some enteric-coated or slow-release preparations may be acceptable. Slow-release capsules containing many small beads may be acceptable for administration via a feeding tube if the intact beads can pass through the tube openings without clogging the tube. Proper dosing is ensured as long as the beads remain intact for administration (not crushed or dissolved) and the complete contents of the capsule are delivered as a single dose[4] (See Tables 14.3 and 14.4).

Any enteral nutrition formula characteristic that decreases gastric emptying, such as high osmolality, high viscosity, or high fat content, can be expected to slow absorption of medication.[2]

Patients should not receive foods containing tyramine while receiving MAO inhibitors (Table 14.9).

To avoid significant vitamin and nutrient depletion associated with laxative use, antibiotics, and bile acid binders, these medications should be limited to short-term use. In most cases the need for supplementation of vitamins has not been adequately studied. Vitamin supplementation may be given if clinical judgment warrants it.[27]

Fed Versus Fasted State

In order to prevent interactions with presystemic binding resulting in reduced drug bioavailability, attention must be given to the fed versus fasted state of the patient.

While it is recommended that some medications be administered to an empty stomach, this is not always practical in an ICU patient receiving continuous tube feedings. A delay in drug absorption generally is not clinically significant. The interaction results in a delayed time to peak drug concentration but not necessarily a decreased amount of drug absorbed.

For many drugs, it is important only that they be administered consistently with or without food. In order to standardize the administration of drugs to an empty stomach, the most common recommendation from pharmaceutical manufacturers is to administer the medication either 1 hour before a meal or 2 hours after a meal.[1] This translates to interruption of continuous feedings 1 hour prior to drug administration and for 1 to 2 hours following administration. For phenytoin specifically, the recommendation is to interrupt the feeding for 2 hours before and after the dose.[14]

Changing to a formula with different nutrient sources may be beneficial. Both fiber and non-fiber containing intact protein formulas demonstrated incompatibilities when tested with numerous different medications. Different protein sources, and the degree of protein hydrolysis in particular, also affect interactions with medications. Hydrolyzed protein and free amino acid formulas appear to demonstrate the greatest stability when mixed with a variety of pharmaceutical preparations[4] (see Table 14.2).

Interactions Affecting Systemic or Physiologic Dispositions

The definition selected describes this type of interaction as occurring after the drug or the nutritional element has entered systemic circulation (i.e., after absorption for enterally or orally administered compounds). It may involve an alteration in cellular or tissue distribution, systemic metabolism or transport, penetration to specific organ/tissues (e.g., across the blood-brain barrier), or other co-factors (e.g., clotting factors) or hormones.

Drug-Nutrient Interaction Pairs

Warfarin and Vitamin K

Vitamin K antagonizes the drug effect while warfarin blocks the formation of active vitamin K-dependent factors (factors II, VII, IX, X).[4] Appropriate anticoagulation with warfarin generally occurs with a vitamin K intake of 300–500 mcg/d from the typical Western diet.[36] The vitamin K content of many enteral formulas was reduced after the initial reports of warfarin resistance.[37]

Vitamin E and Vitamin K

Vitamin E increases the international normalizing ratio (INR) by interfering with vitamin K-dependent clotting factors. Patients should be instructed to limit vitamin E intake to the RDA of 400 mg/d.[36]

Corticosteroids

Corticosteroids alter calcium/vitamin D disposition by affecting osteocalcin and probably parathyroid hormone activities with a resulting risk of osteoporosis.

The recommendation is for calcium and vitamin D replacement for patients on intermittent or chronic steroids.[27]

Valproic Acid (VPA)

This anticonvulsant drug results in decreased carnitine and ammonemia/hepatic encephalopathy without other liver injury. Death has also been reported.[38]

The mechanism of action is the inhibition of the biosynthesis of carnitine and possibly decreased tissue uptake of carnitine. Oral L-carnitine supplementation of special subgroups of patients has been recommended: secondary carnitine deficiency syndromes, symptomatic VPA-associated hyperammonemia, multiple-risk factors for VPA-associated hepatotoxicity, or renal-associated syndromes, infants and young children taking VPA, patients with epilepsy using ketogenic diet who have hypocarnitinemia, patients on dialysis, and premature infants receiving TPN. The recommended dosage is 100 mg/kg/d up to a maximum of 2 g/d orally.[39]

Sinemet (Anti-Parkinson's)

There is reduced drug efficacy with high protein ingestion.[40]

TABLE 14.10

Pyridoxine-Rich Foods to Avoid When Taking Levodopa[1]	
Avocados	Peas
Beans	Pork
Bacon	Sweet potatoes
Beef liver	Tuna

THEOPHYLLINE (BRONCHODILATOR)

There is reduced drug efficacy with high protein intake.[40]

LEVODOPA (DOPAR)

Levodopa is converted to dopamine. Dopamine is deficient in basal ganglia of patients with Parkinson's disease. Pyridoxine can increase the metabolism of levodopa, decreasing the amount available to cross the blood-brain barrier. Patients taking levodopa should avoid pyridoxine-rich foods[1] (Table 14.10).

ISONIAZID (HISTAMINASE INHIBITOR)

Individuals taking isoniazid are particularly sensitive to scombroid fish poisoning. Tuna, mackerel, and salmon are scombroid fish and contain large quantities of histidine. If scombroid fish is not refrigerated properly, bacteria can convert histidine to histamine which is heat stable and not affected by cooking. Symptoms of scombroid fish poisoning may mimic drug allergy to isoniazid; patients may experience facial flushing, abdominal cramps, palpitations, headache, nausea, dizziness, or erythematous and urticarial rash.[1] Patients on isoniazid should be particularly cautious of this reaction. Other histamine-containing foods include sauerkraut and yeast extract.

PHENYTOIN (DILANTIN, ANTI-CONVULSANT), FOSPHENYTOIN (CEREBYX, ANTI-CONVULSANT) AND CARBAMAZEPINE (TEGRETOL, ANTI-CONVULSANT)

Studies of anti-convulsants in general demonstrate lower folic acid levels in treated patients.[26] Drugs deplete folic acid (folate) by inducing hepatic microsomal enzymes leading to an increase in folic acid metabolism, not by decreasing dietary absorption. After a period of chronic therapy, megaloblastic anemia can develop. Practitioners should consider folic acid supplementation with the initial dose of an anticonvulsant to prevent folate deficiency.[41]

METHOTREXATE (ANTINEOPLASTIC, ANTIPSORIATIC, ANTIRHEUMATIC)

This agent is a folic acid antagonist that prevents the conversion of folate to folic acid. It is not compatible with many common ICU medications (e.g., Decadron®, Reglan®, Versed®, Diprivan®, or selected TPN solutions).[42] Physicians should consult a pharmacist prior to administering this agent with any other medications. The recommendation is to replace folic acid for patients on prolonged therapy as 1 mg/d or 7 mg once/wk.[27]

Drug-Nutrient Interactions Involving Alteration of Elimination or Clearance

The definition selected describes these drugs or nutrients as those that are involved in interactions affecting either renal excretion or enterohepatic biliary recirculation of other drugs or nutrients. The mechanisms usually involve the modulation, antagonism, or impairment of renal or enterohepatic transport.[5]

High protein diets have been reported to accelerate hepatic metabolism of certain medications, and a protein-poor diet can decrease renal clearance of medications.[43]

Amphotericin B has been shown to cause renal wasting of potassium and magnesium. In addition, amphotericin B has been implicated in nephrotoxicity exhibited by azotemia, renal tubular acidosis, and nephrocalcinosis.[44]

Many drugs are eliminated via the urine in their pharmacologically active forms and a significant change in urinary pH can alter drug half-life. Depending on the drug's acid dissociation constant (pKa), the half-life of acidic drugs can be extended in acidic urine, whereas the half-life of acidic drugs in alkaline urine is reduced. Similarly, the half-life of basic drugs can be extended in alkaline urine, whereas the half-life of basic drugs in acidic urine is reduced. One example of this can be seen with the anti-coagulant warfarin. Alkaline urine increases the elimination of this basic drug, and acidic urine can decrease the rate of elimination potentiating drug side effects. Large doses of ascorbic acid (vitamin C) yield urine acidification, which in turn affects renal uptake of certain drugs.[2]

Loop diuretics such as bumetanide, ethacrinic acid, and lasix all contribute to an increased urinary excretion of calcium, magnesium, potassium, sodium chloride, ammonium, bicarbonate, and zinc. Loop diuretics exert their effect by inhibiting the reabsorption of electrolytes in the ascending limb of the loop of Henle.[1] Electrolyte disturbances are more likely with higher doses or when used in combination with diuretics of another class, such as thiazide and thiazide derivatives.[27] Drugs in this class that further contribute to losses of magnesium, sodium, potassium, and zinc include chlorothiazide, hydrochlorothiazide, metolazone, and chlorthalidone.

The anti-infective activity of several antibiotics can be affected by foods that make urine acidic or basic, due to increased or decreased urinary elimination. Examples include kanamycin, nalidixic acid, nitrofurantoin, streptomycin, and sulfonamides.[2]

Management of Drug-Nutrient Interactions Involving Altered Renal Clearance

Awareness of the drug's potential to be affected by the pH of the urine is the primary prevention; consultation with the pharmacist is required for possible adjustment of medication dosage. Consultation with the dietitian is also required in order to make dietary adjustments so that drug effects will not be significantly increased or decreased by protein, dairy products, grapefruit juice, vitamin K, etc. (Table 14.11).

TABLE 14.11

Foods That Affect the pH of the Urine[45]

Increase Acidity	
Bacon	Grains
Brazil nuts	Lentils
Breads	Meats
Cakes	Orange juice
Cereals	Pasta
Cheeses	Peanuts/peanut butter
Cookies	Plums/prunes
Corn	Rice
Crackers	Shellfish
Cranberries/juice	Walnuts
Eggs	
Fish	
Fowl/poultry	
Increase Alkalinity	
Beets	Kale
Chestnuts	Molasses
Coconuts	Nuts (except peanuts & walnuts)
Dairy products	Spinach
Fruits (except cranberries, plums, & prunes)	Vegetables (except corn & lentils)

Drugs with a narrow range of therapeutic action should have serum levels monitored closely. Renal function tests should also be closely monitored in the critical care setting or with the use of nephrotoxic agents.

Conclusions

Drug-nutrient interactions are a complex issue for healthcare providers today. New drugs are commonly marketed without complete investigation into their interactions with foods and such dietary supplements as vitamins, herbs, and minerals. Reference studies use formulations of drugs or nutritional products that no longer exist. Enteral formulas undergo modifications regularly to meet a growing need for specialized nutrition. Nonmedicinal or inert ingredients in pharmaceutical preparations previously tested have also changed, and continue to be protected as proprietary information. Use caution when applying information from published compatibility studies to specialized nutrition support today.

It is of utmost importance that healthcare providers consider drug-nutrient interactions in all settings, but especially in the ICU setting. Vulnerable patients who can not verbalize their response to new and potent medications may be subjected to a lack of drug activity, serious side effects, or toxicity. Members of the Nutrition Support Team have a professional responsibility to instill an awareness of the potential for drug-nutrient interactions in their ICU clinician colleagues. In turn, physicians, nurses, dietitians and pharmacists must continually educate themselves and their patients about the effect of food and nutritional supplements on the effectiveness, potential interactions, and toxicity of medications.

Case Study

J. Smith is a 65-year-old African American male who was admitted for a non-healing diabetic foot ulcer on January 15, 2001. His height was 165.1 cm and admission weight was 98 kg. His underlying medical conditions included end-stage renal disease (ESRD) 2° to insulin-requiring type II diabetes mellitus since 1970, chronic renal insufficiency, hypertension, congestive heart failure, and chronic obstructive pulmonary disease. He presented with a tracheostomy placed following a stroke 20 years ago. He underwent a right below-the-knee amputation on January 19th and was recovered in the ICU following surgery. His postoperative course was complicated by a perioperative myocardial infarction, nosocomial pneumonia, corneal infection, heparin-induced thrombocytopenia, cholestatic liver failure, and septic shock, for which he was aggressively treated with antibiotics, vasoactive agents, and fluid resuscitation. His previously stable renal disease further deteriorated and he experienced numerous electrolyte/mineral abnormalities each day. He began daily hemodialysis on his third postoperative day. His medications included Prilosec, Vasotec, insulin, Combivent MDI, Flovent, Diflucan, Hydrocortisone, antibiotic eye drops, Nephrocap, and Phoslo. All medications were renal-adjusted to a GFR <10.

Early enteral feedings were initiated via Dobhoff nasogastric tube with Magnacal Renal (Mead Johnson Nutritionals, Evansville, IN), which contained 800 mg of phosphorus per liter. This 2.0 kcal/cc formula for dialysis patients provided 32 kcal/kg, 1.2 g/kg of protein/d and 100% of RDA for vitamins and minerals. His admission phosphorus level was 1.9 mg/dL (nl 2.7–4.5 mg/dL). He was receiving Phoslo (Calcium acetate, 25% Ca) 667 mg twice a day. Three weeks later his phosphorus levels had risen to 7.7 mg/dL. Tube feedings ran 24 hours a day at 48 cc/h so the patient received a continuous diet containing phosphate and calcium.

Plasma calcium and phosphate exist in a reciprocal relationship. If the calcium level decreases, the phosphate level increases. The ionized plasma calcium level controls the amount of calcium absorbed from the gastrointestinal tract. Vitamin D facilitates its absorption. The majority of dietary phosphate is excreted via the kidney to maintain a normal serum phosphate level. Phosphate excretion by the kidney is directly proportional to the serum phosphate level. Because the kidney is the primary route of phosphate excretion, an elevation of the plasma phosphorus level occurs in ESRD. The rising phosphorus, the impaired conversion of vitamin D to its active metabolite, and the reduced calcium absorption from the GI tract, affect plasma calcium. ESRD will also impair calcium mobilization from bone worsening the hypocalcemia.

Ideally, a low phosphate diet will prevent hyperphosphatemia. However, in some cases phosphate binders are required. These medications bind with the phosphate in the GI tract and are excreted in the feces, thus preventing absorption of the phosphate from the GI tract. Phosphate binders may come in the form of aluminum-containing antacids or calcium salts. Calcium salts, such as calcium carbonate (Os-Cal), are not as effective in phosphate binding and may contribute to hypercalcemia, but aluminum toxicity is a more serious consequence of aluminum-containing antacids. Aluminum accumulation in ESRD results in central nervous system, hematologic, and bone toxicity.

Phosphate binders are typically given three times a day with meals, but with continuous feedings, phosphate binders may need more frequent dosing. Phosphate binders can be given as often as every 2 to 3 hours when a patient is receiving continuous enteral feedings. Due to persistent hyperphosphatemia, Mr. Smith's phosphate binder was changed to Os-Cal liquid (625 mg Ca/2.5 mL) three times a day. Over the next 5 days his serum phosphorus level dropped from 6.1 mg/dL to 5.0 mg/dL. He was then maintained on Os-Cal liquid (1250 mg Ca/5 mL), titrated to a phosphorus level of <5.5 mg/dL, as long as calcium was within normal limits (8.4–10.2 mg/dL). Mr. Smith underwent a gastrostomy with jejunal extension three weeks after his initial surgery.

Because phosphate binders are intended to bind the phosphate in a "meal" they are commonly taken with meals or ordered to be placed in the tube feeding bag. Because of a concern for clumping in the bag or clogging of the feeding tube, we undertook an investigation to see what the characteristics of the feeding were once the medication was added to the administration set. Our results appear in Table 14.12 (McCarthy, unpublished data). While each patient must be looked at individually, it is important to remember that optimal binding will occur if medication administration is temporally related to diet.

In preparation for his transfer, Mr. Smith was placed on an isotonic formula with intermittent dosing of Os-Cal 1250 mg via G-J tube. Mr. J. Smith did fully recover from his surgery and was transported to a rehabilitation center after 62 hospital days.

References

1. Maka DA, Murphy LK. Drug-nutrient interactions: a review. *AACN Clin Issues.* 2000;11:580–589.
2. Williamson JS, Wyandt CM. What the pharmacist should know about food and drug interactions. *Hosp Pharmacist Report.* 1998;Apr: 43–52.
3. *Comprehensive Accreditation Manual for Hospitals. The Official Handbook.* Oakbrook, IL: The Joint Commission on Accreditation of Healthcare Organizations; Update 1999.
4. Rollins CJ. General pharmacology issues. In: Matarese LE, Gottschlich MM, eds. *Contemporary Nutrition Support Practice.* Philadelphia: W.B. Saunders Company; 1998: 303–323.
5. Chan LN. Redefining drug-nutrient interactions. NCP, 2000;15(5):249–252.

TABLE 14.12

Phosphate Binders in Enteral Feeding Products		
Nutritional Formula	Phosphate-Binding Medication Formulation	Characteristics Noted/Recommendation
Immune modulated, high fat, calorically dense (1.5 kcal/cc) ***Oxepa*** (Ross Products Division Abbott Laboratories, Columbus, OH)	**OsCal tablet, 1250 mg Calcium** Crushed with HandiCrush Syringe, mixed w/30 cc warm water, squirted into bag with 480 cc formula, and mixed	Almost immediately a gray sediment appeared at the bottom of the bag. This remained in place for 6 hours and when roller clamp released, no formula flow was noted. No clumping in feeding bag noted. **NOT RECOMMENDED.**
Immune modulated, high fat, calorically dense (1.5 kcal/cc) *Oxepa*	**Calcium Carbonate liquid, 1250 mg Calcium/5 mL**, same as OsCal except liquid	White liquid noted at bottom of bag at 2 hours, returned after gentle agitation, remained there at 6 hours. No clumping of formula in the bag; good flow with release of roller clamp. **RECOMMENDED IF PT REQUIRES CONTINUOUS TF.**
Standard hospital formula, isocaloric, 1.06 kcal/cc ***Isocal HN*** (Mead Johnson Nutritionals, Evansville, IN)	**Aluminum Hydroxide Liquid, 15 mL, 0 mg Calcium**	Mixed thoroughly with formula, no sediment, no clumping. Excellent flow when roller clamp released. Stable for 6 hours. Could be used as alternative preparation if supplemental calcium not desirable. **RECOMMENDED AS ALTERNATIVE.**
Standard hospital formula with fiber, isocaloric, 1.06 kcal/cc ***Ultracal*** (Mead Johnson Nutritionals, Evansville, IN)	**Calcium Carbonate liquid, 1250 mg Calcium/5 mL**	Mixed thoroughly with formula, no sediment, no clumping. No sign of interaction with formula at 4 hours. Calcium carbonate liquid appears to be the best choice for phosphate-binder in the feeding bag. **RECOMMENDED IF PT REQUIRES CONTINUOUS TF.**
Standard hospital formula for fluid-restricted patients; calorically dense, 2.0 kcal/cc ***TwoCal HN*** (Ross Products Division Abbott Laboratories, Columbus, OH)	**Aluminum Hydroxide Liquid, 30 mL, 0 mg Calcium**	Mixed very easily, no precipitation, no clumping noted. 4 hours later flowed slowly, appeared somewhat "thick." **NOT RECOMMENDED.**
Special diet preparation for the renal failure patient receiving dialysis, calorically dense, 2.0 kcal/cc . . . ***MagnaCal Renal*** (Mead Johnson Nutritionals, Evansville, IN)	**OsCal tablet, 1250 mg Calcium** Crushed with HandiCrush Syringe, mixed w/30 cc warm water, squirted into bag with 240 cc formula, and mixed	Noticed gray particles settling in the bottom of the bag right away. 4 hours later did not flow well at all. Liquid did not even reach the chamber. **NOT RECOMMENDED.**

***It is preferred that no medications be added to the TF bag due to the risk of contamination.** Uncertainty about tolerance to therapy and starting and stopping the infusion may lead to an unknown amount of medication delivery. In the case of phosphate binding, the medication must interact with the nutrient meal to begin binding of the phosphate. In this situation, a phosphate binder may be added to the bag to ensure appropriate therapy is rendered for the renal failure patient. Calcium carbonate contains 40% calcium, which is greater than many other preparations. If the patient is receiving RenalCal (Nestle Clinical Nutrition, Wheeling, IL), it is not necessary to add a phosphate binder, as the formula contains no phosphorus. However, enteral therapy with a phosphate-binder may still be prescribed as an intermittent dose to eliminate other GI sources of phosphate. **Intermittent dosing is recommended** and should be used with continuous and intermittent feedings, bolus feedings, or po feedings/normal diet pattern.

6. Keeth CK. Enteral nutrition. In: Hennessy KA, Orr ME, eds. *Nutrition Support Nursing Core Curriculum.* 3rd ed. Silver Spring, MD: American Society of Enteral and Parenteral Nutrition 1996: 20–29.
7. Lumpkin MM. Safety alert: hazards of precipitation associated with parenteral nutrition. *Am J Hosp Pharm.* 1994; 51:1427–1428.
8. Zaccardelli DS, Krcmarik CS, Wolk R, et al. Stability of imipenem and cilastatin sodium in TPN solution. *J Parenter Enteral Nutr.* 1990;14:306–309.
9. Gora ML, Tschampel MM, Visconti JA. Considerations of drug therapy in patients receiving enteral nutrition. *Nutr Clin Pract.* 1989;4:105–110.
10. Engle KK, Hannawa TE. Techniques for administering oral medications to critical care patients receiving continuous enteral nutrition. *Am J Health-Sys Pharm.* 1999;56: 1441–1444.
11. Cutie AJ, Altman E, Lenkel L. Compatibility of enteral products with commonly employed drug additives. *J Parenter Enteral Nutr.* 1983;7:186–191.
12. Altman E, Cutie AJ. Compatibility of enteral products with commonly employed drug additives. *Nutr Supp Serv.* 1984;4:8–17.
13. Burns PE, McCall L, Wirsching R. Physical compatibility of enteral formulas with various common medications. *J Am Diet Assoc.* 1988;88:1094–1096.

14. Splinter MY, Seifert CF, Bradberry JL, et al. Effect of pH on the equilibrium dialysis of phenytoin suspension with and without enteral feeding formula. *J Parenter Enteral Nut.* 1990;14:275–278.

15. Benson DW, Griggs BA, Hamilton F, et al. Clogging of feeding tubes: a randomized trial of a newly designed tube. *Nutr Clin Prac.* 1990;5:107–110.

16. Wilson M, Haynes-Johnson V. Cranberry juice or water? A comparison of feeding tube irrigants. *Nutr Supp Serv.* 1987;7:23–24.

17. Niemiec PW Jr., Vanderveen TW, Morrison JI, et al. Gastrointestinal disorders caused by medication and electrolyte solution osmolality during enteral nutrition. *J Parenter Enteral Nutr.* 1983; 7:387–389.

18. Marcuard SP, Perkins PM. Clogging of feeding tubes. *J Parenter Enteral Nutr.* 1988;12:403–405.

19. Marcuard SP, Stegall KS. Unclogging feeding tubes with pancreatic enzymes. *J Parenter Enteral Nutr.* 1990;14:198–200.

20. Powell KS, Marcuard SP, Farrior ES, et al. Aspirating gastric residuals causes occlusion of small bore feeding tubes. *J Parenter Enteral Nutr.* 1993;17:243–246.

21. Wright B, Robinson L. Enteral feeding tubes as drug delivery systems. *Nutr Supp Serv.* 1986;6:33–48.

22. Golioto M, Lytle J, Jowell P. Re-Establishing Patency of a Small Bore Feeding Tube with Complete Occlusion—A novel use for an ERCP catheter. *Nutr Clin Prac.* 2001;284–285.

23. Sullivan DW, Ford MA, Boyden TW. Grapefruit juice and the response to warfarin. *Am J Health-Sys Pharm.* 1998;55: 1581–1583.

24. Lilja JJ, Kivisto KT, Backman JT, et al. Grapefruit juice substantially increases plasma concentrations of buspirone. *Clin Pharmacol Ther.* 1998;64:655–660.

25. Kirk J. Significant drug-nutrient interactions. *Am Fam Phys.* 1995;51:1175–1182.

26. Melia AT, Koss-Twardy SG, Zhi J. The effect of orlistat, an inhibitor of dietary fat absorption on the absorption of vitamins A and E in healthy volunteers. *J Clin Pharm.* 1996;36:647–653.

27. Ables J, Batz F. Drug influences on nutrient levels and depletion. *Pharm Ltr.* (Web ID # 787144) 2000:1–8.

28. Rivey MP, Schottelius D, Berg MJ. Phenytoin-folic acid: a review. *Drug Intell and Clin Pharm.* 1984;18:292–301.

29. Winter ME. Theophylline. In: Koda-Kimble MA, Young LY, eds. *Basic Clinical Pharmacokinetics.* 3rd ed. Vancouver; Applied Therapeutics, Inc; 1994:405–445.

30. Freeman CD, Klutman NE, Lamp KC, et al. Relative bioavailability of atovaquone suspension when administered with an enteral nutrition supplement. *Ann Pharmaco.* 1998;32:1004–1007.

31. Cathartics and laxatives. In: McEvoy GK, ed. *American Hospital Formulary Service Drug Information 1999.* Bethesda, MD: American Society of Health-System Pharmacists; 1999:2523–2537.

32. Segal S, Kaminski S. Drug-nutrient interactions. *Am Druggist.* 1996;213:42–49.

33. Quinolones. In: McEvoy GK, ed. *American Hospital Formulary Service Drug Information 1999.* Bethesda, MD: American Society of Health-System Pharmacists. 1999: 265–306.

34. Garrelts JC, Godley PJ, Peterie JD, et al. Sucralfate significantly reduces ciprofloxacin concentrations in serum. *Antimicrob Agents Chemother.* 1990;34:931–933.

35. Vincent J, Teng R, Pelletier SM, et al. The bioavailability of nasogastric versus tablet form oral trovafloxacin in healthy subjects. *Am J Surg.* 1998;176 (6A Suppl):23S–26S.

36. *National Research Council. Recommended Dietary Allowances,* 10th ed. Washington, DC: National Academy Press, Washington, D.C., 1989.

37. Kutsup JJ. Update on vitamin K content of enteral products. (Letter) *Am J Hosp Pharm.* 1984;41:1762.

38. Opala G, Winter S, Vance C, et al. The effect of valproic acid on plasma carnitine levels. *Am J Dis Child.* 1991;145: 999–1001.

39. Coulter DL. Carnitine, valproate and toxicity. *J Child Neurol.* 1991;6:7–14.

40. Thomson C, LaFrance R. Pharmacotherapeutics. In: MM Gottschlich, LE Matarese, EP Shronts, eds. *Nutrition Support Dietetics Core Curriculum.* 2nd ed. Silver Spring, MD: American Society of Parenteral and Enteral Nutrition; 1993:433–456.

41. Berg MJ, Stumbo PJ, Chenard CA, et al. Folic acid improves phenytoin pharmacokinetics. 1995;95:352–356.

42. Methotrexate sodium. In: Gahart BL, Nazareno AR. *Intravenous Medications 2001,* 17th ed. St. Louis: Mosby, Inc; 2001:609–612.

43. Williams L, Davis JA, Lowenthal DT. The influence of food on the absorption and metabolism of drugs. *Med Clin North Am.* 77:815–829.

44. Diuretics. In: McEvoy, GK, ed. *American Hospital Formulary Service Drug Information 1999.* Bethesda, MD: American Society of Health-Systems Pharmacists; 1999:2297–2332.

45. Holt, GA. *Food and Drug Interactions: A Health Care Professional's Guide.* Chicago: Precept Press Inc.; 1992.

CHAPTER 15

Nutrition Support in the Critically Ill Diabetic Patient

Polyxeni Koutkia, M.D., Caroline M. Apovian, M.D.

INTRODUCTION 175
BACKGROUND 175
PHYSIOLOGY OF DIABETES MELLITUS AND THE STRESSED STATE 175
Nutritional Assessment of the Critically Ill Diabetic Patient 176
DETERMINING ENERGY REQUIREMENTS 177
Route of Administration 178
GLYCEMIC CONTROL IN THE CRITICALLY ILL DIABETIC PATIENT: A METABOLIC CHALLENGE 178
Goals for Targeted Glycemic Control 179
Avoiding Hypoglycemia 179
Avoiding Hyperglycemia 180
THE DIABETIC PATIENT ON TOTAL PARENTERAL NUTRITION (TPN) 180
THE DIABETIC PATIENT ON ENTERAL NUTRITION 181
NUTRIENT COMPOSITION OF ENTERAL FORMULAS 181
SPECIAL SITUATIONS 181
Intravenous Insulin Therapy for Diabetic Patients with Myocardial Infarction (MI) 181
Management of the Diabetic Patient with Stroke 182
TRANSITIONING FROM INTRAVENOUS TO SUBCUTANEOUS INSULIN 182
Monitoring 183
CONCLUSIONS 183
CASE STUDY 183
Case Discussion 184
REFERENCES 184

Introduction

It is estimated that there are 15.6 million diabetics in the United States, a prevalence of 7.8% in U.S. adults aged 20 and older. An estimated 6 million hospitalizations per year in the United States are accompanied by hyperglycemia.[1] Because the prevalence and the co-morbidity of diabetes in the United States is high, most physicians will be faced with treating hospitalized patients with diabetes.

When the individual with diabetes requires hospitalization, it is necessary to consider two global perspectives. First, what is the effect of the underlying disorder, its treatment, and the hospitalization on overall glycemic control? Second, what is the impact of the acute diabetic state on the outcomes of the pathologic condition?[2] The appropriate nutritional management of diabetics in the stressed state is crucial to successful outcome and decreased length of stay. This chapter discusses the nutritional assessment of the diabetic and special concerns regarding glucose control, nutritional therapy, and monitoring. A case study with nutritional challenges is discussed at the end of the chapter, illustrating the management of the critically ill diabetic patient.

Background

Diabetes mellitus is a metabolic disorder characterized by complete (as in type 1 or insulin-dependent) or relative lack of insulin and insulin resistance (as in type 2). Along with these primary forms of diabetes, impairment of glucose tolerance can arise from other conditions. For the purposes of this chapter, the most relevant secondary form of glucose intolerance is that caused by stress (e.g., infection, trauma, surgery).

Physiology of Diabetes Mellitus and the Stressed State

Provision of appropriate nutrition support in diabetics and patients with stress glucose intolerance requires a working knowledge of glucose regulation. Plasma glucose concentration is normally closely regulated in both the fasting and postprandial periods. In the fasting state, the rate of glucose production by the liver equals the rate of glucose utilization by the brain, peripheral nervous tissue and red blood cells (approximately 2 mg/kg/min or 200 g/d). After a meal, the increase in plasma glucose and insulin suppresses hepatic glucose production and increases peripheral glucose uptake. As the plasma glucose and insulin concentrations decrease after eating, the rate of hepatic glucose production and peripheral glucose uptake revert to basal levels such that glucose production increases while glucose uptake decreases. This buffering system is impaired in patients with diabetes (diabetics have both preprandial and postprandial hyperglycemia). The hyperglycemia is due to excessive hepatic glucose release, impaired glucose uptake, and decreased insulin secretion and action.[3]

When an individual is hospitalized with an acute illness, a generalized stress response is initiated. Elevations occur in counterregulatory hormones, including epinephrine, glucagon, cortisol, and growth hormone. These hormone elevations significantly accelerate catabolism, hepatic gluconeogenesis, and lipolysis. The end result of these processes is an increase in levels of circulating serum glucose, free fatty acids, and ketone bodies. The rise of circulating substrate levels further fuels hyperglycemia and blunts the islet-cell insulin secretory response via the mechanism of glucose toxicity.[4] The diabetic critically ill patient cannot increase insulin secretion and in the diabetic the alteration in glucose metabolism is exaggerated, and glucose levels are even higher.[5]

In addition, acute illness and surgery may also result in acidosis from lactate or ketone body accumulation. Acidosis leads to impairment in peripheral insulin sensitivity, causing additional impairment in carbohydrate metabolism. These events propagate a cycle whereby acute illness induces hyperglycemia, and hyperglycemia subsequently impairs the physiologic response to that illness.[2] The difficulty in achieving glycemic control is further exacerbated by a disruption in typical daily activities, the use of pharmacologic interventions, dramatic changes in dietary intake, decreased activity levels, and difficulty keeping a precise timing for the administration of subcutaneous regular insulin 30 to 45 minutes before meals. All these variables commonly lead to dramatic fluctuations in glucose control during hospitalization.[2]

Nutritional Assessment of the Critically Ill Diabetic Patient

The nutritional assessment and management of the critically ill diabetic patient is similar to that of the non-diabetic. The production of counterregulatory hormones and cytokines, along with altered fluid balance, makes the interpretation of nutritional parameters more difficult during critical illness. During illness, cytokine production causes anorexia, resulting in a decrease in food intake and weight loss. Cytokines also cause hypoalbuminemia from increase in catabolism and altered permeability, allowing albumin to translocate from the intravascular to extravascular space. In addition, cytokines downregulate the albumin gene, which decreases production of albumin by decreasing the rate of mRNA translation.[6]

In severely stressed patients the immobility, anorexia, anabolic inefficiency, and increased catabolism promote the development of malnutrition. The percent weight loss (taking into account the presence of excess fluid along with degree of hypoalbuminemia) and an estimation of the length of time the patient will be unable to eat should determine the need for nutritional intervention. Three principal factors predict the need for nutrition support: current nutritional status (i.e., body composition), the anticipated duration of inadequate nutrient intake, and the presence and degree of stress response.[7]

The purpose of nutrition support in the critically ill patient is to preserve lean muscle mass from protein catabolism that occurs in the stressed state. The principal goals of nutrition support are to (1) provide substrate (protein, carbohydrate, lipid, electrolytes, minerals, and vitamins) for ongoing metabolic functions, (2) maximize protein synthesis and limit protein catabolism, (3) bolster immune function and improve wound healing, (4) improve cardiac and respiratory function by restoring glycogen stores in cardiac and diaphragmatic muscle, (5) correct acid-base and electrolyte disturbances, and (6) potentially modify the systemic inflammatory response.[8]

Serum levels of visceral protein markers such as prealbumin, retinol-binding protein, transferrin, and insulin-like growth factor I (somatomedin C) have commonly been used as indicators of nutritional status. The serum albumin level is a powerful marker of morbidity and mortality and is an accurate marker of stress, but a poor measure of nutritional status.[9] Therefore the albumin level alone should not prompt a nutrition support consult.

Because most critically ill patients have severe inflammatory processes and require nutritional support, it follows that hypoalbuminemia in the ICU is usually associated with the need for nutritional intervention. Exogenous albumin administration may raise serum albumin levels in hypoalbuminemic patients but does not decrease morbidity or mortality.[10] Albumin also can become glycosylated when mixed with hypertonic dextrose solutions, thereby losing many of its functional characteristics.[11]

There are no data to indicate that nutrition support given for less than one week confers any benefit to the patient.[12] It is therefore important to anticipate the estimated time period that the patient will remain unable to eat, and also to plan accordingly when providing nutrition support preoperatively to patients about to undergo elective surgery.

Although the patient's weight and weight change are important, they are affected by critical illness. Critically ill patients generally suffer from increases in total body water from several sources, including cardiac, renal, and hepatic disease, so the patient's weight status should be interpreted accordingly. A weight loss of greater than 10% of usual body weight in the past 3 to 6 months warrants a nutritional assessment. Moderate protein-calorie malnutrition is suggested by a weight loss of 10% to 20% of usual weight, whereas a loss of more than 20% indicates severe malnutrition. A weight loss of up to 10% of usual body weight is typically well-tolerated, and protein stores are generally adequate for up to 7 to 10 days without nutrition support in patients with a moderate systemic inflammatory response.[13]

Determining Energy Requirements

The caloric requirement the diabetic patient can be estimated with the help of formulas such as the Harris-Benedict equation, or by indirect calorimetry. Most studies indicate that needs are met in the ICU by providing 25–35 kcal/kg of ideal body weight. However, predicting energy needs in critical illness can be difficult because of uncertainties about the influence of multiple factors on energy expenditure. Many type 2 diabetics are obese, and assessing requirements of the obese critically ill patient is even more difficult because controversy exists as to whether the ideal body weight (IBW) or an adjusted weight should be used in calculations. One recommendation has been to use a weight halfway between IBW and actual weight in estimating caloric requirements in the obese. Another recommendation uses the obesity-adjusted weight obtained with the following formula: Obesity-adjusted weight = IBW + 0.25 × (actual – IBW).[14]

Strict use of the Harris-Benedict equation multiplied by stress factors can lead to overfeeding, one of the principal errors made in TPN support (discussed elsewhere in this book). In the obese, type 2 diabetic who is critically ill, it is crucial to avoid overfeeding, which can occur if actual body weight is used in calculating energy needs. Overfeeding is potentially harmful for the following reasons: (1) it leads to hyperglycemia, which decreases the neutrophil and macrophage function as well as immunoglobulin opsonization[15] and increases the risks for catheter-related infections and candidemia[16]; (2) it can lead to hepatic steatosis as excessive dextrose calories are increasingly disposed of by nonoxidative pathways, including de novo lipogenesis, whereby the liver directly converts glucose to lipid; and (3) it leads to an increase in the respiratory quotient and lipogenesis, which can compromise patient respiratory function. Therefore, in the severely stressed, obese, type 2 diabetic, indirect calorimetry estimates of energy expenditure are often warranted.

Protein needs for the stressed patient approximate 1.5 grams of protein per kilogram of body weight, and this can be provided as long as hepatic and renal function are normal. Stricter protein restriction may be indicated in the diabetic with overt nephropathy, although for short-term nutrition support this should not be an overriding consideration. There is no proof that branched-chain amino acids (valine, leucine, and isoleucine) enriched in parenteral formulas are beneficial for critically ill patients with sepsis or trauma.[17]

Most critically ill patients do not tolerate, nor do they require, more than 400 g of dextrose/d. Rates of dextrose infusion of 4 mg/kg/min (400 g/d for a 70 kg man) should be considered the upper limit of parenteral dextrose infusion; however, most patients require considerably fewer calories than this. Increasing the rate of the infusion can lead to hyperglycemia and de novo lipogenesis with its complications.[2] When one is calculating the total dextrose calories supplied to a patient, medications and drips using 5% dextrose in water (D_5W) as a vehicle, which can amount to substantial volume and dextrose loads in some ICU patients, should be carefully evaluated and included in the calorie calculations.

Lipids should comprise approximately 30% of total calories and should be provided continuously to avoid high infusion rates. Currently available lipid emulsions in the United States are composed solely of long-chain triglycerides (LCTs) and provide 9 kcal/g. Because they are supplied as 20% emulsions, parenteral lipids are actually less calorie-dense than parenteral dextrose solutions. When administered improperly, lipid emulsions: (1) inhibit the reticuloendothelial system and impair phagocyte function, particularly the Kuppfer cells; (2) worsen oxygenation in the adult respiratory distress syndrome (ARDS); (3) carry an infectious risk when administered separately over a prolonged time (lipid emulsions by themselves serve an excellent culture medium but are bactericidal once mixed with hypertonic dextrose solutions), and (4) promote production of immunosuppressive eicosanoid derivatives.[8] To avoid these untoward effects, the rate of lipid administration for a severely stressed patient should never exceed 0.11 g/kg/h and should remain below 20% of the total calories delivered.

Parenteral lipid administration decreases the de novo lipogenesis and reduces the dextrose requirements of diabetic patients offering potentially better glycemic control. Serum triglyceride levels should be checked periodically after administration of parenteral lipid emulsions and the lipid component of the TPN discontinued if this level rises above 400 to 500 mg/dL. Alternative forms of lipids, including medium-chain triglycerides and omega-3 fatty acids (fish oil), are under investigation for parenteral use.

Route of Administration

Nutritional support may be administered by enteral or parenteral routes. Choosing the appropriate route of nutrition support for a critically ill patient is an important decision predicated on the patient's clinical situation. As is true for any patient, the enteral route is preferred for nutrition support if the gastrointestinal tract is functional. Advantages of enteral nutrition include lower cost, avoidance of catheter complications, especially infection, a more physiologic route, and its trophic effect on gastrointestinal cells. Many critically ill patients have relative or absolute contraindications to enteral feedings. The complications of enteral nutrition include pulmonary aspiration, diarrhea, and intestinal ischemia or infarction.[18] Owing to the seriousness of the last complication, hemodynamically unstable patients with low cardiac outputs and patients on moderate to large doses of alpha agonists should not be fed by the enteral route.[8]

Many seriously ill patients with a functional gut continue to receive TPN. Patients with severe diarrhea, abdominal distention, high nasogastric tube output, gastroparesis, pancreatitis, or unobtainable safe access to the gastrointestinal tract are poor candidates for enteral nutrition and could be supported by total parenteral nutrition. The goals of parenteral nutrition remain supportive in order to (1) improve wound healing, (2) bolster immune function, (3) influence acid-base and mineral homeostasis, and (4) minimize obligate nitrogen loss in the catabolic postinjury state.[8]

Glycemic Control in the Critically Ill Diabetic Patient: A Metabolic Challenge

Studies in the areas of stroke, myocardial infarction (MI), cardiac bypass surgery, wound and nosocomial infections all point to a tremendous potential to reduce morbidity, mortality, lengths of stay, and added costs among hospitalized patients with hyperglycemia (Table 15.1).[15, 19–26] It is essential to identify hyperglycemia at the time of the hospital admission and to implement therapy to achieve blood glucose levels below 200 mg/dL regardless of a patient's primary reason for admission.

An accumulating body of evidence among patients with diabetes, stroke, and MI, and patients undergoing bypass surgery suggests that treatment of hyperglycemia can potentially affect morbidity and mortality (Table 15.1).[15, 19–26] Approximately 75% of admissions of patients with diabetes are attributable to cardiovascular disease.[27] When diabetes is addressed along with other acute problems, outcomes are improved and hospital stays are potentially shorter.

Central, or hepatic insulin resistance is common in severely stressed patients and is characterized by the reduced capacity of insulin to inhibit gluconeogenesis. Peripheral insulin resistance reduces the ability of skeletal muscle from participating fully in the uptake of metabolic fuels. Owing to these factors the dextrose content in the initial TPN solution should be minimal, 50 to 150 g of dextrose per day, depending on whether hyperglycemia is present. TPN should not be initiated until hyperglycemia has been adequately controlled (<200 mg/dL) with either a subcutaneous administered insulin sliding scale or a continuous insulin drip. Once euglycemia has been achieved, the dextrose load can be increased by 50 g/d. Optimal glycemic control is achieved with serum glucose values of 120 to 200 mg/dL. For metabolically labile patients, patients with unpredictable subcutaneous absorption, or patients who require excessive doses of insulin, an accessory insulin infusion is appropriate. Parenterally administered dextrose is best managed with intravenous insulin (regular insulin drip or part of the nutrient admixture), whereas enterally administered dextrose is best managed with subcutaneous insulin administra-

TABLE 15.1

Hyperglycemia Predicts Morbidity and Mortality		
Event	**Reference**	**Comments**
Myocardial infarction	Malmberg et al., 1995	IV insulin administered for glucose on admission >198 mg/dL followed by SQ insulin injections in patients with acute MI resulted in 30% reduction in mortality at 1 year.
	Capes et al., 2000	Meta analysis of 15 studies demonstrated that admission glucose of 108–124 mg/dL increased the in-hospital death rate by 3.9-fold in non-diabetics; the relative risk of death among known diabetic patients with admission glucose values of 124-180 was 1.7.
Stroke	Pulsinelli et al.*, 1983	Admission glucose of >120 mg/dL predicted disability and ability to return to work in diabetic and non-diabetic populations.
	Weir et al., 1997	Admission glucose of 148 mg/dL was an independent risk factor that doubled the mortality risk.
	Jorgenson et al., 1994	Glucose >104 mg/dL correlated linearly with the severity of stroke in hyperglycemic individuals without a diabetes history. Diabetes doubled the mortality risk among patients with stroke.
Bypass surgery	Kalin et al., 1998	IV insulin begun before bypass resulted in hospital mortality rates at non-diabetic levels and 50% lower than national rates for diabetic patients undergoing bypass.
	Furnary et al., 1999	IV insulin begun perioperatively resulted in 60% (n=1500) reduction of sternal wounds.
	Zerr et al., 1997	IV insulin begun perioperatively resulted in 1.5% sternal wounds compared with the rate of 2.4% for controls receiving SQ injections (p<0.02%).
General surgery	Pomposelli et al., 1998	Glucose >220 mg/dL on postoperative day 1 increased the risk of serious infections sixfold.

*Randomized prospective trial
*IV= intravenous; SQ= subcutaneous; MI= myocardial infarction

tion. When one is advancing the dextrose content of TPN, the insulin-dextrose ratio of the previous bag should serve as a guide. Diabetic patients who require TPN often require more than 100% of their usual insulin needs once they receive their calorie goal.[8]

Goals for Targeted Glycemic Control

Among hospitalized patients with hyperglycemia, including patients undergoing surgical procedures, it is desirable to maintain serum glucose levels in the range of 120 to 200 mg/dL. Patients with type 1 diabetes must always receive treatment with insulin because they do not produce any insulin and because withholding it, even for short periods of time, leads rapidly to marked hyperglycemia and diabetic ketoacidosis. Maintenance of glycemic control requires an ongoing assessment of nutritional intake (enteral and parenteral), activity, concomitant medications (e.g., steroids), and blood glucose. Bedside capillary blood glucose monitoring is available in most hospitals and permits rapid and accurate determination of blood glucose levels throughout the day. Such monitoring is imperative for assessing the efficacy of insulin therapy and determining adjustments in insulin. Urine ketone testing is an important adjunct to metabolic monitoring during acute illness and stress. The testing should be done if serum glucose determinations exceed 240 mg/dL.[28] Assays of glycosylated hemoglobin (HbA1c) cannot be used for short-term manipulations of insulin regimes and are not necessary in the acute inpatient settings. However, in the absence of severe anemia, the HbA1c level does provide information about the degree of glycemic control prior to hospitalization.

Avoiding Hypoglycemia

Hypoglycemia can occur in the hospitalized setting for various reasons and should be avoided by intensive monitoring of blood glucose as well as anticipating potential causes. Tube feeds in hospitalized patients are often held for tests and other reasons, and it is important to be aware of potential hypoglycemia in those patients receiving subcutaneous insulin. Frequent causes of hypoglycemia include the abrupt discontinuation of nutrition support, improvement in stressed state, alterations in doses of corticosteroids or sympathomimetic agents or their abrupt withdrawal, renal failure, severe hepatitis, sepsis, and diabetic gastroparesis. Hypoglycemic unawareness is a problem in some hospitalized diabetics, particularly those with longstanding type 1 diabetes mellitus. Because the adrenergic response to hypoglycemia is lost, the typical symptoms of shakiness and palpitations tend not to occur. In addition, neuroglycopenic symptoms such as mental confusion can be impossible to ascertain in patients who are sedated or mechanically ventilated. Therefore, blood glucose levels should be monitored frequently.[29]

Avoiding Hyperglycemia

Causes of hyperglycemia include infection, overfeeding, insufficient insulin, volume depletion and such medications as corticosteroids, β-blockers, thiazide diuretics, narcotics, cyclosporine, and sympathomimetic agents. A common cause of hyperglycemia in the critically ill patient is inadvertent overfeeding when full nutrition support is administered in a patient already receiving dextrose-containing intravenous fluids or a patient already absorbing dextrose during peritoneal dialysis. Hyperglycemia is associated with neutrophil dysfunction, and impaired complement function and may be one of the contributing factors that explain the higher incidence of postoperative wound infections in diabetics than in non-diabetic patients.

The Diabetic Patient on Total Parenteral Nutrition (TPN)

The management of patients with diabetes requiring parenteral nutrition should focus on achieving glucose control and avoiding hyperglycemia or hypoglycemia. Full caloric needs should be approached gradually over several days to avoid blood sugars above 200 mg/dL. Dextrose in TPN should be limited to between 100 and 150 grams on the first day in diabetic patients.[3]

Park and co-workers reported the use of mean insulin doses of 100 ± 8 U/day in type 2 patients who had not previously been treated with insulin. Sixty-seven percent of type 1 patients need an increase in insulin dose, with a mean increase of 22 ± 8 U/day.[30] Insulin can be added directly to the total parenteral nutrition (TPN) bag. Use of this method may require several days to achieve glycemic control. Supplementation with doses of subcutaneous regular insulin every 4 to 6 hours in this setting may frequently lead to erratic control or prolonged periods of hyperglycemia or hypoglycemia.[2]

Gavin has suggested an algorithm for the initial insulin dose added to each liter of TPN. Because in most institutions, standard TPN usually contains 25% dextrose, when delivered at 100 mL/h, it provides 25 g of carbohydrate/h. A total of 2.4 L of TPN is delivered in a 24-hour period (assuming 100 mL/h). The patient's insulin dose requirement is based on the previous insulin regimen used, the degree of stress, and the rate of TPN to be delivered.[31] For example, one can estimate the insulin requirement for a 24-hour period by calculating a basal need of about 1 U/h (alternatively calculated as 0.02 U/h/kg body weight) and adding 2–3 U/h per 25 g carbohydrate delivered. This method allows calculation of an actual daily insulin dose requirement.

If the insulin is to be added to the TPN bag, one must divide by the total number of liters to be delivered to obtain the number of Units of insulin to be added to each bag. This formula takes into account variations in carbohydrate content and delivery rates, allowing a rational way to calculate a starting dose of insulin to add to each bag when using TPN.[2] Alternatively, a separate intravenous insulin infusion can be used to achieve glycemic control and to calculate the 24-hour insulin requirement on TPN. This amount of insulin can subsequently be added directly to the TPN in place of the intravenous infusion. Woolfson demonstrated that 32 of 34 patients achieved glucose target values of 125 to 200 mg/dL within 24 hours of initiation of the above method.[32]

If hypoglycemia (blood glucose <80 mg/dL) develops while a patient is receiving TPN with insulin, dextrose should be given intravenously, either separately or piggybacked into the TPN. The TPN insulin content should be decreased by 30% to 50% to avoid the chance of subsequent episodes of hypoglycemia. Similar reductions in TPN insulin should be administered if blood glucose levels over a 24-hour period are consistently below goal range. Hypoglycemia after abrupt discontinuation of TPN is uncommon unless excessive dextrose calories have been administered. However it is prudent in patients with creatinine levels greater than 2.0 mg/dL, or if TPN contains more than 0.2 units of insulin per gram of dextrose, to monitor glucose levels every 15 minutes for the first hour after discontinuation of TPN. Alternatively, TPN can be discontinued gradually over the last hour of infusion by reducing the rate to approximately 40 cc per hour before discontinuation.

The Diabetic Patient on Enteral Nutrition

Achieving blood glucose control while transitioning a diabetic patient from TPN to enteral nutrition can be a challenge, especially in a patient with gastroparesis diabeticorum and delayed nutrient absorption. While the patient is getting started on tube feeds (generally at a rate of 10–20 cc/h full strength), TPN calories are decreased as is insulin in TPN so that the same insulin-to-dextrose ratio is maintained. In the patient receiving enteral nutrition, short-acting insulin should be used initially until it has been demonstrated that the patient is tolerating the tube feedings well. Use of short-acting insulin alone is also indicated for additional periods of time when there is a possibility that the tube feedings will be interrupted. The use of short-acting insulin alone minimizes the risk of hypoglycemia in these settings. When continuous infusion enteral feeding is used and the rate of delivery has reached 30 mL/h, use of an intermediate-acting insulin preparation, NPH or Lente, may be considered.

If tube feedings are to be administered continuously during the day, McMahon and Rizza recommend a starting dose of intermediate-acting insulin equivalent to one-half of the patient's preadmission morning insulin dose. Intermediate-acting insulin is given in the evening if the tube feeding will continue overnight.[33] In situations in which glycemic control is erratic or difficult during continuous tube feedings, intravenous insulin infusion can be given to achieve control.

When bolus enteral tube feedings are given, the fingerstick blood glucose level should be assessed before the bolus has been delivered to assess the preprandial level of control. Regular insulin before each bolus or twice daily regular insulin mixed with intermediate-acting insulin may logically be used for glycemic management. If blood glucose values during subcutaneous insulin delivery exceed 200 mg/dL when checked every 4 to 6 hours, supplemental doses of regular insulin should be added to the regimen. When a consistent need for supplemental regular insulin doses is demonstrated, the programmed regular and intermediate-acting insulin doses should be raised accordingly every 24 hours until control is achieved. Until the tube feeding regimen is stabilized and blood glucose levels are controlled, frequent fingerstick monitoring and adjustments in the insulin doses as indicated by the glucose values obtained are crucial to achieve adequate glycemic control.[2]

Diabetic patients with gastroparesis present a special challenge when they are tube fed. Most of these patients will tolerate post-pyloric tube feeding when iso-osmolar formulas are used at slow initial rates of 10–20 cc/h and advanced 10–20 cc every 12 hours. Another variable that may affect glucose control in enterally fed patients is whether the feedings are bolus, gravity, or continuous drip. Patients who are fed by gravity or bolus will likely need combined treatment with intermediate and short-acting insulin. Another challenge is the longstanding insulin-dependent diabetic with peripheral and autonomic neuropathy who has also developed diabetic diarrhea. Often these patients cannot be tube fed and are at risk of protein-calorie malnutrition without TPN.[34]

Nutrient Composition of Enteral Formulas

Nutrient composition of the formula in the diabetic patient has been a subject of controversy. Either a standard enteral formula with 50% carbohydrate or a lower carbohydrate formula with 33%–40% carbohydrate can be used in enterally fed diabetics. Some studies suggest that glycemic response to the lower carbohydrate formulas is blunted in comparison with the standard formulas, but outcome studies have yet to be done.[35] In addition, the presence of fiber in enteral formulas has not been shown to have a significant effect on glycemic response.[36] However, the use of fiber-enhanced formulas are beneficial in patients who require tube feeding for prolonged periods of time and in patients who require home enteral feeding.

Special Situations

Intravenous Insulin Therapy for Diabetic Patients with Myocardial Infarction (MI)

The Diabetes and Insulin-Glucose Infusion in Acute MI (DIGAMI) study randomized diabetic patients with probable MI to receive insulin infusion (n=306) or placebo/usual care (n=314). Insulin was administered for at least 24 hours early in the course of the patient's hospitalization to maintain plasma glucose between 7 and 10.9 mmol/L. Thereafter, the insulin treatment group remained on multiple daily injections of subcutaneous insulin for a period of at least 3 months postinfarction, whereas the placebo group was treated with insulin only as needed. The overall in-hospital and 12-month mortality rates were 30% lower in the group that received intravenous insulin therapy than in the group that received conventional therapy.

A subgroup analysis suggested that the individuals who received the most benefit were low-risk patients who had never received insulin before the study. Subsequently published data indicated that the reduction in mortality remained unchanged up to 3.4 years post infarction. The only significant adverse effect during the 34-hour insulin infusion was a higher risk of hypoglycemia, which occurred at a rate of 15% in the intensively treated group.[37]

Despite these encouraging results, another study did not show any benefit of intensive insulin therapy in acute MI. Low-dose glucose and insulin were infused over 24 hours in diabetic patients admitted for MI. No difference was seen in the 35-day incidence of cardiac mortality or reinfarction. This lack of benefit may have occurred because the study patients tended to be at lower risk for complications than the patients in the DIGAMI study.[38]

Management of the Diabetic Patient with Stroke

Special considerations apply to the management of stroke in the patient with diabetes. Guidelines for insulin drip therapy and monitoring are shown in Tables 15.2 and 15.3. Several metabolic abnormalities may mimic the clinical presentation of acute stroke in patients with diabetes. The first of these is hypoglycemia.[39] Diagnosis is established by documentation of low serum glucose level (<35 mg/dL). Appropriate treatment consists of intravenous dextrose infusion and observation. The second clinical setting that can mimic stroke in patients with diabetes is the postictal state. Seizures may be seen in association with hypoglycemic reactions. Localizing signs that suggest a stroke may be seen in the postictal setting and may last up to 48 hours after the event. A hyperosmolar state may present with focal neurologic deficits, which are reversible with correction of hydration and metabolic status.[2]

TABLE 15.2

Guidelines for the Management of the Diabetic Patient with Stroke with Insulin Drip (100 Units of regular insulin in 200 mL of normal saline at 0.5 U/mL)

Begin insulin drip at 0.02 U/kg/h	for perioperative management or maintenance
0.05 U/kg/h	for hyperosmolar state or diabetic ketoacidosis if delay anticipated in getting patient to floor unit
0.10 U/kg/h	for diabetic ketoacidosis intensive care unit
Target blood glucose, 100–180 mg/dL	

Reprinted with permission from Leveton CS, Magee MF. Hospital management of diabetes. In: Vassal J, ed. Endocrinology and Metabolism Clinics of North America. Philadelphia: W.B. Saunders; 2000; 29:745–770.

TABLE 15.3

Blood Glucose Monitoring of the Diabetic Patient with Stroke When Treated with Insulin Drip

Every 1 hour after start of drip, then
Every 1 hour in operating room
Every 1 hour after any change in drip rate
Every 2 hours if no change after two serial 1-hour checks
Every 4 hours if no change after two serial 2-hour checks

In patients with diabetes, relative contraindications to tight control in the setting of stroke include a history of coma or seizures in the presence of hypoglycemia or a concurrent unstable cardiac status, such as acute MI, arrythmias, and acute congestive heart failure. Data collected by Pulsinelli, Jorgenson, and Weir and their colleagues support the observation that outcomes, including stroke severity and mortality, are worse when glucose is less than 120 mg/dL, 108 mg/dL, and 144 mg/dL, respectively. Targeted glycemic control can be attempted in the setting of acute stroke, unless contraindicated.[21–23] In the presence of active cardiac disease, the increased sympathetic nervous system activity that may be associated with a hypoglycemic episode would place the patient at risk for exacerbation of the underlying cardiac condition; therefore, such stress should be avoided.

Transitioning from Intravenous to Subcutaneous Insulin

One of the most confusing areas in inpatient insulin management is transitioning a patient to subcutaneous insulin once they are stabilized on an insulin drip. Not infrequently, diabetic ketoacidosis has occurred following discontinuation of the insulin drip without appropriate administration of subcutaneous regular insulin. It is generally accepted that once patients can tolerate food well, they can be transitioned to subcutaneous insulin. It is often easier to make this transition in the morning (before breakfast) or at dinnertime. In a patient who was previously taking insulin injections, as much as the entire previous morning or evening dosage of regular plus intermediate-acting insulin is administered 30 minutes before discontinuation of the drip to allow time for the onset of action of subcutaneous regular insulin. If only intermediate-acting insulin is to be administered, the drip is discontinued 2 hours later. An injection of regular and NPH insulin may be given at 6 a.m. or approximately 4 p.m. with subsequent discontinuation of the insulin drip at 6:30 a.m. or 4:30 p.m. Following the transition from intravenous to subcutaneous insulin, preprandial and 2-hour postprandial glucose monitoring must be performed for at least 24 hours as well as a 3 a.m. glucose measurement to ensure that the levels remain less than 180 mg/dL. When glycemic control is stable, capillary blood glucose monitoring may be reduced.

It is best to write standard orders for intermediate- and short-acting insulin because it provides the basis for making finer adjustments rather than using the sliding-scale coverage with regular insulin.[2] The daily estimated dose of insulin (0.6 U/kg) is given as two thirds of the insulin in the morning and one third in the evening. If there is inadequate time between insulin injection and mealtime, lispro insulin may be a more suitable option owing to its shorter onset of action (10 to 15 minutes). Overall the most critical element, particularly in the patient with type 1 diabetes, is the administration of subcutaneous insulin before the discontinuation of the intravenous insulin drip.

Monitoring

The monitoring of a diabetic patient on nutrition support requires the same careful consideration of data as does monitoring a non-diabetic patient on nutrition support. These data include daily plasma glucose, electrolytes, magnesium, and phosphorus until stable. Triglyceride levels can be assessed once or twice per week. Hyperglycemia may cause a pseudohyponatremia and hyperkalemia that can result from inadequate insulin coverage and acidosis. Hyperinsulinemia due to refeeding syndrome or exogenous insulin administration causes the intracellular migration of potassium and magnesium, and thus a decrease in their plasma levels. Hyperinsulinemia also stimulates glycolysis, which in turn causes uptake of phosphorus for metabolism and synthesis of adenosine triphosphate and thus a decrease in plasma levels of phosphorus.[40] As previously mentioned, triglyceride levels above 400 mg/dL should prompt discontinuation of the TPN until levels normalize.[40]

Conclusions

The degree of hyperglycemia may be an important predictor of morbidity and mortality among critically ill diabetic patients. Nutrition support of the critically ill diabetic patient requires intensive monitoring to insure glycemic control. Glycemic control should never be sacrificed in order to achieve full caloric needs, and overfeeding should be avoided. Special care should be taken in transitioning the diabetic patient from TPN to enteral feeding. Innovative systems for monitoring glucose and for delivering insulin coupled with new pharmacologic therapy, such as long-acting insulin analogues, may help reduce the morbidity and mortality occurring in the estimated 6 million annual hospitalizations that are accompanied by hyperglycemia in the United States.

Case Study

A 64-year-old woman with history of type 2 diabetes mellitus for 10 years, obesity, asthma, and coronary artery disease was admitted to the intensive care unit (ICU) because of respiratory failure secondary to asthma exacerbation and was intubated shortly thereafter. Her weight on admission was 98.5 kg and the ideal body weight (IBW) was 55 kg with weight loss 5 kg since admission to the hospital (6 days earlier). For sedation, she was placed on a propofol drip. Her hospital course was complicated by an acute coronary event and pneumonia. She was treated with tapering doses of glucocorticoids intravenously for a few days and was then maintained at 20 mg of prednisone daily. The pneumonia was treated with intravenous antibiotics. For glucose control, she was receiving her home doses of insulin (NPH insulin 54 Units subcutaneously every 12 hours and regular insulin by sliding scale every 6 hours). Her serum blood glucose level was persistently high (>350 mg/dL) throughout the day. Careful work-up to evaluate her hyperglycemia revealed that she had urinary tract infection with *Turolopsis glabrata*, and she was treated with antifungals, based on published guidelines.[41]

According to an indirect calorimetry measurement, the patient's REE was 1650 kcal/d. The patient was started on an enteral feeding that was low in carbohydrate (1.5 cal/cc, protein 62.5 g/L, fat 94 g/L, carbohydrate 105.5 g/L) at 40 cc/h because of her respiratory distress. As soon as her respiratory status improved she was switched to a higher protein formula (1.5 cal/cc, protein 82 g/L, fat 68 g/L, carbohydrate 142 g/L) at 40 cc/h. Later she was switched to a more standard formulation with fiber (1 cal/cc, protein 62.5 g/L, fat 28 g/L, carbohydrate 139 g/L) at 60 cc/h, because of diarrhea. Electrolytes were checked daily and pre-albumin once weekly. The subcutaneous insulin regimen that the patient was taking at home was discontinued, and she was started on an insulin drip at 10 U/h. Her blood glucose control started improving the second day on the regular in–sulin drip, with values of 150–200 mg/dL. The in–travenous regular insulin infusion was maintained at 2–4 U/h for 2 weeks. When the stressed state improved, the infections were treated, her asthma exacerbation improved, and she was extubated and started eating; we treated her diabetes mellitus with subcutaneous insulin, 35 U NPH twice daily and sliding scale with humalog insulin before her meals. Her blood glucose levels were between preprandial and postprandial 150–200 mg/dL.

Case Discussion

This diabetic patient had persistent hyperglycemia because of concurrent infections, the stress of being intubated, the history of insulin resistance because of her type 2 diabetes, the steroids, and the continuous tube-feedings providing a carbohydrate load. Her nutrition requirements were 1320–1650 kcal/d (20–25 cal/kg) and protein 99 g (1.5 g/kg). Her enteral feedings were providing the following mg of carbohydrates daily: Oxepa, 105.5 mg; Traumacal, 142 mg; and Promote with fiber, 139 mg. Enteral nutrition provided the metabolic support for this critically ill patient. At the beginning of treatment the intravenous steroids worsened her hyperglycemia. The subcutaneous insulin was not effective probably because of her generalized edema that resulted in poor and erratic absorption. Optimal glycemic control was attained only with an intravenous insulin drip during the stress status. The appropriate treatment of the glucotoxicity permitted the reinstitution of the subcutaneous NPH insulin as soon as the infections were treated. This case illustrates the usefulness of the insulin drip in the management of critically ill diabetic patients receiving nutritional support. Appropriate nutritional and metabolic support as part of the overall ICU schema for critically ill patients may shorten the length of stay in the ICU, decrease morbidity, and improve survival.

References

1. US Center for Health Statistics: 1997 National Hospital Discharge Survey (public use data tape). Washington DC: US Department of Health and Human Services; 1999.
2. Levetan CS, Magee MF. Hospital management of diabetes. *Endocrinol Metab Clin North Am.* 2000;29:745–770.
3. McMahon M, Manji N, Driscoll DF, et al. Parenteral Nutrition in patients with diabetes mellitus: theoretical and practical considerations. *J Parenter Enteral Nutr.* 1989;13: 545–553.
4. Leahy JL, Bonner-Weir S, Weig GC. B-cell dysfunction induced by chronic hyperglycemia. *Diabetes Care.* 1992;15: 442–455.
5. Davies MG, Hagen PO. Systemic inflammatory response syndrome. *Br J Surg.* 1997;84:920–935.
6. Brodsky IG. Hormone, cytokine, and nutrient interactions. In: Shils ME, Olson JA, Shike M, et al, eds. *Modern Nutrition in Health and Disease.* Baltimore: Williams and Wilkins; 1999;44.
7. Stack J, Babineau T, Bistrian B. Assessment of nutritional status in clinical practice. *Gastroenterologist.* 1996; 4:S8.
8. Sternberg JA, Rohovsky SA, Blackburn GL, et al. Total parenteral nutrition for the critically ill patient. In: Grenvik A, Ayres SM, Holbrook PR, et al, eds. *Critical Care,* 4th ed, Philadelphia: W.B. Saunders Company; 2000;80: 898–908.
9. Apovian CM, Still CD, Blackburn GL. Nutrition Support. In: Berger AM, Portenoy RK, Weissman DE, eds. *Principles and Practice of Supportive Oncology.* Philadelphia: Lippincott-Raven; 1998:41.
10. Foley EF, Borlase BC, Dzik WH, et al. Albumin therapy in the critically ill. *Arch Surg.* 1990;125:739–742.
11. Doweiko JP, Bistrian BR. The effect of glycosylated albumin on platelet aggregation. *J Parenter Enteral Nutr.* 1994; 18:516–520.
12. A.S.P.E.N. Board of Directors. Guidelines for the use of parenteral and enteral nutrition in adult and pediatric patients. *J Parenter Enteral Nutr.* 1993;17(Suppl.):S12.
13. Bistrian BR. Nutritional Assessment. In: Goldman L, Bennett JC, eds. *Cecil Textbook of Medicine.* Philadelphia: W.B. Saunders; 2000:225.
14. Cutts ME, Dowdy RP, Ellersieck MR, et al. Predicting energy needs in ventilator-dependent critically ill patients: effect of adjusting weight for edema or adiposity. *Am J Clin Nutr.* 1997;66:1250–1256.
15. Pomposelli J, Baxter JK 3rd, Babineau TJ, et al. Early postoperative glucose control predicts nosocomial infection rate in diabetic patients. *J Parenter Enteral Nutr.* 1998; 22:77–81.
16. Rosmarin D, Wardlaw G, Mirtallo J. Hyperglycemia with high continuous infusion rates of total parenteral nutrition glucose. *Nutr Clin Pract.* 1996;11:151–156.
17. Klein S, Kinney J, Jeejeebhoy K, et al. Nutrition support in clinical practice. Review of published data and recommendations for future research directives. *Am J Clin Nutr.* 1997;66:683–706.
18. Smith-Choban P, Max MH. Feeding jejunostomy: a small bowel stress test? *Am J Surg.* 1988;115:112–117.
19. Malmberg K, Ryden L, Efendic S, et al. Randomized trial of insulin-glucose infusion followed by subcutaneous insulin treatment in diabetic patients with acute myocardial infarction (DIGAMI study). Effects on mortality at 1 year. *J Am Coll Cardiol.* 1995;26:57–65.
20. Capes SE, Hunt D, Malberg K, et al. Stress hyperglycemia and increased risk of death after myocardial infarction in patients with and without diabetes. A systematic overview. *Lancet.* 2000;355:733–778.

21. Pulsinelli WA, Levy DE, Sigsbee B, et al. Increased damage after ischemic stroke in patients with or without established diabetes. *Am J Med.* 1983;74:540–543.
22. Weir CJ, Murray GD, Dyker AG, et al. Is hyperglycemia an independent predictor of poor outcome after acute stroke? Results of a long term follow-up study. *BMJ.* 1997;314:1303–1306.
23. Jorgensen HS, Nakayama H, Raaschou HO, et al. Stroke in patients with diabetes: The Copenhagen Stroke Study. *Stroke.* 1994;25:1977–1984.
24. Kalin MF, Tranbaugh RF, Salas J, et al. Intensive intervention by a diabetes team diminishes excess hospital mortality in patients with diabetes who undergo coronary artery bypass graft [abstract]. *Diabetes.* 1998;47(Suppl 1):A87.
25. Furnary AP, Zerr KJ, Grunkemeter GL, et al. Continuous intravenous insulin infusion reduces the incidence of deep sternal wound infection in diabetic patients after cardiac surgical procedures. *Ann Thorac Surg.* 1999;67:352–362.
26. Zerr KJ, Furnary AP, Grunkemeir GL, et al. Glucose control lowers the risk of wound infection in diabetics after open heart operations. *Ann Thorac Surg.* 1997;63:356–361.
27. Lewis GF. Diabetic dyslipidemia. A case for aggressive intervention in the absence of clinical trial and cost-effectiveness data. *Can J Cardiol.* 1995;11(Suppl C):24–28C.
28. American Diabetes Association. Position statement on urine glucose and ketone determinations. *Diabetes Care.* 1991;14(Suppl 2):39–40.
29. Hoogwerf BJ. Perioperative management of diabetes mellitus: striving for metabolic balance. *Clev Clin J Med.* 1992; 59:447–449.
30. Park RH, Hansell DT, Davidson LE, et al. Management of diabetic patients requiring nutritional support. *Nutrition.* 1992;8:316–320.
31. Gavin LA. Perioperative management of the diabetic patient. *Endocrinol Metab Clin North Am.* 1992;2:457–475.
32. Woolfson AM. An improved method for glucose control during nutritional support. *J Parenteral Enteral Nutr.* 1981; 5:436–440.
33. McMahon MM, Rizza RA. Nutrition support in hospitalized patients with diabetes mellitus. *Mayo Clin Proc.* 1996; 71:587–594.
34. Thomas P, Rogers J, Fish J, et al. Total parenteral nutrition in a patient with severe diabetic diarrhea. *Nutrition.* 1995;11:456–461.
35. Schafer RG, Bohannon B, Franz M, et al. Translation of the diabetes nutrition recommendations for health care institutions. *Diabetes Care.* 1997;20:96–105.
36. Peters AL, Davidson MB. Effects of various enteral feeding products on postprandial blood glucose response in patients with type I diabetes. *J Parenter Enteral Nutr.* 1992; 16:69–74.
37. Malmberg K. Prospective randomized study of intensive insulin treatment on long term survival after acute myocardial infarction in patients with diabetes mellitus: DIGAMI (Diabetes Mellitus, Insulin Glucose Infusion in Acute Myocardial Infarction) Study Group [see comment]. *BMJ.* 1997;314(7093):1512–1515.
38. Ceremuzynski L, Budaj A, Czepiel A, et al. Low-dose glucose-insulin-potassium is ineffective in acute myocardial infarction: Results of a randomized multicenter Pol-GIK trial [see comments]. *Cardiovasc Drugs Ther.* 1999;13:191–200.
39. Bell DHS, Ovalle F. Stroke management in the diabetic patient. *J Crit Ill.* 1999;14(6):309–318.
40. Apovian CM, McMahon M, Bistrian B. Guidelines for refeeding the marasmic patient. *Crit Care Med.* 1990;18: 1030–1033.
41. Rex JH, Walsh TJ, Sobel JD, et al. Practice guidelines for the treatment of candidiasis. Infectious Diseases Society of America. *Clin Infect Dis.* 2000;30:662–78.

CHAPTER

16

Nutrition Support in Respiratory Failure

Mary S. McCarthy, R.N., M.N., C.N.S.N.,
Leonard E. Deal, MAJ., M.C., Chief, ICU Service

INTRODUCTION 187
EFFECTS OF MALNUTRITION ON THE RESPIRATORY SYSTEM 188
Short Term 188
Long Term 188
OVERVIEW OF RESPIRATORY FAILURE 188
Acute Respiratory Failure 188
High Minute Ventilation (V_E) Requirements 189
Considerations for Nutrition Intervention 189
CHRONIC OBSTRUCTIVE PULMONARY DISEASE (COPD) 189
Considerations for Nutrition Intervention 189
ACUTE LUNG INJURY 190
Considerations for Nutrition Intervention 190
ACUTE RESPIRATORY DISTRESS SYNDROME (ARDS) 190
Considerations for Nutrition Support 190
ESTIMATING ENERGY EXPENDITURE IN RESPIRATORY FAILURE 191
Nutritional Assessment 191
NUTRITION SUPPORT IN RESPIRATORY FAILURE 192
Macronutrient Needs 192
Micronutrient Needs 193
ENTERAL NUTRITION (EN) 194
TOTAL PARENTERAL NUTRITION (TPN) 194
CONCLUSIONS 195
CASE STUDY 195
REFERENCES 196

Introduction

Nutritional support is an important adjunct to the care of the pulmonary patient in the Intensive Care Unit (ICU). Malnutrition and respiratory failure are integrally linked. Whether respiratory failure is chronic and a consequence of primary pulmonary disease, e.g., chronic obstructive pulmonary disease (COPD), or occurs as part of the spectrum of acute lung injury ranging from mild pulmonary edema to adult respiratory distress syndrome (ARDS) that results from inflammation, sepsis, or injury, malnutrition is frequently a problem.[1] In addition, the critically ill patient with respiratory failure is especially vulnerable to complications of underfeeding or overfeeding. They generally require intubation and mechanical ventilation and cannot take nutrients by mouth for 7 days or longer. This interval is considered the maximum appropriate interval for lack of nutritional support according to the guidelines published by the American Society for Parenteral and Enteral Nutrition (A.S.P.E.N.).[2] Excessive nutrition may also be deleterious to the patient with respiratory failure as a result of increased carbon dioxide (CO_2) production and subsequent high ventilatory demands on a pulmonary organ system that is already compromised. Whether respiratory failure is acute or chronic, inadequate nutrition leads to further immunocompromise, respiratory muscle wasting, and ventilatory dysfunction that may result in prolonged ventilator dependence or death.

While clinical trials of adequate sample size demonstrating a clear benefit of nutrition support in respiratory failure are lacking, a great deal of optimism surrounds the development of specialized nutrition support with immune-enhancing components. In the last decade, exciting advances in the field of specialized nutrition support have led to improved outcomes for pulmonary patients as measured by ventilator days, morbidity, time in the ICU, and hospital stay. In a healthcare environment where quality is measured by outcomes, the goal of nutritional support for the acute respiratory failure patient should be to provide sufficient energy to meet metabolic and protein requirements, while limiting wasting of respiratory muscles, in order to restore health and baseline pulmonary function. Nutrition support for this high-risk population requires thorough knowledge of the underlying disease process and consideration of the potential benefits and risks of nutrition intervention.

Effects of Malnutrition on the Respiratory System

Short Term

Malnutrition is common in patients with lung disease. The entire muscle mass of the body, including the muscles of respiration, is subject to the catabolic effect of malnutrition. The chronic pulmonary disease patient is apt to develop malnutrition as an adaptive mechanism to decrease oxygen consumption and lower the work of breathing.[3] Medications and co-morbidities further affect appetite, diet selection, and metabolism.

Along with weight loss is a reduction of diaphragmatic muscle mass, contractile strength, endurance, and vital capacity. Muscle weakness occurs in both inspiratory and expiratory muscles. These changes, along with a decreased ability to breathe deeply and effectively cough up secretions, predispose the pulmonary disease patient to atelectasis and pulmonary infection. The reduced ventilatory drive, along with decreased endurance and increased work of breathing, results in progression to acute respiratory failure. The consequences of respiratory muscle weakness and altered ventilatory drive may be failure to wean from the ventilator.[4]

Long Term

Sustained malnutrition alters host immune response and may contribute to chronic or repeated pulmonary infections. Along with diminished cell-mediated immunity are an alteration in immunoglobulin turnover, decreased surfactant production, and decreased ability for repair following lung injury.[4]

Chronic fatigue and hypoxia lead to work and activity restrictions that may have a negative impact on overall quality of life.

Overview of Respiratory Failure

Acute Respiratory Failure

Ventilatory failure most often results from an inability of the respiratory muscles to generate the negative inflation pressure necessary to ovecome the high impedance to ventilation associated with certain parenchymal disorders.[2]

CAUSES[4]

Muscle Weakness

Muscle weakness leading to respiratory failure may be caused by metabolic abnormalities, including hypophosphatemia, hypomagnesemia, hypokalemia, or hypothyroidism. Hypophosphatemia occurs not only from inadequate replacement in total parenteral nutrition solutions, but also from peritoneal dialysis with hypertonic dextrose solutions and insulin provided in the dialysate, as well as aggressive use of aluminum-containing antacids.

Muscle weakness may also be the result of catabolism of the diaphragm, intercostals, and accessory muscle during periods of starvation and stress.

Primary neuromuscular disease, such as multiple sclerosis, can also contribute to muscle weakness.

Lastly, muscle atrophy secondary to passive breathing on the ventilator will contribute to muscle weakness and subsequent respiratory failure.

Insufficient Ventilatory Drive

Metabolic alkalosis from diuretic-induced renal potassium losses and chloride depletion from hydrogen ion losses from the GI tract will reduce oxygen delivery, predispose to arrhythmias, and cause compensatory hypercarbia leading to an insufficient ventilatory drive.

Large doses of narcotic analgesics and/or sedatives will suppress the ventilatory drive.

A lack of hypoxic or hypercapnic sensitivity or central respiratory drive secondary to a cerebrovascular accident will inevitably lead to acute respiratory failure.

Excessive Work of Breathing

Respiratory insufficiency develops as parenchymal lung disease and associated ventilation-perfusion mismatch increase respiratory muscle work to compensate for the reduced efficiency of gas exchange.

Small or obstructed endotracheal tubes will have a negative impact on the work of breathing from the resistance of flow through the tube and the inability to overcome it. Also, the resistance to spontaneous breathing caused by ventilators and tubing circuits may further increase the work of breathing.

Airway obstructions from thick secretions, airway edema, bronchospasm, or foreign bodies in the major airways will contribute to excessive work of breathing.

Dressings or other restraints, as well as pain or anxiety, will all increase the patient's respiratory efforts.

High Minute Ventilation (V_E) Requirements

Ongoing sepsis and inflammation will increase minute ventilation requirements. Critically ill patients require increases in cardiac output and minute ventilation to support the hypermetabolism associated with their illness. This hypermetabolism is common in critical illness and is associated with increases in measured oxygen consumption.

As patients recover from respiratory failure they will often have increases in physiologic dead space, requiring an increased ventilatory reserve to sustain spontaneous ventilation. These patients are prone to develop hypercarbia as a consequence of overfeeding with carbohydrate provided by enteral or parenteral nutrition. During carbohydrate overfeeding, carbon dioxide production can exceed the ventilatory capability of the lung and respiratory muscles, resulting in hypercarbia. Only when carbohydrate intake exceeds energy expenditure does the respiratory quotient (RQ) exceed 1.0 and become clinically significant.[5]

High physiologic dead space ventilation,[4] such as that seen with ARDS, leads to a high minute ventilation as a compensatory effort to offset the life-threatening hypoxemia. Efficiency of ventilation is measured by determination of the ratio of dead space to tidal volume (V_D/V_T). Values of V_D/V_T 0.6 r eflect major increases in physiologic dead space precluding spontaneous ventilation.[5]

Considerations for Nutrition Intervention

In some patients the respiratory muscles account for as much as 50% of total oxygen consumption. In the patient with pulmonary dysfunction, this increased workload can precipitate respiratory distress and result in an inability to wean from mechanical ventilation. Positive-pressure ventilation can be lifesaving in patients with acute severe hypoxemia or worsening respiratory acidosis that is refractory to more conservative measures. When work of breathing becomes intolerable, mechanical ventilation substitutes for the action of the respiratory muscles.[6] Moderate degrees of malnutrition and respiratory muscle weakness may prolong respiratory failure and delay the transition back to spontaneous ventilation.[5]

Chronic Obstructive Pulmonary Disease (COPD)

COPD is a generic term that includes emphysema, bronchitis and chronic asthma. It is caused by an airflow obstruction during expiration secondary to airway smooth muscle contraction, bronchial inflammation and edema, bronchial gland hypertrophy with mucus plugging, loss of elastic recoil, or collapse of the airways and changes in lung volume. Precipitating factors include smoking, air pollution, occupational exposure, repeated respiratory infections, heredity, aging, and allergies.[3]

Causes

Causes of COPD may include:

a. airflow obstruction
b. hyperinflation and airtrapping
c. flattening of the diaphragm
d. increased residual volume

Considerations for Nutrition Intervention

As many as 25% of outpatients with COPD are malnourished and up to 50% of COPD patients admitted to the hospital may have malnutrition.[7] Of critically ill patients with COPD admitted to the ICU with acute respiratory failure, 60% have significant malnutrition.[8] Nutritional depletion in the patient with COPD has been attributed to anorexia and hypermetabolism as a result of the increased work of breathing.[4] Inadequate protein and calorie intake may further contribute to primary lung parenchymal disease, immunocompromise, and respiratory muscle wasting and dysfunction that result in the need for intubation and mechanical ventilation.

Malnourished patients with COPD demonstrate a greater degree of hyperinflation and inspiratory muscle weakness than well-nourished patients with COPD. In patients with underlying COPD, malnutrition may limit the response of the respiratory muscles to the extreme demands of acute respiratory failure.[1] Studies have shown that the abnormalities of respiratory muscle function and endurance may explain the tendency for respiratory failure in malnourished patients with COPD.[9] Researchers in Spain[10] studied energy muscle metabolism in the quadriceps muscle of a group of 12 patients with acute exacerbation of COPD. As compared with controls, the patients had at baseline a reduced content of ATP creatine phosphate and glycose synthase, and an increase in lactate and glycogen phosphorylase concentrations. Nutritional support with enteral nutrition for 8 days was able to restore high-energy phosphate stores in skeletal muscle.

Malnutrition, together with a loss of lean body mass, has been identified as a prognostic variable for greater morbidity and mortality in the patient with COPD, especially those with emphysema. The effects of malnutrition are most easily seen with failure to wean the patient from mechanical ventilation.[4]

Acute Lung Injury

According to the European-American Consensus Conference definition,[11] acute lung injury is a condition involving impaired oxygenation with (1) a ratio of the partial pressure of arterial oxygen to the fraction of inspired oxygen that is 300 mmHg regardless of whether or how much positive end-expiratory pressure (PEEP) is used, (2) detection of bilateral pulmonary infiltrates on frontal chest radiograph, and (3) a pulmonary artery occlusion pressure 18 mmHg or no clinical evidence of elevated left atrial pressure on the basis of the chest radiograph and other clinical data.

Acute lung injury results in an acute change in the gas exchange function of the lung. Injury to the alveolocapillary membrane inevitably disrupts the endothelial barrier, leading to the development of noncardiogenic pulmonary edema through increased vascular permeability. As the air spaces fill with fluid, the gas exchange and mechanical properties of the lung deteriorate.

Causes

Direct insults include aspiration of gastric contents, inhalation of toxic substances, high inspired oxygen, drugs, pneumonitis, pulmonary contusion, or radiation.

Indirect insults include sepsis syndrome, multisystem trauma, shock, pancreatitis, pulmonary embolism, disseminated intravascular clotting, fat embolism, or bypass surgery.

Considerations for Nutrition Intervention

The reversal of respiratory muscle fatigue, which may have a role in precipitating acute ventilatory failure, depends on adequate rest of the respiratory muscles. Positive-pressure ventilation is used to reverse and prevent atelectasis and decrease the work of breathing. Improvements in pulmonary gas exchange and relief from excessive respiratory work provide an opportunity for the lungs and airways to heal.[12] Any metabolic stress, including nutrient administration, will augment CO_2 production and therefore act as a ventilatory stress to a patient with impaired respiratory function.[2]

However, immune-enhancing diets (IEDs) represent a promising strategy to modulate the dysfunctional inflammatory response seen in ALI by preventing the severe delayed immunosuppression that sets the stage for multiple organ failure. While varying results have been reported following prospective clinical randomized trials using immune-enhancing diets, most researchers will agree that the use of IEDs clearly reduces hospital length of stay and days on mechanical ventilation, which has important implications for cost and resource utilization.[13]

Acute Respiratory Distress Syndrome (ARDS)

ARDS is the most severe form of acute lung injury characterized by increasing pulmonary capillary permeability, pulmonary edema, increased pulmonary vascular resistance, and progressive hypoxemia. These abnormalities have been linked to the excessive release of arachidonic acid-derived inflammatory mediators and toxic oxygen radicals from activated macrophages and neutrophils.[14] The definition of ARDS, according to the European-American Consensus Conference, includes the same three components as acute lung injury except the ratio of the partial pressure of arterial oxygen to the fraction of inspired oxygen must be 200 mmHg, r egardless of the level of PEEP. The amount of extravascular water in the lungs of ARDS patients is about three times the upper limit of normal, which is 500 mL.[11]

Causes

Direct insults and indirect insults are the same as for acute lung injury.

Considerations for Nutrition Support

As with acute lung injury, therapeutic goals include to (1) improve oxygen delivery and provide hemodynamic support, (2) reduce oxygen consumption, (3) individualize nutritional support, and (4) optimize gas exchange. All efforts must be directed at discontinuing mechanical ventilation as soon as possible since complications are generally related to duration of support. The ultimate success of the weaning from mechanical ventilation is a result of the interaction between lung function, respiratory muscle strength and endurance, and nutritional state. Nutritional support is essential for weaning from prolonged mechanical ventilation. Patients who respond to nutritional support during mechanical ventilation demonstrate a diuresis as normal oncotic and tonicity relationships are restored. Respiratory muscle strength and endurance also demonstrate improvement.[5]

Attention is now focused on the role of omega-3 fatty acids to aid the immune system by competing with arachidonic acid for cyclo-oxygenase metabolism at the cell membrane. Omega-3 fatty acids, typically found in fish oils, minimize the reaction of T-cells to the inflammatory process. A study of 146 patients with ARDS revealed that patients who received an enteral formula with fish oil experienced improvement in ventilatory status and spent less time on the ventilator and shorter time in the ICU compared with patients who received an isonitrogenous, isocaloric control.[34] Understanding the role of nutritional manipulation in meeting high metabolic rates and controlling inflammation is still in the early stages.

Estimating Energy Expenditure in Respiratory Failure

Nutritional Assessment

Anthropometric measurements and laboratory studies in the patient with prolonged respiratory failure will indicate a reduction in lean body mass and body fat. Once in the ICU these patients are often subjected to an extended fast while resuscitative measures are underway. The patients are unable to ingest sufficient protein and calories to meet hypermetabolic requirements. Clinical studies of critically ill and ambulatory patients support the concept that provision of adequate protein and energy to patients with respiratory disease results in improved muscle strength and endurance.[12] Malnourished patients with COPD have been shown to have an increased ratio of measured-to-predicted resting energy expenditure (REE) relative to nourished patients with COPD and to normal controls. In addition, the malnourished COPD patients had a significantly greater oxygen cost of augmented ventilation than did well-nourished COPD patients or normal controls.[12] In adolescents and young adults with advanced cystic fibrosis, resting energy expenditure has been shown to be approximately 120% of that predicted by the Harris-Benedict equation, while in patients with less advanced disease, REE approximates that calculated by the Harris-Benedict equation.[15]

Predictive Formulas

General versus Population-Specific

While more than 200 equations have been developed for estimating energy expenditure, few are designed for acutely ill patients.[16] Resting energy expenditure (REE) can be based on the formula 25–30 kcal/kg/d for a conservative estimate of calorie need for all critically ill patients. REE can also be calculated with Harris-Benedict equations multiplied by a stress factor of 1.2–2.0. However, the Harris-Benedict equations were developed from indirect calorimetric measurements of energy expenditure in normal-weight, healthy young adults in the early 1900s.[17] Due to the variability in the calculation using stress factors and/or activity factors, indirect calorimetry is recommended for the most precise measurement of REE. Stress factors may manifest differently in patients of different ages, comorbidities, and immunologic status. Owen et al.[18] summed it up by saying that the idea that patients respond in a similar fashion to a given injury or disease state is erroneous because different patterns of inherited metabolic response between patients may lead to differences in energy expenditure despite similar injuries.

The Ireton-Jones energy equations[16] (IJEE) were developed by using a methodology similar to the Harris-Benedict equations but used measurements of energy expenditure from patients requiring enteral and parenteral nutrition support. The equations include considerations for diagnosis, obesity, and ventilatory status, so they are applicable to a wide range of patients. The IJEE is recommended for estimating energy requirements of nutrition support patients because it has been developed and tested on that specific population.[16]

Indirect Calorimetry

Accuracy becomes a greater issue for patients with a greater severity of illness; therefore, indirect calorimetry should be employed if available. Energy expenditure can be determined accurately by measuring oxygen consumption and carbon dioxide production values when standardized testing conditions are maintained. As mentioned previously, the ventilatory failure patient is especially vulnerable to the complications of underfeeding and overfeeding. Underfeeding compromises respiratory function, as evidenced by increased respiratory muscle dysfunction, decreased ventilatory response to hypoxemia and hypercapnia,[19] increased respiratory infection,[20] and delayed weaning.[21] Overfeeding can lead to respiratory insuffiency by creating excess carbon dioxide and increasing minute ventilation, dead space ventilation, and the respiratory quotient.[22] With its portability, documented validity, and ease of use, indirect calorimetry has emerged as the gold standard for determining caloric requirements in the patient who is critically ill and has multisystem organ dysfunction, sepsis, or complicated gastrointestinal tract abnormalities.[23]

Nutrition Support in Respiratory Failure

Nutrition support of patients with respiratory failure should be simple and follow basic concepts utilized in providing nutrition support for other critically ill patients. Traditionally, nutritional support is instituted 3 to 5 days after admission. However, based on a variety of studies performed in animals and humans, it is suggested that earlier nutrient administration is beneficial when compared with the introduction of nutritional support later in the illness. This is especially true in patients who already demonstrate malnutrition and severe stress.[24] The hypermetabolism that may be associated with respiratory failure results in muscle wasting that may be aggravated by bedrest, sedation and neuromuscular blockade. Prolonged ventilator support may result in further deconditioning. In these patients, malnutrition can occur rapidly, both as a result of increased protein catabolism and inadequate nutritional intake.[1]

Dextrose, protein, and fat all yield CO_2 oxidative end-products, with dextrose producing the greatest amount. Excessive dextrose administration can result in increased respiratory quotient (RQ) from lipogenesis. An RQ >1.0 increases O_2 consumption with a resultant increase in work of breathing. Any metabolic stress, even nutrient administration, will augment CO_2 production and act as a ventilatory stress to a patient with impaired pulmonary function.[18] Therefore, nutrient intake must be monitored closely in patients with borderline ventilatory status to prevent increased metabolic demands. Adjusting the proportion of nonprotein calories as fat and carbohydrates may reduce CO_2 production in some patients. The significance of modifying a formula's respiratory quotient through changes in the proportion of total calories as fat and carbohydrate is undetermined in controlled trials.[2]

MACRONUTRIENT NEEDS

Carbohydrate (CHO)

Excessive calories, particularly excessive carbohydrate calories, can result in excessive CO_2 production and increase the ventilatory demand in patients with already compromised pulmonary function. Identification of the potential detrimental effects of excessive CHO intake was initially observed in patients receiving dextrose-based parenteral nutrition solutions. In 1980 Askanazi et al.[27] reported increased $\dot{V}CO_2$, $\dot{V}O_2$, and minute ventilation in patients receiving high glucose loads (100% nonprotein calories). In 1987 Delafosse et al.[28] observed a greater increase in $\dot{V}CO_2$, RQ, and minute ventilation with a 100% glucose-based nonprotein calorie source than with a 50% glucose, 50% lipid prescription. These studies have led to the recommendation to limit CHO calories to 35% to 45% of the parenteral nutrition prescription.

Protein (PRO)

The counterregulatory hormones and proinflammatory cytokines of critical illness cause breakdown of body protein stores. Acidosis, loss of appetite, and inactivity will do the same. Loss of intact protein from structural and functional components of the body is associated with immune dysfunction, increased infection rates, delayed tissue repair, decreased wound healing, and diminished skeletal muscle function.[29] It has long been accepted that 0.8 g of protein/kg body weight/d is adequate for 95% of the population consuming an adequate energy intake that constitutes the recommended dietary allowance. Conditions that predispose the patient to the systemic inflammatory response syndrome (SIRS) are often associated with protein malnutrition from anorexia, motor inactivity, protein anabolic inefficiency, and an increase in protein catabolism. Patients with these conditions require greater amounts of protein than the RDA to achieve complete protein sparing, but the amount of protein provided should not exceed 1.5 g of protein/kg body weight. In severely burned patients, Wolfe et al.[30] demonstrated that protein provided in excess of 1.5 g/kg body weight was converted to urea, when comparing 1.4 g of protein/kg body weight to 2.2 g of protein/kg body weight. The ratio of whole body protein synthesis to catabolism was found to be optimal at 1.4 g of protein/kg body weight. The results of Dr. Ishibashi et al.[31] suggest that a protein intake of 1.2 g/kg of corrected weight (e.g., normally hydrated) or 1.0 g/kg of resuscitated weight was more effective than a lower protein intake in patients with SIRS. There was no further improvement by intakes of 1.5 g/kg of corrected weight. Shaw and Wolfe[32] have found that one way to avoid the potential problem of hyperglycemia, in a population with a very high incidence of hyperglycemia, is to underfeed modestly, but provide higher amounts of protein at a level of maximum utilization, 1.5 g/kg.

Fat

Thirty percent to 40% of nonprotein calories should be provided as fat to minimize hyperglycemia in the face of ongoing gluconeogenesis in hypermetabolic patients, and to minimize CO_2 production in patients with compromised ventilatory function. As a general rule, fat substrate should not exceed 1 g/kg in the patients with severe oxygenation defects and should be provided continuously at rates that do not exceed 30 to 50 mg/kg/h. In 1988, Al-Saady et al.[32] studied the effects of enteral formula modification on 20 mechanically ventilated patients in an ICU. Patients were randomized to receive either a high-fat (55%) or a typical-fat (31%) formula in amounts equal to the estimated energy requirements. The high-fat group showed reductions in $PaCO_2$, tidal volume, and peak inspiratory pressure, whereas the typical-fat formula group showed increases in these variables. Time on mechanical ventilation was 42% less in the high-fat group than in the typical-fat group. The authors concluded that a high-fat formula may reduce ventilatory requirements and therefore reduce the duration of mechanical ventilation.

Lipids play an integral role in cell membrane structure, cholesterol oxidation and transport, and the generation of eicosanoids. Conventional formulas often contain high levels of the omega-6 polyunsaturated fatty acid (PUFA) linoleic acid, which is the precursor of prostaglandin E_2 and other eicosanoids of the arachidonic acid cascade. Recent studies have shown that dietary fatty acids, namely, omega-3 PUFAs, can reduce the severity of inflammatory injury by altering the availability of arachidonic acid in tissue phospholipids. Animal and human clinical studies have shown that nutritional intervention with dietary fish oil containing eicosapentaenoic acid (EPA) can favorably modulate proinflammatory eicosanoid production from arachidonic acid.[34] Similarly, experimental studies have demonstrated that short-term enteral feeding with either fish oil alone or in combination with borage seed oil (gamma-linolenic acid, GLA) promoted rapid replacement of lung and liver macrophage phospholipid arachidonic and linoleic acids with eicosapentaenoic acid (EPA) and dihomo-gamma-linolenic acid (DGLA) within 3 days, whether administered in continuous or cyclic fashion.[35] Immune cells enriched with dietary EPA release lower amounts of arachidonic acid-derived eicosanoids and cytokines upon stimulation in vitro than cells enriched with arachidonic acid. Additionally, the eicosanoids that are formed from EPA tend to be less vasoactive than those derived from arachidonic acid. Thus, supplementation of nutritional formulas with a combination of EPA and GLA should favor an antiinflammatory state and play an important role in governing physiologic responses within the lung.[34]

Micronutrient Needs

Essential nutrients such as potassium, calcium, phosphate and magnesium should be provided in adequate amounts to meet muscle requirements and maintain optimal respiratory muscle force.

Vitamins

Antioxidant vitamins A, C, and E appear to have a favorable impact on immune defenses. Only one "specialized" formula to date has included additional amounts of these antioxidant vitamins. While there is evidence that antioxidants, such as vitamin E, may lower risk in more chronic inflammatory conditions (i.e., coronary artery disease) as yet no evidence supports antioxidant therapy in critically ill patients. We do have documentation of the effects of deficiency of these vitamins,[36] which include:

a. Vitamin A—thymus atrophy, decreased lymphocyte proliferation, decreased immunoglobulin production, and increased bacterial adherence to host epithelium,
b. Vitamin C—decreased locomotion of macrophages, decreased bactericidal capacity of macrophages, and decreased antioxidant capacity,
c. Vitamin E—decreased cell-mediated immunity, decreased immunoglobulin production, and decreased antioxidant capacity.

Minerals and Trace Elements

Changes in trace minerals associated with the stress of illness often include a decrease in serum iron and zinc concentrations and an increase in serum copper. During illness, decreased plasma zinc and iron concentrations may reflect tissue sequestration rather than an actual deficiency. Serum copper levels may increase because of the cytokine-induced stimulation of production of ceruloplasmin, an acute-phase protein and the major copper-binding protein. Hypoalbuminemia can affect interpretation of plasma trace metal levels.

Zinc is 55% albumin-bound, calcium is 50%, and magnesium is 30%. As a result, an apparently low plasma calcium, magnesium, or zinc concentration may be "normal" because of decreased plasma albumin level, and supplementation of these elements may be unnecessary or inappropriate. Algorithms to correct levels based on the albumin level tend to be inaccurate in highly stressed patients.[37]

Copper and manganese should be deleted in the setting of biliary obstruction and liver failure. And while parenteral iron is available in the form of iron dextran, it is not compatible with lipid-containing TPN solutions.[36]

Enteral Nutrition (EN)

When specialized nutrition is necessary, enteral nutrition is preferred over parenteral as EN is less expensive and more physiologic, is less likely to cause hyperglycemia or other metabolic complications, and is better suited for maintenance of the gut barrier and immune function.

Advantages

In most disease states, enteral nutrition is the preferred method of nutritional support. Frequently, critically ill patients have a delay in gastric emptying and impaired colonic motility. Usually the small bowel motility and absorption remain adequate in the majority of patients. A significantly lower incidence of septic morbidity is found in patients fed enterally,[36] along with a decrease in liver dysfunction, hospital length of stay, and costs.[23] In addition, early enteral nutrition decreases catabolism and preserves protein mass, improving nitrogen balance.

The use of nutritional support to modulate the inflammatory response to pulmonary injury via a nutritional pathway has gained a great deal of attention. In general, nutrition support is considered immune stimulating. Although many nutrients modulate immune function, arginine, omega-3 long chain fatty acids, and nucleotides have received the most attention. Arginine is a precursor of nitric oxide and as such participates in the regulation of blood flow and the inflammatory response. Arginine supplementation decreases T-cell dysfunction associated with malignancies and the systemic inflammatory response syndrome. Omega-3 PUFAs are thought to decrease levels of arachidonic acid in cells and thereby eliminate some of the immuno-suppressive mediators associated with the breakdown of arachidonic acid. Omega-3 fatty acids also diminish the production of other cellular mediators that are important in the inflammatory response. This suggests an immunosuppressive role that may be undesirable if prolonged in certain disease states.[24]

Disadvantages

As with any medical therapy, enteral nutrition support is not without potential risks. Potential complications can be classified as technical, metabolic, functional and mechanical. While the respiratory failure patient is not necessarily at increased risk for complications, the resulting aspiration, pneumonitis, or electrolyte abnormalities may be more costly in terms of morbidity.

Total Parenteral Nutrition (TPN)

Advantages

Total parenteral nutrition prescribed appropriately and monitored closely is a safe and effective medical therapy to offset the overwhelming depletion that can occur during critical illness. However, the most important criterion that must be met before deciding to use TPN is that the gastrointestinal (GI) tract be nonfunctional. Dysfunction in the GI tract can be due to abnormal motility, decreased blood flow, or interference in intestinal continuity. With delayed gastric emptying often seen in critical illness, or compromised absorptive capacity resulting in severe diarrhea, the parenteral route is preferred. In the setting of severe hemodynamic instability, blood flow to the intestine may not be sufficient to support digestion and could result in intestinal ischemia. And finally, if appropriate enteral access (e.g., small bowel feedings are indicated) cannot be achieved, the parenteral route is an option.[39] Transition to enteral feedings as soon as possible is a therapeutic imperative.

Disadvantages

TPN impairs the basic immunologic system, altering gut-associated lymphoid tissue (GALT) cell populations and decreasing intestinal and respiratory IgA levels.[40] In addition, TPN impairs established IgA mediated upper respiratory tract immunity to mouse-adapted influenza virus. Both viral-specific and absolute levels of IgA are significantly depressed within the respiratory tract,[40] offering a potential explanation for the increase in pneumonia occurring in critically ill patients receiving TPN. Rats immunized against a virus demonstrated significant levels of IgA within respiratory secretions, such that a subsequent challenge with the virus was almost immediately neutralized with sterilization of the epithelial surface against the virus. When these same animals were fed intravenous nutrition, approximately 50% of the animals lost their respiratory immunity. When fed via the gastrointestinal tract, the animals maintained an effective defense against the virus.[40] Interestingly, a 2% glutamine supplementation in an isocaloric, isonitrogenous TPN solution improved the defense against the virus in the upper respiratory tract but did not provide the protection of either a complex enteral diet or chow. In the animal model of pneumonia, glutamine partially, but not completely, maintained a barrier against the Pseudomonas challenge similar to its effectiveness in maintaining Ig-A mediated antiviral immunity. Glutamine is regarded as a conditionally essential amino acid with an important role in maintaining host defense mechanisms. For patients who are not candidates for enteral feeding, glutamine-enriched TPN may offer benefits in maintaining GALT function and mucosal immunity.[42] Provision of excess lipid calories in parenteral formulations has been associated with alterations in pulmonary function, which could result in altered gas exchange. Studies of critically ill patients yield conflicting results, although the safety of the use of lipid emulsions may be related to underlying lung disease and rate of lipid administration.[1]

Historically, TPN solutions have been implicated as a major cause of catheter-related infections. Current TPN formulas containing synthetic crystalline amino acids have very low pH and therefore a relatively poor growth medium. Lipid solutions have a higher pH and subsequently support a slightly higher level of bacterial/fungal proliferation. Strict quality control measures have eliminated the infusion as a major source of contamination.[39] This is not to say that TPN is without potential mechanical, metabolic, or infectious complications. Mechanical complications typically occur at the time of insertion and include pneumothorax, hemothorax, brachial plexus injury, lymphatic injury, or embolic events. Metabolic complications are related to the derangements in normal metabolism that impair the patient's ability to tolerate the prescribed nutrient load. Excess glucose provision results in hyperglycemia, which affects the cellular transport of potassium and phosphorus and impairs immune response. Hepatic steatosis, cholestasis, and gall bladder disease have been reported but are more common with long-term administration of parenteral nutrition. Excessive carbon dioxide production occurs when excessive non-protein calories are delivered and can prolong mechanical ventilation. Elevation in serum triglyceride level occurs with excessive administration of lipid calories (>2.5 g/kg body weight daily) or when clearance is impaired.[39] Close monitoring of TPN can minimize complications and optimize patient response to therapy.

Conclusions

In the hypermetabolic critically ill patient, moderate degrees of malnutrition and respiratory muscle weakness may prolong respiratory failure and delay the transition to spontaneous ventilation. Repeated measures of indirect calorimetry permit the clinician to evaluate the patient's response to both nutritional and ventilatory support and to make adjustments as the patient's clinical condition changes. Nutritional maintenance with an appropriate mix of substrates appears to significantly influence the success in weaning, and should be provided when prolonged mechanical ventilation is anticipated. The evidence supporting use of specialty pulmonary formulas is limited and inconsistent. It is much more important to avoid overfeeding in general than to concentrate on modifying carbohydrate/fat ratios.[43]

Case Study

J.H. is a 70-year-old female with a past medical history significant for COPD, hypertension, morbid obesity, obstructive sleep apnea requiring CPAP at night, diastolic dysfunction (normal EF), anemia, depression, and hypothyroidism. This admission she presented with acute respiratory failure secondary to multilobar pneumonia versus ARDS, and sepsis. She was electively intubated and placed on synchronized intermittent mandatory ventilation (SIMV) with initial settings of FiO_2 .50, tidal volume 600 mL, positive end-expiratory pressure (PEEP) of 5, pressure support (PS) of 20 and respiratory rate was set at 12 bpm with no spontaneous respirations noted. Her resulting arterial blood gas was pH 7.43, pO_2 102, pCO_2 42, HCO_3 27.7, base excess 3.0 and 98% saturation. A subjective global assessment performed by the registered dietitian gave her an overall rating of "mild malnutrition to well nourished." Her baseline weight was stated as 250 lbs. (113.6 kg) and her current weight was 300 lbs. (136.4 kg). She reportedly gained 50 lbs. (22.7 kg) in the previous 6 months. Her adjusted body weight was calculated to be 88 kg. Her level of activity was extremely limited as she was chair- or bedridden and required assistance with activities of daily living from a visiting health care worker for the past 6 years.

Nutritional support was initiated on hospital day 2 with nasogastric enteral feedings infused by means of an 8 French Dobhoff feeding tube. She received

Oxepa (Ross Products Division, Abbott Laboratories, Columbus, Ohio), an immunonutrition formula for acute lung injury and ARDS, at a goal rate of 50 cc/h for a total of 1800 kcal/d. This provided 74 g protein, 111 g of fat, and 125 g carbohydrate. This low carbohydrate, calorically dense (1.5 cal/mL) formula contains omega-3 fatty acids (EPA, GLA), and antioxidant vitamins A, C, and E. She attained goal rate for feedings in 24 hours and tolerated this well for one week. At that time, having received maximum therapeutic benefit from the immune formula, she was changed to Ultracal (Mead Johnson, Evanston, IL) at 65 cc/h with 22 scoops of ProMod (a powdered protein module) for 1000 kcal (10.5 kcal/kg adj. wt) and 132 g PRO (1.5 g/kg adj. wt). This diet strategy reflected a hypocaloric, high-protein approach to feeding a morbidly obese patient. We used prealbumin levels to assess nutritional status and 24-hour urine urea nitrogen to calculate nitrogen balance.

J.H. did not have a completely smooth course of enteral feeding and required the addition of total parenteral nutrition (TPN) for a short period of time when diarrhea, correlating with a positive stool culture for clostridium difficile (C. diff), prevented caloric goals from being achieved. However, following treatment for the C. difficile colitis she eventually tolerated full enteral feeds again. Various modes of ventilation, to include inverse-ratio, were also required to maximize oxygenation and reduce minute ventilation. Another setback occurred when she developed acute renal failure (BUN 108, Cr 1.5) and a formula modification (RenalCal) was necessary to restrict protein temporarily.

On March 3 the patient had a surgical tracheostomy placed and her pulmonary status gradually improved over the next 3 weeks. The colitis and renal failure resolved. From March 5 to March 18 the patient received hypocaloric, high-protein feedings (1100 kcal/d and 1.5 g/kg/d PRO) and finally achieved a positive nitrogen balance of +2.22 g after a negative measurement of –9.45 g 2 weeks prior (see Table 16.1.)

By March 18 she was tolerating CPAP trials with FiO_2 .40, PS 10, and PEEP 5. Her arterial blood gas at this time revealed pH 7.37, pO_2 85, pCO_2 36, HCO_3 20.8, BE –4.3 and 96% saturation. On March 24 she was successfully weaned to a trach mask and transferred to the stepdown unit 5 days later. Maximum ventilatory support and individualized nutritional support over the course of 52 days in the ICU assisted this patient in her recovery from ARDS, acute renal failure, and several nosocomial infections. The respiratory failure patient who is also morbidly obese presents the greatest challenge to the nutrition support team, who must balance the goals of both nutritional therapy and ventilatory mechanics to protect lean body mass, conserve energy, and promote healing.

References

1. Barton, RG. Nutrition in patients with respiratory failure. *A.S.P.E.N. Proceedings, 23rd Clinical Congress*, San Diego, CA; 1999.
2. A.S.P.E.N. Board of Directors: Guidelines for the use of parenteral and enteral nutrition in adult and pediatric patients. *J Parenter Enteral Nutr.* 1993;17(Suppl):17SA.
3. Kovacevich DS, Dechert RE. Respiratory failure. In: Henessy KA and Orr ME, eds. *Nutrition Support Nursing Core Curriculum.* 3rd ed. Silver Spring, MD: American Society for Parenteral and Enteral Nutrition; 1996:24-1–24-14.
4. Murphy LM, Conforti CG. Nutritional support of the cardiopulmonary patient. *Crit Care Nurs Clin N Am.* 1993; 5:57–64.
5. Benotti PN, Bistrian B. Metabolic and nutritional aspects of weaning from mechanical ventilation. *Crit Care Med.* 1989;17:181–185.
6. Tobin MJ: Mechanical ventilation. *N Engl J Med.* 1994; 330:1056–1061.
7. Braun ST, Keim NL, Dixon RM, et al. The prevalence and determinants of nutritional changes in chronic obstructive pulmonary disease. *Chest.* 1984;86:558–563.

TABLE 16.1

Date	Kcal/d Pro g/kg adj. wt	Prealbumin g/dL	Albumin g/dL	UUN g
11 Feb	1000/Pro 1.5 g/kg	13.0	2.4	-7.01
18 Feb	1250/TBN + trophic feeds 35 cc/h, Pro .8g/kg	24.8	2.9	-10.6
25 Feb	1000/Pro 1.05 g/kg	36.9	3.0	-2.9
4 Mar	1680 (RenalCal) + ProMod for 1.5 g/kg (Pro)	39.5	2.6	-9.45
11 Mar	1000/Pro .6 g/kg	31.8		-16.98
18 Mar	1000/Pro 1.5 g/kg adj. BW	31.8	3.2	**+2.22**

8. Driver AG, McAlvey MT, Smith JL. Nutritional assessment of patients with chronic obstructive pulmonary disease and respiratory failure. *Chest.* 1982;82:568–571.
9. Aguilaniu B, Goldstein-Shapses S, Pajon A, et al. Muscle protein degradation in severely malnourished patients with COPD subject to short-term TPN. *J Parenter Enteral Nutr.* 1992;16:248–254.
10. Planas M, Iglesia R, Gomez JB, et al. Muscle metabolism in patients with chronic obstructive pulmonary disease (COPD). *A.S.P.E.N. Clinical Congress Proceedings, 23rd Clinical Congress.* San Diego, CA. Abstr 73, 1999:52.
11. American Thoracic Society. Round Table Conference: Acute lung injury. *Am J Respir Crit Care Med.* 1998;158: 675–679.
12. Donahoe M, Rogers R. Nutritional assessment and support in COPD. *Clin Chest Med.* 1990;11:487–504.
13. Moore, FA. Effects of immune-enhancing diets on infectious morbidity and multiple organ failure. *J Parenter Enteral Nutr.* 2001;25: S36–S43.
14. Kollef MH, and Schuster DP. The acute respiratory distress syndrome. *N Engl J Med.* 1995;332:27–37.
15. Field S, Kelly SM, Macklem FT. The oxygen cost of breathing in patients with cardiorespiratory disease. *Am Rev Respir Dis.* 1982;126:9–13.
16. Ireton-Jones CS, Jones JD. Should predictive equations or indirect calorimetry be used to design nutrition support regimens? Predictive equations should be used. *Nutr Clin Prac.* 1998;13:141–145.
17. Harris JA, Benedict FG. *Biometric Studies of Basal Metabolism in Man.* Washington, DC: Carnegie Institution, publication 270, 1919.
18. Owen OE, Colliver JA, Schrage JP. Adult human energy requirements. *Front Clin Nutr.* 1993;2:1–8.
19. Doekel R, Zwillich CW, Scoggin C, et al. Clinical semistarvation. Depression of hypoxic ventilatory response. *N Engl J Med.* 1976;295:358–361.
20. Niederman M, Merrill W, Ferranti R, et al. Nutritional status and bacterial binding in the lower respiratory tract in patients with chronic tracheostomy. *Ann Intern Med.* 1984;100:795–800.
21. Mattar JA, Velasco IT, Esgaib AS, et al. Parenteral nutrition (PN) as a useful method for weaning patients from mechanical ventilation (MV). *J Parenter Enteral Nutr.* 1978;2:50.
22. Liposkey JM, Nelson LD. Ventilatory response to high caloric loads in critically ill patients. *Crit Care Med.* 1994; 22:796–802.
23. McClave SA, Spain DA. Should predictive equations or indirect calorimetry be used to design nutrition support regimens? Indirect calorimetry should be used. *Nutr Clin Prac.* 1998;13:141–145.
24. Zaloga G, Ackerman M. A review of disease-specific formulas. *AACN Clinical Issues in Critical Care Nursing.* 1994; 5:421–435.
25. Kudsk KA, Croce MA, Fabian TC, et al. Enteral versus parenteral feeding. *Ann Surg.* 1992;215:503–513.
26. Malone AM. Is a pulmonary enteral formula warranted for patients with pulmonary dysfunction? *Nutr Clin Prac.* 1997;12:168–171.
27. Askanazi J, Rosenbaum SH, Hyman AI, et al. Respiratory changes induced by the large glucose loads of total parenteral nutrition. *JAMA.* 1980;243:1444–1447.
28. Delafosse B, Bouffard Y, Viale JP, et al. Respiratory changes induced by parenteral nutrition in postoperative patients undergoing inspiratory pressure support ventilation. *Anesthesiology.* 1987;66:393–396.
29. Ziegler TR, Gatzen C, Wilmore DW. Strategies for attenuating protein-catabolic responses in the critically ill. *Annu Rev Med.* 1994;45:459–480.
30. Wolfe RR, Goodenough RD, Burke JF. Response of protein and urea kinetics in burn patients to different levels of protein intake. *Ann Surg.* 1983;197:163–171.
31. Ishibashi N, Plank LD, Sando K, et al. Optimal protein requirements during the first two weeks after onset of critical illness. *Crit Care Med.* 1998;26:1529–1535.
32. Shaw J, Wolfe RR. An integrated analysis of glucose, fat, and protein metabolism in severely traumatized patients: studies in the basal state and the response to total parenteral nutrition. *Ann Surg.* 1989;209:63–72.
33. Al-Saady NM, Blackmore CM, Bennett ED. High fat, low carbohydrate, enteral feeding lowers $PaCO_2$ and reduces the period of ventilation in artificially ventilated patients. *Intensive Care Med.* 1989;15:290–295.
34. Gadek JE, DeMichele SJ, Karlstad MD, et al. Effect of enteral feeding with eicosapentaenoic acid, γ-linolenic acid, and antioxidants in patients with acute respiratory distress syndrome. *Crit Care Med.* 1999;27:1409–1420.
35. Palombo JD, DeMichele SJ, Boyce PJ, et al. Effect of short-term feeding with eicosapentaenoic and gamma-linolenic acids on alveolar macrophage eicosanoid synthesis and bactericidal function in rats. *Crit Care Med.* 1999; 27:1908–1915.
36. Hulsewe KW, van Acker BA, von Meyenfeldt MF, et al. Nutritional depletion and dietary manipulation: effects on the immune response. *World J Surg.* 1999;23:536–544.
37. McMahon MM, Farnell MB, Murray MJ. Nutritional support of critically ill patients. *Mayo Clin Proc.* 1993;68:911–920.
38. Moore FA, Feliciano DV, Andrassy RJ, et al. Early enteral feeding, compared with parenteral, reduces postoperative systemic complications. *Ann Surg.* 1992;216:172–183.
39. Evans NJ. The role of total parenteral nutrition in critical illness: Guidelines and recommendations. *AACN Clin Iss in Crit Care Nurs.* 1994;5:476–484.
40. Kudsk K, Li J, Renegar KB. Loss of upper respiratory tract immunity with parenteral feeding. *Ann Surg.* 1996; 223:629–638.
41. Li J, King BK, Janu PG, et al. Glycyl-L-glutamine-enriched total parenteral nutrition maintains small intestine gut-associated lymphoid tissue and upper respiratory tract immunity. *J Parenter Enteral Nutr.* 1997:22:31–36.
42. King BK, Li J, Kudsk K. A temporal study of TPN-induced changes in GALT and muscosal immunity. *Surgical Infection Society Proceedings.* Pittsburgh, PA; April 30–May 3, 1997.
43. Talpers SS, Romberger DJ, Bunce SB, et al. Nutritionally associated increased carbon dioxide production. Excess total calories vs. high proportion of carbohydrate calories. *Chest.* 1992;102:551–555.

CHAPTER

17 Nutrition Support in the Patient with Hepatic Failure

James J. Pomposelli, M.D., Ph.D., David L. Burns, M.D., C.N.S.P.

INTRODUCTION 199

GENERAL GUIDELINES: NUTRITION SUPPORT IN THE PATIENT WITH LIVER FAILURE 200
- Patient Evaluation 200
- Route of Administration 201
- Patient Specific Formula: Total Parenteral Nutrition 201

CALCULATING PATIENT SPECIFIC REQUIREMENTS FOR HEPATIC FAILURE 202
- Caloric Requirements 202
- Protein Requirements 202
- Carbohydrate Requirements 202
- Lipid Requirements 203

FLUID RESTRICTED ICU PATIENT: USING MAXIMALLY CONCENTRATED SOLUTIONS 204

METABOLIC ISSUES 204
- Phosphorus 204
- Diabetic Patients with Liver Failure 204
- Type I Diabetic Patients Receiving TPN 205
- Type II Diabetic Patients Receiving TPN 205
- Starting Insulin in TPN 205

ACID/BASE ISSUES 206

CONCLUSIONS 206

REFERENCES 206

Introduction

The liver is the most important metabolic organ for orchestrating physiologic processes essential for a well-nourished state. Patients who develop hepatic failure can be divided into two broad categories, acute or fulminant and chronic liver failure. Fulminant hepatic failure is defined as an acute process that destroys the majority of functioning liver mass, which results in rapid deterioration of metabolic processes, coma, and death within 7 days. Examples of etiologies resulting in fulminant hepatic failure include acute viral hepatitis B and less commonly hepatitis A, toxic exposure such as drug overdose, or a failed liver transplant. Obviously, the goals of nutrition support in the patient with fulminant hepatic failure differ significantly from those in treating patients recovering on the surgical ward or at home. Chronic liver failure and cirrhosis can result from a variety of causes and include chronic viral hepatitis (B and C), alcohol and drug-induced diseases, metabolic and genetic diseases (Wilson's, alpha-1 antitrypsin deficiency, etc.), vascular diseases (Budd Chiari syndrome), and trauma. Regardless of the etiology, cirrhosis is associated with protein-energy malnutrition in the majority of patients. Nutrition support in these patients can be complicated by the presence of portosystemic encephalopathy that is exacerbated by protein administration. Therefore, careful monitoring of patients with cirrhosis during nutrition support with adjustment of medical regimen to control encephalopathy is warranted.

In the malnourished patient without major metabolic stress, provision of adequate protein and calories above energy expenditure results in positive nitrogen balance and appropriate body mass gain. In patients with liver failure, the hormonal *milieu* will not support anabolism regardless of intake.[1] Attempts to replete the malnourished metabolically stressed live-failure patient with substrate in excess of energy expenditure leads to hyperglycemia, increased complications, and nullifies any benefit of feeding.[2,3] The goals of nutrition support in the patient with liver failure are to support the metabolic response to injury and infection by providing adequate protein and energy equivalent to, or slightly less than energy expenditure.[4,5]

As a rule, the enteral route of administration is favored over the parenteral route for nutrition support.[6,7] However, many patients with liver failure are unable to tolerate enteral feedings, or have underlying maldigestion due to impaired absorption that limits effective enteral support. In these situations, total parenteral nutrition (TPN) is a safe and efficacious means of nutrition support and provides the opportunity to correct fluid and electrolyte disturbances and improve acid/base status while providing a vehicle for medication administration.[8–10] The ability to compound a total nutrient admixture (TNA) containing substrate and medications can help to avoid excessive volume administration that can lead to increased morbidity and mortality.[11]

In this chapter, practical guidelines for the safe and efficacious administration of nutrition support in the patient with hepatic failure will be reviewed. Calculation of substrate requirements are standardized regardless of route of administration (enteral vs. parenteral) and can be used on the intensive care unit or general surgical or medical ward as well. Recommendations for prescribing nutrition support for the diabetic patient with liver failure will also be explored.

Specialty formulas containing substrates such as glutamine, arginine, omega-3 fatty acids (fish oil), structured lipids, or branched-chain amino acids have been shown to be efficacious in certain clinical applications.[12–16] Branched-chain amino acids have been shown in some studies to be beneficial in patients with liver disease, although their impact on improving the outcome of the majority of patients with hepatic failure is still uncertain. Liver replacement through transplantation remains the "gold standard" therapy for liver failure and provides the best opportunity to improve metabolic and nutritional parameters.

General Guidelines: Nutrition Support in the Patient with Liver Failure

The goals of nutritional therapy in the patient with liver failure are to support hepatocellular function and improve altered nutrient metabolism and absorption. The objective is to preserve lean body mass while supporting the metabolic response to injury and infection.[17] Multiple conditions predispose to malnutrition in patients with acute or chronic liver disease. Symptomatically these include chronic nausea, diarrhea, anorexia, and early satiety with associated weight loss. In addition, the use of unpalatable "restrictive" diets limiting fluid and sodium in patients with ascites, or protein for those patients with portosystemic encephalopathy, contribute to malnutrition. Alcoholic liver disease is commonly associated with a history of poor dietary habits and an increased risk of protein-calorie malnutrition with micronutrient deficiencies of folate, thiamine, and magnesium. Coexistent pancreatic insufficiency or depletion of the bile salt pool in cholestatic liver disease can result in steatorrhea and fat-soluble vitamin deficit. Inflammatory bowel disease in association with sclerosing cholangitis contributes to malnutrition through malabsorption of fats, fat-soluble vitamins, vitamin B_{12}, and diarrheal losses of zinc.

The decision to start nutrition support is based on clinical subjective and objective parameters. The relationship between chronic liver disease and malnutrition is well established. Patients with severe alcoholic hepatitis in the V.A. Cooperative Study had a 100% prevalence of protein-calorie malnutrition.[18] DiCecco et al.[19] found that 74 consecutive patients with end-stage liver disease referred for transplantation all had evidence of malnutrition.

Patients with acute hepatic failure (i.e., acetaminophen overdose) are generally well nourished and do not have a pre-hospital history of weight loss. Thus, patients without protein-calorie malnutrition will tolerate 5 to 7 days of *nil per os* (NPO) before initiating nutrition support. Patients who will predictably not eat for 7 days (severe encephalopathy, spontaneous bacterial peritonitis, etc.) or those with underlying malnutrition should start nutrition support sooner since nitrogen loss is cumulative and debilitating. Withholding nutrition support and inducing a cumulative caloric deficit of over 10,000 kcal has been associated with survival disadvantage.[20] In addition, nitrogen losses from catabolic illness can rapidly lead to organ dysfunction and poorer outcome.[21] Early enteral feeding may reduce septic complications by maintaining gut barrier function and immunocompetence.[22] However, attempts to replete the malnourished live-failure patient with calories above energy expenditure can result in severe hyperglycemia, reticuloendolthelial system (RES) blockade, and increased infection.[3,23–25]

Patient Evaluation

Nutritional assessment of the patient with hepatic insufficiency can be difficult, and multiple nutritional parameters may be invalid (Table 17.1). History of recent weight loss from the usual body weight is easy to obtain but may be inaccurate due to the presence of significant ascites or peripheral edema. Further, the recent use of diuretics may spuriously increase the perceived pre-hospital weight loss. Weight loss greater than 10% from usual body weight is associated with moderate risk for in-hospital complications; greater than 20% body weight loss is associated with severe risk.[26–28] Patients suffering from moderate to severe malnutrition (>15% body weight loss) should be started on nutrition support immediately through enteral supplementation or parenteral nutrition.

Accurate nutritional assessment can generally be accomplished with a paucity of labs and clinical exam. Albumin, transferrin, and pre-albumin are all exclusively produced by the liver and correlate well with malnutrition risk and hospital outcome. In the setting of acute or chronic hepatic dysfunction there is impaired humoral protein production, thus invalidating these "classical" assessment parameters (Table 17.1). Triceps skin-fold measurement, serum transferrin, and albumin can be used to calculate the Prognostic Nutritional Index (PNI), which predicts the risk of complications for general surgical patients during hospitalization.[29] This model, however, has been invalidated in end-stage liver disease patients undergoing hepatic transplantation.[19]

In patients with liver failure, "subjective global assessment" has been shown to have a very high concordance with surgical morbidity and mortality after orthotopic liver transplantation.[30,31,32]

TABLE 17.1

Nutrition Assessment in Liver Disease

Parameter	Invalidation
Weight	Edema, ascites, and diuretic therapy
Anthropometry	Edema, inter-observer variability
Creatinine-Height Index	Renal insufficiency
Albumin, Transferrin, Pre-albumin	Impaired hepatic production
Delayed type hypersensitivity	Non-nutritional impairment
Nitrogen balance	Renal insufficiency
Bioelectric impedance	Ascites

Route of Administration

Enteral nutrition support is the preferred route of nutrient administration. Enteral therapy is "physiologic" and supports gut enterocyte nutrition that helps maintain small intestinal villous integrity. While providing nutrition to the enterocyte and the patient, enteral feeding provides antigenic stimulation to the gut-associated lymphoid tissue and is a stimulus for biliary secretion of IgA. These factors maintain the barrier against translocation of luminal bacteria to the portal circulation.[33] Enteral therapy is also associated with decreased infectious complications as compared to parenteral support and is more cost-effective.[20] Specialized "immune enhancing" formulas containing fish oil, glutamine, arginine, and RNA can be provided enterally to attenuate the systemic inflammatory response and may improve outcome in critically ill patients.[15]

Enteral support can be provided orally as a supplement or via an enteral feeding tube. Soft feeding tubes are generally well tolerated, easy to place, and very useful for both nutrition support and drug delivery.[34] Alternatively patients intolerant to intragastric feeding or at high risk for aspiration may benefit by placement of a nasojejunal tube. These tubes can be placed in the post-pyloric position at the patient's bedside with the aid of pro-kinetic agents such as metoclopramide. Alternatively, nasojejunal tubes can be placed quickly and safely endoscopically with rapid achievement of goal nutrition.[35]

Rapid advancement of tube feeding rate can lead to intolerance with diarrhea, metabolic abnormalities, and patient discomfort. Generally slowing the rate of administration or selecting a lower osmolarity formula can ameliorate problems. Critically ill patients with liver failure may be intolerant to enteral nutrition support, particularly those with an ileus or bowel obstruction, or those on high-dose pressors. Parenteral nutrition can attenuate the impact of inadequate enteral intake while helping to correct metabolic abnormalities.[36] For these reasons, both the parenteral and enteral modes of nutrition are complimentary and not in discord as suggested by some.[37]

Patient Specific Formula: Total Parenteral Nutrition

Many hospitals offer "standardized" TPN order forms to prescribe parenteral nutrition. Most TPN order forms will allow for customized parenteral nutrition solutions for specific patient needs. Patients with liver failure have a multitude of physiologic and metabolic alterations that are best served by "patient specific" TPN formulation.[20] The decision to use standard or patient specific TPN solutions is impacted by the patients fluid status. Use of standardized formulas should be restricted to the stable patient with no evidence of fluid overload and who requires maintenance fluid administration only. Patients with hyponatremia and fluid overload fluid are best treated with maximally concentrated TPN solutions. Regardless of route of administration (enteral versus parenteral), calculating the substrate needs of the patient with liver failure are standardized.

Calculating Patient Specific Requirements for Hepatic Failure

Caloric Requirements

Many patients with liver failure are cachectic and have low levels of serum albumin. When providing nutrition support, the clinician needs to resist the urge to provide substrate at levels significantly above energy expenditure with the implausible goal of creating an anabolic state. Provision of calories significantly above energy expenditure will result in hyperglycemia, increase septic complications, and nullify any benefit of feeding.[2,3]

In a study by Hunter et al.,[38] energy expenditure (EE, kcal/d) was measured utilizing a metabolic cart in critically ill patients with a variety of illnesses including liver failure. Measured energy expenditure was then compared to estimates of resting energy expenditure (REE) using the Harris-Benedict equation or an empiric formula of 22 kcal/kg/d. Nearly perfect concordance between measured, Harris-Benedict equation and the empiric formula of 22 kcal/d was seen (1382 kcal, 1324 kcal, and 1370 kcal respectively).[38] Therefore, it has been our practice to limit calories to 22–25 kcal/kg/d using pre-hospital (dry) weight to avoid the complications of overfeeding and hyperglycemia.

Not uncommonly, the stable patient with liver disease suffers from morbid obesity due to inactivity and continued oral intake. In these patients, energy availability is not generally a problem since each pound of adipose contains 3500 kcal of energy. Therefore, energy restriction to 1500 kcal/d is routinely used to encourage mobilization of native fat stores.[39] Adequate protein is required to maintain lean body mass and to preserve organ function.

Protein Requirements

The recommended daily allowance (RDA) for protein to support health and growth in the "normal" individual is approximately 0.8 g/kg/d.[40] Critically ill patients require approximately twice this amount at 1.5 g/kg/d using prehospital (dry) weight.[28] Provision of protein above 2 g/kg/d is expensive, will lead to increased ureagenesis, and will not improve outcome.[41] As a rule, protein requirements for the hospitalized patient are 1.5 g/kg body weight/d. In the patient with severe liver disease and hepatic encephalopathy, restriction to 1.0 g/kg body weight/d is reasonable to avoid exacerbating increased ammonia production. Severe protein restriction, which was common practice to avoid hepatic encephalopathy in the past, compounds nutritional deficits and should be avoided. More aggressive medical management of encephalopathy can usually overcome any additional derangement induced by increased protein intake and ammonia production. The use of branched-chain amino acid formulas to correct hepatic encephalopathy is controversial. In a meta-analysis by Naylor et al., branched-chain amino acids provided parenterally did significantly reduce the incidence of encephalopathy but was not associated with any survival advantage.[42] Given the high cost of branched-chain amino acid formulas and questionable benefit, their use should be reserved for patients with intractable encephalopathy.

Correction of body weight in patients with massive ascites should be performed to avoid excessive protein administration. Estimate of total body water in the patient with anasarca is difficult. In these situations, obtaining the patient's "usual" body weight before the development of ascites can be helpful.

Protein requirement for the obese patient requires adjustment for excess body weight above ideal body weight (IBW). Protein needs are based on estimates of lean tissue weight (muscle, organs, and bone) and ignore the relatively metabolically stable adipose mass. A variety of estimates of IBW are available.[43] In our experience, using the simple formula of 110 lbs. for the first 5 feet of height, plus 3 pounds for every inch above that for women and 5 pounds for men is easy to remember and relatively reliable for the "average" sized patient.

Excess body weight is calculated as the current "dry" weight minus the IBW. Excess weight in the obese patient contains approximately 75% adipose and 25% lean tissue. Therefore, calculation of protein needs in the obese is based on the IBW plus 25% of the excess weight. For example, a 100 kg patient who should weigh 60 kg has 40 kg excess weight. Therefore, the weight used for calculating protein requirement would be 70 kg (60 kg plus 25% of excess weight).

Carbohydrate Requirements

Patients in fulminant hepatic failure require a steady infusion of glucose to avoid hypoglycemia. The observation of hypoglycemia in a patient with fulminant hepatic failure (not receiving insulin) is usually a premorbid event. After glucose reserves from muscle and liver glycogen have been depleted, the inability to manufacture glucose from skeletal muscle suggests that the degree of liver failure is so severe that survival without liver transplantation is doubtful. Infusion of

10% dextrose will usually avoid life-threatening hypoglycemia, but immediate liver transplantation provides the best chance for survival. Provision of other nutrients is generally not necessary since the metabolic machinery for processing such substrates has already been severely incapacitated. Death from cerebral edema usually occurs within a few days; therefore appropriate cerebral pressure monitoring and medical management is required until a suitable organ for transplantation can be found.

In the chronic liver-failure patient, gluconeogenesis is impaired secondary to decreased hepatic glycogen stores. In the patient with normal hepatic function, glycogen mobilization can support cerebral glucose requirements for approximately 36 to 48 hours. In the setting of cirrhosis, glycogen stores are rapidly depleted providing substrate for glucose production for 10–12 hours. Because glycogen stores are impaired, there is accelerated gluconeogenesis from skeletal muscle, resulting in further protein catabolism.

The clinician prescribing nutrition support to the patient with hepatic failure needs to resist the temptation of trying to aggressively replete substrate with the impractical goal of producing anabolism. Careful calculation of glucose requirement is needed to avoid iatrogenic complications related to hyperglycemia.[3] When feeding a patient enterally, excessive feeding will lead to intolerance with diarrhea, bloating, and possibly vomiting. Because the gut provides a "gate-keeper" role, major complications related to excessive tube-feed administration are generally kept to a minimum. With total parenteral nutrition however, there are no means of regulation and the patient is forced to assimilate the entire substrate load. Therefore, the clinician needs to be aware of the maximal disposal rate of glucose to avoid overfeeding.

In the patient with "normal" liver function, the oxidation rate of glucose is approximately 5 mg/kg/min/d.[44,45] In other words, a typical 70 kg reference patient has a maximal disposal rate of glucose of approximately 500 grams per day.[45] Administration of glucose above this level will result in severe hyperglycemia, lipogenesis, and increased carbon dioxide production.[46] Patients with liver failure can have alterations in glucose homeostasis; therefore, careful monitoring of serum glucose is warranted to avoid complications associated with hyperglycemia. Using the preset guideline of 22–25 kcal/kg/d for energy requirement, glucose should be provided at a rate that will not exceed the maximal oxidation rate of glucose. To minimize carbohydrate load, lipid administration can be used as an alternate source of energy.

LIPID REQUIREMENTS

Lipid can be an important component of nutrition support. Many enteral feeding formulas provide a wide range of lipid dosages from a variety of sources for fatty acids. When prescribing TPN, many hospitals compound "3 in 1" TPN solutions containing amino acids, dextrose, and lipid. Other hospitals favor "piggyback" lipid administration as a separate infusion. Authors favoring piggyback lipid infusion cite possible increased infection risk with TPN solutions hanging for up to 24 hours and criticize the use of multi-dose lipid vials used for compounding TPN.[47] Currently, there are no prospective randomized trials to confirm increased infection risk with TPN compounded with lipid. Indeed, an argument can be made that piggyback lipid administration increases risk of line infection since the central line is violated two additional times daily to hang and remove single doses of lipid.[48]

The Federal Drug Administration (FDA) has approved lipid emulsions for parenteral administration prepared from either soybean oil or a combination of soybean and safflower oil. These preparations are primarily designed to provide an adequate amount of the essential fatty acids, and linoleic and linolenic acids. Since essential fatty acid deficiency takes approximately 5 to 6 weeks to develop with no intake of linoleic or linolenic acid, this is not likely to become an issue for most patients with liver failure except in those who are most severely malnourished. Therefore, a short course of "fat free" TPN is perfectly reasonable and may be desirable in patients with ascites and requiring fluid restriction (see "Fluid Restricted Patient," page 204). An additional advantage of TPN containing lipid emulsion is the ability to replace dextrose calories that may be useful in avoiding hyperglycemia in the diabetic liver-failure patient.[49] Experimental lipid formulas from a variety of sources are currently under study and may provide additional benefits in certain disease states such as liver failure.[50–53] Chemically engineered "designer" structured lipids may improve both immunologic and protein kinetic parameters compared to currently available formulas.[54–56] The increased cost and problems with shelf-life stability have hampered the development of these compounds.

Patients with liver failure and cirrhosis have lost much of their reticuloendothelial system and are at increased risk for infection. Large doses of parenteral lipid can result in reticuloendothelial system (RES) blockade in both animals and humans.[57,58] This problem is exacerbated by rapid piggyback infusion techniques and is ameliorated by slower continuous infusion. In general, lipid administration should not exceed 1 g/kg/d using prehospital (dry) weight and should be given over 24 hours if possible. When compounding a total nutrient admixture (3 in 1), the minimum dose of lipid should be 20 g/L or final concentration of the solution of 2%. More dilute lipid formulas are unstable in the presence of hypertonic dextrose and amino acids and result in the lipid emulsion "cracking," which is the separation of the lipid emulsion into oil and water.[48,59]

Fluid Restricted ICU Patient: Using Maximally Concentrated Solutions

For many patients with liver failure who are in the ICU, the need for fluid restriction will preclude providing optimal protein and calories. Establishment of enteral feedings, even at a low dose, can be beneficial and should be pursued. Patients on high-dose vasopressors or those with massive ascites and fluid retention may be intolerant to enteral feedings and can be maintained on TPN. In these situations, nutrition support utilizing maximally concentrated solutions provides the best opportunity to avoid further salt and fluid overload while providing necessary substrate for anabolism. Additionally, certain medications can be compounded within the TPN bag to avoid further fluid overload.

Patients with severe salt and water overload who cannot tolerate enteral diets should be given 1 liter of a maximally concentrated TPN solution. Theoretically, infinite combinations of maximally concentrated solutions can be compounded, but many do not adequately meet the metabolic needs of the patient. The amino acid stock solution provided by the pharmacy will somewhat dictate the amount of protein and dextrose that can be provided in any solution (Table 17.2). For example, typical amino stock solutions contain either 10% (100 g/L) or 15% (150 g/L) amino acids. Therefore, if you wish to limit total volume to 1 liter and provide 100 grams of protein, no additional volume will be available for dextrose if the pharmacy stocks only 10% amino acids.

In our practice for the fluid-restricted patient, we favor the use of a combination of 7% amino acids with 21% dextrose when a 10% amino acid stock solution is available. In pharmacies providing 15% stock amino acid solution, we favor the use of 10.5% amino acids with 21% dextrose. One liter of these formulas provides adequate protein for the majority of patients and 210 grams of dextrose for nitrogen sparing. Although counter intuitive, lipid is omitted since the stock solution of dextrose (70%) is more calorically dense than the stock solution of lipid (20%) (2.4 kcal/cc vs. 2.0 kcal/cc respectively). Adding lipid emulsion will only add more fluid while decreasing caloric density.

TABLE 17.2

Commonly Available Pharmacy Stock Solutions and Their Caloric Densities

Stock Solution	Caloric Density (kcal/cc)
Amino Acid 10% or 15%	4 kcal/cc, 6 kcal/cc respectively
Dextrose 70%	2.38 kcal/cc
Lipid Emulsion 10% or 20%	1.1 kcal/cc, 2.0 kcal/cc respectively

Metabolic Issues

Phosphorus

Hypophosphatemia has been sporadically reported after major liver resection and in cases of fulminant liver failure.[60,61] Some authors have proposed that hypophosphatemia may contribute to the development of liver failure.[62]

Acute severe hypophosphatemia results in numerous clinical manifestations that are shown in Table 17.3. Hypophosphatemia-induced alterations in neurologic, hematologic, immunologic, respiratory, cardiac, and muscular systems have been observed and can contribute to complications. Cardiac manifestations include reversible cardiomyopathy and depressed vascular response to vasopressors that improve with phosphorus repletion.[63]

Patients with liver failure, especially fulminant hepatic failure, are at risk for developing severe hypophosphatemia (<1.0 mg/dL). Careful monitoring and correction of depleted levels may improve outcome. Provision of phosphorus at 60 mmol/day as part of TPN reduces the incidence of severe hypophosphatemia induced by major liver resection and may be of benefit to the patient with hepatic failure-induced hypophosphatemia.[64]

Diabetic Patients with Liver Failure

The major goal of nutritional support in the diabetic patient is to avoid hyper- or hypoglycemia.[65] One area of confusion when starting nutrition support in the diabetic patient is the amount of insulin to be administered. Patients on enteral tube feedings should be covered with long-acting NPH insulin with sliding scale for episodes of hyperglycemia. Any sliding-scale

TABLE 17.3

Clinical Manifestations of Severe Hypophosphatemia	
Hematologic:	Reduced red cell 2,3DPG Hemolytic anemia Platelet dysfunction
Immunologic:	Impaired leukocytic chemotaxis Impaired phagocytosis Impaired bacterial killing
Cardiac:	Reversible cardiomyopathy Depressed vascular responses to vasopressors
Neurologic:	Paresthesia Confusion Seizures Ataxia Intention tremor Coma
Respiratory:	Acute respiratory failure Hyper or hypoventilation
Endocrine:	Glucose intolerance Functional hypoparathyroidism
Renal:	Hyperchloremic metabolic acidosis Hypermagnesuria Hypercalciuria Hypophosphaturia

2,3DPG = 2,3-diphosphoglycerate.

insulin administered within a 24-hour period should be added to the total dose of NPH administered the next day. "Stop insulin" orders need to be written for any gastrointestinal intolerance that interrupts enteral feedings. Coverage of hyperglycemia is provided using sliding-scale regular insulin with appropriate adjustment in NPH insulin dose the next day until euglycemia is obtained (all serum glucose values <220 mg/dL).

For patients prescribed TPN, a simple insulin algorithm has been developed to avoid potential problems with blood sugar control in diabetic patients. The important concepts are to start slowly with a moderate dose of dextrose, obtain euglycemia with parenteral insulin in the bag of TPN (not with secondary drips), coverage of hyperglycemia with sliding-scale insulin, and then gradual advancement of calories to goal levels. Patients receiving parenteral nutrition must have carefully and individually tailored prescriptions of insulin. The major goal is to avoid hyperglycemia (>220 mg/dL), which is associated with increased risk of infection and likelihood of adverse outcomes.[3]

Type I Diabetic Patients Receiving TPN

TPN should be started with only 100 g dextrose/d with advancement of calories only when euglycemia is obtained (all blood glucose values for 24 hours <220 mg/dL) with parenteral insulin in the bag. Once euglycemia is obtained, calories and insulin should be increased proportionally. Replacing some of the calories in the TPN bag with lipid is usually helpful in glucose control. The amount of insulin to start with is reviewed below.

Type II Diabetic Patients Receiving TPN

TPN should be initiated with 200 grams dextrose/day and advance calories only when euglycemia is obtained (all blood glucose values for 24 hours <220 mg/dL) with parenteral insulin in the bag. Use of secondary insulin drips should not be used. If blood sugar control is difficult with relatively low doses of dextrose, the TPN bag should be discontinued. Cover blood glucose levels over 200 with sliding-scale insulin. The amount of insulin to start with is reviewed below.

Starting Insulin in TPN

The dose of insulin needed to achieve euglycemia can be predicted by the patient's usual dose of insulin at home.[66] Use of parenteral insulin/prehospital insulin ratio developed by Hongsemeier et al. predicts that all diabetic patients (Type I and II) on average will require twice their usual insulin dose while receiving TPN, and no patient will require less than his or her usual home dose of insulin. Therefore, a Type II diabetic requiring 70 units of total insulin at home is predicted to require at least 70–140 units of parenteral insulin while on TPN. For patients with severe metabolic stress, the dose may be even higher. When prescribing insulin in TPN, only regular insulin should be used. The equation for calculating insulin dose for TPN is as follows:

$$\frac{\text{Initial Parenteral Insulin Dose (IPI)}}{\text{Prehospital Insulin Dose (PHI)}} = \frac{\text{Initial Parenteral Calories (IPC)}}{\text{Basal Energy Expenditure (BEE)}}$$

$$\text{Solving for IPI} \qquad \text{IPI} = \frac{\text{IPC} \times \text{PHI}}{\text{BEE}}$$

Remember: IPC = Initial Parenteral Calories calculated for the first bag of TPN (including protein, lipid, and dextrose 100 or 200 grams for first day).

BEE = use 25 kcal/kg usual body or "dry" body weight.

Check blood sugars Q 6 hours and cover hyperglycemia with regular insulin sliding scale. A typical sliding scale is shown in Table 17.4.

TABLE 17.4

Typical Sliding Scale of Regular Insulin for Blood Sugar Control		
Blood Glucose:	0–200 mg/dL	0 units regular insulin
	201–250 mg/dL	3 units regular insulin
	251–300 mg/dL	6 units regular insulin
	301–350 mg/dL	9 units regular insulin
	351–400 mg/dL	12 units regular insulin
	>400 mg/dL	Call MD

On consecutive days, add any sliding-scale insulin that was given over the previous 24 hours to the next bag of TPN. When euglycemia is maintained (all blood glucose values <220 mg/dL), increase calories and insulin in a proportionate fashion.

Acid/Base Issues

Patients with chronic liver failure are often maintained on diuretic therapy to control ascites and peripheral edema. A consequence of chronic diuretic therapy is the disturbance in normal acid/base status with the development of metabolic alkalosis. Metabolic alkalosis is defined as the removal of acid or the addition of base to the patient's blood. Alkalemia is defined as a blood pH above 7.45. Metabolic alkalosis is the most common acid/base disturbance encountered in patients with liver failure and relates to the liberal use of diuretics and citrate administration in blood products. Steroid use is also a common cause of metabolic alkalosis but is rarely clinically significant. Since alkalemia is poorly tolerated compared to acidemia (significant mortality seen with pH >7.55), it is not a simple academic exercise to correct this derangement.[67] Fortunately, the vast majority (>90%) of metabolic alkalosis are chloride sensitive and easily correctable. Using TPN as a vehicle, chloride can be delivered in one or more of three forms: sodium chloride, potassium chloride and hydrochloric acid 0.1N (100 mEq/d max; lipid free TPN only).

To correct metabolic alkalosis, calculate the base excess or acid deficit and correct one-half of this over the next 24 hours with additional chloride. Many hospitals use "standard" electrolyte formulations, which have equivalent amounts of chloride and acetate or gluconate. Acetate and gluconate are metabolically equivalent to bicarbonate and thus cancel the effect of chloride on an equal molar basis. Therefore, to correct metabolic alkalosis, acetate and gluconate should be minimized.

Although less commonly seen, metabolic acidosis is seen in patients with liver failure and coexisting renal failure or with increased fixed acid production. The usual acid production rate is approximately 1 mEq/kg/d but can rise to as much as 3 mEq/kg/d in critically ill patients. It is important to note that for every 6-mEq decline in serum total CO_2, the buffering capacity of the blood is halved. Therefore, any patient with measured bicarbonate less than 20 mEq/L should be corrected regardless of a "normal" pH. Calculate the base deficit in mEq and replace one-half over the next 24 hours. The most commonly used forms of base used in TPN are sodium acetate, calcium gluconate, and potassium acetate.

Conclusions

Nutrition support in the patient with hepatic failure can be a life-saving treatment modality, an important adjunct to the multidisciplinary approach to the critically ill patient. The metabolic disturbances induced by liver failure make traditional assessment of nutritional status difficult. Whenever possible, the enteral route of administration is favored over parenteral nutrition support. Attempts to aggressively replete the malnourished liver-failure patient with energy and substrate above energy expenditure are likely to lead to complications and nullify any benefit of feeding. For the patient intolerant to full enteral nutrition, combination feeding with parenteral nutrition may provide the benefits of enteral nutrition while affording the ability to correct metabolic disturbances and may serve as a vehicle to administer medications. Communication with the hospital pharmacy is vital in avoiding potentially lethal interactions and to improve the outcome of nutrition support.

References

1. Dahn MS, Lange P. Hormonal changes and their influence on metabolism and nutrition in the critically ill. *Intensive Care Med.* 1982;8:209–213.
2. Pomposelli JJ, Bistrian BR. Is total parenteral nutrition immunosuppressive? *New Horiz.* 1994;2:224–229.
3. Pomposelli JJ, Baxter JK 3rd, Babineau TJ, et al. Early postoperative glucose control predicts nosocomial infection rate in diabetic patients. *J Parenter Enteral Nutr.* 1998; 22:77–81.
4. Christman JW, McCain RW. A sensible approach to the nutritional support of mechanically ventilated critically ill patients. *Intensive Care Med.* 1993;19:129–136.
5. Tayek JA, Blackburn GL. Goals of nutritional support in acute infections. *Am J Med.* 1984;76:81–90.

6. Waddell LS, Michel KE. Critical care nutrition: routes of feeding. *Clin Tech Small Anim Pract*. 1998;13:197–203.
7. Moore EE, Moore FA. Immediate enteral nutrition following multisystem truama: a decade perspective. *J Am Coll Nutr*. 1991;10:633–648.
8. Driscoll DF, Baptista RJ, Mitrano FP, et al. Parenteral nutrient admixtures as drug vehicles: theory and practice in the critical care setting. *Dicp*. 1991;25:276–283.
9. Echenique MM, Bistrian BR, Blackburn GL. Theory and techniques of nutritional support in the ICU. *Crit Care Med*. 1982;10:546–549.
10. Bistrian BR. Dietary treatment in secondary wasting and cachexia. *J Nutr*. 1999;129(1S Suppl):290S–294S.
11. Lowell JA, Schifferdecker C, Driscoll DF, et al. Postoperative fluid overload: not a benign problem [see comments]. *Crit Care Med*. 1990;18:728–733.
12. Bistrian BR. Enteral nutrition: just a fuel or an immunity enhancer? *Minerva Anesthesiol*. 1999;65:471–474.
13. Cerra FB, Lehmann S, Konstantinides N, et al. Improvement in immune function in ICU patients by enteral nutrition supplemented with arginine, RNA, and menhaden oil is independent of nitrogen balance. *Nutrition*. 1991;73: 193–199.
14. Man-Fan Wan J, Kanders BS, Kowalchuk M, et al. Omega 3 fatty acids and cancer metastasis in humans. *World Rev Nutr Diet*. 1991;66:477–487.
15. Kenler AS, Swails WS, Driscoll DF, et al. Early enteral feeding in postsurgical cancer patients. Fish oil structured lipid-based polymeric formula versus a standard polymeric formula. *Ann Surg*. 1996;223:316–333.
16. Benotti PN, Blackburn GL, Miller JD, et al. Role of branched-chain amino acids (BCAA) intake in preventing muscle proteolysis. *Surg Forum*. 1976;27(62):7–10.
17. Wilmore DW. Postoperative protein sparing. *World J Surg*. 1999;23:545–552.
18. Mendenhall CL, Moritz TE, Roselle GA, et al. A study of oral nutrition support with oxandrolone in malnourished patients with alcoholic hepatitis: Results of a Department of Veterans Affairs cooperative study. *Hepatolgy*. 1993;17: 564–576.
19. DiCecco SR, Wieners EJ, Wiesner RH, et al. Assessment of nutritional status of patients with end-stage liver disease undergoing liver transplantation. *Mayo Clin Proc*. 1989;64: 95–102.
20. Driscoll DF, Blackburn GL. Total parenteral nutrition 1990. A review of its currect status in hospitalized patients, and the need for patient-specific feeding. *Drugs*. 1990;40: 346–363.
21. Kudsk KA, Mirtallo JM. Nutritional support of the critically ill patient. *Drug Intell Clin Pharm*. 1983;17:501–506.
22. Moore FA, Moore EE, Jones TN, et al. TEN versus TPN following major abdominal trauma—reduced septic morbidity. *J Trauma*. 1989;29:916–922; discussion 922–923.
23. Frankenfield DC, Smith JS, Cooney RN. Accelerated nitrogen loss after traumatic injury is not attenuated by achievement of energy balance [see comments]. *J Parenter Enteral Nutr*. 1997;21:324–329.
24. Sobrado J, Moldawer LL, Pomposelli JJ, et al. Lipid emulsions and reticuloendothelial system function in healthy and burned guinea pigs. *AM J Clin Nutr*. 1985;42:855–863.
25. Jensen GL, Mascioli EA, Seidner DL, et al. Parenteral infusion of long- and medium-chain triglycerides and reticuloendothelial system function in man. *J Parenter Enteral Nutr*. 1990;14:467–471.
26. Bistrian BR, Blackburn GL, Hallowell E, et al. Protein status of general surgical patients. *JAMA*. 1974;230:858–860.
27. Tan YS, Nambiar R, Yo SL. Prevalence of protein calorie malnutrition in general surgical patients. *Ann Acad Med Singapore*. 1992;21:334–338.
28. Wilmore DW. Catabolic illness. Strategies for enhancing recovery. *N Engl J Med*. 1991;325:695–702.
29. Dempsey DT, Buzby GP, Mullen JL. Nutritional assessment in the seriously ill patient. *J Am Coll Nutr*. 1983;2: 15–22.
30. Pikul J, Sharpe MD, Lowndes R, et al. Degree of preoperative malnutrition is predictive of postoperative morbidity and mortality in liver transplantation. *Transplantation*. 1994;57:469–472.
31. Driscoll DF, Palombo JD, Bistrian BR. Nutritional and metabolic considerations of the adult liver transplant candidate and organ donor. *Nutrition*. 1995;11:255–263.
32. Hirsch S, de Obaldia N, Petermann M, et al. Subjective global assessment of nutritional status: further validation. *Nutrition*. 1991;71:35–37; discussion 37–38.
33. Kotani J, Usami M, Nomura H, et al. Enteral nutrition prevents bacterial translocation but does not improve survival during acute pancreatitis. *Arch Surg*. 1999;134:287–292.
34. Boyes RJ, Kruse JA. Nasogastric and nasoenteric intubation. *Crit Care Clin*. 1992;8:865–878.
35. Burns D, Schaeffer D, Bosco J. Nutritional assessment of endoscopically placed nasojejunal feeding tubes. *Gastrointest Endosc*. 1995;41:263–269.
36. DeBiasse MA, Wilmore DW. What is optimal nutritional support? *New Horiz*. 1994;2:122–130.
37. Wernerman J. Enteral or parenteral nutrition? Pro-parenteral. *Acta Anaesthesiol Scand Suppl*. 1997;110:148–150.
38. Hunter DC, Jaksic T, Lewis D, et al. Resting energy expenditure in the critically ill: estimations versus measurement. *Br J Surg*. 1988;75:875–878.
39. Ireton-Jones CS, Francis C. Obesity: nutrition support practice and application to critical care. *Nutr Clin Pract*. 1995;10:144–149.
40. Palombo JD, Blackburn GL. Human protein requirements. *ASDC J Dent Child*. 1980;47:277–280.
41. Cerra FB, Benitez MR, Blackburn GL, et al. Applied nutrition in ICU patients. A consensus statement of the American College of Chest Physicians. *Chest*. 1997;111: 769–778.
42. Naylor CD, O'Rourke K, Baker JP. Parenteral nutrition with branched-chain amino acids in hepatic encephalopathy. A meta-analysis. *Gastroenterology*. 1989;97:1033–1042.

43. Cutts ME, Dowdy RP, Ellersieck MR, et al. Predicting energy needs in ventilator-dependent critically ill patients: effect of adjusting weight for edema or adiposity. *Am J Clin Nutr.* 1997;66:1250–1256.

44. Guenst JM, Nelson LD. Predictors of total parenteral nutrition-induced lipogenesis. *Chest.* 1994;105:553–559.

45. Nygren J, Thorell A, Efendic S, et al. Site of insulin resistance after surgery: the contribution of hypocaloric nutrition and bed rest. *Clin Sci (Colch).* 1997;93:137–146.

46. Yamamoto T. Metabolic response to glucose overload in surgical stress: energy disposal in brown adipose tissue. *Surg Today.* 1996;26(3):151–157.

47. Moro ML, Maffei C, Manso E, et al. Nosocomial outbreak of systemic candidosis associated with parenteral nutrition. *Infect Control Hosp Epidemiol.* 1990;11:27–35.

48. Driscoll DF, Baptista RJ, Bistrian BR, et al. Practical considerations regarding the use of total nutrient admixtures. *Am J Hosp Pharm.* 1986;43:416–419.

49. Watanabe Y, Sato M, Abe Y, et al. Fat emulsions as an ideal nonprotein energy source under surgical stress for diabetic patients. *Nutrition* 1995;11:734–738.

50. Ball MJ, White K. Metabolic effects of intravenous medium- and long-chain triacylglycerols in critically ill patients. *Clin Sci.* 1989;76:165–170.

51. Pomposelli JJ, Flores E, Hirschberg Y, et al. Short-term TPN containing n-3 fatty acids ameliorate lactic acidosis induced by endotoxin in guinea pigs. *Am J Clin Nutr.* 1990;52:548–552.

52. Pomposelli JJ, Flores EA, Blackburn L, et al. Diets enriched with N-3 fatty acids ameliorate lactic acidosis by improving endotoxin-induced tissue hypoperfusion in guinea pigs. *Ann Surg.* 1991;213:166–176.

53. Ling PR, Istfan NW, Lopes SM, et al. Structured lipid made from fish oil and medium-chain triglycerides alters tumor and host metabolism in Yoshida-sarcoma-bearing rats. *Am J Clin Nutr.* 1991;53:1177–1184.

54. Bellantone R, Bossola M, Carriero C, et al. Structured versus long-chain triglycerides: a safety, tolerance, and efficacy randomized study in colorectal surgical patients. *J Parenter Enteral Nutr.* 1999;23:123–127.

55. Sierra P, Ling PR, Istfan NW, et al. Fish oil feeding improves muscle glucose uptake in tumor necrosis factor-treated rats. *Metabolism.* 1995;44:1365–1370.

56. DeMichele SJ, Karlstad MD, Bistrian BR, et al. Enteral nutrition with structured lipid: effect on protein metabolism in thermal injury. *Am J Clin Nutr.* 1989;50:1295–1302.

57. Hamawy KJ, Moldawer LL, Georgieff M, et al. The Henry M. Vars Award. The effect of lipid emulsions on reticuloendothelial system function in the injured animal. *J Parenter Enteral Nutr.* 1985;9:559–565.

58. Mascioli EA, Babayan VK, Bistrian BR, et al. Novel triglycerides for special medical purposes. *J Parenter Enteral Nutr.* 1988;12:127S–132S.

59. Driscoll DF, Newton DW, Bistrian BR. Precipitation of calcium phosphate from parenteral nutrient fluids. *Am J Hosp Pharm.* 1994;51:2834–2836.

60. Pinson CW, Daya MR, Benner KG, et al. Liver transplantation for severe Amanita phalloides mushroom poisoning. *Am J Surg.* 1990;159:493–499.

61. George R, Shiu MH. Hypophosphatemia after major hepatic resection. *Surgery.* 1992;111:281–286.

62. Nanji AA, Anderson FH. Acute liver failure: a possible consequence of severe hypophosphatemia. *J Clin Gastroenterol.* 1985;7:338–340.

63. Zazzo JF, Troche G, Ruel P, et al. High incidence of hypophosphatemia in surgical intensive care patients: efficacy of phosphorus therapy on myocardial function. *Intensive Care Med.* 1995;21:826–831.

64. Pomposelli JJ, Pomfret EA, Burns DL, et al. Life-threatening hypophosphatemia after right hepatic lobectomy for liver donor adult transplantation. *Liver Transpl.* 2001;7:637–642.

65. McMahon M, Manji N, Driscoll DF, et al. Parenteral nutrition in patients with diabetes mellitus: theoretical and practical considerations. *J Parenter Enteral Nutr.* 1989;13:545–553.

66. Hongsermeier T, Bistrian BR. Evaluation of a practical technique for determining insulin requirements in diabetic patients receiving total parenteral nutrition [see comments]. *J Parenter Enteral Nutr.* 1993;17:16–19.

67. Driscoll DF, Bistrian BR, Jenkins RL, et al. Development of metabolic alkalosis after massive transfusion during orthotopic liver transplantation. *Crit Care Med.* 1987;15:905–908.

CHAPTER

18 Nutrition Support in Acute Renal Failure

Pamela Charney, M.S., R.D., C.N.S.D., David Charney, M.D., F.A.C.P.

INTRODUCTION 209

CAUSES OF ARF 209

DIALYTIC THERAPY AND NUTRITION 210

NUTRITION ASSESSMENT IN ARF 212

DETERMINING REQUIREMENTS IN ARF: ENERGY AND PROTEIN 213

DETERMINING REQUIREMENTS IN ARF: VITAMINS AND MINERALS 213

NUTRITION SUPPORT IN ACUTE RENAL FAILURE 214

INITIATING AND MONITORING NUTRITION SUPPORT 215

CONCLUSIONS 216

REFERENCES 216

Introduction

Acute renal failure (ARF) is often defined as abrupt decrease or cessation of normal renal function, often associated with azotemia and significant decline in urine output. Patients with ARF also may have other metabolic disturbances due to the integral role of the kidney in maintaining normal homeostatic mechanisms. Morbidity rates for patients with ARF have continued to be high in spite of advances in the care of critically ill patients.[1] Critically ill patients with ARF often have significant co-morbidities affecting nutrition therapy.[2] While controversial, appropriate medical nutrition therapy may be a vital part of managing these often complicated patients. However, delivery of nutrients may be made difficult due to electrolyte disturbances, fluid imbalances, and significant azotemia unless adequate dialytic therapy is provided.

Causes of ARF

Acute renal failure is defined as an abrupt decline in renal function. This usually manifests itself as an elevation of the BUN and serum creatinine levels, at times with a decrease in the patient's urine output. Each instance of acute renal failure can be separated into one of three general etiologies: pre-renal, intrinsic renal, and post-renal acute renal failure (Table 18.1).

Pre-renal acute renal failure is defined by a decrease in renal perfusion. This is not synonymous with volume depletion, although a decrease in circulating blood volume (for example, bleeding, gastrointestinal fluid losses with emesis or diarrhea, or overdiuresis) can certainly be a cause of this. Renal blood flow can also be diminished in conditions with renal arteriolar vasoconstriction, such as in sepsis or hepatorenal syndrome, or with arterial obstruction, such as with aortic dissection. Certain edematous conditions, such as congestive heart failure, cirrhosis, or nephrotic syndrome, result in a decreased effective arterial blood volume and decreased renal perfusion. Last, toxic effects from certain medications, such as nonsteroidal anti-inflammatory agents or ACE inhibitors, may affect intrarenal hemodynamics.

Post-renal acute renal failure is defined by obstruction to urine flow. This can occur at various levels of the urinary system. Tumor lysis syndrome can result in the obstruction of large numbers of renal tubules from deposition of uric acid and calcium-phosphate precipitates. Ureteral obstruction can occur with retroperitoneal fibrosis or intra-abdominal masses such as lymphomas. Unilateral ureteral obstruction will not usually cause acute renal failure, unless there is preexisting renal insufficiency. Bladder outlet obstruction can be caused by prostatic hypertrophy, for example.

Intrinsic renal disease can also be broken down into general categories. Acute glomerulonephritis can result from either primary renal diseases, such as post-infectious glomerulonephritis or a rapidly progressive (crescentic) glomerulonephritis, or a systemic disease, such as systemic lupus erythematosus or Henoch-

TABLE 18.1

Causes of Acute Renal Failure	
Examples	
Pre-renal	
Volume depletion	Bleeding, GI losses, overdiuresis
Renal vasoconstriction	Sepsis, hepatorenal syndrome
Renal arterial obstruction	Aortic dissection
Volume excess/decreased effective arterial blood volume	Cirrhosis, nephrotic syndrome, congestive heart failure
Medication effects	ACE inhibitors, NSAIDs
Renal	
Acute glomerulonephritis	Postinfectious GN, idiopathic RPGN, lupus nephritis
Acute interstitial nephritis	Allergic medication reaction
Acute tubular necrosis	Hypotension, hypoxia, toxic injury (rhabdomyolysis, intravenous contrast)
Post-renal	
Tubular obstruction	Tumor lysis syndrome
Ureteral obstruction	Retroperitoneal fibrosis
Urethral obstruction	Prostatic hypertrophy

Schonlein purpura. Acute interstitial nephritis may occur, often resulting from an allergic reaction to a medication. The most common etiology for intrinsic renal acute renal failure is acute tubular necrosis (ATN). This can be due to hypotensive or hypoxic injury, such as with sepsis or cardiac arrest, or toxic injury, such as with rhabdomyolysis (myoglobinuria), intravenous contrast agents, or gentamicin nephrotoxicity.

Dialytic Therapy and Nutrition

Although this list of differential diagnoses may seem daunting, the major distinctions between various types of acute renal failure involve three factors: is it easily reversible, is dialytic therapy being used, and is the patient catabolic. Obviously, if the renal failure is reversible in a timely fashion, the renal dysfunction becomes a moot point and nutrition therapy can be guided by the remaining morbid conditions. Dietary restrictions (protein, fluid, phosphate, and potassium, for example) become more important in a patient with ongoing renal failure in whom the attempt is made to avoid dialysis; these issues will be discussed in more detail later in the chapter. However, the use of renal replacement therapy allows for a more generalized approach to the nutritional treatment of the patient, with the dialytic therapy being adjusted in order to allow optimization of this treatment. An extremely important factor in both adjusting the nutrition therapy and the question of dialysis is whether the patient is catabolic. Certain patients, such as those with acute renal failure from intravenous contrast during an elective radiologic procedure, may not show much catabolism. Formation of uremic toxins is slow, and a short period with reduced nutritional intake is not of much risk to the overall health. In these patients, an attempt may be made to avoid dialysis if possible, and protein and nutrient intake may be significantly restricted. At the opposite end of the spectrum, a patient with a closed head injury on high doses of corticosteroids can be intensely catabolic; in such a patient, restriction of protein intake would be detrimental and avoidance of dialysis may be impossible.

A number of renal therapies are possible in a patient with acute renal failure.[3] Conservative management, with protein, fluid, and electrolyte restriction and avoiding dialysis, can reasonably be attempted in non-catabolic patients while awaiting a return of renal function. Studies have shown that it is necessary to ensure adequate caloric intake in the face of protein restriction in order to maintain nitrogen balance (Table 18.2).

In all renal replacement therapies, the patient's blood is brought into contact with a manufactured dialysate fluid, separated by a semipermeable membrane. Changes in fluid and solutes during these treatments are accomplished by both diffusive (concentration gradient driven) and convective (pressure driven) forces, and are affected by a number of factors. The first of these factors is the permeability of the membrane to a given substance. Dialyzer membranes are extremely permeable to water and small solutes such as sodium, potassium, and urea; they are impermeable to cells. Different membranes have varied degrees of permeability to moderate-size molecules, such as plasma proteins. Solute flux across the membrane depends as well

TABLE 18.2

Impact of Dialysis Modality on Nutrition

Modality	Time/Rx	Frequency	Common in ARF	Maximum Fluid Removal (L)	Protein Losses	Amino Acid Losses	Glucose Load
Intermittent HD	4-5 hours	3-7/week	Yes	2/hour	Low	Moderate	Mild
PD	24 hours	Daily	No	4/day	Moderate	Moderate	High
SCUF	24 hours	Daily	No	1/hour	Low	Low	None
CAVH/ CVVH	24 hours	Daily	Yes	1/hour	Moderate	Moderate	None-mild
CAVHD/ CVVHD	24 hours	Daily	Yes	1/hour	Moderate	Moderate	None-mild

on the concentration gradient created by the composition of the dialysate. If removal of excess solute is desired, the dialysate concentration of that concentration is manufactured to be low; a common example of this would be the removal of excess potassium by decreasing the dialysate concentration of potassium, creating a gradient across the dialyzer membrane. In some instances, the patient is deficient in solute and the dialysate concentration is higher than that found in the patient's blood, allowing for repletion; examples of this include bicarbonate and calcium. Certain solutes are not present in abnormal concentration, and the dialysate is created to have a neutral gradient. However, the situation allows for inadvertent losses due to the concentration gradient created by omission of solutes in the dialysate fluid. This can include water-soluble vitamins and amino acids; protein losses can vary depending on the permeability of dialyzer membrane. Removal of a substance by dialysis also depends on the accessibility of the patient's solute load to the circulating blood. An excellent example of this is the renal failure patient overloaded with phosphate. In addition to problems with membrane permeability due to a large radius of hydration, the majority of the body phosphate load is intracellular and does not easily equilibrate with the pool in the circulating blood. Therefore, it is difficult to effect efficient removal of the phosphate load with dialysis. Lastly, the hydrostatic pressure applied by the dialysis machine will affect the amount of convective losses; this is mostly used for water and sodium removal from the overloaded patient.

The most familiar dialytic treatment for acute renal failure is intermittent hemodialysis. During this treatment, the patient undergoes dialysis for typically four or more hours, 3 to 7 times a week. The procedure involves high blood and dialysate flows and is quite efficient. The majority of the removal of solutes occurs via diffusive losses, with fluid removal being accomplished by convection (ultrafiltration). Ultrafiltrate is the fluid that is removed from the blood volume by passing across the dialyzer membrane; it is composed of water and solutes to which the dialyzer membrane is permeable. Overall control of the patient's serum chemistries and fluid balance can be excellent. Unfortunately, the efficiency results in relatively marked changes in fluid status and chemical balance over a short period of time, often causing hemodynamic instability in otherwise tenuous patients. The peak and trough effect of an intermittent therapy can require some restrictions on fluid or nutrient intake between dialysis sessions, in order to prevent excessive build-up during the interdialytic period.

Continuous hemodialytic methods have evolved to avoid the peak and trough effect as well as the hemodynamic instability that can result from intermittent therapies.[4] There are various permutations on the basic premise of a slower blood and dialysis flow as well as the use of convective forces to a higher degree than in intermittent hemodialysis. Slow continuous ultrafiltration (SCUF), continuous arteriovenous hemofiltration (CAVH) or hemodiafiltration (CAVHD), and continuous venovenous hemofiltration (CVVH) or hemodiafiltration (CVVHD) are essentially quite similar.[5] Blood is delivered at a slower flow rate to the dialyzer, driven by either arterial pressure (arteriovenous) or via a blood pump (venovenous). Large amounts of ultrafiltrate are removed, with the procedure being performed continuously at the ICU bedside. In SCUF, the ultrafiltrate is not replaced. In hemofiltration, the fluid removed is replaced with a specialized intravenous fluid designed to contain those electrolytes needed by the patient, without the uremic toxins and electrolytes present at elevated levels in the serum. Over time, by dilution, the levels of the unwanted solutes (such as urea and potassium) decrease as desired without change in others (such as sodium). Unfortunately, the dialyzer membrane is only selective with regard to molecular size; therefore, significant losses of essential smaller solutes, such as amino acids and water-soluble vitamins, can occur inadvertently during this process. In hemodiafiltration, all of the above occurs, with the addition of diffusive losses by allowing a relatively low flow of dialysate through the dialyzer.

Another method of renal replacement therapy, peritoneal dialysis, is used infrequently in acute renal failure. It is also a continuous therapy, thus both less efficient and less prone to hemodynamic instability. In this method, manufactured dialysate is instilled into the peritoneal cavity and allowed to dwell for a period of hours, then drained and replaced with fresh fluid. Rather than a manufactured dialyzer membrane, this type of dialysis uses the peritoneal membrane and walls of the capillaries lining the membrane as the semipermeable barrier between blood and dialysate. Important factors to note from a nutrition standpoint are the glucose used in the dialysate and the permeability of the peritoneal membrane to protein. Rather than hydrostatic pressure to effect ultrafiltration, peritoneal dialysate has a high glucose concentration to manufacture oncotic pressure. A significant portion of this glucose can be absorbed during the peritoneal dialysis, affecting serum glucose concentrations and caloric intake. In addition, the peritoneal membrane is much more permeable than manufactured dialysis membranes to large proteins such as albumin; this can result in marked protein losses into the dialysate and needs to be factored into protein requirements.

Nutrition Assessment in ARF

It is generally accepted that individuals with ARF are at increased risk for development of nutrition-related complications. Fiaccadori[5] et al. investigated the relationship between nutritional status and outcome in patients with ARF. They found a high level of severe malnutrition, as determined by Subjective Global Assessment (42% of patients with ARF were severely malnourished) along with significantly higher morbidity from a variety of causes when compared to patients with ARF who were identified as having normal nutritional status. Poor nutritional status was also associated with a significant increase in hospital length of stay.[6] Nutrition assessment of the patient with ARF would be similar to that of any other critically ill patient. If possible, a diet history should be obtained in order to determine adequacy of intake prior to illness. Patients with pre-existing chronic conditions such as diabetes mellitus, HIV/AIDS, or chronic renal failure may have had restricted intake, which may accelerate development of nutrient deficiencies. Medication use, including prescribed, over the counter, and herbal/alternative therapies should be reviewed, as many medications can affect renal function.

The use of serum protein levels in nutrition assessment of critically ill patients has become controversial. There is a well known relationship between serum albumin levels and long-term survival in patients with end-stage renal disease receiving dialytic therapy.[7] It is also known that levels of albumin and prealbumin decrease as a part of the acute phase response. Stress or trauma leads to a re-prioritization of hepatic protein synthetic levels and rates, with changes to some extent depending on the severity of the insult. For these reasons, levels of hepatic transport proteins do not provide information on nutritional status, but may act as prognostic indicators in patients with ARF. C-reactive protein is a positive acute phase protein and acts as a component of the immune response. Levels may provide an indication of the severity of the stress response.[8] The dialytic process is felt to induce a mild acute phase response that may further cloud interpretation of serum protein levels, particularly in patients with ARF.[9] Serum prealbumin levels may provide a monitor of response to feeding in critically ill patients. Since prealbumin is degraded in the healthy kidney, levels may be slightly higher in patients with ARF. However, trends in prealbumin levels can still be followed in individual patients.

Weight loss can be an important prognostic indicator in many patient populations. Assessment of body weight may be hampered in the critical care setting by lack of information concerning usual weight, as well as fluid administration combined with decreased urine output leading to falsely elevated weight measurements. In the critical care setting, increased protein catabolism combined with decreased synthetic capabilities can lead to significant loss of lean body mass that can be masked by fluid retention. Uremia and metabolic acidosis may lead to accelerated loss of lean body mass.[10] Excessive fluid retention can mask loss of lean body mass; it should be remembered that 1 L of excess fluid adds 1 kg to body weight. Whenever possible, the patient's dry weight (weight without edema) should be monitored and changes in weight assessed in terms of fluid status, intake, and clinical condition. In an intensive care setting, daily weights should be followed. Weight changes of more than .5 kg/d should be investigated carefully.

Determining Requirements in ARF: Energy and Protein

Stress, injury, or trauma can lead to alterations in energy requirements, depending on the severity of the insult. Several equations have been developed to estimate energy requirements in critically ill patients. However, as all of the equations currently in use have limitations in critical care. The most accurate determination of energy requirements in this population remains indirect calorimetry. It is most probable that ARF per se does not lead to significant alterations in energy requirements. Energy expenditure was measured using indirect calorimetry in 29 patients with acute renal failure. Patients who had ARF with septicemia had significant increases in energy expenditure (1.28 ± 0.04 vs 0.96 ± 0.02 kcal/min/1.73m^2) when compared to control subjects. Subjects with ARF without sepsis had energy expenditures that were not different from control subjects.[11] Similar results were found in a group of critically ill post-operative patients with and without ARF.[12] The increase in energy expenditure in these patients was most likely a function of underlying critical illness rather than ARF.

Both carbohydrate and lipid metabolism are altered by ARF. Hyperglycemia can be seen in critically ill patients due to peripheral insulin resistance as well as increased hepatic gluconeogenesis.[13] Insulin resistance is felt to be a post-receptor defect, as insulin binding to receptors is normal.[14,15] However, because insulin is mainly degraded by the healthy kidney, insulin levels may be increased in the patient with ARF. Lipid metabolism is also significantly impaired in ARF. Typically, levels of very low density lipoproteins and low density lipoproteins are elevated while cholesterol and HDL cholesterol levels are decreased.

Critical illness can lead to significant catabolism and increased protein requirements. Traditional therapy of ARF included a mild to moderate protein restriction in hope of minimizing accumulation of nitrogenous waste products to avoid the need for dialysis. With improvement in delivery of dialytic therapy and the development of continuous renal replacement therapies (CRRT), protein restrictions have become much less necessary. Continuous hemodiafiltration allowed for provision of more than 2 g protein/kg in a group of critically ill patients with multiple organ failure. Urea nitrogen removal by dialytic therapy was no different from critically ill patients without renal failure.[16] There may be further loss of protein and amino acids during dialytic therapy due to permeability of the dialysis membrane to small molecules and peptides.[17] Individual amino acid losses during CRRT may be important to note as one study found that glutamine, arginine, lysine, and proline made up more than 50% of the amino acids lost during CRRT in a group of critically ill children. Additionally, intake of 1.5 g of protein/kg was not sufficient to maintain nitrogen balance in this study group.[18] These results indicate that protein restriction is not warranted during continuous dialytic therapy in critically ill patients.

Several other factors involved in ARF can lead to alterations in protein metabolism. Inflammatory mediators of the stress response can lead to significant increases in protein catabolism and alterations in protein synthesis as a result of circulating inflammatory mediators.[19] Changes in protein synthesis and degradation appear to vary depending on the severity of injury. The presence of metabolic acidosis can lead to increased protein catabolism. Price et al. found increased activity of proteolytic enzymes in rats with ARF that was stimulated by acidosis.[20] Several studies have shown a relationship between the degree of metabolic acidosis and uremia in patients with chronic renal failure.[21,22,23] Correction of acidosis can lead to improvements in protein synthesis.[24]

Determining Requirements in ARF: Vitamins and Minerals

There has been much interest recently concerning the role of the antioxidant nutrients in acute illness. Metnitz[24] et al. investigated the effects of critical illness and ARF on levels of several of the antioxidant nutrients as well as markers of lipid peroxidation. They found decreased levels of ascorbate, carotene, and selenium in patients with multiple organ failure with and without ARF. All of the patients with ARF were receiving dialytic therapy. Plasma levels of tocopherol were decreased only in patients with multiple organ failure. There was no difference in levels of catalase and superoxide dismutase in either group when compared to a group of healthy control subjects. However, levels of malondialdehyde, a marker of lipid peroxidation, were significantly increased in both groups of patients, with a higher level found in the ARF patients. All patients were receiving parenteral nutrition with addition of standard amounts of vitamins and minerals. While these results indicate the potential need for higher levels of these nutrients during critical illness, it would be difficult to recommend additional supplementation in critically ill patients with ARF, as the subjects with

ARF all had a higher multiple organ failure score.[25] Levels of the fat-soluble vitamins were depressed in eight patients with ARF when compared to levels in 28 healthy control subjects. Vitamin K levels were found to be normal to elevated, with a wide range noted. While the authors recommended re-evaluation of recommended vitamin requirements for patients with ARF,[26] it should be noted that it is difficult to determine if the changes found in these studies were due to ARF per se, or as a result of critical illness.

Electrolyte control can be problematic in management of the critically ill patient with ARF.[27] Under normal circumstances, the kidney is integral in maintaining serum levels of sodium, phosphorus, potassium, and magnesium. Calcium and phosphorus are also affected by parathyroid hormone. Tissue destruction and cell lysis can also release potassium, magnesium, and phosphorus, leading to further increases in serum levels. It is imperative to monitor electrolyte levels and adjust feedings accordingly. Patients who are receiving CRRT may require electrolyte supplementation, while the patient who is not receiving dialytic therapy may require electrolyte-free fluids until levels stabilize.

The use of L-carnitine in acutely ill patients with renal failure remains controversial. Carnitine is an amine compound required for transport of long chain fatty acids into the mitochondria for oxidation and ultimate production of ATP by oxidative phosphorylation. Carnitine is normally considered to be non-essential in the diet of adult humans, as it can be readily synthesized in the liver from the amino acids lysine and methionine. There may be a requirement for carnitine supplementation in the sick premature neonate due to immature hepatic synthetic capability. Others have reported the development of carnitine deficiency in patients on long term TPN, although the mechanism responsible is unknown.[28] It has also been reported that serum carnitine levels decrease to less than 80% of normal immediately following hemodialysis in patients with end-stage renal disease[29]; however, the significance of this is unknown, as others have reported a rapid return to normal levels within hours of dialysis. Carnitine levels can be increased by supplementing intravenous L-Carnitine[30]; however, it is unknown if improving levels improves outcome, as levels are normal in patients with ARF.[31] As carnitine is a small molecule, its removal by dialysis is extremely efficient. Caution should be used in interpretation of serum carnitine levels, as 90% of the body's carnitine content is found intracellularly.[32] More research is needed regarding the role of carnitine in critically ill patients with ARF before recommendations can be made regarding supplementation in this population.

Nutrition Support in Acute Renal Failure

It is difficult to evaluate the role of special amino acid solutions in ARF, as many of the original studies compared different levels of protein intake using essential amino acids or a mixture of essential and non-essential amino acids, or to infusion of hypotonic dextrose alone.[33,34] Many of the early specialized solutions did not include the amino acids now thought to be "conditionally" essential in the critically ill population, such as arginine, glutamine, and possibly cysteine. Most catabolic patients with ARF can be safely fed with enteral and parenteral solutions containing a mixture of both essential and non-essential amino acids.

There may be some evidence that enteral feeding is beneficial in recovery from ARF or in protection from renal ischemic injury. Rats who were fed enterally for 7 days prior to and for 3 days following ischemic acute renal failure had higher creatinine clearance than rats who were fed an isocaloric, isonitrogenous parenteral diet, potentially indicating a role of enteral feeding in recovery from ARF.[35] Enteral feeding may be protective against ARF by its role in improving renal blood flow following ischemic injury. Enteral feeding of a peptide-based diet was shown to significantly improve survival, renal plasma flow, and glomerular filtration rate in rats with rhabdomyolysis. The mechanism for this protection against ARF is unknown, although the role of protein feeding and specific amino acids has been implicated.[36] There are currently no human studies available investigating the role of enteral feeding in preventing or lessening the severity of ARF. Of interest, there have been reports of renal impairment in patients on long term TPN[37,38]; however, the role of nutrition support in ARF is unknown.

The use of parenteral lipid solutions with a mixture of long chain fatty acids (LCFA) and medium chain fatty acids (MCFA) has been advocated for some critically ill patients. MCFA offer some theoretical advantages to LCFA in that they are cleared more rapidly by lipoprotein lipase, do not require carnitine transport for oxidation, and more rapid oxidation. Because metabolism of LCFA can be altered by renal failure, the use of MCFA would allow provision of concentrated lipid calories while minimizing metabolic abnormalities caused by excessive LCFA. However, when MCFA and LCFA were compared in critically ill patients with acute renal failure, there was no difference in clearance rates in a fat elimination test. Metabolic clearance of both lipid emulsions was significantly reduced compared to normal controls.[38]

Initiating and Monitoring Nutrition Support

The decision to initiate enteral or parenteral nutrition support in patients with acute renal failure should be guided by an evaluation of the cause and current management of ARF. Patients who are only mildly hypercatabolic or with minimal changes in renal function will most likely recover renal function with no long-term consequences. ARF in these patients is not an indication for specialized nutrition support. However, in critically ill patients with ARF who are metabolically unstable, it would be imperative to initiate nutrition support in order to avoid nutrition-related complications of critical illness.

Indications for enteral and parenteral nutrition support in ARF are no different from any other critically ill population. It is felt by most that enteral nutrition is safer and more cost-effective, and may lead to fewer serious complications than parenteral nutrition. A considerable body of evidence leads to the conclusion that enteral nutrition can support gut integrity. For these reasons, enteral nutrition is preferred in patients with at least minimally functional GI tracts.

There are literally hundreds of different enteral formulas available for use in feeding patients with ARF. Choice of formula should be guided by clinical condition, fluid and electrolyte status, and adequacy of dialytic therapy. Patients who are not being dialyzed or are otherwise fluid restricted may be fed using a calorically concentrated formula. These formulas most often contain 2 cal/mL with a reasonable amount of protein, often ranging from 70–80 g/L. If electrolyte control is problematic, several formulas are available that contain reduced amounts of potassium and phosphorus (Table 18.3). However, use of these formulas should be accompanied by close monitoring, as recovery of renal function may lead to normalization of electrolyte status and the need for additional supplementation. Careful evaluation of patient status and electrolyte levels should be made before using restricted formulas, as there is a subset of patients with ARF who may become hypophosphatemic or hypokalemic. If a fluid restriction is not indicated, most standard enteral formulas are appropriate for use.

Enteral feeding can be initiated at 1/4 to 1/2 of goal rate in most patients with ARF and advanced according to tolerance to goal rates, usually within 24 to 48 hours. Advancement of feedings should be guided by signs and symptoms of intolerance, such as abdominal distension, unacceptable gastric residuals, or diarrhea unresponsive to standard medical therapy. As renal function improves, fluid intake may be increased. Daily monitoring of electrolyte levels is recommended until the patient is stable, at which point frequency of electrolyte measurement can be decreased.

Parenteral nutrition should be initiated with close monitoring of fluid and electrolyte status along with frequent monitoring of glucose levels. Insulin can be added to PN solutions in order to maintain blood glucose levels less than 200 mg/dL. Choice of PN solution should be guided by the patient's underlying condition. A balanced solution containing lipids and dextrose either as part of a three-in-one solution or a separate infusion of lipid emulsion is appropriate. As hyperglycemia can be problematic in this population, it would be appropriate to utilize moderate amounts of dextrose in the initial formulation. A conservative recommendation would be to initiate PN with 175–200 g dextrose with amounts advanced to keep blood glucose levels at desired levels.

TABLE 18.3

Comparison of Enteral Formula Categories*

Nutrient	Regular Diet	Standard 2 kcal/cc	Renal 2 kcal/cc	Low Protein Renal 2 kcal/cc
Protein (g/L)	60-80 g/d	75–90	70–75	25–35
Fat (g/L)	varies	90–100	95–100	90–100
Na (mg/L)	2000-4000 mg/d	800–1400	800–1000	0–800
K (mg/L)	2500-3000 mg/d	1600–2000	850–1100	0–1200
P (mg/L)	1000-1200 mg/d	1000–1300	700–800	0–800
Mg (mg/L)	varies		200–220	0–200
Ca (mg/L)	800-1200 mg/d	1000–1300	1100–1400	0–1400

*All values are averaged from several commercially available formulas and are meant to allow comparison between categories.

Conclusions

Patients with ARF continue to have high rates of morbidity and mortality despite advances in the care of critically ill patients. Nutrition support of the patient with ARF presents significant challenges to the nutrition support team. It is imperative that patients with ARF who are critically ill and hypercatabolic be identified as soon as possible so that appropriate nutrition therapy can be initiated. Enteral nutrition should be utilized whenever possible in patients with at least minimally functional GI tracts. Parenteral nutrition should be initiated when enteral nutrition cannot provide substrate to support metabolic processes. Careful attention should be given to monitoring of fluid and electrolyte status, as these patients can have severe abnormalities in levels of several electrolytes along with difficult fluid status.

References

1. Nolan CR, Anderson RJ. Hospital-acquired acute renal failure. *J Am Soc Nephrol.* 1998;9:710–718.
2. Star R. Treatment of acute renal failure. *Kidney Int.* 1998; 54:1817–1831.
3. Manns M, Sigler MH, Teehan BP. Continuous renal replacement therapies: an update. *Am J Kidney Dis.* 1998;32: 185–207.
4. Forni LG, Hilton PJ. Continuous hemofiltration in the treatment of acute renal failure. *New Eng J Med.* 1997;336: 1303–1309.
5. Fiaccadori E, Lombardi M, Leonardi S, et al. Prevalence and clinical outcome associated with preexisting malnutrition in acute renal failure: a prospective cohort study. *J Am Soc Nephrol.* 1999;10:581–593.
6. Owen WF. Nutritional status and survival in end-stage renal disease patients. *Min Elec Metab.* 1998;24:72–81.
7. Gabay C, Kushner I. Acute-phase proteins and other systemic responses to inflammation. *N Engl J Med.* 1999; 340:448–454.
8. Riella MC. Malnutrition in dialysis: Malnourishment or uremic inflammatory response? *Kidney Int.* 2000;57:1211–1232.
9. Lim VS, Kopple JD. Protein metabolism in patients with chronic renal failure: role of uremia and dialysis. *Kidney Int.* 2000;58:1–10.
10. Schneeweiss B, Graninger W, Stockenhuber F, et al. Energy metabolism in acute and chronic renal failure. *Am J Clin Nutr.* 1990;52:596–601.
11. Soop M, Forsberg A, Thorne A. Energy expenditure in postoperative multiple organ failure with acute renal failure. *Clin Nephrol.* 1989;31:139–145.
12. May RC, Clark AS, Goheer MA. Specific defects in insulin-mediated muscle metabolism in acute uremia. *Kidney Int.* 1985;28:490–497.
13. Smith D, DeFronzo RA. Insulin resistance in uremia mediated by postbinding defects. *Kidney Int.* 1982;22:490–497.
14. Riella MC. Nutrition in acute renal failure. *Renal Failure* 1997;19:237–252.
15. Frankenfield DC, Reynolds HN, Wiles CE, et al. Urea removal during continuous hemodiafiltration. *Crit Care Med.* 1994;22:407–412.
16. Navarro JF, Mora C, Leon C, et al. Amino acid losses during hemodialysis with polyacrylonitrile membranes: effect of intradialytic amino acid supplementation on plasma amino acid concentrations and nutritional variables in nondiabetic patients. *Am J Clin Nutr.* 2000;71:765–773.
17. Maxvold NJ, Smoyer WE, Custer FR, et al. Amino acid loss and nitrogen balance in critically ill children with acute renal failure: a prospective comparison between classic hemofiltration and hemofiltration with dialysis. *Crit Care Med.* 2000;28:1161–1165.
18. Wilmore DW. Catabolic illness: strategies for enhancing recovery. *N Engl J Med.* 1991;325:1161–1165.
19. Price SR, Reaich D, Marinovic AC, et al. Mechanisms contributing to muscle wasting in acute uremia: activation of amino acid catabolism. *J Am Soc Nephrol.* 1998;9:439–443.
20. Bergstrom J, Alvestrand A, Furst P. Plasma and muscle free amino acids in maintenance hemodialysis patients without protein malnutrition. *Kidney Int.* 1990;38:104–114.
21. Williams B, Hattersley J, Layward E, et al. Metabolic acidosis and skeletal muscle adaptation to low protein diets in chronic uremia. *Kidney Int.* 1991;40:779–786.
22. Ballmer PE, McNurlan MA, Hulter HN, et al. Chronic metabolic acidosis decreases albumin synthesis and induces negative nitrogen balance in humans. *J Clin Invest.* 1995; 95:39–45.
23. Lim VS, Yarasheski KE, Flanigan MJ. The effect of uraemia, acidosis and dialysis treatment of protein metabolism: a longitudinal leucine kinetic study. *Nephrol Dial Transplant.* 1998;13:1723–1730.
24. Metnitz PGH, Fischer M, Bartens C, et al. Impact of acute renal failure on antioxidant status in multiple organ failure. *Acta Anaesthesiol Scand.* 2000;44:236–240.
25. Druml W, Schwarzenhofer M, Apsner R, Horl WH. Fat-soluble vitamins in patients with acute renal failure. *Miner Electrolyte Metab.* 1998;24:220–226.
26. Wolk R. Micronutrition in dialysis. *Nutr Clin Prac.* 1993;8: 267–277.
27. Palombo JD, Schnure F, Bistrian BR, et al. Improvement of liver function tests by administration of L-Carnitine to a carnitine deficient patient receiving home parenteral nutrition: a case report. *J Parenter Enteral Nutr.* 1987;11:88–92.
28. Bartel LL, Hussey JL, Shrago E. Perturbation of serum carnitine levels in human adults by chronic renal disease and dialysis therapy. *AJCN.* 1981;34:1314–1320.
29. Evans AM, Faull R, Fornasini G, et al. Pharmacokinetics of L-carnitine in patients with end-stage renal disease undergoing long-term hemodialysis. *Clin Pharmacol Ther.* 2000;68:238–249.

30. Druml W. Nutritional support in acute renal failure. In: Mitch WE, Klahr S, eds. *Handbook of Nutrition and the Kidney.* 3rd ed. Philadelphia: Lippincott-Raven; 1998:213–236.

31. Boehm KA, Helms RA, Christensen ML, et al. Carnitine: a review for the pharmacy clinician. *Hosp Pharm.* 1993;9: 847–850.

32. Feinstein EI, Kipple JD, Silberman H, et al. Total parenteral nutrition with high or low nitrogen intakes in patients with acute renal failure. *Kidney Int.* 1983;26:S319–S323.

33. Abel RM, Beck CH, Abbott WM, et al. Improved survival from acute renal failure after treatment with intravenous essential L-amino acids and glucose: results of a prospective double blind study. *N Engl J Med.* 1973;288:695–699.

34. Mouser JF, Hak EB, Kuhl DA, et al. Recovery from ischemic acute renal failure is improved with enteral compared with parenteral nutrition. *Crit Care Med.* 1997;25:1748–1754.

35. Roberts PR, Black KW, Zaloga GP. Enteral feeding improves outcome and protects against glycerol-induced acute renal failure in the rat. *Am J Respir Crit Care Med.* 1997;156:1265–1269.

36. Mokaurzel A, Ament ME, Buchman AL. Renal function of children receiving long term parenteral nutrition. *J Pediatr.* 1991;119:864–868.

37. Buchman AL, Ament ME, Moukarzel A. The impairment of renal function is associated with long term parenteral nutrition. *J Parenter Enteral Nutr.* 1993;17:438–444.

38. Druml W, Fischer M, Sertl S, et al. Fat elimination in acute renal failure: long-chain vs medium-chain triglycerides. *Am J Clin Nutr.* 1992;55:468–472.

CHAPTER 19

Nutritional Aspects of Cardiac Disease

Karl V. Hakmiller, M.D., Mylan C. Cohen, M.D., M.P.H.

INTRODUCTION	219
PREVALENCE	219
CARDIAC METABOLISM	220
ACUTE MYOCARDIAL INFARCTION	220
CONGESTIVE HEART FAILURE	221
CARDIAC CACHEXIA	222
ELECTROLYTE/METABOLIC ABNORMALITIES	223
HYPOKALEMIA	223
HYPERKALEMIA	223
HYPOMAGNESEMIA	223
HYPOCALCEMIA	224
HYPOPHOSPHATEMIA	224
SELENIUM	224
THIAMINE	224
NUTRITIONAL ASSESSMENT	225
NUTRITIONAL RECOMMENDATIONS	225
CARDIAC COMPLICATIONS OF REFEEDING	225
MONITORING PATIENTS WITH CARDIAC DISEASE DURING NUTRITION THERAPY	226
CONCLUSIONS	226
REFERENCES	226

Introduction

The past century has witnessed significant advances in the treatment of acute and chronic illness, including a 50% reduction in coronary artery disease mortality over the last four decades. Despite this progress, or perhaps because of it, cardiovascular disease remains one of the most important causes of morbidity and mortality in Western society.[1] The aging of the population, dietary shifts towards higher fat intake, a more sedentary lifestyle, and continued significant use of tobacco products, combined with the ability of the modern physician to intervene and treat very complex medical conditions, have resulted in more patients with cardiac disease and increasingly complex cardiac problems.

Nutritional and lifestyle changes have been the foundation for cardiovascular care in the outpatient setting but are likely equally important in the hospitalized patient. Acutely ill patients with cardiac disease are frequently faced with nutritional, hemodynamic, metabolic, and neuroendocrine challenges that stress the cardiovascular system.[2–6] Recent evidence has suggested that some patients with acute and chronic myocardial decompensation benefit greatly from careful attention to metabolic and nutritional support. [7–15] The careful practitioner in the modern era should recognize these relationships to be able to provide the best care for his or her patients. It is the purpose of the following discussion to outline recent information concerning nutritional and metabolic factors related to cardiovascular disease. To do so, we will focus on the most common cardiac problems including unstable angina (UA), acute myocardial infarction (MI), and congestive heart failure (CHF), as well as systemic conditions that frequently complicate these problems, including diabetes mellitus, advanced age, renal failure, and metabolic abnormalities.

Prevalence

Cardiac disease is common. Unstable angina accounts for more than 1 million hospital admissions in the United States annually. Acute myocardial infarction accounts for an additional 1.5 million admissions to the hospital, with approximately 30% dying from this diagnosis. Sequelae of these acute events can include CHF, with more than 400,000 to 700,000 new cases diagnosed each year in the United States.[1] Crude prevalence (unadjusted for age) for heart failure ranges from 3 to 20 individuals per 1000, with a prevalence of 30 to 130 individuals per 1000 for those over 65 years of age.[16] Two to three million Americans have CHF at any given time, and this diagnosis represents the leading hospital discharge diagnosis in patients over 65 years old. CHF directly or indirectly contributes to the death of 250,000 patients per year.[16,17]

Cardiac Metabolism

The normally functioning heart requires a constant supply of oxygen and other fuels obtained primarily from the coronary circulation. The delivery of oxygen and fuel sources must be flexible enough to meet the heart's constantly changing energy requirements.[18] Basal requirements of the human heart include the generation of approximately 35 kg of adenosine triphosphate (ATP) daily.[14]

The heart has been termed an "omnivore" because of its capability of using fatty acids, glucose, and other fuel sources depending on changing environmental conditions.[19] A hierarchy of preference of fuel selection favors fatty acids over glucose metabolism.[20] During the fasting state, circulating levels of fatty acids are high and these are used preferentially for oxidative metabolism. This fatty acid metabolism suppresses glucose oxidation resulting in glucose being converted to glycogen. However, in conditions of increased carbohydrate intake resulting in increased glucose and insulin levels, the balance is shifted to glucose oxidation as the primary cardiac fuel. This glucose metabolism, in turn, directly suppresses fatty acid oxidation. Under extreme conditions of a very high fat diet, circulating triglycerides may become the major fuel source for the myocardium. Triglycerides can be broken down to fatty acids that then enter the fatty acid oxidation pathway. During periods of acute, aerobic exercise, lactate becomes a major fuel source and is transported into myocytes for oxidation.[21,22] Lactate produced during exercise in turn inhibits both the oxidation of glucose and free fatty acids (FFA).[18,20,21,22] In situations of starvation or diabetic ketoacidosis, ketone bodies may also contribute significantly to the energy metabolism of the myocardium.[18]

During periods of acute stress, such as ischemia or starvation, there is yet another shift in the heart's preferred metabolic pathway. The limited supply of oxygen occurring during myocardial ischemia triggers a change from predominately FFA metabolism to glucose metabolism.[18] After an acute ischemic event, even with adequate reperfusion, the energy substrate preference may not return immediately to pre-ischemic conditions. A persistent change in energy utilization favoring glucose metabolism may occur that is independent of availability of FFA as a fuel source.[18,23,24]

Acute Myocardial Infarction

Over the past 40 years, there has been an explosion of knowledge related to the understanding of the pathophysiology and treatment of acute coronary syndromes, including MI. Multiple strategies designed to achieve early reperfusion through the use of thrombolytics, aspirin, primary angioplasty, and glycoprotein IIb/IIIa inhibitors have been employed and are undergoing continued study. The focus of nutritional and metabolic interventions has been directed predominately at primary and secondary preventive strategies in coronary artery disease. Lipid reduction and diabetic control have deservedly received much attention and have a great impact on the incidence of initial and recurrent MI. In the acute setting, the concept of metabolic protection or using metabolic substrates for therapy of the ischemic myocardium, which was described more than 35 years ago, has received renewed attention.

Sodi-Pallares et al. reported in 1962 that the systemic administration of a glucose-insulin-potassium (GIK) solution shortened the ECG evolution of an acute MI, reduced ventricular ectopy, and improved early survival following acute MI.[11] This early work was based on the metabolic principal that insulin stimulates potassium reuptake through the activation of the Na^+K^+ ATPase pump and that insulin increases glucose uptake required for glycolytic energy production, the preferred energy pathway in acutely ischemic myocardium. Studies using isolated heart muscle with experimentally created ischemia suggested that GIK solutions decrease infarct size, increase high-energy phosphate levels, and improve ventricular function.[11] Recently proposed additional protective effects of GIK protocols include the ability to minimize both ischemically induced systolic and diastolic dysfunction and to decrease "no-reflow" phenomena after percutaneous reperfusion. These effects may result from increased transport of Ca^{++} into the sarcoplasmic reticulum, improved sodium homeostasis, and restoration of rapidly depleting glycogen reserves.[12,13]

More recently, several large-scale studies have supported the observations made by Sodi-Pallares. The

Diabetes-Insulin-Glucose in Acute Myocardial Infarction (DIGAMI) and Estudios Cardiologicos Latinoamerica (ECLA) trials, as well as a meta-analysis by Fath-Ordoubadi and Beatt of nine smaller trials, suggest that metabolic therapy with GIK type protocols have a potential to significantly reduce mortality associated with acute MI.[7–10]

The DIGAMI study group evaluated mortality in diabetic patients with acute MI. Patients were treated with a glucose-insulin infusion acutely and then aggressively followed using multidose subcutaneous insulin therapy for 3 months (Table 19.1). In the glucose-insulin treatment group there was a trend toward decreased mortality at 3 months that became statistically significant at one year (29% relative reduction in mortality, p=0.027). Subgroup analysis identified a greater benefit in patients without previous insulin therapy and at low cardiovascular risk (in-hospital mortality decreased 58%, p=0.05; 1-year mortality decreased 52%, p=0.02).[8,9]

TABLE 19.1

DIGAMI Protocol[2]	
Infusion: 500 mL 5% glucose with 80 IU of soluble insulin (~1 IU/6 mL)	
Start with 30 mL/h. Check blood glucose after 1 hour. Adjust infusion rate according to protocol and aim for blood glucose of 7 to 10 mmol/L (126-180 mg/dL).	
Blood glucose should be checked after 1 hour if infusion rate has been changed otherwise every 2 hours.	
If the initial decrease in blood glucose exceeds 30%, the infusion rate should be left unchanged if blood glucose is >11 mmol/L (196 mg/dL) and reduced by 6 mL/h if blood glucose is within the target range of 7 to 10.9 mmol/L (126-196 mg/dL).	
If blood glucose is stable and ≤10.9 mmol/L after 10 p.m., reduce infusion rate by 50% during the night.	
Blood Glucose Level and Insulin Titration	
>15 mmol/L (270 mg/dL)	Give 8 IU of Insulin as bolus and increase infusion rate 6 mL/h.
11 to 14.9 mmol/L (198-268 mg/dL)	Increase infusion by 3 mL/h.
7 to 10.9 mmol/L (126-196 mg/dL)	Leave infusion rate unchanged.
4 to 6.9 mmol/L (72-124 mg/dL)	Decrease infusion rate by 6 mL/h.
<4 mmol/L (<72 mg/dL)	Stop infusion for 15 min. Test glucose every 15 min until glucose above 7 mmol/L. In the presence of symptoms of hypoglycemia, administer 20 mL of 30% glucose intravenously. The infusion is restarted with an infusion rate decreased by 6 mL/h when blood glucose >7 mmol/L (125 mg/dL).

The ECLA study group evaluated a GIK protocol in patients admitted within 24 hours of the onset of symptoms of an acute MI. Patients were randomized to either high- or low-dose GIK protocols (Table 19.2) or placebo in addition to standard therapy including various reperfusion strategies. There was a two-thirds reduction in mortality for the GIK infusion arm compared to placebo. The absolute mortality risk decreased from 15.2% to 5.2% (p=0.008). The survival benefit persisted in the high-dose GIK plus reperfusion group out to 1 year.[7]

Finally, Fath-Ordoubadi and Beatt reported the results of their meta-analysis of nine earlier trials of GIK protocols including four trials that used a high-dose GIK regimen. These trials were performed in the pre-thrombolytic era. Mortality appeared to be reduced by 28% overall and by 48% in the trials using the high-dose GIK regimen.[10]

These results suggest that metabolic therapy at the time of acute MI may have benefits comparable to thrombolysis. The results of ECLA and DIGAMI also suggest that the benefits of GIK protocols may be additive to thrombolytic therapy in reducing mortality after reperfusion.

Congestive Heart Failure

Often occurring as a result of coronary artery disease, but frequently a manifestation of other systemic illness, CHF is a common presenting illness or comorbid condition seen in the intensive care unit. Given improved technologies leading to greater survival in coronary artery disease, the increased prevalence in CHF has been termed "the ironic failure of success."[25] Until recently, the major focus of therapy has been on the hemodynamic abnormalities associated with heart failure. More recently a greater appreciation of the neurohormonal response to the failing heart has led to improved understanding of the problem and more effective therapies.[2,3,6,26] Fifty percent of patients with CHF, however, are also malnourished to some de-

TABLE 19.2

ECLA Protocol[1]
High-Dose GIK Infusion
25% glucose, 50 IU soluble insulin per liter and 80 mmol KC/L at an infusion rate of 1.5 mL/(kg· h) over 24 hours.
Low-Dose GIK Infusion
10% glucose, 20 IU soluble insulin per liter and 40 mmol KC/L at an infusion rate of 1.0 mL/(kg· h) over 24 hours.

gree.[27] Furthermore, cachexia is recognized as an independent predictor of higher mortality in patients with chronic heart failure.[28] Recently performed small trials focusing on nutritional support and the manipulation of the putative causes of cachexia in patients with chronic heart failure may point to another therapeutic avenue for this group of patients.[29,30]

The concept of mechanical failure of the heart has been well described.[2,6,26,31,32] Often mechanical failure is defined as either right heart failure (inadequate emptying of the venous reservoirs) or left heart failure (reduced ejection of blood under pressure into the aorta and pulmonary artery). Frequently these entities coexist and lead to the cardinal signs and symptoms of heart failure including pulmonary and peripheral edema, dyspnea, orthopnea, paroxysmal nocturnal dyspnea, and jugular venous distention.[26]

It is clear that neurohormonal responses associated with compensation for a failing heart also contribute to the symptoms and mortality associated with chronic CHF. Salt and water retention, vasoconstriction, and sympathetic nervous system stimulation are initially compensatory mechanisms driven by neurohormonal reflexes leading to increased pre-load, maintenance of blood pressure, and cardiac output.[2,6,33] Over a period of time, however, these compensatory mechanisms become detrimental to the failing heart.[2]

The mainstay of therapy for the management of CHF has included a search for a correctable cause, sodium restriction, angiotensin converting enzyme (ACE) inhibition, beta-blocker therapy, diuretic therapy, digoxin therapy, and oxygen therapy. In heart failure, both decreased renal perfusion and increased beta-adrenergic stimulation lead to angiotensin-related effects including vasoconstriction, increased sympathetic tone, and increased aldosterone production, leading to increased retention of sodium and water. Sympathetic stimulation occurs early in the course of heart failure as a compensatory mechanism and may initially impart a survival benefit. Increased sympathetic tone leads to beta-adrenergic receptor mediated sinus tachycardia and increased inotropy as well as alpha-adrenergic receptor mediated peripheral vasoconstriction. Over time, cardiac beta-receptors are down regulated. Thus any positive inotropic effect from increased sympathetic tone only partially compensates for the failing heart.[2,31,34] Recognition of the role played by the renin-angiotensin system and sympathetic nervous system effects in the development of CHF have led to treatment regimens including ACE inhibitors and beta blockers that have demonstrated significant reductions in mortality.[2,33–37] A recent study with spironolactone to reduce aldosterone production has also shown a beneficial effect in patients with severe heart failure.[38]

Another beneficial hormonal response to chronic heart failure includes the production of atrial natriuretic peptide (ANP), brain natriuretic peptide (BNP), and C-type natriuretic peptide. Circulating levels of natriuretic peptides increase with increasing atrial pressure. Natriuretic peptides vasodilate, inhibit aldosterone secretion, and act as a diuretic. Unfortunately the protective effects of natriuretic peptides are often overcome by the tendency toward vasoconstriction and sodium retention generated by the Renin-angiotensin system.[39]

Cardiac Cachexia

Wasting in association with chronic heart failure has been recognized since antiquity.[4] In the modern era, various criteria have been used to define cachexia in heart failure. Definitions have included body fat content <29% (women) or <27% (men), <80%–85% of ideal body weight or a documented weight loss of at least 10% of lean tissue.[4,40] A more practical approach has been proposed: the diagnosis of "clinical cardiac cachexia" may be applied to "*patients with CHF of at least 6 months duration without signs of other primary cachectic states (e.g., cancer, thyroid disease, or severe liver disease) . . . and when weight loss (over a 6-month period) of >7.5% of previous normal weight is 'observed'.*"[4] The choice of a >7.5% weight loss is arbitrary and the degree of weight loss that most closely correlates with impaired survival is currently being studied.[4] Nevertheless, it is clear that cardiac cachexia is associated with impaired survival. Mortality in cachectic patients is high, having been demonstrated at 18% at 3 months, 29% at 6 months, 39% at 12 months, and 50% at 18 months in one study.[28]

The etiology of cachexia in heart failure is unclear. Mechanisms including cellular hypoxia with increased catabolism, dietary malabsorbtion due to gut edema or decreased perfusion, decreased dietary intake, loss of nutrients through the urinary or digestive tracts, and increased resting metabolic rate have been proposed and all may play a role.[4,41,42,43,44] Evaluation over the past 30 years has failed, however, to identify a single mechanism behind the etiology of cachexia. More recently, the presence of increased levels of tumor necrosis factor alpha (TNF-alpha) have been identified in patients with cardiac cachexia.[45,46] High levels of TNF-alpha have subsequently been confirmed as one of the strongest predictors of weight loss.[47] Other predictors of cachexia may include elevated norepinephrine,

epinephrine, aldosterone, renin activity, and cortisol levels.[4]

A careful weight history should be included in the initial and follow-up evaluations of the patient with heart failure. Dietary consultation should be considered in all cardiac patients. Cardiac rehabilitation should be considered to reverse peripheral muscle atrophy, improve peripheral blood flow, and increase exercise capacity.[4] Intensive nutritional support is particularly important when surgery is contemplated. Otaki found that patients with cardiac cachexia who received preoperative nutritional support for 5 to 8 weeks before cardiac surgery had a lower mortality (17 vs. 57%, p=<.05) compared to those who did not receive support.[15]

Electrolyte/Metabolic Abnormalities

Abnormalities of electrolytes, occurring as a component of heart failure from decreased renal perfusion or drug therapy, are frequent complications in the treatment of cardiac disease.

Hypokalemia

Hypokalemia (<3.0 mEq/L) is a common finding in patients with CHF. Drugs, including loop and thiazide diuretics, may cause a kaliuresis leading to abnormally low serum potassium levels. Diuresis can cause a metabolic alkalosis that drives the intracellular transfer of potassium in exchange for hydrogen ions resulting in an extravascular hypokalemia.[48] Although symptoms of hypokalemia occur when the potassium is less than 3 mEq/L, symptoms are more frequent with a level below 2.7 mEq/L. Cramps, weakness, ileus, nausea, and other nonspecific symptoms may occur.[49] Hypokalemia rarely causes life-threatening arrhythmias by itself. However, hypokalemia may potentiate arrhythmias in the setting of acute MI or in the presence of digitalis therapy. Electrocardiographic changes associated with hypokalemia include prominent U waves, flattened or inverted T waves, and nonspecific ST changes.[49] Oral replacement with 80–120 mEq/d in divided doses for mild to moderate potassium depletion is preferred. Intravenous replacement with less than 100–150 mEq/d (10 mEq/h) if necessary can be given.[48,49,50]

Hyperkalemia

The effects of hyperkalemia depend upon the rate of potassium rise. With a rapid rise in potassium levels, life-threatening tachyarrhythmias may develop, whereas slower changes in potassium may produce bradyarrhythmias. Drugs that impair cellular uptake or renal disposal of potassium such as ACE inhibitors, spironolactone, and digitalis may be associated with the development of hyperkalemia.[51,52] Metabolic acidosis and the development of renal insufficiency are frequent comorbid factors in the development of hyperkalemia.[53] The cardiotoxic effects of hyperkalemia are enhanced in the presence of hypocalcemia, acidosis, and hyponatremia.[49] Signs and symptoms of hyperkalemia are limited primarily to muscle weakness and abnormalities of the cardiac conduction system. Electrocardiographic changes include T wave changes at levels between 5.5–6.5 mEq/L, while at levels greater than 7.0 loss of P waves and widening of the QRS complex occur.[50]

Muscle weakness generally does not begin until levels are greater than 8 mEq/L.[49] The aim of management is to correct both the hyperkalemia and its underlying cause. In general, potassium levels of 5.5 to 6.5 mEq/L can be treated with potassium restriction and potassium exchange resins (e.g., Kayexelate). For potassium >6.5 mEq/L the clinical situation needs to be assessed. Calcium gluconate infusion will be immediately effective and should be followed by glucose-insulin therapy and sodium bicarbonate to shift potassium intracellularly. Treatment with glucose and insulin infusions will start to have an effect in 10–30 minutes. Sodium bicarbonate will lower potassium levels within a hour.[49]

Hypomagnesemia

Magnesium is predominately an intracellular cation and as such, serum magnesium may not correlate well with total body content of magnesium. Serum magnesium may actually be normal despite the presence of magnesium deficiency. The etiology of this disorder is multifactorial and includes disorders of decreased magnesium intake, increased gastrointestinal and renal loss, and miscellaneous entities such as acute pancreatitis and severe burns. Signs and symptoms of hypomagnesemia usually correlate with serum levels of magnesium of less than 1 mEq/L and include anorexia, nausea, altered mentation, carpal and pedal spasm, both supraventricular and ventricular arrhythmias, and prolonged QT interval. Treatment is empiric as the size of the magnesium deficit is hard to estimate. In severe deficiency not more than 100 mEq should be given in any 12-hour period. The rate of intravenous infusion should not exceed 1 mEq/min. Because magnesium is renally excreted, caution must be exercised when magnesium is administered in the presence of renal insufficiency.[49]

Hypocalcemia

Hypocalcemia and its symptoms are related to duration, level, and rate of development. The etiology is diverse but includes malnutrition, hyperphosphatemia, hypoparathyroidism, vitamin D deficiency, magnesium deficiency, acute pancreatitis, various drugs, neoplastic disorders, and renal disease. Acute hypocalcemia may cause decreased cardiac contractility and prolongation of the QT interval. Acutely, treatment can begin with calcium gluconate 10% in 100 cc of D5W administered over 15 minutes followed by intravenous calcium gluconate 10% titrated to maintain a serum calcium of 8 to 8.5 mg/100 mL. Oral calcium supplements can then be started. The maximum rate of calcium gluconate infusion should not exceed 2 mL/min, or not greater than 0.5 mL/min if a patient is receiving digoxin.[49]

Hypophosphatemia

Most of the causes of acute hypophosphatemia are related to shifts of phosphorus into cells. Situations that stimulate glycolysis such as glucose and insulin administration, acute respiratory alkalosis, and epinephrine administration shift phosphorus intracellularly. Profound hypophosphatemia (<1 mg/dL) may result from inadequate intake in patients on hyperalimentation without phosphorus supplementation, refeeding in protein-calorie malnutrition, the recovery phase of severe burns, prolonged treatment with phosphate-binding antacids (aluminum hydroxide), or alcoholism. Symptoms of severe hypophosphatemia include rhabdomyolysis, hemolytic anemia, platelet dysfunction, neurologic dysfunction, muscle weakness, respiratory failure, and congestive cardiomyopathy. Hypophosphatemia specifically leads to decreased left ventricular stroke work, which is reversible with phosphate repletion.

Because phosphorus is predominately an intracellular ion, serum levels may not accurately predict the size of the deficit or response to phosphorus therapy. Therapy for hypophosphatemia therefore is empiric, requiring close monitoring of phosphorus and other electrolytes including specifically calcium, potassium, and sodium. Oral phosphorus replacement may be used in moderate hypophosphatemia (>1 mg/dL) with an initial dose of 1–2 grams of elemental phosphorus. Parenteral replacement may be required in severe hypophosphatemia (<1 mg/dL) and can be achieved with 2.5 to 5.0 mg phosphorus/kg body weight given over 6 hours with a maximum of 7.5 mg phosphorus/kg for patients with normal renal function. Contraindications to IV therapy include hypercalcemia, renal insufficiency, and severe tissue necrosis.[49]

Selenium

Selenium deficiency can occur in patients receiving parenteral nutrition for prolonged periods of time. It has been associated with the development of a dilated cardiomyopathy, muscle weakness, and even death. Congestive symptoms may be prevented or alleviated with appropriate selenium supplementation. Recommended dietary allowances for selenium range between 50–75 mg/d for an adult.[50,51]

Thiamine

Thiamine deficiency in the United States results predominately from decreased thiamine absorption caused by alcoholism. In developing countries that rely on polished rice as a staple, decreased dietary intake of thiamine plays a greater role. Other chronic illnesses such as diabetes and cancer as well as treatments such as long-term parenteral nutrition without thiamine replacement and diuretic therapy have been associated with thiamine deficiency.[54] Furthermore, co-administration of furosemide and digoxin decreases thiamine uptake by cardiac cells.[54]

Symptoms of early thiamine deficiency are nonspecific and include anorexia, irritability, and weight loss. Advanced thiamine deficiency has been classically characterized as predominately involving the cardiovascular system (wet beriberi or beriberi heart disease) or the nervous system (dry beriberi). The diagnostic criteria for "wet beriberi" include: (1) 3 months of documented dietary deficiency of thiamine, (2) associated peripheral neuritis, (3) enlarged heart with normal sinus rhythm (usually tachycardia), (4) non-specific ST and T wave changes, and (5) therapeutic response to thiamine replacement. "Wet beriberi" causes profound peripheral vasodilation and, as a result, high-output failure. Diagnostic testing with urinary thiamine excretion or transketolase activity coefficient may be used, but a therapeutic trial of thiamine, which provides rapid improvement within 24–48 hours, may be regarded as supportive evidence for this diagnosis. Treatment includes 50–100 mg of thiamine administered intravenously or intramuscularly daily for several days followed by oral replacement of 5–10 mg daily.[50]

Nutritional Assessment

As in many acute conditions, the nutritional assessment of the cardiac patient begins with the development of a detailed metabolic and nutritional profile.[55] Deficiency of a single nutrient or metabolic deficiency rarely occurs; rather multiple deficiencies are the norm. An assessment of a patient's nutritional status should be made based on multiple pieces of information, including dietary history, anthropomorphic measurements, laboratory measurements, and clinical exam.[55,56,57,58] Edema associated with cardiac failure may complicate this assessment and it is best to establish this nutritional profile after edematous fluid has been reduced or eliminated.

A detailed dietary history may be difficult to obtain from certain patient sub-groups including those who are acutely ill, elderly or demented. Poverty, social isolation, dysphagia, nausea, poorly fitting dentures, impaired short-term memory, complicated drug therapy, depression, and alcoholism all increase the risk for malnutrition and metabolic abnormalities.[50] Certain key questions and clues from the medical and social history may alert the physician to nutritional deficiencies. Incorporating a team approach using a clinical dietician further improves this assessment.[56]

Anthropomorphic measurements including height, weight, body-mass index, triceps skin fold thickness and mid-arm muscle area at one point in time may be useful indicators of nutritional status and have been used extensively in cross-sectional and prospective analyses.[50,59] Amount and rate of weight loss may be more indicative of risk for malnutrition. Triceps skin fold estimates the body's stored fat reserves and mid-arm muscle area is used to estimate lean body muscle mass.[50]

A number of laboratory measurements have been used to assess nutritional status and, while useful, have to be interpreted carefully as they may be influenced by other non-nutritional conditions. Commonly, hemoglobin, serum protein, albumin, pre-albumin, urinary creatinine excretion, creatinine-height index, lymphocyte count, and impaired delayed hypersensitivity reaction have been used. The value of any one parameter in predicting outcome is unproven and each should be viewed in the context of all the other clinical data available.[50,53]

Nutritional Recommendations

Planning nutritional replacement for the malnourished cardiac patient should involve the following: (1) careful estimation of energy requirements using the indirect calorimetry, Harris-Benedict equation, or thermodilution technique (Fick Method) [54,60,61]; (2) minimization of fluid retention; (3) aggressive repletion of nitrogen, phosphorus, potassium, and magnesium; and (4) careful assessment of weight changes.

Most hospitalized patients do not require replacement of calories greater than their estimated basal requirement based on their usual weight. The most commonly used formula for determining energy requirements is the Harris-Benedict equation.[55,60,61] In ambulatory patients, the basal requirements are estimated at two-thirds of total caloric need. The Harris-Benedict equation may underestimate the basal metabolic requirement by 10%–20% in malnourished patients and overestimate in the obese.[55,60,61,62]

Protein needs are affected by many factors including metabolic rate, caloric intake, nutritional status, age, and body protein reserves. During acute physiologic stress the goal of nutritional therapy is directed at supplying enough protein to maintain the accelerated rate of protein synthesis. The optimal therapeutic range of protein supplementation to offset nitrogen losses during this period is narrow. In normal individuals approximately 8% of the required calories are provided as protein while the hypermetabolic patient may require 16%–20% to maintain a positive nitrogen balance. A ratio of 1 to 1.5 g of protein/kg ideal body weight/d with a nitrogen-to-calorie ratio of 1:120 to 1:150 is desirable. A ratio of 1:200 in patients with cardiac cachexia may be preferable.[50]

With parenteral replacement glucose is the principal energy source. For the acutely ill patient with cardiac disease, it is best to deliver the glucose solution in a slow, gradual manner with careful attention to amount of volume and sodium concomitantly infused. While infusion rates of 4 mg/kg/min may be desirable, starting out at the endogenous hepatic glucose production rate of 2 mg/kg/min and titrating upward may decrease stress on a compromised heart.

Cardiac Complications of Refeeding

The normal physiologic response to nutritional replacement may actually transiently worsen cardiac function. Refeeding stimulates the sympathetic nervous system leading to increased heart rate, oxygen consumption, increased sodium re-absorption, and arrhythmias. Mobilization of electrolytes intracellularly, especially phosphorous, may precipitate an acute drop in serum levels leading to life-threatening arrhythmias, respiratory failure and neurological changes.[63] A hyper-insulinemic state caused by the administration of hypertonic glucose may cause further sodium retention, as insulin is a potent antidiuretic hormone. In patients with pre-existing cardiac disease, refeeding, therefore, may predispose patients to CHF and sudden death.[50]

Right-sided CHF may be difficult to distinguish from benign refeeding edema. The cause of benign refeeding edema is unclear but may be related to changes in renal sodium excretion, increased serum insulin, and poor venous tone. Treatment for this condition includes compression stockings, elevation of dependent areas, and modest sodium restriction.[50]

Monitoring Patients with Cardiac Disease during Nutrition Therapy

Routine monitoring of nutritional and metabolic parameters after an initial nutritional assessment in cardiac patients in the intensive care unit is essential. This should include daily evaluation of weight, fluid balance, and electrolytes (including, as deemed necessary, magnesium, phosphorus, and calcium). In an era in which GIK/DIGAMI protocols are being considered for adjuvant treatment for acute myocardial ischemia, this issue will assume a greater role. Periodic reassessment of nutritional status including additional laboratory investigation with albumin and pre-albumin should be considered. Coordination with a clinical dietician early in the course of the illness is recommended. In patients with significant electrolyte abnormalities, evidence of ischemia or significant cardiomyopathy at baseline, serial electrocardiograms and telemetry monitoring should be considered. QT prolongation has been associated with severe malnourishment and patients with QT prolongation should undergo continuous monitoring during the initial stages of nutritional therapy in the hospital.[51,64] In patients with evidence of significant malnutrition, 2D echocardiography should be considered to assess cardiac function. Hemodynamic monitoring with Swan-Ganz catheters may be useful in differentiating low- versus high-output heart failure and benign refeeding edema versus right heart failure as well as directing treatment for CHF.[50]

Conclusions

Careful attention to the nutritional and metabolic parameters associated with the acutely ill cardiac patient is essential to effective management. This is particularly important in patients in whom cachexia is part of the syndrome. Nutritional therapy, like all therapies, is not without risks. Understanding these risks as well as treatment options is essential to provide clinically effective nutritional and metabolic therapy for patients with cardiac disease.

References

1. American Heart Association. *2000 Heart and Stroke Statistical Update*. Dallas, TX; 1999.
2. Packer M. The neurohormonal hypothesis: a theory to explain the mechanism of disease progression in heart failure. *J Am Coll Cardiol.* 1992;20:248–254.
3. Schrier RW, Abraham WT. Mechanisms of Disease: hormones and hemodynamics in heart failure. *N Eng J Med.* 1999;341: 577–585.
4. Anker SD, Coats AJS. Cardiac cachexia: a syndrome of impaired survival and immune and neuroendocrine activation. *Chest.* 1999;115:836–847.
5. Anker SD, Rauchbaus M. Heart failure as a metabolic problem. *Eur J Heart Failure.* 1999;1:127–131.
6. Heart Failure Society Guidelines: A model of consensus and excellence. *J Cardiac Failure.* 1999;5:358–382.
7. Diaz R, Paolasso EA, Piegas LS, et al. Metabolic modulation of acute myocardial infarction: the ECLA glucose-insulin-potassium pilot trial. *Circulation.* 1998;98:2227–2234.
8. Malmberg K, Ryden L, Efendic S, et al. Randomized trial of insulin-glucose infusion followed by subcutaneous insulin treatment in diabetic patients with acute myocardial infarction (DIGAMI Study): effect on mortality at 1 year. *J Am Coll Cardiol.* 1995;26:57–65.
9. Malmberg K, for the DIGAMI (Diabetes Mellitus, Insulin Glucose Infusion in Acute Myocardial Infarction) Study Group. Prospective randomized study of intensive insulin treatment on long term survival after acute myocardial infarction in patients with diabetes mellitus. *Br Med J.* 1997; 314:1512–1515.
10. Fath-Ordoubadi F, Beatt KJ. Glucose-insulin-potassium therapy of treatment of acute myocardial infarction: an overview of randomized placebo-controlled trials. *Circulation.* 1997;96:1152–1156.
11. Sodi-Pallares D, Testelli M, Fishleder F, et al. Effects of an intravenous infusion of a potassium-glucose-insulin solution on the electrocardiographic signs of myocardial infarction. *Am J Cardiol.* 1962;9:166–181.
12. Apstein CS. Glucose-insulin-potassium in acute myocardial infarction: the time has come for a large, prospective trial. *Circulation.* 1997;96:1074–1077.
13. Lazar HL. Enhanced preservation of acutely ischemic myocardium and improved clinical outcomes using glucose-insulin-potassium (GIK) solutions. *Am J Cardiol.* 1997;80(3A):90A-93A.
14. Taegtmeyer H. Energy metabolism of the heart: from basic concepts to clinical applications. *Curr Prob Cardiol.* 1994;19:59–113.

15. Otaki M. Surgical treatment of patients with cardiac cachexia: an analysis of factors affecting operative mortality. *Chest.* 1994:105:1347–1351.
16. Cowie MR, Mosterd DA, Wood DA. The epidemiology of heart failure. *Eur Heart J.* 1997:18:208–225.
17. Kannel WB, Ho K, Thom T. Changing epidemiological features of cardiac failure. *Br Heart J.* 1994;72:S3–9.
18. Opie, L. *The Heart Physiology, from Cell to Circulation.* 3rd Ed., Philadelphia: Lippincott-Raven. 1998:295–302.
19. Taegtmeyer H. Carbohydrate interconversions and energy production. *Circulation.* 1985;72(suppl IV):1–8.
20. Taegtmeyer H, Goodwin G, Doenst T, et al. Substrate metabolism as a determinant for post-ischemic functional recovery of the heart. *Am J Cardiol.* 1997;80:3A-10A.
21. Zorzano A, Sevilla L, Camps M, et al. Regulation of glucose transport, and glucose transporters expression and trafficking in the heart: studies on cardiac myocytes. *Am J Cardiol.* 1997;80: 65A-76A.
22. Halestrap A, Wang X, Poole R, et al. Lactate transport in heart in relation to myocardial ischemia. *Am J Cardiol.* 1997;80:17A-25A.
23. Barger P, Kelly D. Fatty acid utilization in the hypertrophied and failing heart: molecular regulatory mechanisms. *Am J Med Sci.* 1999:318:36–42.
24. Lopashuk GD. Alterations in fatty acid oxidation during reperfusion of the heart after myocardial ischemia. *Am J Cardiol.* 1997;80:11A-16A.
25. Beamish RE. Heart failure: the ironic failure of success. *Can J Cardiol.* 1994;10:603.
26. Katz AM. Cardiomyopathy of overload: a major determinant of prognosis in congestive heart failure. *N Engl J Med.* 1990;322:100–110.
27. Carr JG, Stevenson LW, Walden JA, et al. Prevalence and hemodynamic correlates of malnutrition in severe congestive heart failure secondary to ischemic or idiopathic cardiomyopathy. *Am J Cardiol.* 1989; 3:709–713.
28. Anker SD, Ponikowski P, Varney S, et al. Wasting as independent risk factor for mortality in chronic heart failure. *Lancet.* 1997;349:1050–1053.
29. Mann DL, Young JB. Basic mechanisms in congestive heart failure: recognizing the role of proinflammatory cytokines. *Chest.* 1994;105:897–904.
30. Bozkurt B, Torre-Amione G. TNF antagonism in heart failure. *Circulation.* 2001;103:1044–1047.
31. Opie L. Compensation and overcompensation in congestive heart failure. *Am Heart J.* 1990;120:1552–1557.
32. Anand IS, Ferrar R, Kalra GS, et al. Edema of cardiac origin: studies of body water and sodium, renal function, hemodynamic indexes, and plasma hormones in untreated congestive cardiac failure. *Circulation.* 1989;80:299–305.
33. Krum H. Sympathetic activation and the role of betablockers in chronic heart failure. *Aust NZ J Med.* 1999;29: 418–427.
34. Cody RJ. The sympathetic nervous system and the renin angiotensin aldosterone system in cardiovascular disease. *Am J Cardiol.* 1997;80(9B):9J-14J.
35. Ahjalmarson A, Goldstein S, Fagerberg B, et al. Effects of controlled-release metoprolol, hospitalization and well being in patients with heart failure. *JAMA.* 2000;283:1295–1397.
36. CIBIS Investigators, The cardiac insufficiency bisoprolol study II (CIBIS II): a randomized trial. *Lancet.* 1999;353: 9–13.
37. Richardson M, Cockburn N, Cleland J. Update of recent clinical trials in heart failure and myocardial infarction. *Eur J Heart Failure.* 1999;1:109–115.
38. Pitt B, Zannad F, Remme WJ, et al. (RALES Investigators). The effect of spironolactone on morbidity and mortality in patients with severe heart failure. *N Eng J Med.* 1999;34:709–717.
39. Chen H, Burnett J. The natriuretic peptides in heart failure: diagnostic and therapeutic potentials. *Proc Assoc Am Physicians.* 1999;111:406–416.
40. Freeman LM, Roubenoff R. The nutritional implications of cardiac cachexia. *Nutr Rev.* 1994;52:340–347.
41. Pittman JG, Cohen P. The pathogenesis of cardiac cachexia. *N Eng J Med.* 1964;271:403–409, 453–460.
42. Anker SD, Ponikowski PP, Clark AL, et al. Cytokines and neurohormones relating to body composition alterations in the wasting syndrome of chronic heart failure. *Eur Heart J.* 1999:20:683–693.
43. Poehlman ET, Scheffers J, Gottlieb SS, et al. Increased resting metabolic rate in patients with congestive heart failure. *Ann Intern Med.* 1994;121:860–862.
44. Riley M, Elborn JS, McKane WR, et al. Resting energy expenditure in chronic heart failure. *Clin Sci.* 1991;80:633–639.
45. Levine B, Kalman J, Mayer L, et al. Elevated circulating levels of tumor necrosis factor in severe chronic heart failure. *N Engl J Med.* 1990;323:236–241.
46. McMurray J, Abdullah I, Dargie H, et al. Increased concentrations of tumor necrosis factor in "cachectic" patients with severe chronic heart failure. *Br Heart J.* 1991;66:356–358.
47. Anker SD, Chua TP, Ponikowski P, et al. Hormonal changes and catabolic/anabolic imbalance in chronic heart failure and their importance of cardiac cachexia. *Circulation.* 1997;96:526–534.
48. Gennari FJ. Current concepts: hypokalemia. *New Eng J Med.* 1998;339:451–458.
49. Kammerer WS, Gross RJ, eds. *Medical Consultation: The Internist on Surgical, Obstetric and Psychiatric Services*, 2nd ed. Baltimore: Williams & Wilkins; 1990:209–229.
50. Wyngaarden J, Smith L, Bennett JC eds. *Cecil Textbook of Medicine*, 19th ed. Philadelphia: WB Saunders; 1996:517, 518, 1148–1158, 1172.
51. Holben DH, Smith AM. The diverse role of selenium within selenoproteins: a review. *J Am Diet Assoc.* 1999;99: 836–843.
52. Perazella MA, Mahnensmith RL. Hyperkalemia in the elderly: drugs exacerbate impaired potassium homeostasis. *J Gen Intern Med.* 1997;12:646–656.

53. Acker CG, Johnson JP, Plevsky PM, et al. Hyperkalemia in hospitalized patients: causes, adequacy of treatment, and results of an attempt to improve physician compliance with published therapeutic guidelines. *Arch Int Med.* 1998; 158:917–924.
54. Seligman H, Halkin H, Rauchfleisch S, et al. Thiamine deficiency in patients with congestive heart failure receiving long term furosemide therapy: a pilot study. *Am J Med.* 1991;91:151–155.
55. Fung E. Estimating energy expenditure in critically ill adults and children. *AACN Clin Issues.* 2000;11:480–497.
56. Gales B, Gales M. Nutritional support teams: a review of comparative trials. *Ann Pharmacother.* 1994;28:227–235.
57. Souba W. Nutritional support. *N Eng J Med.* 1997;336: 41–48.
58. Bistrian BR, Blackburn GL, Vitale J, et al. The prevalence of malnutrition in general medical patients. *JAMA.* 1976;235:1567–1570.
59. Frankenfield DC, Muth ER, Rowe WA. The Harris-Benedict studies of human basal metabolism: history and limitations. *J Am Diet Assoc.* 1998;98:439–445.
60. Williams SR, Jones E, Bell W, et al. Body habitus and coronary heart disease in men: a review with reference to methods of body habitus assessment. *Eur Heart J.* 1997;18: 376–393.
61. Flancbaum L, Choban PS, Sambucco S, et al. Comparison of indirect calorimetry, the Fick method, and predictive equations in estimating the energy requirements of critically ill patients. *Am J Clin Nutr.* 1999;69:461–466.
62. Ahmad A, Duerksen DR, Munroe S, et al. An evaluation of resting energy expenditure in hospitalized, severely underweight patients. *Nutrition.* 1999;15:384–388.
63. Kohn MR, Golden NH, Shenker IR. Cardiac arrest and delerium: presentations of the refeeding syndrome in severely malnourished adolescents with anorexia nervosa. *J Adolesc Health.* 1998;22:239–243.
64. Swenne I, Larsson P. Heart risk associated with weight loss in anorexia nervosa and eating disorders: risk factors for QTC interval prolongation and dispersion. *Acta-Pediatr.* 1999;88:304–309.

CHAPTER

20

Nutritional Support of Trauma Patients

Rosemary A. Kozar, M.D., Ph.D., Margaret M. McQuiggan, M.S., R.D., C.S.M., Frederick A. Moore, M.D.

INTRODUCTION 229

ENTERAL ROUTE PREFERRED 230

IMMUNE ENHANCING DIETS 231

ENTERAL NUTRITION PROTOCOL 232
- Rationale 232
- Patient Selection 233
- Enteral Access 233
- Formula Selection 234
- Feeding Protocol 235
- Monitoring Tolerance and Managing Intolerance 235
- Nutritional Assessment 237
- Co-Morbid Disease Assessment 237
- Patient Specific Goals 238

TOTAL PARENTERAL NUTRITION 238

ACUTE RENAL FAILURE 239

MONITORING RESPONSE TO SUPPORT 239

COMPLICATIONS 240
- Refeeding Syndrome 240
- Hyperglycemia 240
- Catheter Related Sepsis 240
- Jejunostomy-Related Complications 240
- Nonocclusive Bowel Necrosis 240

CONTROVERSIES 241
- Bioimpedance 241
- Hypocaloric Feeding 241
- Glutamine Supplementation 241

CASE STUDY 241

REFERENCES 242

Introduction

In the early 1970s, a new syndrome of multiple organ failure (MOF) emerged in trauma intensive care units (ICUs) as a result of the ability to keep patients alive with advanced technology.[1] A consistent association was noted between MOF and late nosocomial infections, and it was concluded that MOF occurred primarily as a result of uncontrolled infection.[2,3] At the same time other investigators noted that MOF patients were prone to develop acute protein malnutrition as a result of persistent hypermetabolism,[4] which compromised the immune response and increased the risk of late MOF-associated nosocomial infections. Thus, it was proposed that early administration of exogenous substrates to meet the increased metabolic demands would prevent or slow the development of acute protein malnutrition and improve patient outcome.

At this time total enteral nutrition (TEN) was preferred over total parenteral nutrition (TPN) because it was less expensive, safer, and more convenient. The gut was thought to be a dormant organ early after severe trauma and thus initiation of TEN was delayed until the gut was clearly functioning. However, by the late 1970s a better understanding of shock resuscitation provided the rationale for earlier nutritional support (Chapter 2). By the early 1980s, TPN had become widely available and safer. Additionally, central venous catheterization had become routine in ICU patients. TPN was promoted to be a great advance in perioperative care and early administration (preferably preoperatively) was widely practiced.[5,6] Thus, TPN became the preferred route in severely injured ICU patients. However, by the mid-1980s research offered compelling physiologic advantages favoring TEN. Substrates delivered enterally appeared to be better utilized[7,8] and did not produce the hyperglycemia associated with TPN.[9,10] In animal models comparing TEN to TPN, TEN prevented gut mucosal atrophy, attenuated the stress response, maintained immunocompetence, and preserved gut flora.[11–17] Moreover, the gut became recognized as metabolically active, immunologically important, and bacteriologically decisive in critically ill patients.[18–20] Thus, by the end of the 1980s there was a renewed interest in TEN. Over the decade of the 1990s considerable amount of information concerning the relationship between nutritional support, gut function and MOF emerged.[21,22] As a result, an alternative paradigm has been proposed (Figure 20.1). Following a traumatic insult patients are resuscitated into a state of hyperinflamation (now called systemic inflammatory response syndrome [SIRS]), which if severe, can precipitate early MOF. As time proceeds, certain aspects of SIRS are downregulated to minimize autogenous tissue injury. This counter anti-inflammatory response (CARS) results in delayed immunosuppression, which, when severe, can contribute to late MOF-associated infections. Simultaneously, for a variety of reasons (i.e., ischemia/reperfusion; laparotomy; standard ICU therapies including H_2 antagonists, narcotics and broad spectrum antibiotics; and disuse of the gut) the gut becomes dysfunctional. This is characterized by progressive ileus, colonization of the normally sterile upper gut, increased mucosal permeability, and decreased local gut immunity. Depressed gut immunity worsens systemic immunosuppression. Additionally, gut flora disseminate systemically by aspiration or translocation to become the pathogens that cause late infection. In addition to preventing acute protein malnutrition, early TEN (most recently with immune enhancing diets) appears to promote normal gut function and enhance systemic immune responsiveness, thereby preventing nosocomial infections.

The purpose of this chapter is to briefly review: (1) clinical trials supporting the early use of the enteral route, (2) trauma trials supporting the use of immune enhancing diets in high risk patients, (3) our current enteral nutrition protocol, and (4) complications and controversies relevant to trauma ICU patients.

Enteral Route Preferred

There were three single institutional prospective randomized controlled trials (PRCTs) and one meta-analysis published in the late 1980s and early 1990s that had a significant impact on clinical practice in trauma ICUs[9,23–25] (Table 20.1). The first study was published in 1986.[23] Trauma patients requiring an emergency laparatomy with abdominal trauma index (ATI) >15 were randomized. The study group (n=31) received early TEN (within 12 hours post-operatively) via needle catheter jejunostomy (NCJ), and the control group (n=32) received delayed TPN, which was started on day 6 if oral intake was inadequate (30% received TPN). Patients who received the early TEN

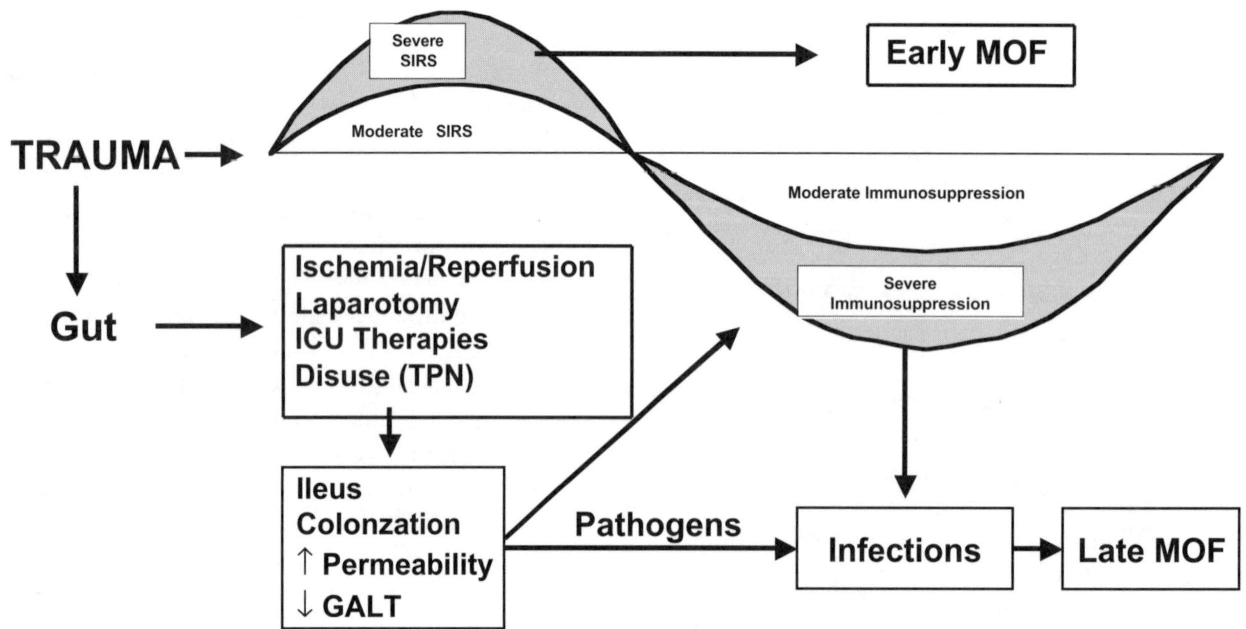

Figure 20.1

Conceptual Framework for the Role of the Gut in Late MOF. MOF=Multiple Organ Failure

TABLE 20.1

Septic Morbidity of TEN vs. TPN			
Moore et al.[23] 1986	**TEN**	**No nutrition first 5 days**	**p value**
Number of patients	31	32	
Major infections	3 (9%)	9 (29%)	<0.05
Moore et al.[9] 1989	**TEN**	**TPN**	
Number of patients	29	30	
Major infections	1 (3%)	6 (20%)	<0.05
Minor infections	4 (14%)	5 (17%)	NS
Kudsk et al.[24] 1992	**TEN**	**TPN**	
Number of patients	51	45	
Major infections	8 (14%)	14 (38%)	<0.05
Minor infections	4 (8%)	10 (22%)	NS
Meta analysis			
Moore et al.[25] 1992	**TEN**	**TPN**	
Number of patients	118	112	<0.05
Infectious complications	19 (16%)	39 (35%)	

had better nitrogen balance, higher lymphocyte counts, and fewer major infections. In a second follow-up study by the same group published in 1989, patients found to have an ATI of 15 to 40 were randomized to receive early TEN via a NCJ (n=29) or early TPN (n=30), which was formulated to be comparable to the enteral diet.[9] Despite a slight advantage in protein-caloric intake with TPN, there was no significant difference in nitrogen balance. In regards to clinical outcome, there was a significant decrease in the incidence of major infections (one [3%] patient in the TEN group versus six [20%] in the TPN group). A different group of investigators confirmed these observations in a trial published in 1992.[24] Patients with an ATI >15 were randomized to receive early TEN via NCJ or Witzel jejunostomy (<24 hrs, n=51) or early TPN (n=45) with a comparably formulated TPN solution. Patients randomized to receive TEN experienced significantly fewer major septic complications than did patients receiving TPN (TEN=14% vs. TPN=38%). Additionally, TPN patients experienced a significantly higher incidence of catheter related sepsis (TEN=2% vs. TPN=14%). In the same year a meta-analysis was published that combined data from eight PRCTs (six published, two not published) conducted to assess the nutritional equivalence of TEN compared to TPN in high-risk trauma and/or postoperative patients.[25] The same enteral formula was compared to similar TPN formulations, and septic complications were recorded prospectively by similar definitions. The eight studies contributing data enrolled 230 patients; 118 were randomized to TEN and 112 to TPN. One or more infections developed in twice as many TPN as TEN patients (TPN=35% vs. TEN=16%). When patients with catheter-related sepsis were removed from the analysis, a significant difference in infections between groups remained (TEN=16% vs. TPN=35%). Taken together, the above PRCTs provide convincing evidence that TEN is preferred to TPN in patients sustaining major torso trauma.

Immune Enhancing Diets

The above-described PRCTs documenting improved outcomes with enteral nutrition utilized elemental formulas. More recent trials suggest that additional benefits can be achieved by utilizing polymeric immune enhancing diets (IEDs). IEDs include a variety of potential immune enhancing agents, though the individual contributions of each have not been well investigated. Glutamine is acknowledged to be the preferred fuel of the enterocyte, and stimulates lymphocyte and monocyte function.[26] It also promotes protein synthesis and is a precursor for nucleotides as well as glutathione. Arginine is a semi-essential amino acid that promotes collagen synthesis required in wound healing and increases the number of total lymphocytes as well as the proportion of helper T cells. It also is a powerful secretagogue, increasing the production of growth hormone, prolactin, somatostatin, insulin, and glucagon. Additionally, arginine is the chief precursor of nitrous oxide[27] and has been shown to enhance delayed cutaneous hypersensitivity and lymphocyte blastogenesis.[28] Although traditional enteral products contain a high proportion of omega-6 polyunsaturated fatty acid (PUFA), diets with a low omega-6 PUFA and high omega-3 PUFA content more favorably alter the fatty acid composition of membrane phospholipids toward reduced inflammation.[29] Finally, nucleotides (purines and pyrimidines) are needed for DNA and RNA synthesis and may be necessary in stressed states to maintain rapid cell proliferation and responsiveness.[30] In the setting of increased demand, most tissues can increase intracellular de novo synthesis of nucleotides. Lymphocytes and enterocytes, however, rely on increased salvage from the extracellular pool which may be depleted during stress.

There are currently a number of commercially available formulas that contain two or more of these agents. Two formulas have been to shown in clinical studies to improve patient outcome (principally reduced infections and improved wound healings). The others have not been adequately tested and are dissimilar enough from the tested formulas that no conclusions can be made about their use in trauma patients. At present, there are 18 published PRCTs that have tested the efficiency and safety of IEDs in a variety of clinical settings.[31] Sixteen (89%) have demonstrated improved patient outcome with the use of IEDs. These data have been analyzed by meta-analysis and demonstrate improved patient outcome.[32–34] Five of these studies have been performed in trauma patients (Table 20.2).[35–39] The first study by Brown et al.[35] documented that patients who received the IED had fewer nosocomial infections (16% vs. 56%) than those randomized to the standard enteral diets (SED). This study, however, has several methodologic flaws including (1) non-specific entry criteria, (2) TEN was started late (IED=3.5 days vs. SED=5.0 days), and (3) patients who received the IED had more jejunostomy tubes and were fed earlier. The second study, a multicenter study by Moore et al.[36] showed a reduction in intra-abdominal abscesses (IED=0% vs. SED 11%) and MOF (IED=0% vs. SED=11%) in patients receiving the IED. This study has been criticized because the control group received Vivonex TEN® (Sandoz Nutrition, Minneapolis, MN), which had a lower nitrogen content than the IED. This concern was addressed in a follow-up by Kudsk et al.[37] who used the same IED but the control diet was isonitrogenous and polymeric. The results showed a similar reduction in intra-abdominal abscess (IED=6% vs. SED=35%) as well as a decrease in days of therapeutic antibiotic usage and length of hospital stay. The fourth study by Mendez et al.[38] failed to demonstrate any outcome improvement and suggested that the IED may exacerbate organ failure. This study had several methodologic flaws including (1) TEN was started late, (2) there was a 25% dropout rate, and (3) the IED and SED groups were not comparable. The IED patients were a decade younger (IED=25 vs. SED=35 years) and prior to starting TEN, they had a higher incidence of ARDS (IED=31% vs. SED=14%). The last study by Wei-

TABLE 20.2

Immune Enhancing Diets

Author Evaluable	# enrolled/ with IED	Study IED Outcome	Control SED	Results	Improved
Brown[35] 1994	41/37 (Isonitrogenous)	Noncommercial ↓ Late Infection	Polymeric	↑ Immunity	? Yes
Moore[36] 1994	105/98 ↓ IAI	Immun-Aid ↓ MOF	Elemental	↑ Immunity Yes	
Kudsk[37] 1996	37/35 (Isonitrogenous)	Immun-Aid ↓Antibiotics	Polymeric ↓ Length of stay	↓ Infections Yes	
Mendez[38] 1997	59/43	Noncommercial	Polymeric	↑ ARDS	No
Weimann[39] 1998	32/39 (Isonitrogenous)	Impact ↓ MOF	Noncommercial	↓ SIRS ? Yes	

PRCTs=prospective randomized controlled trials; IED=immune enhancing diet; SED=standard enteral diet; IAI=intra-abdominal infections; ARDS=acute respiratory distress syndrome; SIRS=systemic inflammatory response syndrome; MOF=multiple organ failure.

mann et al.[9] demonstrated a decrease in the number of days of SIRS and a decrease in MOF. Analysis of these individual studies provides convincing evidence that IEDs provide additional benefits compared to SEDs in patients sustaining major torso trauma.

Enteral Nutrition Protocol

RATIONALE

The above studies demonstrate that trauma patients benefit from receiving early TEN. Unfortunately, the majority of clinicians today lack specific training and experience in administering TEN. Current feeding protocols were empirically developed in centers to perform studies in specific subgroups of high-risk patients. When clinicians apply these protocols to broader groups of patients, not surprisingly they are less successful. But more disturbingly, there are case reports of nonocclusive bowel necrosis that suggest that early TEN may be harmful to certain patients. The clinical presentation of this devastating complication is similar to neonatal necrotizing enterocolitis (NEC). Like NEC, the pathogenesis of nonocclusive bowel necrosis is undoubtedly multifactorial. However, the consistent association with TEN indicates that inappropriate administration of nutrients into a dysfunctional gut plays a pathogenic role. A clinical protocol to provide early TEN with multidisciplinary input was therefore devised at our university-based teaching hospital and initiated in 1997.[40] The protocol markedly streamlines the decision-making process related to enteral feeding, decreases delay time in the initiation and advancement of feedings, and is a multi-disciplinary learning tool.

PATIENT SELECTION

Identification of patients who are candidates for nutritional support is based on the American Society for Parenteral and Enteral Nutrition's (A.S.P.E.N.) guidelines.[41] Potential candidates are identified within the first day of ICU admission and early enteral nutrition begun in high risk patients.

ENTERAL ACCESS (FIGURE 20.2)

Clinical experience and experimental evidence demonstrate that gastric motility is frequently attenuated after severe injury, particularly in neurologic injury.[42–44] Studies specifically addressing the optimal site for enteral feedings in trauma patients in general are limited.[45] Based on a review of the literature and our experience, we believe that to achieve adequate amounts of

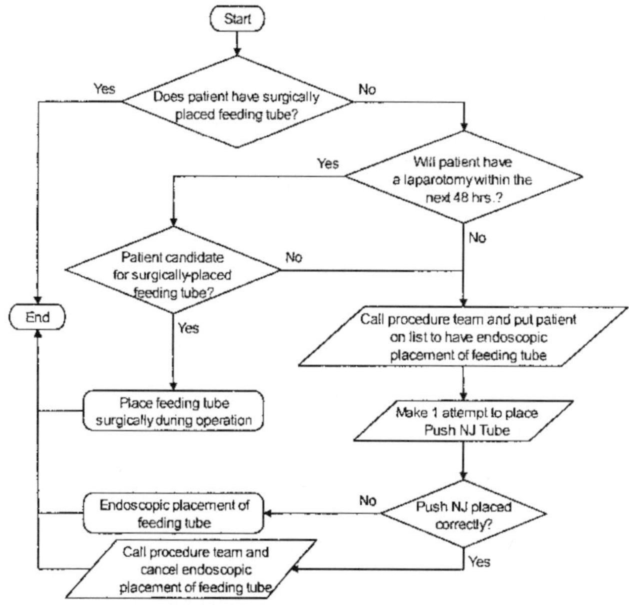

Figure 20.2

Enteral Feeding Access

early TEN, it is best delivered into the proximal small intestine. We have developed a protocol to ensure early jejunal access (Table 20.3). Enteral feeding access should be obtained at the time of initial laparotomy. We believe that the needle catheter jejunostomy (NCJ) is the preferred method of access and use a commercially available kit that contains a silastic 7 French catheter.[46] If the patient undergoes an abbreviated laparotomy with a temporary abdominal closure, the NCJ can be placed during a subsequent operation, ideally within the first 48 hours after injury. Critically injured patients who do not undergo immediate laparotomy have a nasojejunal (NJ) tube placed, preferably in the first 24 hours after injury. This procedure is first attempted by the bedside nurse who is permitted one chance to blindly place a "Push" NJ tube (Corpak Medsystems, Wheeling, IL). This is successful in approximately half of cases. The ICU Procedure Team is consulted in the failures to place the NJ tube endoscopically.[47] This commonly requires less than 10 minutes to complete. The technique involves passage of an 8 French nasobiliary drainage catheter (Wilson, Winston-Salem, NC) through the biopsy channel of a flexible endoscope that has been advanced into the duodenum.[48] Nasojejunal feeding can be done indefinitely, but if the need for long-term access becomes apparent, it will be converted into a jejunal extension tube through a percutaneous endoscopic gastrostomy (PEG-J). An occasional patient may have a contraindication to upper gastrointestinal endoscopy. Examples of such patients include those with penetrating trauma to the pharynx or cervical esophagus, or massive hemorrhage following complex maxillofacial/mandibular fractures. In such patients a jejunostomy tube can be easily placed laparoscopically.

FORMULA SELECTION

Our criteria for selection of general formula for nutritional support (Table 20.3) are as follows:

Immune Enhancing Diet

Patients who have sustained major torso trauma and who are at known risk for septic complications and MOF. Usage is limited to 10 days after which a polymeric, high-protein formula is used. Approximately 15% of our patients receive IEDs.

Polymeric High-Protein Formula

Patients who do not meet the criteria for IEDs who have normal gut digestive and absorptive capacity and are believed to have increased nitrogen requirements

TABLE 20.3

Enteral Nutrition Protocol

Formula Selection

A. **Immune Enhancing Diet:** These formulas should be used in patients sustaining major torso trauma who are at known risk for major septic complications and MOF:

*IEDs are limited to a 10-day usage period.

1. Combined flail chest/pulmonary contusion anticipated to require prolonged mechanical ventilation.
2. Major abdominal trauma defined by an Abdominal Trauma Index >18.
3. Two or more of the following:
   a. >6 unit transfusion requirement
   b. Major pelvic fracture (e.g. acetabular fx, vertical shear, open fx)
   c. Two or more long bone fractures
4. Non-trauma patients whom the attending surgeon believes to be at risk for major septic morbidity, e.g.,
   a. Moderately malnourished patients (albumin <3.5 g/dL) undergoing major elective procedures of the esophagus, stomach, pancreas (with or without duodenum), hepatobiliary tree or abdominal-perineal resection.
   b. Severely malnourished patients (albumin <2.8 g/dL) undergoing colonic, sigmoid, and proximal rectal anastamosis.

B. **Polymeric High Protein Formula:** These formulas should be used in patients who do not meet the criteria for immune-enhancing diets but have normal digestive and absorptive capacity of the GI tract and are believed to have increased nitrogen requirements due to the presence of:

1. Major torso trauma
2. Major head injuries
3. Major upper GI surgery
4. Obese patients with moderate calorie need, but high protein needs.

C. **Elemental Formulas:** These should be used in patients who have:

1. Proven intolerance to the first formula used
2. Not been fed enterally starting hospital day #7
3. Pancreatitis
4. Short gut
5. High output distal colonic or ileal fistula
6. Persistent,severe diarrhea >48 hours while on polymeric formula
7. $PrCO_2$ >70 but <90 for greater than 8 hours.
8. Moderate distention >24 hours and/or girth increase >2 inches Maintain elemental feeding minimum 72 hours. Reinstate polymeric once all parameters are improved and $PrCO_2$ <70 3 72 hours.
9. At the discretion of the attending physician.

D. **Renal Failure Formula:** Renal failure requiring intermittent hemodialysis degree of injury may merit dilution of formula to 3/4 strength to reduce viscosity and the addition of Promod (protein powder) to meet protein needs.

Formula	Kcal/cc	g protein/L
Immune-enhancing (Impact)	1.0	68
Polymeric high protein (Promote)	1.0	62
Elemental (Vivonex)	1.0	45
Renal (Nepro)	2.0	70

Feeding Protocol

A. After resuscitation is complete (as defined by the resuscitation protocol), start full strength formula 15 cc/h and if no moderate or severe symptoms exist advance to the rate of tube feeding as follows:

- 30 cc/h (720 cc/d) at 12 hours
- 45 cc/h (1080 cc/d) at 24 hours
- 60 cc/h (1440 cc/d) at 36 hours
- 60 cc/h rate should be maintained for at least 24 hours to assure tolerance.
- After waiting period, the rate will be advanced by 15 cc/h every 12 hours until the targeted goal is reached.

due to major torso and/or head injuries. A modular protein component may be added to the polymeric high-protein formula for use in the morbidly obese patient. Approximately 65% of our enterally fed patients receive a polymeric high-protein formula.

Elemental Formulas

Patients who are intolerant to a polymeric formula or who have not received enteral feeds for the first week postinjury are candidates for an elemental formula. Approximately 10% of our patients meet these criteria.

Renal Failure Formula

A concentrated, reduced electrolyte formulation is selected for use only in patients requiring intermittent hemodialysis. Often a modular protein component is added to the prepared, commercially available renal formula because commercially available renal products do not include sufficient protein for the critically injured patient.

Feeding Protocol

Once resuscitation is judged to be complete and enteral access has been obtained, 15 cc/h of full-strength formula is started and advanced by 15 cc/h every 12 hours if no moderate or severe symptoms of intolerance exist to a set goal of 60 cc/h. To assure tolerance, this rate is maintained for 24 hours and then advanced by 15 cc/h every 12 hours to a patient-specific targeted goal. This protocol is based upon a previous analysis of prospectively collected data from trauma patients requiring emergency laparotomies that were randomized in a series of clinical trials.[49] The control patients (n=52) received no early nutrition. The study patients (n=71) had a NCJ placed at laparotomy and had an elemental diet started within 12 hours postoperatively at 25 cc/h. This was advanced by 25 cc/h every 12 hours to a goal rate of 125 cc/h if no significant intolerance was observed. When questioned on a daily basis, half of the control group (receiving no TEN) experienced GI complaints of which 76% were graded minor and 24% were moderate. In contrast, 83% of the group receiving early TEN had GI complaints of which 39% were minor, 42% moderate, and 19% severe. Most of these symptoms occurred as feedings were advanced to the higher rates. At that time, the goal was to meet the patients' metabolic demands by 72 hours. We now, however, believe that early positive caloric balance is not necessary and may be harmful. We, therefore, have lowered the initial goal to 60 cc/h and only advance to the patient-specific goal after a 24-hour waiting period. We recently prospectively analyzed our incidence of enteral tolerance in a group of 17 severe torso trauma patients requiring shock resuscitation.[50] Early tolerance (during advancement of enteral feeds to a goal of 60 cc/h) was good in 14 patients and poor in 3, whereas late tolerance (after standard goal rate met) was good in 11, moderate in 1, and poor in 3 patients. Two additional patients never achieved goal rate feeds and were started on TPN. Overall, 88% (15 patients) of these severely injured patients were successfully maintained on early enteral nutrition using our standardized protocol.

Monitoring Tolerance and Managing Intolerance

Tolerance parameters are assessed and documented on an enteral tolerance flow sheet by the bedside ICU nurse every 12 hours and are reviewed by the ICU team daily. The decision to advance feeding is based on objective data. Specific criteria to identify and manage intolerance (Table 20.4) have also been developed and are managed per our protocol. Our current indicators of intolerance are vomiting, abdominal distention or cramping/tenderness, diarrhea, high nasogastric tube output, elevated $PrCO_2$ (regional PCO_2), and medication contraindications. Symptoms are graded as mild, moderate, or severe. Mild symptoms of intolerance, such as mild abdominal distention or diarrhea (one to two diarrheal stools per 12-hours) are managed by a physical exam at the time of onset of symptoms and in 6 hours, with the current rate of feeding being maintained. Moderate symptoms are managed based on the particular symptom. For distention, tube feeds are stopped and the patient assessed for evidence of small bowel obstruction. A gastric tonometer is inserted and the patient re-examined in 6 hours. If distention remains moderate, an elemental formula is begun. Moderate diarrhea (3 to 4 diarrheal stools per shift) is managed by maintaining current feeding rate (but not increasing) and repeat exam in 6 hours. A moderate elevation in $PrCO_2$, which we define as between 70–90 mmHg for 8 hours, prompts changing to an elemental diet. Finally, severe distention is managed by stopping all tube feeds, increasing intravenous fluid administration, and evaluating the patient for possible nonocclusive bowel necrosis. While for severe diarrhea (>4 per shift), tube feeds are reduced by 50%, antidiarrheal medications are added, and the patient is evaluated for possible *Clostridium difficile*. A severe elevation in $PrCO_2$ (>90 for 8 hours) prompts a discontinuation of feeds and reevaluation in 6 hours. Vomiting is man-

TABLE 20.4

Grading and Management of Intolerance to Enteral Nutrition			
Indicator	**Severity**	**Definition**	**Treatment**
Vomiting	Occurrence	1-4+ times/12 h	■ Place NG suction catheter, check function ■ Check existing NG function ■ Decrease TF infusion rate by 50%
Abdominal distention and/or cramping or tenderness (if detectable)	Mild	Hx and/or PE	■ Maintain TF infusion rate ■ Re-examine in 6 hours
	Moderate	Hx and/or PE	■ Stop TF infusion ■ Order AP supine KUB x-ray —assess for small bowel obstruction if SBO, notify primary team ■ Place gastric tonometer NG catheter —replace existing NG catheter if not gastric tonometer ■ Re-examine in 6 hours if moderate distension for >= 24 hours, switch to elemental for 72 hours
	Severe	Hx and/or PE	■ Stop TF infusion ■ Set IV fluid infusion rate = 250 mL/h ■ Consider CBC, lactate, ABG, Chem7, CT scan abdomen
Diarrhea	Mild	1-2 × per shift or 100-200 cc/12 h	■ Maintain or increase TF infusion rate per protocol
	Moderate	3-4 × per shift or 200-300 cc/12 h	■ Maintain TF infusion rate ■ Re-examine in 6 hours
	Severe	>4 × per shift or >300 cc/12 h	■ Decrease TF infusion rate by 50% ■ Give Diphenoxylate/Atropine (Lomotil) 10 cc q 6 h via feeding tube ■ Review MAR: note antibiotic, other GI drugs ■ Order stool studies: fecal leukocytes, toxin assays ■ If persistent (with Diphenoxylate/Atropine) >48 h, switch to elemental feeding
High NG output	(measured)	>1200 cc/12 h	■ Check existing xray for post-pyloric placement of feeding tube if >48 h since last xray, order KUB if not tube post-pyloric, hold TF order new feeding tube placement ■ Check NG aspirate for glucose if glucose present and feeding tube post-pyloric, hold TF and reassess in 12 hours retest NG aspirate for glucose 12 hours
$PrCO_2$ If patient is in permissive hypercapnia ($PaCO_2$ >50 mmHg) use $PrCO_2$ - $PaCO_2$ gap, otherwise use $PrCO_2$ reading.	Moderate	70 mmHg <$PrCO_2$ <= 90 mmHg for >= 8 h (only 2 or fewer measurements not in this range) or $PrCO_2$ - $PaCO_2$ gap = 30-50 mmHg	■ Change to elemental diet at present rate and advance as per protocol ■ If already on elemental diet, continue to advance as per protocol
	Severe	$PrCO_2$ >90 mmHg for >= 8 h (only 2 or fewer measurements not in this range) or $PrCO_2$ - $PaCO_2$ gap >50 mmHg	■ Stop TF infusion ■ Re-evaluate in 6 hours If $PrCO_2$ is moderate, start elemental formula at 15 mL/h and advance per protocol If $PrCO_2$ is still severe, begin Gatorade and 15 cc/h
Medication Contraindications	inotropic agents (e.g., Dobutamine, Milranone, Dopamine <= 5 mcg/kg)		■ Re-assess in 6 hours
	paralytics (i.e., Neuromuscular blockade drip for mechanical ventilation)		■ Begin elemental diet at 15 cc/h ■ Re-assess in 24 hours
	Norepinepherine >0.1 µg/kg/min Epinepherine >0.1 µg/kg/min	Phenylepherine >1 µg/kg/min Dopamine >5 µg/kg	■ Begin Gatorade at 15 cc/h ■ Re-assess in 24 hours

aged by ensuring adequate gastric decompression and decreasing the tube feed infusion rate by half. High nasogastric output (>1200 cc/12 h) is treated by verifying postpyloric placement of the feeding tube and checking the nasogastric aspirate for glucose. Any amount of glucose is considered abnormal and tube feeds are held. Finally, feeds are continued if inotropic agents are required while vasopressors mandate tube feeds to be discontinued, and Gatorade is begun at 15 cc/h. If continuous paralytics are needed, the patient is then begun on an elemental diet at 15 cc/h.

Nutritional Assessment

A nutritional assessment is made by a registered dietician within 72 hours of admission. Physical assessment of the patient includes evaluation of changes in body composition, edema, wound healing, nutrient composition of fluid losses through wounds or drains, and review of the lab and medication profile. Height and pre-admission weights are obtained and information on chronic disease, medications, previous dietary restrictions, drug, and tobacco patterns is elicited.

Co-Morbid Disease Assessment

Comorbid conditions may be present in up to 20% of severely injured patients[51] and will influence the patient's specific nutritional goal (Table 20.5).

Advanced Age

In adult ICU patients, loss of lean body mass may approach 1% per day and is accelerated in the elderly because baseline lean body mass is low. Both early nutritional intervention and early mobilization may slow this process. Additionally, in males, circulating levels of testosterone decline approximately 100 ng/dL per decade of aging. In the setting of a poor anabolic response to nutritional support, hormonal status should be assessed. Replacement of testosterone in elderly, hypogonadal men is associated with increased protein synthesis and muscle strength.[52]

TABLE 20.5

Comorbid Conditions that Influence Nutritional Support

Comorbid Condition	Global Nutritional Assessment	Action
Advanced Age	Reduced muscle mass	Early nutrition intervention, weight bearing and resistance activity.
	Decreased serum creatinine masks declining renal functionformulas.	Measure creatinine clearance. Reduced electrolyte.
	Decline in testosterone in aging males	Assess hormonal status. Administer oxandrolone.
Obesity	Increased risk of aspiration	Post-pyloric feeding.
	Increased insulin resistance	Hypocaloric feedings. Indirect calorimetry. Insulin protocol.
	Increased infectious morbidity	Tight glucose control. Strict catheter site hygiene.
	Decreased substrate mobilization in elderly obese	Assure positive nitrogen balance when hypocaloric regimens are used.
Diabetes Mellitus Type 2	Increased insulin resistance	Hypocaloric feedings (if obese); indirect calorimetry; insulin protocol; limit dextrose in TPN to 5 mg/kg/min.
	Increased infectious morbidity	Tight glucose control. Strict catheter site hygiene.
	Gastroparesis	Post-pyloric feeding; avoid high-fat intragastric feedings.
Liver Disease	Urine urea nitrogen, prealbumin, and transferrin are inaccurate indicators of nutritional status.	Limit use of these parameters, use indirect calorimetry.
	Chronic severe malnutrition	Anticipate refeeding syndrome.
	Hepatic encephalopathy	Limit protein if needed to assess neurologic status or to aid in ventilator weaning.

Obesity

Trauma patients with a body mass index >31 have an eight-fold higher rate of mortality following blunt trauma, frequently due to pulmonary complications.[53] To minimize the risk of aspiration, post-pyloric enteral feeds are recommended. Various feeding strategies have been employed in the obese, critically ill patient.[54] We feed 20–25 kcal and 1.75 g/protein/kg of adjusted weight. Sequential monitoring is essential. Assessment parameters, medication profile (e.g., insulin needs), wound healing, and clinical evidence of overfeeding are used to refine predictions. Indirect calorimetry is a useful adjunct.

Diabetes Mellitus

Due to high incidence of unsuspected gastroparesis, we routinely administer post-pyloric TEN. If the gastric route is used, high-fat diets should be avoided. To minimize hyperglycemia, we utilize an insulin protocol (Table 20.6), hypocaloric feeds if the patient is obese, and limit dextrose in TPN.

Liver Disease

Patients with underlying liver disease present a challenge in nutritional assessment. Urine urea nitrogen (UUN) may poorly reflect total nitrogen losses while prealbumin and transferrin may be decreased due to poor synthetic function of the liver. Indirect calorimetry may be a better indicator of nutritional needs. These patients are often severely malnourished and are thus at risk for the refeeding syndrome. Hepatic encephalopathy may occur secondary to multiple non-nutritional factors such as electrolyte and pH abnormalities, hypoxia, hypercapnia, sepsis, drugs, GI bleeding and azotemia.[55] We do not restrict protein unless encephalopathy adversely affects ventilator weaning or assessment of neurological function.

TABLE 20.6

Insulin Protocol

If any blood sugar (BS) >200 mg/dL, begin every 4 hour fingerstick BS.

If BS 0–60 mg/dL	Give 50 mL D50 and recheck BS in 15 minutes.
If BS 61–150 mg/dL	0 units regular insulin SQ
If BS 151–200 mg/dL	5 units regular insulin SQ
If BS 201–250 mg/dL	10 units regular insulin SQ
If BS 251–300 mg/dL	15 units regular insulin SQ
If BS >300 mg/dL	20 units regular insulin SQ Call physician and begin an insulin infusion.

TABLE 20.7

Nutritional Goals in Trauma Patients

Admit weight	Total kcal/kg	Protein
80–120% IBW	30	1.75 g/kg
>120% IBW using adjusted weight	20–25 kcal/kg	1.75 g/kg
<80% IBW	40 kcal/kg	1.75 g/kg

PATIENT SPECIFIC GOALS

Patient-specific nutritional goals are initially based on body weight (Table 20.7). We use the actual body weight when the patient is $\leq$120% of ideal body weight and an adjusted body weight for patients >120% employing the formula:

$$\text{Adjusted weight} = [(\text{Actual weight} - \text{Ideal weight}) \times 25\%] + \text{Ideal body weight}$$

Initially, protein is provided at 1.5–1.75 g/kg actual or adjusted body weight. Goals are adjusted to reflect comorbid conditions.

Total Parenteral Nutrition

With the widespread use of enteral nutrition, the indications for TPN have narrowed. It is employed in less than 10% of feeding days in our Shock Trauma ICU, using the criteria outlined in Table 20.8. A full discussion of TPN in metabolically stressed patients can be found in other chapters. In brief, we do not use specialty amino acid solutions including high branch chain amino acids, hepatic failure (low aromatic amino acids), or renal formulations (high essential amino acids). When delivered isonitrogeneously, these solutions

TABLE 20.8

Indications for TPN

1. When enteral access cannot be obtained (rare instance)
2. Feeding into the small bowel is not feasible:
   Massive small bowel resection refractory to enteral feeds
   High output fistula after failure of elemental diet
3. Splanchnic hypoperfusion:
   Active shock resuscitation
   High dose vasopressors
   Intermittent hemodialysis associated with hypotension
4. Enteral nutrition fails to meet nutritional requirements.
   (We define this as ICU day 8 and <60% of calories delivered enterally.)

are 15 to 20 times the cost of standard amino acids and have not been shown to improve nutritional status or outcome.[56]

If enteral access is delayed or hemodynamic status prevents early enteral nutrition, we do not advocate early TPN unless the patient is severely malnourished. Routine TPN may be associated with worse outcomes than no nutrition in patients with normal to moderate malnutrition.[40]

In planning TPN, we use the kcal plus protein goals outlined in Table 20.5. A standard 10% amino acid solution is used unless hemodialysis necessitates the use of a concentrated 15% solution. Dextrose is limited to 5 mg/kg/min to prevent hyperglycemia hepatic steogenesis and hypercapnea. A modest fat load of 1 ≤ g/kg is included in the TPN as a total nutrient admixture, which is infused over 24 hours to minimize potential reticuloendothelial dysfunction.[57] Standard doses of multivitamins and trace elements are included daily. Vitamins K and B_{12} are included weekly.

Acute Renal Failure

Approximately 1% of trauma patients will have underlying chronic renal insufficiency[58] and, for a variety of reasons, trauma places patients at high risk for acute renal failure. Nutritional support of hypermetabolic trauma patients with renal failure is challenging. We treat these patients with continuous venous-venous hemodialysis (CVVHD). Intermittent hemodialysis is reserved for those whose hypermetabolism has resolved. Although more labor-intensive, CVVHD is better tolerated from a hemodynamic perspective and allows for greater volume, urea, and electrolyte clearance. As a result, TPN with high fluid volumes and high protein loads can be used. With enteral support, standard isotonic, normal-electrolyte solutions are employed. The usage of high volume post-filter dextrose solutions can deliver considerable dextrose calories (approaching 300 gm daily) and should be considered as part of the total kilocalories.[59] Hyperglycemia often results and thus we discourage the use of D5 post-filter.[60] Additionally, 10% of daily infused amino acids and 75 grams of dextrose are dialyzed off during continuous dialysis.[60,61] Assessment of nutritional needs is difficult. Measurements of urine urea nitrogen (UUN) become less reliable when creatinine clearance is below 50 mL/minute. Standard assessment parameters such as prealbumin and transferrin have limited utility in the acute stages of renal failure. Also, renal failure has variable effects on energy expenditure.[62,63] Indirect calorimetry, if feasible, is recommended. Kilocalorie level should match needs and increasing kilocalorie loads are associated with a decreased protein catabolic rate.[64] An estimate of protein catabolic rate can be obtained during intermittent dialysis by urea kinetic modeling.[65] We provide 30–35 kcal/kg actual or adjusted weight and 1.6–1.8 g of protein/kg in the patient with continuous dialysis. Once the patient transitions to intermittent hemodialysis, a specialty renal enteral formula is employed with the addition of a modular protein component.

Monitoring Response to Support

Although total urinary nitrogen is a better indicator of nitrogen losses in the critical care setting,[66] UUN is more readily-available. A weekly 12-hour UUN is obtained in all patients with creatinine clearance >50 mL/min, without cirrhosis or acute spinal cord injury. Patients with spinal cord injury and paralysis are excluded from UUN measurements since obligatory losses are generally extraordinary regardless of the level of support and persist for up to seven weeks post-injury.[67] One may estimate the protein needs of the patient by:

$$[24\text{h UUN (g)} + 2 \text{ g N insensible losses} + 5] \times 6.25 = \text{amount of protein (g)}$$

All patients also have a C-reactive protein obtained within 72 hours of admission and then weekly as well as weekly serum prealbumin. C-reactive protein is a sensitive acute phase reactant that increases from a normal level near zero to 20 to 30 within 48 to 72 hours of injury. It can be used as an indicator of the severity of injury, inflammation, and sepsis. Only when this level begins to decline, can the liver begin to synthesize constitutive proteins such as albumin, prealbumin, and transferrin. Once the level falls below 10–15 mg/dL, a prompt increase in prealbumin typically occurs. If not, the clinician is prompted to reevaluate the adequacy of the support regimen or investigate other factors that may thwart anabolism. Prealbumin is an accessible and inexpensive indicator of anabolic activity. A half-life of 2 to 4 days increases its utility in the critical care setting. Once the acute phase response has subsided, increases in prealbumin are typically 0.5–1.0 mg/dL daily in the patient with adequate support.

Indirect calorimetry is obtained on an as needed basis and may be performed on the mechanically-ventilated patient with an FiO_2 <60% and PEEP <10. Studies are helpful (1) when overfeeding would be undesirable (as in diabetes or COPD), (2) when underfeeding would be especially detrimental (renal failure, large wounds), (3) in patients whose physical or clinical factors promote energy expenditure deviant from normal, (4) when drugs are used that may significantly alter energy expenditure (paralytic agents, beta-blockers, corticosteroids), (5) in patients who do not respond as expected to calculated regimens, and (6) when body habitus makes energy expenditure predictions challenging (morbid obesity, quadriplegia).[68]

Complications

Refeeding Syndrome

Refeeding syndrome can occur with rapid and excessive feeding of patients with severe malnutrition due to starvation, alcoholism, delayed support, anorexia nervosa, and insufficient intracellular ions.[69] As a result of ion fluxes into the cell with refeeding, serum phosphate, magnesium, potassium, and calcium levels can drop precipitously. Due to blunted basal insulin secretion, severe hyperglycemia may arise. Symptoms include cardiac arrhythmias, confusion, respiratory failure, and even death. This can be prevented by initiating TPN at approximately two-thirds of the required goal, predominantly by decreasing dextrose kcal. Then, carbohydrate kcal can be gradually increased over the next 5 days while anticipating and correcting electrolyte abnormalities. Exogenous insulin may be required.

Hyperglycemia

Critical illness is accompanied by increased plasma counter regulatory hormone levels that have multiple effects on glucose homeostasis. The end result is hyperglycemia with resistance to insulin. Other factors that contribute to "stress diabetes" include obesity, SIRS, advanced age, exogenous steroids or catecholamines, increased free fatty acids, and nutritional support (TPN > TEN). The resulting hyperglycemia can adversely affect outcome through several mechanisms including glycosuria and inappropriate diuresis, increased risk of infection (by impairing neutrophil and immunoglobulin function), and exacerbation of cerebral edema. We therefore aggressively control glucose levels (Table 20.6).

Catheter Related Sepsis

The pathogenesis of catheter-related sepsis (CRS) is multifactorial.[70] The indwelling catheter becomes contaminated and, over time, the bacteria or yeast proliferate, resulting in heavy local colonization, which then seeds the blood, resulting in bacteremia and signs of systemic sepsis. The catheter may have been contaminated at the time of insertion; later, due to skin colonization; or hub contamination may have occurred during catheter manipulation.[70–71] Preventive measures should focus on catheter insertion, care, and removal and are addressed in Chapter 12.

Jejunostomy-Related Complications

The largest study examining the safety of NCJs in patients undergoing major elective and emergency abdominal operations documented an incidence of major complications of 1% and minor complications of 1.7%.[73] When feeding jejunostomy-related complications in trauma patients were recently reviewed by Holmes et al.,[74] the overall major complications rate was 4% (9/122). However, the majority of complications occurred in patients with a Witzel tube jejunostomy (10%), with only a 2% rate with NCJs. In fact, the only difference between patients with and without major complications was the type of feeding access. Major complications included small bowel perforation, volvuli with infarction, intraperitoneal leaks, and nonocclusive small bowel necrosis. The first three of these complications can be minimized by improved technique and the latter minimized by more judicious feeding.

Nonocclusive Bowel Necrosis

Failure to recognize and appropriately manage intolerance can lead to a rare but frequently fatal condition known as nonocclusive bowel necrosis. Though clinical reports are derived from retrospective case reports, the consistent association of nonocclusive bowel necrosis with enteral nutrition implicates the inappropriate administration of nutrients into a dysfunctional gut. The incidence ranges from 0.3% to 8.5% with a mortality frequently in excess of 50%.[75,76] We recently published a review of 13 cases of nonocclusive bowel necrosis from among 4311 patients admitted to our Surgical or Neurological ICUs from 1993 through 1998, for an incidence of 0.3%.[77] No specific gastrointestinal symptoms associated with this entity were identified, though distention was common and occurred late in the course. Patients who had a gastric tonometer in place during advancement of enteral feeds and went on to develop nonocclusive bowel necrosis were noted to have a pH <7.30, suggesting tonometry may be a useful tool for monitoring intolerance. Additional symptoms associated with nonocclusive bowel necrosis are abdominal pain and tenderness, vomiting and high nasogastric output, all frequently encountered indicators of intolerance. There are no accurate indicators of impending bowel necrosis at this time.

The precise etiology of nonocclusive bowel necrosis remains unclear. Though a number of hypotheses have been proposed to explain its development, all are based on the premise that secondary gut mucosal hypoperfusion somehow plays a role. Hypotheses have included an increase in the metabolic demand of an already metabolically stressed gut or abdominal distention, leading to mucosal hypoperfusion due to either hyperosmolar formulas or bacterial overgrowth. It may well be that intolerance is manifested by a wide spectrum of symptoms ranging from mild abdominal distention, vomiting, or diarrhea to full thickness necrosis and death if not promptly recognized. The premise for nonocclusive bowel necrosis may be set early in the patients postinjury course but only after exposure to escalating volumes of enteral nutrients can such an extreme example of injury become manifest.

Controversies

Bioimpedance

Bioelectrical impedance analysis is a relatively inexpensive, portable and easy-to-use technology which determines the amount of body fat, body cell mass, total body water, and extracellular water. Intracellular dehydration parallels the loss of body protein and total body potassium.[78] Thus, the ability to measure and influence cellular hydration may be an important tool. The accuracy of bio-impedance analysis has been validated in a number of studies[79] and in various populations. The use of bioimpedance in critical care patients for monitoring body composition changes as they relate to various forms of nutrition support merits further investigation.

Hypocaloric Feeding

In an effort to lessen infectious complications associated with overfeeding of carbohydrates, the use of hypocaloric TPN has been proposed. However, a recent study failed to show a difference in infectious complications when a standard feeding regimen was compared to a hypocaloric feeding regimen (70 g protein and 1000 kcal) in hospitalized patients requiring TPN.[80] However, it was proposed that aggressive control of hyperglycemia in patients on the standard regimen was responsible for the lack of a higher rate of infections.

While controversial, hypocaloric feeding in the obese patient has also been suggested to lessen infectious complications secondary to hyperglycemia. Comparable nitrogen balance is achieved in this patient population when hypocaloric feeds are administered.[81–83] General recommendations are to provide a high-protein (2 g/kg IBW/d) but low nonprotein caloric (15 kcal/kg/d) diet. Monitoring for clinical evidence of overfeeding (hypercapnea, hyperglycemia, insulin resistance, hypertriglyceridemia, diarrhea, and distention) is used to refine predictions.

Glutamine Supplementation

Increasing evidence supports the addition of glutamine to standard amino acid intravenous solutions for use in critical care. The provision of 25 g L-glutamine to TPN has been associated with decreased hospital costs and improved survival,[84] which may be due to maintenance of skeletal muscle glutamine reserves, maintenance of glutathione production in the liver and intestinal mucosa, and preservation of gut barrier function.

Anabolic Compounds

Growth hormone therapy has been shown to exert a positive impact on trauma patients.[85,86] However, a multicenter European trial employing growth hormone early after cardiac surgery, abdominal surgery, multiple trauma (8% of study group), and respiratory failure in patients of average age 60, demonstrated significantly higher mortality and morbidity in the treated group.[87] The impact of establishing a more defined patient population and initiating therapy later after injury remains to be determined.

Oxandrolone (Oxandrin) is a synthetic testosterone analog with high anabolic and relatively low androgenic potential. It preserves body cell mass in burn patients, restores muscle mass in AIDS, and accelerates wound healing. Gervasio et al.[88] administered 10 mg twice daily to trauma patients with ISS ≥25 beginning within 5 days of admission and lasting up to 28 days. There was no significant difference in length of hospital stay, ICU length of stay, frequency of pneumonia, sepsis, ARDS, or MOF. No studies are reported evaluating the use of Oxandrin in patients who are no longer in acute phase response but demonstrate failure to become anabolic.

Case Study

The patient is a 51-year-old female who sustained a self-inflicted gunshot wound to the chest and abdomen. She arrived to the emergency room hypotensive, with a blood pressure of 90 mm Hg. A trauma ultrasound was negative for fluid in the abdomen but did reveal a pericardial effusion. She was taken to the operating room for a pericardial window and an exploratory laparotomy. There was a large stellate laceration to the right lobe of the liver with active bleeding. The middle hepatic vein was repaired, a hepatorraphy was performed and the liver was packed. Approximately 6 hours later she returned to the operating room with continued bleeding and abdominal compartment syndrome. The left hepatic artery was ligated with cessation of bleeding. A temporary abdominal closure was performed and the patient returned to the Surgical Intensive Care Unit for further resuscitation. She received approximately 21 units of blood in the first 24 hours post injury. She returned to the operating room on the third postinjury day for removal of packs, repair of diaphragm, needle catheter jejunostomy, and placement of a small bowel manometer. Immediately postoperatively she was begun on Impact at 15 cc/h and advanced per our protocol. Baseline $PrCO_2$ prior to initiation of tube feeds was 53 mmHg with a $PaCO_2$ of 35 mmHg. As feeds were advanced, there was a progressive increase in $PrCO_2$ which peaked in the low 100s as feeds reached 60 cc/h. The $PrCO_2$ remained greater than 90 mmHg for 8 hours, mandating that feeds be discontinued and Gatorade be started at 15 cc/h (as per protocol). There were no additional associated signs or symptoms of intolerance other than mild abdominal distention. With the cessation of Impact, $PrCO_2$ returned to baseline over the next 36 hours. The patient returned to the operating room for attempted fascial closure on postinjury day 5, now 36 hours after Impact had been discontinued. The bowel was pink and viable. Postoperatively she was begun on Vivonex that was advanced to goal without difficulty. Approximately 2 weeks later she developed a fever, elevated white blood cell count, and mild right lower quadrant pain. A CT scan of the abdomen revealed pneumatosis of the cecum and right colon. Enteral feeds were discontinued and broad spectrum antibiotics begun, with the presumed diagnosis of early nonocclusive bowel necrosis. Over the next 4 days, symptoms resolved and repeat CT scan showed resolution of the pneumatosis. Feeds were restarted and the patient had no further abdominal problems.

References

1. Baue AE. Multiple, progressive, or sequential systems failure. A syndrome of the 1970s. *Arch Surg*. 1975;110:779–81.
2. Eisman B, Beart R, Norton L. Multiple organ failure. *Surg Gynec Obstet*. 1977;144:323–326.
3. Fry DE, Pearlstein L, Fulton RL, et al. Multiple organ failure: the role of uncontrolled infection. *Arch Surg*. 1980; 115:136–140.
4. Border JR, Chenier R, McMenamy RH, et al. Multiple systems organ failure: muscle fuel deficit with visceral protein malnutrition. *Surg Clin North Amer*. 1976;56:1147–1159.
5. Cerra FB, Mazuski JE, Chute E, et al. Branched chain metabolic support. A prospective, randomized, double-blind trial in surgical stress. *Ann Surg*. 1984;199:286–291.
6. Detsky AS, Baker JP, O'Rourke K, et al. Perioperative parenteral nutrition: a meta-analysis. *Ann Intern Med*. 1987;197:195–203.
7. Picone VA, LeVeen HH, Glass P. Prehepatic hyperalimentation. *Surgery*. 1980;87:263–271.
8. Enrione EB, Gelfand MJ, Morgan D, et al. The effects of rate and route of nutrient intake on protein metabolism. *J Surg Res*. 1986;40:320–328.
9. Moore FA, Moore EE, Jones TN. TEN versus TPN following major abdominal trauma-reduced septic morbidity. *J Trauma*. 1989;29:916–924.
10. McArdle AH, Palmason C, Morency I. A rationale for enteral feeding as the preferred route for hyperalimentation. *Surgery*. 1981;90:616–623.
11. Mochizuki H, Trocki O, Dominioni L. Mechanism of prevention of postburn hypermetabolism and catabolism by early enteral feeding. *Ann Surg*. 1984;200:297–306.
12. Kudsk KA, Carpenter G, Peterson SR. Effect of enteral and parenteral feeding in malnourished rats with hemoglobin—*E. coli* adjuvant peritonitis. *J Surg Res*. 1981;31: 105–111.
13. Alverdy J, Chi HS, Sheldon GF. The effect of parenteral nutrition on gastrointestinal immunity. *Ann Surg*. 1985; 202:681–690.
14. Birkhahn RH, Renk CM. Immune response and leucine oxidation in oral and intravenous fed rats. Am J Clin Nutr. 1984;39:45–53.
15. Meyer J, Yurt RW, Dehaney R. Differential neutrophil activation before and after endotoxin infusion in enterally vs. parenterally fed volunteers. *Surg Gyn Obstetr*. 1988;67:50–58.
16. Lowry SF. The route of feeding influences injury responses. *J Trauma*. 1990;330 (suppl):20–22.
17. Kudsk KA, Li J, Renegar KB. Loss of upper respiratory tract immunity with parenteral feeding. *Ann Surg*. 1996; 223:629–638.
18. Border JR, Hassett J, LaDuca J, et al. The gut origin septic states in blunt multiple trauma (ISS=40) in the ICU. *Ann Surg*. 1987;206:427–436.
19. Wilmore DW, Smith RJ, O'Dwyer ST, et al. The gut: a central organ after surgical stress. *Surgery*. 1988;104:917–928.
20. Page CP. The surgeon and gut maintenance. *Am J Surg*. 1989;158:485–496.
21. Moore FA. The role of the gastrointestinal tract in postinjury multiple organ failure. *Am J Surg*. 1999;178:449–453.

22. Hassoun HT, Kone BC, Mercer DW, et al. Postinjury mutiple organ failure: the role of the gut. *Shock*. 2001;15: 1–10.

23. Moore EE, Jones TN. Benefits of immediate jejunal feeding after major abdominal trauma—a prospective randomized study. *J Trauma*. 1986;26:874–883.

24. Kudsk KA, Croce MA, Fabian TC, et al. Enteral versus parenteral feeding: effects on septic morbidity following blunt and penetrating abdominal trauma. *Ann Surg*. 1992; 215:503–514.

25. Moore FA, Feliciano DV, Andrassy RJ, et al. Early enteral feeding, compared with parenteral, reduces postoperative septic complications—the results of a meta-analysis. *Ann Surg*. 1992;216:62–69.

26. Wilmore DW, Shabert JK. Role of glutamine in immunologic responses. *Nutrition* 1998;14:618–626.

27. Salzman AL. Nitric oxide in the gut. *New Horizons*. 1995; 3:33–45.

28. Barbul A, Lazarou SA, Efron DT. Arginine enhances wound healing and lymphocyte immune responses in humans. *Surgery*. 1990;108:331–342.

29. Alexander JW, Saito H, Ogle CK, et al. The importance of lipid type in the diet after burn injury. *Ann Surg*. 1986; 204:1–13.

30. Van Buren CT, Kulkarni A, Fanslow WC, et al. Dietary nucleotides, a requirement for helper/inducer T lymphocytes. *Transplantation*. 1985;40:694–706.

31. Moore FA. Effects of immune-enhancing diets on infectious morbidity and multiple organ failure. *J Parenter Enteral Nutr*. 2001;25:S36–S43.

32. Heys SD, Walker LG, Smith I, Eremin O. Enteral nutrition supplementation with key nutrients in patients with critical illness and cancer. *Ann Surg*. 1999;229:467–477.

33. Beale RJ, Bryg DJ, Bihari DJ. Immunonutrition in the critically ill: A systematic review of clinical outcome. *Crit Care Med*. 1999;27:2799–2805.

34. Heyland DK, Novak F, Drover JW, et al. Should immunonutrition become routine in the critically ill patient? Accepted for publication by *JAMA*.

35. Brown RO, Hunt H, Mowatt-Larssen CA, et al. Comparison of specialized and standard enteral formulas in trauma patients. *Pharmacotherapy*. 1994;14:314–320.

36. Moore FA, Moore EE, Kudsk KA, et al. Clinical benefits of an immune-enhancing diet for early postinjury enteral feeding. *J Trauma*. 1994;37:607–615.

37. Kudsk KA, Minard G, Croce MA, et al. A randomized trial of isonitrogenous enteral diets following severe trauma: an immune-enhancing diet reduces septic complications. *Ann Surg*. 1996;224:531–543.

38. Mendez C, Jurkovich GJ, Garcia, et al. Effects of an immune-enhancing diet in critically injured patients. *J Trauma*. 1997;42:933–941.

39. Weimann A, Bastian L, Bischoff WE, et al. Influence of arginine, omega-3-fatty acids and nucleotide-supplemented enteral support on systemic inflammatory response syndrome and multiple organ failure in patients after severe trauma. *Nutrition*. 1998;14:165–172.

40. McQuiggan MM, Marvin RG, McKinley BA, et al. Enteral feeding following major torso trauma: from theory to practice. New Horizons. 1999;7:131–140.

41. A.S.P.E.N. Board of Directors. Guidelines for the use of parenteral and enteral nutrition in adult and pediatric patients. *J Parenter Enteral Nutr*. 2002 (in Press).

42. Ott L, Young B, Phillips R, et al. Altered gastric emptying in the head-injured patient: relationship to feeding intolerance. *J Neurosurg*. 1991;74:738–742.

43. Saxe J, Legerwood A, Lucas C, et al. Lower esophageal sphincter precludes safe gastric feeding after head injury. *J Trauma*. 1994;37:581–586.

44. Moore FA, Cocanour CS, McKinley B, et al. MMCs exist after trauma and predict enteral tolerance. *J Trauma*. In press.

45. Kortbeek JB, Haigh PI, Doig C. Duodenal versus gastric feeding in ventilated blunt trauma patients: a randomized controlled trial. *J Trauma*. 1994;37:581–586.

46. Delaney H, Carnevale N, Garvey J. Jejunostomy by needle catheter technique. *Surgery*. 1973;73:786–790.

47. Marvin RG, Moore FA, Cocanour CS, et al. Implementation of a procedure team improves utilization and reduces cost for critically ill patients in the ICU. J *Trauma*. 1998; 44:425.

48. Reed RL, Eachempati SR, Russell MK, et al. Endoscopic placement of jejunal feeding catheters in critically ill patients by a "push" technique. *J Trauma*. 1998;45:388–393.

49. Jones TN, Moore FA, Moore EE, et al. Gastrointestinal symptoms attributed to jejunostomy feeding after major abdominal trauma—a critical analysis. *Crit Care Med*. 1989;17:1146–1150.

50. Kozar RA, McQuiggan MM, Von Maszewski M, et al. Enteral tolerance following severe trauma is reliably achieved using a standardized protocol. *J Surg Res*. 2001; 100:292–293.

51. Sauaia A, Moore FA, Moore EE, et al. Multiple organ failure can be predicted as early as 12 hours after injury. *J Trauma*. 1998;45:291–303.

52. Urban RJ, Bodenburg YH, Gilkison C. Testosterone replacement in elderly men increases skeletal muscle strength and protein synthesis. *Am J Physiol*. 1995;269(5 Pt1): E820–826.

53. Smith-Choban P, Weireter LJ, Maynes C. Obesity and increased mortality in blunt trauma. *J Trauma*. 1991;31: 1253–1257.

54. Ireton-Jones CS, Francis C. Obesity: nutrition support practice and application to critical care. *Nutr Clin Pract*. 1995;10:144–149.

55. Gomez G, Jacobson LE, Asensio JA, et al. Pre-existing liver disease in the trauma patient. *Critical Care Med*. 1994; 10:555–556.

56. Heyman MB. General and specialized parenteral amino acid formulations for nutrition support. *J Am Diet Assoc*. 1990;90:401–408.

57. Jensen G, Mascioli E, Seidner D. Parenteral infusion of long and medium chain triglycerides and reticuloendothelial system function in man. *J Parenter Enteral Nutr*. 1990; 14:467–471.

58. Cacheco R, Milham FH, Wedel S. Management of the trauma patient with pre-existing renal disease. *Crit Care Clin*. 1994;10:523–526.
59. Monaghan R, Watters JM, Clancey SM. Uptake of glucose during continuous arteriovenous hemofiltration. *Crit Care Med*. 1993;21:1159–1163.
60. Frankenfield DC, Reynolds HN, Badellino MM. Glucose dynamics during continuous hemodiafiltration and total parenteral nutrition. *Intensive Care Med*. 1995;21:1016–1022.
61. Maxvold NJ, Smoyer WE, Custer JR, et al. Amino acid loss and nitrogen balance in critically ill children with acute renal failure: a prospective comparison between classic hemofiltration and hemofiltration and dialysis. *Crit Care Med*. 2000;28:1161–1165.
62. Schneeweiss B, Graninger W, Stockenhuber F. Energy in a randomized study. *AJCN*. 1990;53:977–978.
63. Soop M, Forsberg E, Thome A. Energy expenditure in postoperative multiple organ failure with acute renal failure. *Clin Nephrol*. 1989;31:139–145.
64. Macias WL, Alaka KJ, Murphy MH. Impact of the nutritional regimen on protein catabolism and nitrogen balance in patients with acute renal failure. *J Parenter Enteral Nutr*. 1996;20:56–62.
65. Kosanovich JM, Dumler R, Horst M. Use of urea kinetics in the nutritional care of the acutely ill patient. *J Parenter Enteral Nutr*. 1985;9:165–168.
66. Konstantinides FN, Konstantinides NN, Li JC. Urinary urea nitrogen: too sensitive for calculating nitrogen balance studies in surgical clinical nutrition. *J Parenter Enteral Nutr*. 1991;15:189–193.
67. Rodriguez DJ, Clevenger FW, Osler TM, et al. Obligatory negative nitrogen balance following spinal cord injury. *J Parenter Enteral Nutr*. 1991;15:319–322.
68. McClave SA, Snider HL. Understanding the metabolic response to critical illness: factors that cause patients to deviate from the expected pattern of hypermetabolism. *New Horizons*. 1994;2:139–146.
69. Faintuch J. The refeeding syndrome: a review. *J Parenter Enteral Nutr*. 1990;14:667–668.
70. Pearson ML. Guideline for prevention of intravascular device-related infection. *Am J Infect Control*. 1996;24:262–293.
71. Bjornson HS, Colley R, Bower RH, et al. Association between microorganism growth at the catheter insertion site and colonization of the catheter in patients receiving total parenteral nutrition. *Surgery*. 1982;92:720–727.
72. Salzman MB, Isenberg HD, Shapiro JF, et al. Prospective study of the catheter hub as the portal of entry for microorganisms causing catheter-related sepsis in neonates. *J Infect*. 1993;167:487–490.
73. Myers JG, Page CP, Stewart RM, et al. Complications of needle catheter jejunostomy in 2,002 consecutive applications. *Am J Surg*. 1995;170:547–551.
74. Holmes JH, Brundage SI, Hall RA, et al. Complications of surgical feeding jejunostomy in trauma patients. *J Trauma*. 1999;47:1009–12.
75. Scaife Cl, Saffle JR, Morris SE. Intestinal obstruction secondary to enteral feedings in burn trauma patients. *J Trauma*. 1999;47:859–863.
76. Munshi I, Steingrub JS, Wolpert L. Small bowel necrosis associated with early postoperative tube feeding in a trauma patient. *J Trauma*. 2000;49:163–165.
77. Marvin RG, McKinley BA, McQuiggan M, et al. Nonocclusive bowel necrosis occurring in critically ill trauma patients receiving enteral nutrition manifests no reliable signs for early detection. *Am J Surg*. 2000;179:7–12.
78. Finn PJ, Plank LD, Clark MA. Progressive cellular dehydration and proteolysis in critically ill patients. *Lancet*. 1996;347:654–656.
79. Lipkin EW, Bell S. Assessment of nutritional status: the clinician's perspective. *Clin Lab Med*. 1993;13:329–369.
80. McCowen KC, Friel C, Sternberg J, et al. Hypocaloric total parenteral nutrition: effectiveness in prevention of hyperglycemia and infectious complications—A randomized clinical trial. *Crit Care Med*. 2000;28:3606–3611.
81. Dickerson RN, Rosato EF, Mullen JL. Net protein anabolism with hypocaloric parenteral nutrition in obese stressed patients. *Am J Clin Nutr*. 1986;44:747–755.
82. Burge JC, Goon A, Choban PS. Efficacy of hypocaloric total parenteral nutrition in hospitalized obese: a prospective, double-blind randomized trial. *J Parenter Enteral Nutr*. 1994;18:203–207.
83. Smith-Choban P, Burge JC, Scales D. Hypoenergetic nutrition support in hospitalized obese patients: a simplified method for clinical application. *Am J Clin Nutr.* 1997;66: 546–550.
84. Griffiths RD, Jones C, Palmer TE. Six month outcome of critically ill patients given glutamine-supplemented parentral nutrition. *Nutrition*. 1997;13:295–302.
85. Jeevanandamm M, Begay CK, Shahbazian LM, et al. Altered plasma cytokine and total glutathione levels in parenterally fed critically ill trauma patients with adjuvant recombinant human growth hormone (rhGH) therapy. *Crit Care Med*. 2000;28:324–329.
86. Peterson SR, Holaday NJ, Jeevanandam M. Enhancement of protein synthesis efficiency in parenterally fed trauma victims by adjuvant recombinant human growth hormone. *J Trauma*. 1994;36:726–735.
87. Takkala J, Ruokonen E, Webster NR. Mortality associated with growth hormone treatment in critically ill adults. *NEJM*. 1999;341:785–792.
88. Gervasio JM, Dickerson RN, Swearingen J, et al. Oxandrolone in trauma patients. *Pharmacotherapy*. 2000;20: 1328–1334.

CHAPTER

21 Nutritional Considerations in the Severely Burned Patient

Bruce Friedman, M.D., F.C.C.P., F.C.C.M., C.N.S.P.,
Scott A. Deppe, M.D., F.A.C.P., F.C.C.M., F.C.C.P.

INTRODUCTION 245
METABOLIC AND PHYSIOLOGIC RESPONSES TO THERMAL INJURY 245
PHARMACOKINETICS IN BURN INJURY 246
INITIAL ASSESSMENT AND EVALUATION 246
NUTRITIONAL SUPPORT FOR THE SEVERELY BURNED PATIENT 247
Macronutrient Support 247
ENTERAL NUTRITION FORMULAS 248
EARLY NUTRITIONAL SUPPORT (24-96 HOURS) 248
ADJUNCTIVE NUTRITION SUPPORT 249
Micronutrients Support 249
VITAMINS A/C/E 250
SELENIUM/ZINC 250
CHROMIUM/IRON 251
ARGININE/GLUTAMINE/ORNITHINE 251
ENTERAL FEEDING IN BURN PATIENTS 252
Special Complications 252
FUTURE DIRECTIONS 252
Testosterone Analogs 252
MOLYBDENUM 253
MELATONIN 253
INTERLEUKIN-11 (rhIL-11) 253
CONCLUSIONS 253
REFERENCES 254

Introduction

The metabolic stress associated with traumatic injury causes an initial hypercatabolic response, corresponding to the severity of the physiologic insult. Burn trauma is one of the most severe physiologic insults and thus consistently produces one of the most devastating responses to metabolic stress.[1] The initial metabolic rate is low, with a crescendo following resuscitation, reaching a peak at about 7 days post injury.[2] This response, once initiated, continues until the burn wounds are closed. This chapter will briefly review the metabolic, physiologic, and pharmacokinetic responses to burn injury, followed by an in-depth discussion of the various nutritional and metabolic techniques currently used to diagnose and treat nutritional deficits in serious thermal injury. Future directions of burn nutritional support will be discussed.

Metabolic and Physiologic Responses to Thermal Injury

The hypermetabolic response to burn injury is the product of both evaporation (heat loss from burn wounds) and intense beta-adrenergic stimulation.[3–6] Thermoregulation is maintained at a febrile set point of both core and surface temperatures.[7] In terms of oxygen consumption and basal metabolic rate (BMR), these values increase in a linear fashion based on total body surface area (TBSA) burned until the burn size reaches approximately 40% TBSA. However, in 50% or greater TBSA burned patients, these rates reach and plateau at about twice the normal rates.[3–4] Baseline tachycardia and tachypnea are commonly seen in the seriously burned patient and levels may remain elevated, even after adequate resuscitation. Confounding factors include inhalational injury, associated trauma, and underlying medical disease states.

The hypercatabolic response to burn injury appears to be hormonally mediated and begins to manifest itself by muscle wasting as early as 24 hours after the insult. Catecholamine and glucagon excess are likely mediators of the calorigenic response.[1,3,4] Glucagon secretion inhibits the pancreatic secretion and peripheral activity of insulin.[8,9] The release of glucocorticoids is increased,[1,8,10] leading to hyperglycemia. This hyperglycemia may be initially beneficial, supplying needed energy for wound healing, acute phase protein synthesis, and maintenance of the cellular immune system.[10] Other effects of these hormonal secretions include sodium retention, leukocytosis, and potassium loss.[11] This gluconeogenic response requires pyruvate, lactate, glycerol, and amino acids. The predominant fuel sources are alanine and other amino acids supplied by muscle breakdown in the absence of protein nutritional support. During significant traumatic stress, this hyperglycemic, gluconeogenic response is not suppressed by the administration of exogenous insulin.[12–15] Experimentally and clinically it has been demonstrated that synthesis rates and thus nitrogen balance can be maintained with proper nutritional support.[1,16]

Pharmacokinetics in Burn Injury

Many physiologic changes of burn trauma have an impact on pharmacologic and nutritional interventions. Thermal injuries as small as 10% to 15% TBSA can lead to significant changes in renal, hepatic, and cardiovascular functions and cause marked reductions in plasma protein concentrations.[1,17] Renal function may be decreased acutely by hypotension, hypovolemia, hemoglobinuria, and myoglobinuria. Following resuscitation, the glomerular filtration rate rises as high as two times the normal rate and may remain elevated for a considerable period of time.[17–20] The rise is less in elderly patients, proportional to age. Hypoproteinemia may decrease the half-life of various renal excreted and protein bound agents even further.[21,22]

Likewise, early hepatic changes result from shock and hypovolemia, but more significant changes occur later as a result of sepsis and other complicating factors. After resuscitation, increased hepatic blood flow and the aforementioned increase in gluconeogenesis with protein turnover commonly occur.[23] Transaminase elevations are seen. Oxidation, reduction, demethylation, hydroxylation are routinely impaired while conjugation reaction remain unchanged.[17,18,24] This may lead to shortening of the half-life and efficacy of various analgesics and benzodiazepines.[25,26] Cardiovascular changes are also biphasic, and following resuscitation the hypermetabolic phase increases the cardiac output, leading to an increased metabolism of therapeutic drugs and nutritional substrates. This effect may be delayed or even absent in the geriatric patient.[1,17–19,27]

Initial Assessment and Evaluation

Initial nutritional assessment of the burn injured patient is based on the percentage and severity of the burn injury. Other factors of importance include patient age, inhalational injury, presence of associated injuries and disease states, and baseline nutritional status. The first goal of treatment is volume resuscitation and is accomplished using the Parkland formula as a guide.[28,29] Initial intravenous fluids used are crystalloid, specifically Ringers lactate solution. By general consensus, colloid-containing solutions are not usually indicated in the first 12 hours post burn.[1,28] Some argue the need for colloid solutions somewhere in the resuscitation phase to combat a sometimes precipitous drop in colloid osmotic pressure and predictable edema in nonburned tissue.[30] In the burn unit of the chapter's authors, a 5% albumin solution is usually begun along with resuscitative fluid at a continuous infusion rate after about 12 to 18 hours of initial resuscitation. Hypertonic saline solutions have also been advocated for use during initial resuscitation, but are not widely used in the United States.[31] A baseline prealbumin level and albumin level only have utility if drawn prior to the beginning of volume resuscitation.[32,33]

The use of indirect calorimetry for metabolic monitoring may have some use in the critically burned patient, but only after initial stabilization has been achieved.[28] It is indeed accurate in establishing a resting energy expenditure (REE) and to assess the effects of feeding on the respiratory quotient. For accuracy, indirect calorimetry requires an intubated patient on an oxygen concentration of 60% or less.[34,35] It is the authors' opinion that the use of indirect calorimetry should be reserved for difficult or puzzling cases, where the patient does not appear to be appropriately responding to the nutritional regimen being administered.

Once nutritional support is aggressively underway, a weekly prealbumin level and at least a weekly albumin level are helpful to assess the adequacy of nutritional support.[36] Routine measurements of nitrogen balance are often inaccurate in the burned patient due to protein loss from wounds and various effects of surgical interventions including blood loss, administration of fresh frozen plasma, and tissue debridement.

Since the goal of nutritional support is to limit the loss of somatic and visceral protein substrates, early nutrition and ongoing assessment of this nutrition are mandatory. Specific modalities of nutritional support are discussed below.

Nutritional Support for the Severely Burned Patient

Macronutrient Support

Protein

Paramount in the discussion of macronutrient support of the burned patient is protein administration. In burn injury, like other forms of severe stress, the major source of energy utilized comes from oxidation of protein.[8] The protein breakdown in trauma is often massive, largely supplied from skeletal muscle stores.[37] There appears to be some increase in the synthesis of protein, but this cannot compete with the overwhelming catabolism of protein.[38] Because the largest energy expenditure comes from protein, a major goal of burn injury nutritional support is to replace the somatic and visceral protein loss.[28,39] In major burn trauma, protein loss exceeds 2 g/kg/d[10] and is compounded by protein loss in burn wounds.

Protein breakdown without appropriate replacement leads to loss of essential amino acids including leucine and isoleucine (branched chain amino acids—BCAA).[8,10] Studies in critically ill patients show that replacement with protein high in BCAA improves somatic and visceral protein synthesis, nitrogen retention, and may improve immune competence through increasing visceral protein stores.[40,41] Oligopeptide formulas may demonstrate the most efficient enteral absorption, as compared to intact proteins or amino acids, particularly in protein-depleted patients with decreased colloid osmotic pressure.

It is the recommendation of the authors to institute high biological value protein support at a rate of at least 1.5 to 2.0 g/kg/d, early after burn trauma. This may be either in the form of enteral (preferred)[28,42–44] or parenteral amino acids, or a combination of both routes when enteral nutrition alone is inadequate to meet metabolic needs. In our experience, enteral nutrition is usually begun in the first 12 hours following burn injury, and most patients usually have reached baseline nutritional goals within 72 hours. High BCAA support should be reserved for the occasional patient who remains catabolic despite adequate conventional protein delivery.

Carbohydrates

As explained previously, metabolic stress in burn trauma is characterized by hyperglycemia and elevation of plasma insulin levels. Studies show a proportional relationship between hyperglycemia and the severity of stress.[45–47] The hormonal environment in serious stress promotes gluconeogenesis and peripheral insulin resistance with obligate proteolysis, ketogenesis, and lipolysis.[10,28] Many studies demonstrate the detrimental effects of carbohydrate overfeeding, including excessive carbon dioxide production,[48–50] diminished lipolysis,[51] and fatty liver syndrome.[52] Glucose should be limited in burn injury patients, both by the parenteral and enteral routes, in favor of higher protein and fat ratios to promote better protein synthesis and limit nutritional therapy morbidity.

Fats

The amount of fat calories needed to prevent essential fatty acid insufficiency is about 250 kcal/d if the fat is supplied by fat emulsion. Since the nonprotein calories should be limited in carbohydrate administration, there is an imperative need to supply significant calories as fat. In some unique situations lipid can be used to supply up to 70% of the nonprotein calorie needs. The actual amount of lipid used in more routine burn settings must be tailored based on carbon dioxide production, triglyceride levels, and the degree of hyperglycemia, with consideration of existing pulmonary and hepatic diseases that may be present.

There are problems with supplying lipid parenterally as fat emulsion. Many studies demonstrate potential complications including decreased T-lymphocyte responsiveness,[53] reticuloendothelial system dysfunction,[54] and increased Prostaglandin E_2,[55–57] and hepatic dysfunction.[58] Alexander et al., has researched the effects of enteral versus parenteral nutrition in animals and humans suffering from burn injury.[42,59–61] Enteral nutrition is associated with significantly less septic morbidity and mortality, even with the use of standard enteral nutrition formulations. Equally important, substrate modifications, particularly in the area of fat calories, provide additional beneficial effects specifically related to immuno-modulation.[60–62]

The type of fat utilized may have significant effect on immunocompetence in critically ill patients. It appears that fish oil, high in the omega-3 fatty acids, specifically eicosapentenoic acid, exerts a beneficial effect.[57,62–66] These positive effects are reported in studies where formulas are also supplemented with arginine, nucleotides, and glutamine.[63,66–68]

Specific enteral nutritional formulas are available that can be tailored to meet the needs of individual burn patients. Safflower oil is also high in omega-3 polyunsaturated fatty acids, but the bioavailability of the omega-3 substrates may be limited due to lack of human enzymatic activity in the gut. Another fat substrate, medium-chain triglycerides, may also provide safe and efficiently utilizable fat by both enteral and parenteral routes.[69–71] Medium-chain triglycerides are ketogenic, have specific enteral receptors for transport, and do not appear to be detrimental to the immune system. Again, there are feeding formulas that can provide nutrients tailored to the specific needs of burn trauma patient. Some of these formulations are briefly discussed below. It is beyond the scope of this chapter to discuss specific enteral formulas in detail.

Enteral Nutrition Formulas

Iso-osmolar formulas, with or without fiber, are generally well tolerated, but lack the high levels of protein necessary to meet nutritional requirements of severe burn stress. The use of these enteral feedings requires additional supplementation with proteins, such as whey. Other formulations may contain proteins in the form of oligopeptides and medium-chain triglycerides as a portion of the fat calories, but again, absolute protein content is lacking. There are higher protein formulas in which the protein supplied is in the form of oligopeptides or amino acids ("elemental" or "semi-elemental") that may better meet the nutritional requirements of burn stress. Additional feedings supply high levels of protein including BCAA as well as medium-chain triglycerides. Finally, some high protein formulas promote immunocompetence through the addition of fish oil, nucleotides, and arginine.

Kudsk et al., in a carefully done study with few design flaws, compared the effects of an immune enhanced enteral formulation with those of an isocaloric, isonitrogenous control diet in 33 severely injured trauma patients. Those receiving the immunonutrition had significantly few hospital days and major infections (i.e., nosocomial pneumonias, intraabdominal abscess) than the control group.[72] However, Saffle et al. compared the effects of an immune-enhanced enteral product with those of a standard high protein diet in thermally injured patients with relatively large TBSA burns (21%–40%).[73] No differences in mortality, length of stay or infectious process were found. At this point, the use of enteral immune-enhanced diets in burn patients appears promising but remains controversial.[74]

Early Nutritional Support (24–96 Hours)

It is accepted as a standard of care to provide enteral nutrition as the primary source of nutrition support in the burn patient. Enteral nutrition in comparison to parenteral nutrition improves blood flow to the gastrointestinal tract, preserves gut function by maintaining gut integrity, minimizes bacterial translocation related to gut mucosal atrophy, decreases costs of nutrient delivery, and reduces nosocomial infections.[75] In contrast to parenteral nutrition, enteral routes are easier and safer to use with a vastly lower complication rate.[76]

Despite common concerns about postburn gastroparesis and colonic ileus, immediate intragastric and subsequent post-pyloric feedings within the first 6 to 18 hours of acute burn injury has been shown to be safe and effective.[77,78] Early enteral feeding within 48 hours may also significantly reduce length of stay and reduce the hypermetabolic response to injury.[79,80]

Enteral nutrition is not always possible because tubes can be obstructed or dislodged. In addition, feedings can be interrupted for various medical procedures and delivery of medication. This practice has been shown to consistently reduce reaching overall nutritional goals by as much as 50%. By providing post-pyloric feedings, enteral nutrition can be provided safely and efficaciously throughout nearly all operative procedures. They are well-tolerated and this practice results in increased caloric intake and decreased wound infections.[81,82]

After stabilization of the acute burn with volume resuscitation and appropriate early surgical intervention and debridement, the primary goal of nutrition support is the reintroduction of protein and non-protein calories to begin wound healing. It is also critical to convert from catabolism to anabolism. In the acute phase of burn injury one cannot always provide the adequate amount of calories to the burn patient with enteral nutrition alone. Providing protein and calorie requirements solely by the enteral route in the face of gastric dysmotility and intolerance is often difficult to accomplish. A slow introduction of enteral feedings in the critically ill burn patient is crucial to ultimately attaining feeding goals. In order to do this, a combination of parenteral and enteral nutrition support in the critically ill burn is recommended. Enteral feeding is slowly introduced over a 3-to-4-day period as the gut tolerates. This will provide the maximal amount of protein and calories, but the absorption remains unclear. In order to provide the substantial protein needs required by the burn patient, a combination of enteral and parenteral feeding best meets the nutrition needs of the early phases of burn injury.

These authors have found that exceeding 100 cc/h of enteral feedings, even at goal, will, in most patients, cause significant problems with gastric motility, poor absorption, colonic dysmotility and intolerance of the feedings. This emphasizes again the need for combination parenteral and enteral feeding in the early phases of the burn injury.

Many of the complications related to parenteral nutrition are due to the need for central access. Central access is non-problematic in the burn patient since resuscitation from a volume standpoint is critical in the very early phases of the burn injury, and the vast majority of patients will require a central line. The central line is not placed primarily for parenteral nutrition, eliminating the complication of line placement as a problem in provision of hyperalimentation. At these authors' institution, a high-branch chain amino-acid enhanced, micronutrient enriched, electrolyte solution specifically designed nutritional formula is started within the first 24 hours. The parenteral nutrition (PN) allows fluid, electrolyte and divalent ion manipulations. Divalent ions, such as magnesium, calcium, and phosphorous, are quite variable in the acute phases of injury. The PN allows provision of these important organ modifying divalents. We can also adjust the electrolytes and the acid base modifiers, such as acetate, to allow for internal control of fluids from a tonicity standpoint by modifying the PN. Insulin can be provided for the hyperglycemia commonly seen in the acute phases of injury secondary to the overproduction of catecholamines that induce insulin resistance and intolerance.

The parenteral formulation is modified over 5 to 7 days depending on the visceral protein stores. It is also highly dependent on enteral feeding tolerance. Once the visceral protein stores are responding well to the enteral feedings and/or the BUN is not climbing, the PN is slowly tapered. The micronutrients and the electrolytes, however, can be maintained through the acute phases of the burn injury and subsequently into the later phases in order to provide these necessary adjuncts until the patient is well into an oral phase of nutritional support. Therefore, although increased mortality with the use of total parenteral nutrition in severe burn injuries has been reported,[83] it has been these authors' experience that a modified parenteral nutrition formula in conjunction with enteral feeding may be very beneficial to a severely burned patient.

Adjunctive Nutrition Support

MICRONUTRIENTS SUPPORT

Micronutrients are found in small quantities in all tissues. They are essential for maintaining homeostasis and cellular function and ultimately for survival. Data are continuing to accumulate suggesting that marked deficiencies in key micronutrients occur during severe stress response as a result of increased losses, accelerated consumption from hypermetabolism, and inadequate exogenous replacement. This will further amplify injury-induced metabolic derangements and fuel hypercatabolism. Adjunctive nutrition support with oxygen free radical modifiers appears essential in the severely burned patient.[84]

The micronutrients and trace elements include vitamin C, vitamin A, vitamin E, selenium folate, zinc, chromium, and iron as well as key amino acids such as glutamine, arginine, and ornithine alpha-ketoglutarate. Critical illness, especially burn injury, necessitates increased nutritional requirements associated with the resulting hypermetabolic state. Although mineral metabolism clearly is affected by illness, the precise requirements for micronutrients is not yet defined.

These micronutrients are key components of an anti-oxidant defense network that is significantly impaired in acute injury states such as burns and trauma. Extracellular and intracellular generation of cellular and membrane toxic oxygen free radicals occur in the early phases of injury and shock. This network of exogenous and endogenous anti-oxidants that includes vitamins A, C, E, zinc, selenium, glutathione, arginine, etc., have significant modulatory influences on cytokine production as well as intracellular modifications in macrophages, neutrophils, and wound healing matrices such as fibroblast and collagen formation.

Hammarqvist investigated skeletal glutathione depletion in critically ill patients and demonstrated that oxidative stress in muscle is reflected in decreased glutathione levels, leading to increased susceptibility of early tissue oxidative damage.[85] Impaired amino acid transport, the most difficult process to overcome in nutrition support of the critically ill, was prominent in this study and contributed to catabolism. This decrease impairs the defense of muscle against oxygen free radicals and contributes to the loss of balance between protein synthesis and protein degradation characteristic of protein catabolism. This suggests a clinical role for oxygen free radical scavengers and micronutrients to aid in maintaining normal amino acid transport.

Galley, in patients with sepsis syndrome, demonstrated early elevations in xanthine oxidase activity, high free radical concentrations, and indications of free radical damage (lactate) as well as ascorbyl radical concentrations that were increased, reflecting rapid endogenous vitamin C losses.[86] Vitamin C and its metabolites are depleted early in acute injury, indicating an early role for exogenous micronutrient supplementation.[87] Plasma concentrations of cytokines, along with antioxidant vitamins, have been shown to predict multiorgan failure in patients at risk. Borrelli et al. clearly demonstrated that a decrease in vitamin C, overall zinc pool, and poor availability of vitamin E correlated significantly with multi-organ failure,[88] indicating an association with trauma and a need for antioxidant replacement.

Human and animal studies have shown that supplementation of antioxidants reduce the inflammatory response via the oxygen free-radical defense network. In a rat-burn model, Demling prevented altered cell energetics, reflected by lowered catalase levels, by providing an anti-oxidant oral cocktail.[89] This included vitamin C, N-acetylcysteine, and glutathione. Maderazo gave blunt trauma patients a combination of vitamins E and C and demonstrated significant improvement in neutrophil locomotion with anti-oxidants.[90] Combination therapy was better than either alone and improved over placebo. Roche et al. measured plasma concentrations of vitamin C and tocopherols immediately after extensive adult burn injuries (TBSA >20%) and showed a marked reduction endogenously.[91] Berger et al., in major burns, measured marked decreases in plasma levels of copper, iron, selenium, and zinc with a corollary rise in ferritin and ceruloplasmin.[92] By increasing intravenous copper selenium and zinc during the first 7 days after burn injury, rapid return of these depressed levels occurred. Supplementation of these key micronutrients also resulted in fewer medical complications, higher available blood leukocytes, and decreased length of stay.[92]

Data on micronutrient supplementation in burns and other injured patients are encouraging but not yet fully understood. The significance of these alterations may have an impact on infectious complications, wound healing, and ultimate mortality in burn injury. Based on available data, certain recommendations can be considered, as noted below; however, further research in this area is clearly warranted.

Vitamins A/C/E

The major cellular antioxidant systems include glutamine, alpha-tocopherol (vitamin E), ascorbate (vitamin C), B-carotene (vitamin A) and numerous enzymes and their respective trace mineral co-factors. These micronutrients are all physiologic modulators of oxidative stress and, hence, oxygen free radicals. Other important properties include immunomodulation, restoration of mucosal surfaces by blocking lipid peroxidation, improving while blood cell chemotaxis, and inhibiting apoptosis.[93–96] Supplementation with vitamins A, C, and E is associated with an improvement in antioxidant defenses as assessed by ex vivo tests in both animal[97] and human sepsis[98] and burn studies.[91,99,100] Based on available data the biochemical effects of vitamins A, C, and E may have significant clinical benefit to the burn patient in combination with an aggressive nutrition support plan. Recommendations for these and other vitamin/micronutrient supplementations can be found in Table 21.1.

Selenium/Zinc

Trace elements such as selenium and zinc along with copper have been studied extensively in burns and other critically ill patients. Levels are decreased in trauma, sepsis, and burns.

Selenium in small amounts is needed for tissue oxygenation and protection against lipid peroxidation. It is a key co-factor in glutathione peroxides reactions, important for protection from oxygen radicals, as well as modulator to the arachidonic acid cascade.[101] Major loss of selenium occurs through the dermis, due to thermal destruction of skin, which contains substantial amounts of selenium by weight; removal of eschar; loss through wound exudates; and as a result of the antagonistic relationship between selenium and silver.[102,103] Selenium deficiency occurs in patients with burns,[104] trauma,[105] and sepsis. Forceville et al. demonstrated that early low selenium levels correlated with high APACHE scores, SIRS/shock, and morbidity (ventila-

TABLE 21.1

Acute Burn Intensive Care Rally-Pack	
*IV	*Oral
200 µg Selenium 8000 mg Vitamin C (taper 4-6 g over 7 days) 20–25 mg Zinc MVI ⊕ Trace Elements Chromium 100–300 µg Thiamine 100 mg Folate 5-20 mg	Vitamin E 400 IU QD Chromium 200 µg Zinc 220 mg PO QD MVI/Pre-natal Vitamins Selenium 200 µg PO QD Vitamin C 1000 mg PO BID Vitamin A 10,000 IU QD

*Adjust for Renal Function

tor associated pneumonia, multi-organ failure), and mortality was three times higher.[106]

Zinc, like selenium, is an essential cofactor in multiple metalloenzyme reactions. It is a key micronutrient in DNA/RNA synthesis with immunomodulatory properties. Decreased serum zinc levels occur in response to physiologic stress resulting from losses, dilution, redistribution and the acute phase reaction.[107] Metallothioneins bind zinc; during the stress response, serum zinc becomes less available due to transfer into visceral organs by these metal-binding proteins.[107] Zinc levels in burn patients are acutely lowered as evidenced by hyperzincuria, probably due to postburn elevation of endogenous protein catabolism.[108] As much as 5% to 10% of total body zinc content is lost during the first 7 days after burn injury.[109] Low leukocyte zinc levels have been demonstrated during the acute postburn period in patients with more than 30% TBSA correlating with impaired wound healing.[110]

Chromium/Iron

Chromium deficiency results in glucose intolerance through insulin resistance. It potentiates the action of insulin in vitro and in vivo via an ill-defined chromium nicotinic acid complex.[111,112] Chromium uptake is increased in neutrophils of patients with burn injuries. Neutrophils of fatal burn victims incorporated less chromium than did those from survivors.[112] Chromium supplementation should be given when burn patients are at risk for glucose intolerance and are chromium deficient. Timing of repletion is usually in the acute burn injury phase or correlated with a secondary insult such as shock, ARDS, or septicemia. Supplementation should be coordinated with insulin replacement, enteral feeding formula, and renal function, and can substantially lower baseline insulin requirements in selected patients.[110]

Iron is important in energy metabolism because of its structural role in oxygen-carrying proteins, and is intimately linked to the oxidative enzymes such as catalase, various dehydrogenases, and glutathione peroxidase. In the acute phase response, cytokines cause a rise in serum ferritin. Free uncomplexed iron appears to be increased after burns and trauma and can be harmful. This process correlates with consistently low iron profiles in critically ill patients, despite elevations in ferritin.[113] A delicate balance exists between immune stability and microbial overgrowth when endogenous iron stores and availability are altered by acute injury. Early supplementation of iron should be avoided in burn injuries to reduce the generation of super-oxide radical formation via the Haber-Weiss-Fenton reaction. If activated, lipid peroxidation increases, and membrane and macromolecular damage ensue increasing the risk of apoptosis and microorganism overgrowth. Eventually iron stores will need supplementation in burn patients with heavy blood losses or pre-existent deficiencies. Timing is critical and can be best defined by measuring RBC zinc-protoporphyrin. If this iron marker is low or normal, then, despite other measures of iron, iron stores remain available. If elevated, iron replacement should be considered, either parenterally (preferred) or enterally (later in recovery phase).

Other micronutrients may also play an adjunctive role in major burn injury. We have yet to establish the doses and best method of delivery of these microminerals in critically ill and burn populations. The antioxidant "rally pack" used at the authors' center is given in Table 21.1. This includes the key micronutrients for wound healing and re-establishing the antioxidant defense network. Further research into trace element requirements in burns and critically ill patients is clearly needed.

Arginine/Glutamine/Ornithine

Arginine and glutamine have been classified as conditionally indispensable during stress states, suggesting that endogenous synthesis of these amino acid micronutrients may be inadequate to support tissue maintenance or regeneration. Arginine improves nitrogen balance, wound healing, and immune function. Supplementation with arginine in an injured animal model and in burn patients promoted nitrogen balance.[114,115]

Glutamine supplementation may also be beneficial to burn patients. Glutamine appears to maintain the mucosa of the intestine, reversing the rapid turnover of enterocytes and possibly decreasing the incidence of bacterial translocation.[116] In the first few days of post-burn injury, free-glutamine in skeletal muscle declines over 50%. Glutamine has also been found to enhance the bacteriocidal activity of neutrophils from burn patients.[117,118] Although we provide both enteral arginine (two standard packets/d) and glutamine (30–40 g/d) to our major burns, optimal levels remain to be determined. Newer formulations combining micronutrients, glutamine, arginine, and other oxygen radical modifiers such as N-acetylcysteine are now being marketed.

Recently, Coudray-Lucas[119] evaluated ornithine supplementation in severely burned patients. Both glutamine and arginine are generated by ornithine. In this study ornithine alpha-ketoglutarate at 20 g/d in divided doses was enterally provided in a prospective randomized double-blind trial versus isonitrogenous controls. Arginine and proline were generated along with increases in growth hormone and somatomedin-C. They demonstrated improved healing time, significant increases in prealbumin, and marked decreases in myofibrillar breakdown as measured by 3 methyl-histidine/creatinine ratio. This study suggests that alternate micronutrient provision may re-establish arginine and possibly glutamine levels at a more appropriate biochemical position.

Enteral Feeding in Burn Patients

Special Complications

One major drawback to enteral nutrition is the possibility of multiple interruptions due to surgical/OR needs, multiple procedures, and transportation. McClave evaluated critically ill patients for adequacy of enteral delivery.[120] Only 51.6% of patients studied reached their nutritional goals. Feedings were stopped for OR and procedures, need for supine positioning, intolerance, ileus, and high residuals (>200 mL). Our center has essentially been able to avoid most of the feeding stoppages by placing a dual lumen single tube to provide post-pyloric feeding. This combination tube provides a gastric port for low intermittent suction (reducing paresis problems) and medicine dispensing as well as a post-pyloric jejunal port for feeding only. We can now provide feeding during all surgical and other procedures with impunity. These tubes are safe and have been left in place for 6 weeks or more without complications.

Intolerance to feeding may be an early sign of sepsis in burn patients. Gastroparesis is a common finding in burn patients, as is dysmotility in both the small and large bowel. Promotility agents such as metoclopramide and erythromycin, when initiated early in burn injury, may alter this problem. However, due to the significant need for pain management with narcotics, dysmotility and ileus remain common.

Recently, oral naloxone has been shown to reverse opioid associated constipation in critically ill and oncologic patients. Its use reduced the need for laxatives, and was not associated with systemic narcotic withdrawal signs.[121] Neostigmine has been successfully used to treat acute colonic pseudo-obstruction. A 2 mg intravenous slow-push dosage is most commonly employed. A rapid response ensues in most patients.[122] We have successfully used this therapy in multiple burn patients to relieve colonic ileus. Nurses should be made aware that the response is usually quite dramatic, and patients should be monitored closely as cardiac side effects are reported.

Unfortunately, oral naloxone is not readily available in the USA. However, in a very recent publication, Taguchi, et al.[123] tested a new opioid antagonist with limited oral absorption (ADL8-2698) in postoperative abdominal surgery patients. Faster recovery of gastrointestinal function was found in the treatment group. Hospital stay was decreased, and the agent did not readily cross the blood-brain barrier, suggesting little to no antagonism of systemic narcotic effects. This may be a very worthwhile compound to study in burn patients to reduce gut dysmotility.

Future Directions

Testosterone Analogs

The limiting factor to restoration of anabolism in the hypermetabolic state is the ability to promote effective amino acid transport and synthesis. We can provide all the enteral support possible as well as oxygen free radical modifiers; however, if we cannot reverse catabolism or improve transport, visceral protein stores will not be restored and wound healing will be impaired.

Testosterone analogs have been used for controlling post injury catabolism. Oxandrolone is an orally administered synthetic anabolic steroid used as an effective adjunctive therapy to provide weight gain and restore muscle mass in several catabolic illnesses[124,125] as well as in chronic wounds.[126] Demling and DeSanti[127,128] have shown in burn patients receiving adequate calories and protein intake, elevated visceral protein stores are more rapidly achieved and oxandrolone can increase weight gain post-burn along with strength and endurance. No significant complications were noted with the drug administration.

Subsequently, Demling compared the anabolic effects of oxandrolone to human growth hormone 7 to 10 days after severe burn injury.[129] Earlier work using recombinant human growth hormone in burn patients; however, demonstrated improved wound healing[130] when compared to oxandrolone, human growth hormone caused significant hyperglycemia and was more costly. Liver dysfunction was not seen with either intervention and wound healing was significantly improved with both agents. However, growth hormone showed a significant increase in metabolic rate as compared to oxandrolone. The anti-catabolic effects were comparable, and no major toxicities were noted.

In a double-blind, randomized, placebo-controlled trial, our burn center has recently evaluated the effects of 20 mg/d of oxandrolone in acute burn injury beginning in the acute phase. Preliminary data show a significant difference in restoration of visceral protein stores by prealbumin and UUN markers at days 21 and 28; statistical analysis is pending final review. (Personal communication BF.) Larger studies and dose response studies in the acute burn population are needed. Dosing studies to see if anabolism can be reached earlier in acute injury with higher doses of this analog should be considered.

Very recently, Ferrando et al.[131] from the Galveston, Texas, burn center evaluated the role of long-acting testosterone in a severely burned population (>70% TBSA). Six patients were elegantly evaluated for the effects of a depo-testosterone injection (200 mg IM/wk × 2) 2 weeks from the acute injury. Protein synthetic efficiency increased two-fold, and protein breakdown decreased two-fold, resulting in a net amino acid balance and amelioration of muscle catabolism. This could be a safe and inexpensive modality to promote anabolism after severe burn injury. Larger studies in various burn sizes, as well as the role of testosterone in females, need to be conducted.

Molybdenum[132,133]

Molybdenum is a trace metal that is considered essential because it is part of a complex that is required for three oxidative network enzymes that include xanthine oxidase, aldehyde oxidase, and sulfite oxidase. These enzymes function by transferring an oxygen atom from water to a variety of compounds. Xanthine oxidase catalyzes the oxidation of the purines, xanthine and hypoxanthine, to uric acid. The metabolism of methionine and cystine are dependent on sulfite oxidase to transform sulfite to sulfate. The significance of this essential trace metal remains in its involvement with these amino acids and their transport. It would be interesting to look at the effects of parenterally administered molybdenum in acute burn injuries and measure its effects on protein transport and anti-catabolism. Standard doses are 100–150 mcg/d in a normal diet. In acute injury, we might consider providing 300–500 mcg/d and follow protein kinetics and overall response. Toxicity has only been associated with reduction of copper levels due to an antagonism between molybdate and copper. Minimal research in critically ill or burn patients has been done with this unique trace element.

Melatonin[134]

Melatonin is a neuroendocrine substance principally secreted from the pineal gland. From a nutritional standpoint, it may provide two important foci for acutely injured patients. Both in vitro and in vivo studies have shown that melatonin is a potent scavenger of hydroxyl and other oxygen-centered radicals.[135] Comparing melatonin to mannitol, glutamine, and vitamin E, it was more effective in protecting against oxidative change.[136] Melatonin may also augment the immune response through T-lymphocyte, cytokine IL-4, and IL-10 independent mechanisms.[137] These two unique properties of melatonin should be explored as potential nutritional adjuncts in acutely burned patients. Melatonin along with myriad alternative herbal medicines such as coenzyme Q-(ubiquitin), which may play a key role in amino-acid transport and anabolism,[138] and Echinacea, with its purported immune enhancing properties, should certainly be explored in a more scientific manner in the burn patient.

Interleukin-11 (rhIL-11)

Interleukin-11 is a bone marrow stroma derived hematopoietic multifunctional cytokine derived from many cell and tissue types. Initial activity of this compound was hematopoietic manifested by thrombopoiesis in humans. However, further studies have demonstrated activity in protection and restoration of gastrointestinal mucosa, major effects as an immunomodulating agent and activity in bone metabolism. All of these properties would seem beneficial to the acutely burned patient.

IL-11 can reduce endotoxemia and its hemodynamic consequences in a rabbit sepsis model,[139] and reduce proinflammatory cytokine production during SIRS in vivo in a murine model of endotoxemia independent of IL-10 or IL-6.[140] IL-11 improved survival and reduced bacterial translocation and bone marrow suppression in a murine burns model (32% TBSA).[141] Further human studies of IL-11 from a nutrient standpoint are warranted. IL-11 may also have the ability to help maintain normal platelet counts, which has been associated with increased survival,[142] and improve gastrointestinal absorption of nutrients by restoring the intestinal cytoarchitecture.

Conclusions

Nutrition support is a critical adjunct to the overall treatment plan of the critically injured burn patient. Introducing early nutrition and adjunctive modifiers is paramount in the acute phase of a burn injury. The proper mix of protein and non-protein calories should be emphasized. Overfeeding must be avoided in order to reduce substantial risks for organ dysfunction. Protein supplementation and subsequent restoration of the visceral protein stores are an essential part of burn nutrition. The main goal is the conversion from hypercatabolism to anabolism in a timely manner. Various manipulations of parenteral, enteral and oral routes, along with appropriate modifiers, can aid in reaching these goals.

Future efforts will be aimed at improving amino acid transport by manipulating nutritional parameters through molecular biological techniques. Discovery of more precise methods for measuring nitrogen losses from wounds could facilitate this process. Future research is needed to determine specific nutritional requirements, especially of micronutrients and other oxygen free radical modifiers and nutrition adjuncts. Nutrition practices, when used in combination with appropriate clinical support, surgical interventions, and a preventive intensive care protocol, may substantially reduce lengths of stay, morbidities, and mortalities resulting from burns.

References

1. Krob MJ, Deppe SA, Thompson DR. Burn injury. *Crit Care Med.* 1992;57:781–788.
2. Wilmore DW. Metabolic changes after burn injury. In: Boswick JA, ed. *The Art and Science of Burn Care.* Rockville, MD: Aspen Systems; 1987:137.
3. Wilmore DW. Metabolic changes in burns. In: Artz CP, Moncrief JA, Pruitt BA, eds. *Burns: A Team Approach.* Philadelphia: WB Saunders; 1979:120.
4. Wilmore DW, Long JA, Mason AD Jr, et al. Catecholamines: mediator of the hypermetabolic response to thermal injury. *Ann Surg.* 1974;180:653.
5. Wolfe RR, Desai MH, Herndon DN. Metabolic responses to excision therapy. In: Boswick JA Jr, ed. *The Art and Science of Burn Care.* Rockville, MD: Aspen Systems; 1987:145.
6. Aulick LH, Handar EH, Wilmore DW, et al. The relative significance of thermal and metabolic demands on burn hypermetabolism. *J Trauma.* 1979;19:559.
7. Wilmore DW, Orcutt TW, Mason AD Jr, et al. Alterations in hypothalamic function following thermal injury. *J Trauma.* 1975;15:697.
8. Freund HR. Nutritional support of the trauma patient. *Probl Crit Care.* 1987;1:651.
9. Aulick LH, Wilmore DW, Mason AD Jr. Mechanism of glucagon calorigenesis. *Fed Proc.* 1976;35:401.
10. Deppe SA. Metabolism in starvation, illness, and injury. *Probl Crit Care.* 1988;2:547.
11. Bessey PQ, Watters JM, Aoki TT, et al. Combined hormonal influence stimulates the metabolic response to injury. *Ann Surg.* 1984;200:264.
12. Shamoon H, Hendler R, Sherwin RS. Synergic interactions among anti-insulin hormones in the pathogenesis of stress in humans. *J Endocrinol Metab.* 1981;52:1235.
13. Wolfe RR, Allsop JR, Burke JF. Glucose metabolism in man: responses to intravenous glucose infusion. *Metabolism.* 1979;28:1031.
14. Cerra FB, Siegel JH, Coleman B, et al. Septic autocannibalism: a failure of exogenous nutritional support. *Ann Surg.* 1980;192:570.
15. Long CL, Kinney JM, Geiger JW. Nonsuppressibility of gluconeogenesis by glucose in septic patients. *Metabolism.* 1976;25:193.
16. Herman VK, Clark D, Wilmore DW, et al. Protein metabolism: effects of disease and altered intake on the stable ^{15}N curve. *Surg Forum.* 1980;31:92.
17. Martyn JAJ. Clinical pharmacology and therapeutics in burns. In: Martyn JAJ, ed. *Acute Management of the Burned Patient.* Philadelphia: WB Saunders; 1990:180.
18. Arturson G. The oxygen-releasing capacity in patients with severe skin burns. *Injury.* 1970;1:226.
19. Aikwa N, Martyn JAJ, Burke JP. Pulmonary artery catheterization and thermodilution cardiac output determinations in critical burn management. *Am J Surg.* 1978;135: 811.
20. Herrin JT. Renal function in burns. In: Martyn JAJ, eds. *Acute Management of the Burned Patient.* Philadelphia: WB Saunders; 1990:239.
21. Loriat P, Roha J, Baillet A, et al. Increased glomerular filtration rates in patients with major burns and its effect on the pharmacokinetics of tobramycin. *N Engl J Med.* 1978; 299:915.
22. Martyn JAJ, Greenblatt DJ, Abernathy DP. Increased cimetadine clearance in burn patients. *JAMA.* 1986:253:1288.
23. Demling RH. *Burns. N Engl J Med.* 1985;313:1389.
24. Williams RL. Drug administration in hepatic disease. *N Engl J Med.* 1986;315:1616.
25. Martyn JAJ, Greenblatt DJ, Quinby WC. Diazepam kinetics following burns. *Anesth Analg.* 1983;62:293.
26. Perry S, Inturrisi CE. Analgesia and morphine disposition in burn patients. *J Burn Care Res.* 1983;4:276.
27. Moncrief JA. Burns. *N Engl J Med* 1973;288:444.
28. Hansbrough JF, Field TO, Dominic W, et al. Burns. Critical decisions. *Probl Crit Care.* 1987;1:595.
29. Baxter CR, Shires T. Physiological response to crystalloid resuscitation of severe burns. *Ann NY Acad Sci* 1986;150: 874.
30. Demling RH: Fluid resuscitation. In: Boswick JA Jr, eds. *The Art and Science of Burn Care.* Rockville, MD: Aspen Publishing; 1987:189–202.
31. Monafo WW, Chuntrasakul C, Ayvazian VH. Hypertonic saline solutions in the treatment of burn shock. *Am J Surg* 1973;126:778.
32. Pleban WE. Prealbumin: A biochemical marker of nutritional support. *Connecticut Med.* 1989;53:405.
33. Erstad BL. Serum albumin concentrations: who needs them? *Ann Pharmacol.* 1992;26:1134.

34. Weissman C, Kemper M, Askanazi J, et al. Resting metabolic rate of the critically ill patient: measurement versus predicted. *Anesthiol.* 1986;64:673.

35. Bursztein S, Elwyn DH, Askanazi J, et al, eds. *Energy Metabolism, Indirect Calorimetry, and Nutrition.* Baltimore, MD: Williams and Wilkens; 1989.

36. Tuten MB, Wogt S, Dasse F, et al. Utilization of prealbumin as a nutritional marker. *J Parenter Enteral Nutr.* 1985; 9:709.

37. Long CL, Birkhahn RH, Geiger JW, et al. Contribution of skeletal muscle to protein expenditure following injury. *J Clin Nutr.* 1981;34:1087.

38. Long CL, Jeevanandam M, Kim BM, et al. Whole body protein synthesis and catabolism in septic man. *J Clin Nutr.* 1977;30:1340.

39. Duke JH, Jorgenson SB, Long CL, et al. Contribution of protein to calorie expenditure following injury. *Surgery.* 1970;68:168.

40. Cerra FB, Upson D, Angelico R, et al. Branched chains support postoperative protein synthesis. *Surgery.* 1982;92: 192.

41. Cerra FB, Mazuski JE, Chute E, et al. Branched chain metabolic support: a prospective, randomized, double blind trial in surgical stress. *Ann Surg.* 1984;199:286.

42. Alexander JW, MacMillan BG, Stinnett JD, et al. Beneficial effects of aggressive protein feeding in severely burned children. *Ann Surg.* 1980;182:505.

43. Kudsk KA, Croce MA, Fabian, et al. Enteral versus parenteral nutrition feeding: effects on septic morbidity following blunt and penetrating trauma. *Ann Surg.* 1992; 215:503.

44. Moore FA, Moore EE, Jones TN, et al. TEN versus TPN following major abdominal trauma—reduced septic morbidity. *J Trauma.* 1989;29:916.

45. Clowes GHA, O'Donnell TF, Blackburn GL, et al. Energy metabolism and proteolysis in traumatized and septic man. *Surg Clin North Am.* 1976;56:1169.

46. Cerra FB, Siegel JH, Border JR, et al. Correlations between metabolic and cardiopulmonary measurements in patients after trauma, general surgery and sepsis. *J Trauma.* 1979;19:621.

47. Birkhahn RH, Long CL, Fitkin DL, et al. A comparison of the effects of skeletal trauma and surgery on the ketosis of starvation in man. *J Trauma.* 1981;21:513.

48. Robin AP, Askanazi J, Cooperman A, et al. Influence of hypercaloric glucose infusions on fuel economy in surgical patients. A review. *Crit Care Med.* 1981;9:680.

49. Barrocas A, Tretola T, Alonso A. Nutrition and the critically ill pulmonary patient. *Resp Care.* 1983;28:50.

50. Covelli HD, Black JW, Olsen MS, et al. Respiratory failure precipitated by high carbohydrate loads. *Ann Intern Med.* 1981;95:579.

51. Carpentier VA, Askanazi J, Elwyn DH, et al. The effect of carbohydrate on the lipolytic rate in depleted patients. *Metabolism.* 1980;29:974.

52. Hall RI, Grant JP, Ross LH, et al. Pathogenesis of hepatic steatosis in the parenterally fed rat. *J Clin Invest.* 1984;74: 1658.

53. Fisher SW, et al. Diminished bacterial defenses with interloped. *Lancet.* 1980;2:819.

54. Hamawy KJ, Moldawer LL, Georgieff M, et al. The effect of lipid emulsions on reticuloendothelial system function of the injured animal. *J Paren Ent Nutr.* 1985;9:559.

55. Hamberg M, Jonsson CE. Increased synthesis of prostaglandins in the guinea pig following scald injury. *Acta Physiol Scand.* 1973;87:240.

56. Kinsella JE, Lokesh B, Broughton S, et al. Dietary polyunsaturated fatty acids and eicosanoids: potential effects on the modulation of inflammatory and immune cells: an overview. *Nutrition.* 1990;6:24.

57. Lee TH, Hoover RL, Williams JD, et al. Effect of dietary enrichment with eicosapantaenoic acids on the in vitro neutrophil and monocyte leukotriene generation and neutrophil function. *N Engl J Med.* 1985;312:1217.

58. Sheldon GF, Petersen SR, Sanders R. Hepatic dysfunction during hyperalimentation. *Arch Surg.* 1978;64:134.

59. Alexander JW. Nutrition and infection. New perspectives for an old problem. *Arch Surg.* 1986;121:966.

60. Alexander JW, Gottschlich MM. Nutritional immunomodulation in burn patients. *Crit Care Med.* 1990;18(2): S149.

61. Alexander JW, Saito H, Trocki O, et al. The importance of lipid type in the diet after burn injury. *Ann Surg.* 1986; 204:1.

62. Gottschlich MM, Jenkins M, Warden GD, et al. Differential effects of three enteral dietary regimens on selected outcome variables in burn patients. *J Paren Ent Nutr.* 1990;14:225.

63. Daly JM, Lieberman MK, Goldfine J, et al. Enteral nutrition with supplemental arginine, RNA, and omega-3 fatty acids inpatients after operation: Immunologic, metabolic, and clinical outcome. *Surgery.* 1992;112:56.

64. Cerra FB, McPherson JP, Konstantinides N, et al. Enteral nutrition does not prevent multiple system organ failure (MSOF) after sepsis. *Surgery.* 1988;104:727.

65. Cerra FB, Lehman S, Konstantinides N, et al. Effect of enteral nutrition on in vitro tests of immune function in ICU patients: a preliminary report. *Nutrition.* 1990;6:84.

66. Cerra FB, Lehman S, Konstantinides N, et al: Improvement in immune function in ICU patients by enteral nutrition supplemented with arginine, RNA, and Menhaden oil is independent of nitrogen balance. *Nutrition.* 1991;7: 193.

67. Barbul A. Arginine: biochemistry, physiology, and therapeutic implications. *J Paren Ent Nutr.* 1986;10:227.

68. Alverdy JC. Effects of glutamine supplemented diets on the immunology of the gut. *J Paren Ent Nutr.* 1990;14: S109.

69. Bach AL, Babayan VK: Medium-chain triglycerides. An update. *Am J Clin Nutr.* 1982;36:950.

70. Babayan VK. Medium-chain triglycerides and structural lipids. *Lipids.* 1987;22:47.

71. Mascioli EA, Bistrian BR, Babayan VK. Medium-chain triglycerides as unique nonglucose source in hyperalimentation. *Lipids.* 1987;22:421.

72. Kudsk KA, Minard G, Croce MA. A randomized trial of isonitrogenous enteral diets after severe trauma. An immune enhancing diet reduces septic complications. *Ann Surg*. 1996;224:S31–J43.

73. Saffle JR, Wiebke G, Jennings K. A randomized trial of immune-enhancing enteral nutrition in burn patients. *J Trauma*. 1996;38:A102.

74. Martindale RG, Cresci GA. Use of immune-enhancing diets in burns. *J Parenter Enteral Nutr*. 2001;25:S24–S26.

75. Saito H, Trocki O, Alexander JW, et al. The effect of route of nutrient administration on the nutritional state, catabolic hormonal secretion, and gut mucosal integrity after burn injury. *JPEN*. 1987;11:4–7.

76. Rodriguez D. Nutrition in patients with severe burns: state of the art. *J Burn Care Rehabil*. 1996;17:62–70.

77. McDonald WS, Sharp CW, Deitch EA. Immediate enteral feeding in burn patients is safe and effective. *Ann Surg*. 1991;213:177–83.

78. Hansbrough WB, Hansbrough JF. Success of immediate introgastric feeding of patient with burns. *J Burn Care Rehabil*. 1993;14:512–516.

79. Garrel DR, Davignon I, Lopez D. Length of care in patients with severe burns with or without enteral nutrition support: a retrospective study. *J Burn Care. Rehabil*. 1991; 12:85–90.

80. Mochizuki H, Alexander JW. Mechanism of prevention of post burn hypometabolism and catabolism by early enteral feeding. *Ann Surg*. 1984;200:297–310.

81. Jenkins ME, Gottschlich MM, Warden GD. Enteral feeding during operative procedures in thermal injuries. *J Burn Care Rehabil*. 1994;15:199–205.

82. Heyland DW, Drover JW, MacDonald S. Effect of post pyloric feeding or gastroesophageal regurgitation and pulmonary micro-aspiration: Results of a randomized controlled trial. *Crit Care Med*. 2001;29:1495–1501.

83. Herndon DN, Barrow RE, Stein M. Increased mortality with intravenous supplemental feeding in severely burned patients. *J Burn Care Rehabil*. 1989;10:309–313.

84. Ziv G, DeBiasse MA, Demling RH. Essential micronutrients and their response to burn injury. *J Burn Care Rehabil*. 1996;17:264–71.

85. Hammargvist F, Luo J, Cotgreave IA, Wernerman J. Skeletal glutathione depletion in critically ill patients. *Crit Care Med*. 1997;25:78–84.

86. Galley HF. Xanthine oxidase activity and free radical generation in patients with sepsis syndrome. *Crit Care Med*. 1996;24:1649–1653.

87. Schorah CJ, Downing C, Piripitsi A. Total vit C, ascorbic acid and dehydroascorbic acid concentrations in plasma of critically ill patients. *Am J Clin Nutr*. 1996;63:760–765.

88. Borrelli E, Roux-Lombard P, Grau GE. Plasma concentrations of cytokines, their soluble receptors, and antioxidant vitamins can predict development of multiple organ failure in patients at risk. *Crit Care Med*. 1996;24:392–397.

89. LaLonde C, Demling R. Antioxidants prevent the cellular deficit produced in response to burn injury. *Burn Care Rehabil*. 1997;17:379–383.

90. Maderazo EG, Wornock CL, Hickingbotham N. A randomized trial of replacement antioxidant vitamin therapy for neutrophil locomotory dysfunction in blunt trauma. *J Trauma*. 1991;31:1142–1150.

91. Rock CL, Dechert RE, Khilnani R, Rodriguez JL. Carotenoids and antioxidant vitamins in patients after burn injury. *J Burn Care Rehabil*. 1997;18:269–278.

92. Berger MM, Cavadini C, Chiolero R, Guinchard S. Influence of large intakes of trace elements on recovery after major burns. *Nutrition*. 1994;10:327–334.

93. Krinsky N. Antioxidant functions of carotenoids. *Free Rad Biol Med*. 1989;7:617–635.

94. Rook JC. Biologic characteristics of the antioxidant micronutrients, vitamin C, vitamin E and the carotenoids. *J Am Diet Assoc*. 1996;96:693–702.

95. Semba RD. Vitamin A, immunity and infection. *Clin Infec Dis*. 1994;19:489–499.

96. Tengerdy RP. The role of vitamin E in immune response and disease resistance. *Ann NY Acad Sci*. 1990;587:24–33.

97. Till GO, Friedl HP, Ward PA. Antioxidant treatment in experimental thermal injury. *Adv Exp Med Biol*. 1990; 264:543–549.

98. Preiser JC, Gussum AV, Beme J. Enterol feeding with a solution enriched with antioxidant vitamins A, C, and E enhances the resistance to oxidative stress. *Crit Care Med*. 2000;28:3828–3832.

99. Nguyen TT, Cox CS, Traber DL, Herndon DW. Free radical activity and loss of plasma antioxidants, vitamin E, and sulfhydryl groups in patients with burns. *J Burn Care Rehabil*. 1993;14:602–609.

100. Gottschlich MM, Warden GD. Vitamin supplementation in the patient with burns. *J Burn Care Rehabil*. 1990;11: 275–279.

101. Webster NR, Nunn JF. Molecular structure of free radicals and their importance in biological reactions. *Br J Anesthesia*. 1988;60:98–108.

102. Molokhia A, Portnoy B, Dyer A. Neutron activation analysis of trace elements in skin. *Br J Dem*. 1979;101:567–572.

103. Runyan J, Diploch AT, Cawthorne MA. Vitamin E and stress, nutritional effects of dietary stress with silver in vitamin E deficient chicks and rats. *Br J Nutr*. 1968;22:165–182.

104. Hunt DR, Lane HW, Beesinger D. Selenium depletion in burn patients. *JPEN*. 1984;8:695–699.

105. Berger M, Chidero R, Dirren H. Copper, selenium, and zinc. Status and balances after major trauma. *J Trauma*. 1996;40:103–109.

106. Forceville X, Dominque V, Gazit R. Selenium, systemic immune response syndrome, sepsis and outcome in critically ill patients. *Crit Care Med*. 1998;26:1536–1544.

107. Singh A, Smoak BL, Patterson KY. Biochemical indices of selected trace minerals in men: effect of stress. *Am J Clin Nutr*. 1991;53:126–131.

108. Boosalis MG, Mcall JT. Serum zinc response in thermal injury. *J Am Coll Nutr*. 1988;7:69–76.

109. Berger MM, Cavadini C, Bart A. Cutaneous zinc and copper losses in burns. *Burns*. 1992;18:373–380.

110. Lennard ES, Bjornson AB, Petering HG. An immunologic and nutritional evaluation of burn neutrophil function. *J Surg Res.* 1974;16:286–298.

111. Mertz W. Chromium in human nutrition: a review. *J Nutr.* 1993;123:626–633.

112. Davis JM, Illner H, Dineen P. Increased chromium uptake in polymorphia nuclear leukocytes from burned patients. *J Trauma.* 1984;24:1003–1009.

113. Henry A. Body iron stores in critically ill patients. Significance of serum ferritin. *J Int Care Med.* 1989;15:171–178.

114. Barbul A. Arginine biochemistry, physiology, and therapeutic implications. *JPEN.* 1986;10:227–235.

115. Saito H, Mocki O, Wang S. Metabolism and immune effects of dietary arginine supplementation after burn. *Arch Surg.* 1987;122:784–790.

116. Zapata-Sirvent RL, Hansbrough JF, Ohare MM. Bacterial translocation in burned mice after administration of various diets including fiber and glutamine enriched enteral formulas. *Crit Care Med.* 1994;22:690–695.

117. Furst P, Abers S, Stehle P. Evidence for a nutritional need for glutamine in catabolic patients. *Kidney Int.* 1989;36: 287–295.

118. Ogle CK, Ogle JD, Moo IX. Effect of glutamine on phagocytosis and bacterial killing by normal and pediatric burn patient neutrophils. *JPEN.* 1994;18:128–132.

119. Coudray LC. Ornithine alpha-ketoglutarate improves wound healing in severe burn patients: a prospective randomized double-blind trial versus isonitrogenous controls. *Crit Care Med.* 2000;28:1772–1776.

120. McClae SA. Enteral tube feeding in the ICU: factors impeding adequate delivery. *Crit Care Med.* 1999;27:1252–1256.

121. Meissner W, Schmidt U, Hartmann M. Oral naloxone reverses opioid-associated constipation. *Pain.* 2000;84:105–109.

122. Purec R, Sanders MD, Kimney MB. Neostigmine for the treatment of acute colonic pseudo-obstruction. *N Engl J Med.* 1999;341:137–141.

123. Taguchi A, Sharma N, Saleem R. Selective postoperative inhibition of gastrointestinal opioid receptors. *N Engl J Med.* 2001;345:935–940.

124. Berger J, Poll L, Hall C. Oxandrolone in AIDS-washing myopathy. *AIDS.* 1996;10:657–666.

125. Fox M, Minor A. Oxandrolone: a potent anabolic steroid. *J Clin Endocrinol Metab.* 1962;22:921–940.

126. Demling R, DeSanti L. Closure of the non-healing wound corresponds with correction of weight loss using the anabolic agent oxandrolone. *Ostwal Mgt.* 1998;44:58–68.

127. Demling RH, DeSanti L. Use of anticatabolic agents for burns. *Curr Opin Crit Care.* 1996;2:182–200.

128. Demling RH, DeSanti L. Oxandrolone, an anabolic steroid, significantly increases the role of weight gain in the recovery phase after major burns. *J Trauma.* 1997;43:47–51.

129. Demling RH. Comparison of the anabolic effects and complications of human growth hormone and the testosterone analog, oxandrolone, after severe burn injury. *Burns.* 1999;25:215–221.

130. Fleming RYD, Ruten RL, Jabor F. Effect of recombinant human growth hormone on catabolic hormones and free fatty acids following thermal injury. *J Trauma.* 1992;32: 698–704.

131. Ferrando AA, Sheffield-Moore W, Hamdon DN. Testosterone administration in severe burns ameliorates muscle catabolism. *Crit Care Med.* 2001;29:1936–1942.

132. Sandesai VM. Molybdenum: an essential trace element. *NCP.* 1993;8:277–281.

133. Baumgartner TG. Trace elements in clinical nutrition. *NCP.* 1993;8:251–263.

134. Brzezinski A. Melatonin in humans. *N Engl J Med.* 1997; 336:186–195.

135. Tan DX, Chen LD, Doeggler B. Melatonin. A potent, endogenous hydroxyl radical scavenger. *Endoc J.* 1993;1:57–60.

136. Reiter RJ. The role of the neurohormone melatonin as a buffer against macromolecular oxidative damage. *Neurochem Int.* 1995;27:453–460.

137. Maestroni GJ. The immunoendocrine role of melatonin. *J Pineal Res.* 1993;14:1–10.

138. Fischer JE. Mechanism, mechanism, mechanism. *JPEN.* 1996;20:319–324.

139. Misral BR, Ferranti TJ, Keith JJ. Recombinant human interleukin-II prevents hypotension in LPS treated anesthetized rabbits. *J Endotoxin Res.* 1996;3:297–305.

140. Trepicchio WL, Bozza M, Pedra HG. Recombinant Interleukin-II attenuated the inflammatory response through downregulation of proinflammatory cytokine release and nitric oxide production. *J Immnol.* 1996:157:3627–3634.

141. Schindel D, Maze R, Liu Q. Interleukin-II improves survival and reduces bacterial translocation and bone marrow suppression in burned mice. *J Pediatric Surg.* 1997:32:312–315.

142. Vandersehueren S, Weeralt AD, Molbran M. Thrombocytopenia and prognosis in intensive care. *Crit Care Med.* 2000;28:1871–1876.

CHAPTER

22 Nutritional Considerations in Severe Brain Injury

John R. Vender, M.D., Gail A. Cresci, M.S., R.D., L.D., C.N.S.D., Mark R. Lee, M.D., Ph.D.

INTRODUCTION	259
MANAGEMENT AND TREATMENT OF INTRACRANIAL PRESSURE	260
METABOLIC RESPONSE TO SEVERE BRAIN INJURY	260
Hypermetabolic State	261
Obligatory Nitrogen Excretion	261
Hyperglycemia	261
Acute Phase Response	262
Serum Protein Response	262
NUTRITIONAL SUPPORT	262
Gastric Motility and Emptying	262
Enteral versus Parenteral Nutrition	263
Methods of Enteral Access	263
Prokinetic Therapy	264
INFECTION AND NUTRITION	264
Immune Function	264
NUTRITION AND HEAD INJURY IN THE PEDIATRIC PATIENT	264
CONCLUSIONS	265
REFERENCES	265

Introduction

Head injury is a major cause of morbidity and mortality in the United States. The incidence of head injury is approximately 200/100,000 population/year. This translates into approximately 500,000 people per year that require medical attention. Of these patients, 40,000 to 50,000 die from their injuries. The most common population affected is between 15 and 24 years of age with secondary, smaller peaks in infants and the elderly. Males outnumber females 2–3:1. Epidemiologically, half of all head injuries are the result of motor vehicle accidents, while up to 15% are due to gunshot wounds or other penetrating trauma.

Two types of injuries are associated with brain trauma: primary injury and secondary injury. A primary injury occurs as a result of direct injury to the brain tissue. This can lead to irreversible brain damage because of direct mechanical cell disruption.[1] Craniocerebral trauma can cause a concussion, a contusion, an intracranial hemorrhage, or diffuse axonal injury, which is a sheering of the brain tissue with disruption of the axons. Secondary, or delayed, injuries occur after the traumatic event and lead to further brain damage. Intracranial pressure (ICP) can increase as a result of intracranial and/or systemic causes. Intracranial causes include delayed bleeding or hematoma formation, cerebral edema, or seizures. Systemic causes of elevated ICP are hypoxia, hypo- and hypertension, hypercapnia, hyperthermia, hypoglycemia and excitotoxicity.[2] Hypoxia and hypotension are the most significant possible systemic secondary insults. A systolic blood pressure <90 mmHg and a PaO_2 <60 mmHg greatly increases morbidity and mortality.[1] Endotracheal intubation and mechanical ventilation protect the airway and ensure adequate oxygenation.

Head injuries are characterized by the Glasgow Coma Score (GCS) of the patient at admission. Patients with a GCS of 13–15 have a mild head injury and represent the largest group. Patients with a mild head injury typically have a benign clinical course with minimal or no long-term sequella. Moderate head injury (GCS 8–12) accounts for approximately 20% of all patients. This population is much more heterogeneous and complex. Up to 20% of patients with a moderate head injury will deteriorate to severe brain injury during their hospital admission. Roughly 15% of patients present with a severe brain injury (GCS 3–7). In spite of advances in emergency medicine, rapid transport systems, critical care medicine, and trauma neurosurgery, the prognosis for the severely brain injured patient remains poor. Prevention programs, such as Think First, improved safety legislation including seatbelt laws, and stricter drunk driving legislation, have had a positive impact on the number of patients injured per year. Also, the development of the "trauma center" where multiple specialties are available to simultaneously treat the brain-injured patient has had a positive impact on outcome.[3]

Numerous factors that influence the outcome of the brain injury patient are beyond the control of the clinician. A myriad of variables, including severity of the initial injury, presence of multisystem injuries, the availability and arrival time of paramedical and transport personnel, age, general medical condition, and alcohol use affect the patient's outcome. However, in spite of these factors, up to 40% of the ultimate morbidity and mortality from head injury occurs during the patient's hospitalization. Numerous pathologic mechanisms continue to be delineated. The general care of severely brain-injured patients has been reviewed by the Joint Committee on Trauma and Critical Care of the American Association of Neurological Surgeons and the Congress of Neurological Surgeons. These organizations have provided a generalized framework for the management of such patients. Although these guidelines represent the "best information available," very few care recommendations are rendered with absolute scientific certainty.[3]

Management and Treatment of Intracranial Pressure

As many as 50% of patients with severe head injury will develop elevated ICP. A normal or acceptable ICP ranges between 5–20 mmHg. Controlling the ICP has been shown to improve outcome. Management of increased ICP may include positioning to increase venous drainage, placement of intraventricular catheters to drain cerebrospinal fluid (CSF) and measure intracranial pressure, sedation, and drug therapy. Medications used to reduce ICP include osmotic diuretics, loop diuretics, carbonic anhydrase inhibitors, corticosteroids, and barbiturates. Mannitol, an osmotic agent, lowers blood viscosity and decreases extracellular fluid volume through diuresis. It can cause profound electrolyte disturbances and hyperosmolarity, and can compound acute renal failure. Furosemide can be used along with mannitol in cases with persistent elevation of ICP; a fluid restriction may also be instituted. When using these agents, serum osmolarity, urine-specific gravity, fluid balance, and renal function should be carefully monitored. Steroids historically have been administered to treat elevated ICP, but this approach is no longer recommended as no benefit has been shown with steroid administration. Steroids are known to increase nitrogen excretion by as much as 30% during the first week of head injury.[1] Barbiturates have been known to exhibit cerebral protective and ICP lowering effects. High-dose barbiturate therapy may be instituted after failure of maximal medical and surgical therapies. Barbiturates are known to alter vascular tone, suppress metabolism, and inhibit free radical mediated lipid peroxidation; barbiturates indirectly decrease gastric motility. Moderate hypothermia (30°C–32°C) is being evaluated as another alternative for ICP control and neuroprotection. Chronic hyperventilation, once a mainstay of therapy, correlates with worse outcomes and should be avoided. Episodic hyperventilation may be required to attenuate refractory ICP spikes secondary to plateau waves or patient manipulation. A possible role for mild hyperventilation is also being investigated.[3]

Propofol has become a popular sedative in critical care units for management of ICP due to its rapid onset and quick recovery.[1] Propofol is an intravenous sedative hypnotic agent processed in a soybean oil-in-water emulsion that delivers 1.1 kcal/mL. Propofol should be adjusted according to the patient's condition, response, vital signs, and blood lipid profile, as hypertriglyceridemia can develop.[1] Propofol's lipid content delivers extra calories that can substantially increase daily calories and caution should be made to avoid overfeeding when nutrition support is provided. When parenteral nutrition is provided, total lipid infusion should not exceed 1 g/kg/d. With enteral feeding, a formulation that is low in fat and high in protein should be provided.

Metabolic Response to Severe Brain Injury

Brain injury triggers a cascade of local and systemic metabolic responses. Metabolic responses are initiated by interacting changes in the level of different hormones. The central nervous system (CNS) plays an important role in the initiation of these changes. Also, several afferent stimuli from the wound; responses to changes of blood volume, pH, and osmolality concentration; hypoxia; anxiety; and sepsis contribute to the systemic metabolic responses. Anterior pituitary and sympathetic nervous system activation increases secretion of catecholamines from the adrenal medulla and sympathetic nerve endings.[1] Catecholamines stimulate the entire body and activate secretion of adrenocorticotropic hormone from the pituitary.[1,2] The extent of the hypermetabolic and hypercatabolic responses is directly proportional to the sympathetic and adrenal responses stimulated by the severity of the injury.

Hypermetabolic State

The metabolic response to brain injury has been widely studied.[2,4–11] Estimated energy requirements vary from 140% to 200% above normal for the first 3 weeks post injury.[12] A hypermetabolic state occurs at least partially related to an increase in catabolic hormones and cytokines, neuroepinephrine, and other counter regulatory hormones such as glucagon and cortisol.[1,5,9,13] Factors related to brain injury that appear to have direct impact on energy expenditure include the patient's temperature, catecholamine levels, severity of injury, resting muscle tone, spontaneous muscle activity, certain medications, and fluctuations in intracranial pressure.[14,15] Minimal elevations are seen in patients managed with musculoskeletal blocking drugs[16]; patients sedated pharmacologically also have lower metabolic rates.[10,16] However, these rates remain elevated above non-injured controls. Energy expenditure may be at control levels in brain-dead patients or patients receiving barbiturates with induced pharmacologic coma. Highest levels, reaching 250% of controls, are reported in patients with decerebrate or decorticate posturing.[14] Although various factors can elevate energy expenditure, such as steroid administration, craniotomy, infection, medications, and nutritional support, the impact on metabolic rate is nominal and the elevations noted appear directly attributable to the brain injury.[16] The duration of the hypermetabolic state is variable. It reportedly lasts from 1 week up to 1 year after injury.[2] Because of this duration, even patients who have recovered and are in rehabilitation facilities may be hypermetabolic and at risk for ongoing malnutrition.

Portable, bedside monitoring units capable of providing indirect calorimetry provide the most efficient method of determining energy expenditure. If this technology is not available, predictive formulas have been described (see Chapter 4). Clifton et al. have developed a nomogram for estimating the resting energy expenditure (REE) based on neurological function, medical therapy, heart rate, and time from injury.[17]

Obligatory Nitrogen Excretion

The metabolic response to traumatic brain injury also includes a period of excessive catabolism characterized by a marked increase in protein turnover. This is attributable to increased levels of catabolic hormones and cytokines resulting in urinary nitrogen excretion rates in excess of 25–30 g/d.[2] Physiologically this breakdown is necessary to meet the increased metabolic demands of the tissue (see Chapter 2). Early and aggressive institution of nutritional support can reduce the negative nitrogen balance[18-20]; however, patients rarely achieve a neutral or positive nitrogen balance until 2 to 3 weeks post-injury.[19] Wilson et al.[15] describe a relationship between nitrogen balance and the GCS on admission. Patients with a GCS of 3–8 have the most significant deficit. This hypercatabolic state results in the breakdown of skeletal, visceral, and immunologic proteins. In their series, low urine creatinine is associated with negative nitrogen balances purportedly due to catabolism of nonskeletal muscle tissue.[15] This can rapidly result in multisystem organ dysfunction, impaired immunosurveillance, and impaired wound healing. Increased nitrogen excretion is found in head-injured patients even when the REE is near baseline with gradual weight loss resulting despite nutrition support.[1] Patients with brain injury require at least 1.5–2.0 g/protein/kg body weight daily.[1]

Hyperglycemia

Hyperglycemia, a well-known component of the "stress response" to injury, can have significant deleterious effects on the neuron. Experimental studies have demonstrated that blood glucose levels greater than 200 mg/dL are neurotoxic. The mechanism for the in-vivo toxicity of hyperglycemia is unclear. This may be mediated through excitotoxic pathways or may be secondary to tissue acidosis or increased lactate levels in the neurophil. Hyperglycemia after injury may be mediated by an increase in circulating serum catecholamines and an increase in endogenous glucose production by the liver. The overall result is an elevation of glucose levels in the extracellular spaces. The degree of hyperglycemia correlates with the severity of the brain injury.[15] Patients with levels over 200 mg/dL were shown to have a worse neurologic outcome.[21] It is not clear if this is due to the greater severity of head injury versus hyperglycemia as a separate risk factor. Serum glucose levels can be controlled with insulin administration, pharmacologic agents, and growth factors. IGF–1 has a significant hypoglycemic effect[15] and has been demonstrated to cause significant reductions in serum glucose levels in brain-injured patients. Reduction of serum hyperglycemia, however, has not been conclusively shown to result in improved outcomes.

Acute Phase Response

Beginning immediately after head injury and extending for at least several weeks, the acute-phase response to stress results in increased hepatic production of the acute-phase proteins such as fibrinogen, alpha-1-acid, glycoprotein, c-reactive protein, and ceruloplasmin,[2,22] In order to accomplish this, a corresponding decrease in hepatic visceral protein (albumin, prealbumin) synthesis occurs. A significant decrease in serum zinc and iron levels, increased copper levels, and fever associated with leukocytosis also are characteristic of the acute-phase response.[22] Fever in the absence of detectable infection is associated with the acute-phase response and is inversely related to the Glasgow Coma Score.[15]

Most of the alterations in micronutrients normalize by 3 weeks after injury. However, zinc levels are noted to be profoundly depressed in head injury patients[22,23] with the levels directly correlating with GCS.[15] These low serum zinc concentrations are associated with significant elevated urinary zinc levels, peaking on post-injury day 7.[23] Zinc, as well as copper and iron, exhibits various roles in immune function. The concentration of plasma zinc decreases after trauma, infection, or anaphylaxis due to the acute-phase response. The cause of post-injury zinc loss is not well understood, but beneficial effects of supplementation have been demonstrated.[1,24,25] Zinc supplementation (12 mg/day) has been associated with improved serum protein concentrations and improved rate of neurologic recovery.

Serum Protein Response

Most brain injury patients are healthy and well nourished prior to their injury. Therefore, decreased serum, visceral, and skeletal protein, as well as the significant hypoalbuminemia seen for the first two to three weeks post injury are attributable to the brain injury, the hypercatabolic state, and the acute-phase response as described earlier. The degree of hypoalbuminemia has been correlated with neurological outcome at 3-month follow-up.[26] Aggressive supplementation of protein and albumin via either parenteral or enteral routes has been evaluated.[27] In spite of aggressive, early replacement, serum albumin levels tend to decrease during the patient's hospitalization, suggesting multiple contributory mechanisms of hypoalbuminemia. Decreased albumin, as well as other visceral proteins, secondary to the acute-phase response and hepatic reprioritization of visceral protein synthesis, as well as increased vascular permeability and subsequent intravascular loss, has been implicated. Some contradictory data indicating that albumin synthesis is actually increased in head-injured patients suggest that increased vascular permeability may be the primary mechanism of hypoalbuminemia. Therefore monitoring serum albumin levels does not provide adequate assessment of the patient's nutritional status but rather demonstrates the severity of the acute-phase response responsible for the vascular permeability abnormalities. A more appropriate method of using visceral proteins as part of the nutrition assessment would be to monitor both visceral protein levels and acute-phase reactants together (e.g., prealbumin and C-reactive protein) to determine the switch from a catabolic to anabolic state (see Chapter 3).

Nutritional Support

Gastric Motility and Emptying

The gastrointestinal system is significantly affected by brain injury. Stress gastritis, impaired gastric motility, delayed gastric emptying, and gastroesophageal sphincter dysfunction are common sequella after even isolated head injuries. The degree of dysfunction and time to recovery correlate with the severity of the head injury. An abnormal, biphasic response of initial hypermotility followed by delayed emptying has been described.[28] A correlation exists between daily maximum intracranial pressure measurements and time to tolerance of feeding.[13] No correlation exists, however, between return to normal feeding tolerance and return of bowel sounds.[13] The degree of gastric feeding intolerance correlates directly with mortality in patients even when controlling for severity of illness.[29–31] Normal feeding tolerance is not achieved for approximately 2 weeks after severe brain injury.[28,32] This delayed gastric emptying and impaired gastrointestinal motility may be related to increased sympathetic tone resulting from an injury-related stress state, hormone and hormonal-releasing factor effects, cytokines, or transient vagal nerve dysfunction.[13] Opioid and non-opioid sedation, widely used in the management of severe brain-injury, was questioned as a possible contributor to impaired gastric emptying. This was evaluated[29] and no significant difference was identified in gastric emptying when morphine was avoided.

Saxe et al.[33] have demonstrated the presence of lower esophageal sphincter dysfunction in patients with head injury. This can potentially lead to significant risk of emesis and aspiration when gastric feeding is the selected mode of enteral nutrition. This is particularly the case in someone unable to protect his or her airway as with absent gag reflex and/or diminished cough reflex and gastroparesis. Significantly reduced pressure gradients between the gastric and the esophageal space were identified throughout the first week post-injury. Patients with a GCS up to 12 exhibited decreased lower esophageal sphincter tone. A return toward a normal pressure gradient of more than 20 mm Hg occurs when patients recover to a GCS 12.

Swallowing abnormalities are present in up to 61% of severe traumatic brain injury patients.[34] The greater the severity of injury (as determined by GCS, CT scan results), including mid-line shift, brain stem pathology, operative procedures, and Rancho Los Amigos (RLA) Scale of Cognitive Functioning Level II levels, the greater the incidence of abnormal swallowing and aspiration.[34]

Enteral versus Parenteral Nutrition

There is extensive evidence that the institution of early nutritional support, particularly via the enteral route, enhances outcome in the brain-injury patient.[35–37] Delays of up to 3 weeks prior to achieving maximum enteral caloric intake are not acceptable in these hypercatabolic patients. Therefore, due to the hypermetabolic state of the patient and the need to achieve optimal nutritional support rapidly after injury, total parenteral nutrition (TPN) may be required. Combination therapies for nutritional support are often employed.[38] In this manner, TPN supplies the required nutrition, particularly protein, while enteral feeding is instituted at low volumes to support the intestinal brush-border. Enteral feeding can then be advanced as tolerated while weaning TPN to meet, but not exceed, nutrient requirements. Early arguments against parenteral nutrition focused on the presumption that TPN led to an increase in cerebral edema and intracranial pressure elevations. When this was studied directly, no differences in intracranial pressure were noted between TPN-fed and enterally-fed patient groups.[39] Another concern regarding the use of TPN is the higher risk of hypergylcemia when TPN is used. Attention to the amount of carbohydrate provided in the solution as well as other contributing factors (e.g., steroid administration, sepsis, overfeeding) can minimize the incidence of hyperglycemia. These concerns are not as significant as the clear benefit of early institution of nutritional support.

Methods of Enteral Access

Various modes of enteral feeding in brain injured patients have been evaluated to include nasogastric, post-pyloric (blind, endoscopic, fluoroscopic assistance), percutaneous endoscopic gastrostomy (PEG), PEG with jejunal extension (PEG/J), and surgical gastrostomy and jejunostomy tubes.[40,41] Although gastric and colonic motility are impaired after brain injury, small bowel motility is relatively preserved. This makes the jejunum a logical site for the delivery of enteral nutrition in the early post-injury period.

There are multiple methods reported for placing bedside nasoenteric feeding tubes,[42–49] all report approximately 80%–95% success. However, without dedicated nutrition support team members or staff to place the devices, success may not be as great. Blind nasoenteric tube placement was achieved in only 43% of patients in one series[36]; the rest remained intragastric. Without a standard protocol for placing nasoenteric devices, multiple patient repositionings and radiographic studies may be required. This not only may increase the cost of gaining access and delay feeding, but also many patients are unstable with labile intracranial pressures or have significant cervical spinal injuries and cannot tolerate the procedure. Endoscopic access to the jejunum, when available, can facilitate the transpyloric placement of the feeding tube and minimize the time and manipulation required for blind passage.[50] Ott et al.[40] demonstrated that early enteral feeding is best achieved with endoscopic placement of small bowel feeding tubes compared to blind passage. They reported establishment of full strength enteral feeds by a mean of 4.9 days post-injury compared to 11.5 days in the nasogastric tube fed patients. Aspiration rate of 14% versus 22% respectively was also identified between these modes of enteral access.

Frequently, head-injured patients require more permanent enteral feeding access due to a prolonged recovery and rehabilitation or overall diminished neurological function, making them unable to self-consume adequate nutrition. Findings support that gastric enteral feeding is best achieved in patients who have improved to a GCS 12, [33] or after several weeks when gastric motility and gastroesophageal sphincter function has returned to normal. When comparing a nasogastric tube to a PEG, the PEG offers the advantages of increased patient comfort, decreased risk of sinusitis or nasal erosion, and less risk of tube migration with subsequent intraesophageal feeding. Also, intragastric feeding eliminates the risk of a tube placed across the gastroesophageal junction, which may increase the tendency toward G-E regurgitation, reflux, and aspiration.[15] A PEG, unlike open gastrostomies, carries a lower morbidity and cost as it does not require general anesthesia and can usually be inserted at the bedside in the critical care unit, thus obviating need for transport of the critically ill patient to the operating room or radiology suite. Early enteral feeding following traumatic brain injury has been shown to be safe and well-tolerated when provided via PEG.[52,53] D'Amelio et al.[51] evaluated early (<7 days) versus late (>7 days) placement of tracheotomy and PEG tube for enteral nutrition. Early PEG placement was associated with only a 5% aspiration risk without any significant pneumonitis reported.

Prokinetic Therapy

Upper gastric motility is mediated through numerous mechanisms. These include intrinsic enteric neuronal and paracrine control with autonomic, endocrinologic, and central nervous system modulation. Derangements at any level can therefore result in motility abnormalities. Due to alterations in gastric motility following traumatic brain injury, prokinetic therapy is often sought. The use of exogenous agents to enhance gastric motility has usually focused on metoclopramide. This agent, however, has drawbacks in the brain-injured patient due to its central dopaminergic blocking activity. Cisapride is a prokinetic agent that does not have these centrally mediated side effects[53]; however, it was recently removed from the market by the FDA in the United States secondary to cardiac side effects; it is currently still available in Europe.

Infection and Nutrition

Immune Function

Impaired immune function is present in most patients with severe brain injury. Infection rates of 50% to 75% have been reported.[15,54] The likelihood of infection correlates with the GCS. The high infection rate, however, is associated with low mortality emphasizing the need for a high index of suspicion, careful surveillance, early diagnosis, and aggressive treatment. Helling et al. reported a 41% incidence of pulmonary infections, with gram-negative organisms predominating, in their patients.[54] The presence of chest trauma was identified as an additional factor resulting in a significantly greater likelihood of subsequent pulmonary infections.

Presumed mechanisms for infection include depressed consciousness and impaired cough and gag reflexes, resulting in impaired airway clearing and airway protection. Low pressure, high volume cuffed endotracheal tubes significantly lower the incidence of aspiration pneumonia.[55] In addition to mechanical factors, most patients with head injury demonstrate significant defects in cell-mediated immunity. Most patients tested for delayed type cutaneous hypersensitivity were anergic for up to several weeks after injury.[15,56–58] The anergy rate is proportional to the severity of injury.[59] In addition, interleukin-2 (IL-2) production, IL-2 receptor production, absolute CD4 count, T-lymphocyte responsiveness, and IFN-gamma production are also decreased in the serum of severely head-injured patients.[15,60] T-cell expression and Helper T-cell expression are also decreased, resulting in a decreased CD4/CD8 ratio.[15] This reduction is most prominent during the first 4 days post-injury, which correlates to the highest incidence of infection.[15,57] Hoyt et al.[56] reviewed 27 patients with a mean GCS of 6.75 within 24 hours of injury and at subsequent weekly intervals. They described a reduction in the proliferative response of T-cells to mitogen stimulation that was accompanied by decreased expression of early and late activation antigens. B-cell and polymorphonuclear leukocyte functions were unaffected.

Institution of early parenteral nutrition can have a positive impact on measurable immunologic function parameters in head-injured patients such as an increase in the CD4 surface antigens as well as an increase in the proliferative response to Con A stimulation.[61] Although there is evidence that early nutritional support with TPN helps improve measurable parameters of immune function, TPN, in some studies, is associated with higher infection rates when compared to enteral nutrition when similar nitrogen and caloric loads are considered.[15] Enteral nutrition may be more effective than parenteral nutrition in enhancing immune function in several ways. These include the maintenance of gastrointestinal mucosal integrity, reduction of septic morbidity, and decreased bacterial translocation across the gut wall.[61] Supplementation of specific nutrients (e.g., arginine, omega-3 fatty acids, glutamine, nucleic acids) has been shown to enhance immunologic function[62–65] (see Chapter 32).

Nutrition and Head Injury in the Pediatric Patient

Significantly less research has been performed on the metabolic and nutritional derangements precipitated by severe brain injury in children. Up to 75% of pediatric trauma patients have a concomitant neurological injury. Trauma is the leading cause of death in children. Most of the reported trauma mortalities in children are associated with significant cerebral injuries.[66] Children manifest a similar hypermetabolic, hypercatabolic cascade associated with cytokine release, altered hormonal activity, and elevations in adrenaline and counter regulatory hormones.[67] In the child, there is often a more limited supply of nutritional substrate and lower energy reserves when compared to adults. This increases the vulnerability of the child to these metabolic stressors, thereby increasing morbidity and mortality rates in children.[67,68] Children referred for rehabilitation have significantly decreased body cell mass suggestive of significant muscle wasting.[69]

Conclusions

Significant nutritional derangements are associated with severe brain injury. If not addressed aggressively, these derangements can exacerbate the hypermetabolic and hypercatabolic state present in these patients and result in increased secondary brain injury. Aberrant nutritional status can also result in impaired immune function and increased susceptibility of the neuron to excitotoxcity. Hypercatabolism, if not reversed or minimized, will adversely affect other organ systems as well. In order to minimize infection risk, ongoing neuronal insult, and multisystem organ failure, aggressive nutritional support must be considered as part of the initial management of the head injured patient.

Early identification of patients requiring nutrition support should be made. Once the patient is hemodynamically stable, small bowel enteral access should be attempted so that early enteral feeding may begin. If enteral access is not successful or enteral feeding is not tolerated, then TPN should be provided to meet nutrient requirements.

A high-protein formulation should be utilized to potentially provide 1.5–2.0 g of protein/kg body weight. Total calories should be provided as indicated via measured energy expenditure or predictive equations realizing the patient's hypermetabolic state.[70] Caution should be made to avoid overfeeding calories and carbohydrate to maintain blood glucose levels 180 mg/dL. Fat should be provided at <1 g/kg/d with consideration of lipid-based medications. A combination of long-chain (omega-3 and omega-6) and medium-chain triglycerides should be provided (see Chapter 32). The patient's electrolytes, osmolality, fluid balance, renal and liver function should be monitored closely in accordance with his or her medical management.

References

1. Varella L, Fastremski C. Neurological impairment. In: Gottschlich M, ed. *The Science and Practice of Nutrition Support*. Dubuque, IA: Kendall/Hunt; 2001:421–444.
2. Pepe J, Barba C. The metabolic response to acute traumatic brain injury and implications for nutritional support. *J Head Trauma Rehabil.* 1999;14:462–474.
3. Bullock R, Chestnut R, Clifton G, et al. *Guidelines for the Management of Severe Head Injury*. New York: Brain Trauma Foundation; 1996:517–523.
4. Liebert M. Nutritional support of brain-injured patients. *J Neurotrauma*. 1996;13:721–729.
5. Loan T. Metabolic/nutritional alterations of traumatic brain injury. *Nutrition*. 1999;15:809–812.
6. Planas M. Enteral nutrition in intensive care medicine. *Med Intensiva*. 1994;18:381–385.
7. Taylor S, Fettes S, Jewkes C, et al. Prospective, randomized, controlled trial to determine the effect of early enhanced enteral nutrition on clinical outcome in mechanically ventilated patients suffering head injury. *Crit Care Med*. 1999;27:2525–2531.
8. Woodward S. Nutritional support for head-injured patients. *Professional Nurse*. 1996;11:290–292.
9. Chiolero R, Schutz Y, Lemarchand T, et al. Hormonal and metabolic changes following severe head injury or noncranial injury. *J Parenter Enteral Nutr.* 1989;13:5–12.
10. Chiolero R, Revelly J, Tappy L. Energy metabolism in sepsis and injury. *Nutrition*. 1997;13(Suppl):45S-51S.
11. Raurich J, Ibanex J. Metabolic rate in severe head trauma. *JPEN*. 1994;18:521–524.
12. Sunderland PM, Heilbrun MP. Estimating energy expenditure in traumatic brain injury: comparison of indirect calorimetry with predictive formulas. *Neurosurg*. 1992; 31:246–253.
13. Mogilner AY, Golfinos JF. Nutrition in the patient with severe head injury. In, Cooper PR, Golfinos JG, eds. *Head Injury*. 4th ed. New York: McGraw-Hill; 2000:517–523.
14. Young B, Ott L, Phillips R, et al. Metabolic management of the patient with head injury. *Neurosurg Clin N Am*. 1991;2:301–320.
15. Wilson RF, Tyburski JG. Metabolic responses and nutritional therapy in patients with severe head injuries. *J Head Trauma Rehabil*. 1998;1:11–27.
16. Clifton G, Robertson C, Grossman R, et al. The metabolic response to severe head injury. *J Neurosurg*. 1984;60: 687–696.
17. Clifton G, Robertson C, Choi S. Assessment of nutritional requirements of head-injury patients. *J Neurosurg*. 1986; 64:895–901.
18. Gadisseux P, Ward J, Young H, et al. Nutrition and the neurosurgical patient. *J Neurosurg*. 1984;60:219–232.
19. Twyman D, Young A, Ott L, et al. High protein enteral feedings: a means of achieving positive nitrogen balance in head injured patients. *J Parenter Enteral Nutr.* 1985;9:679–684.

20. Bivins B, Twyman D, Young B. Failure of nonprotein calories to mediate protein conservation in brain-injured patients. *J Trauma.* 1986;26:980–985.
21. Young B, Ott L, Dempsey R, et al. Relationship between admission hyperglycemia and neurological outcome of severe brain-injured patients. *Ann Surg.* 1989;210:466.
22. Young A, Ott L, Beard D, et al. The acute-phase response of the brain-injured patient. *J Neurosurg.* 1988;69:375–380.
23. McClain M, Twyman D, Ott L, et al. Serum and urine zinc response in head-injured patients. *J Neurosurg.* 1986; 64:224–230.
24. Young B, Ott L, Kasarskis E, et al. Zinc supplementation is associated with improved neurologic recovery rate and visceral protein levels of patients with severe closed head injury. *J Neurotrauma.* 1996; 13:25–34.
25. Hennig B, Wang Y, Ramasamy S, et al. Zinc protects against tumor necrosis factor-induced disruption of porcine endothelial cell monolayer integrity. *J Nutr.* 1993;123: 1003–1009.
26. McClain C, Henning B, Ott L, et al. Mechanisms and implications of hypoalbuminemia in head-injured patients. *J Lab Clin Med.* 1988;69:386–392.
27. Borzotta A, Pennings J, Papasadero B, et al. Enteral versus parenteral nutrition after severe closed head injury. *J Trauma.* 1994;37:459–468.
28. Ott L, Young B, Phillips R, et al. Altered gastric emptying in the head-injured patient: Relationship to feeding intolerance. *J Neurosurg.* 1991;74:738–742.
29. McArthur C, Gin T, McLaren I, et al. Gastric emptying following brain injury: effects of choice of sedation and intracranial pressure. *Inten Care Med.* 1995;21:573–576.
30. Kao C, ChangLai S, Chieng P, et al. Gastric emptying in head-injured patients. *Am J Gastroenterology.* 1998;93: 1108–1112.
31. Kirby D. As the gut churns: feeding challenges in the head-injured patient. *J Parenter Enteral Nutr.* 1996;20:1–2.
32. Norton J, Ott L, McClain C, et al. Intolerance to enteral feeding in the brain-injured patient. *J Neurosurg.* 1988;68: 62–66.
33. Saxe J, Ledgerwood A, Lucas C, et al. Lower esophageal sphincter dysfunction precludes safe gastric feeding after head injury. *J Trauma.* 1994;37:581–586.
34. Mackay L, Morgan A, Bernstein B. Factors affecting oral feeding with severe traumatic brain injury. *J Head Trauma Rehabil.* 1999;14:435–447.
35. Sacks G, Brown R, Teague D, et al. Early nutrition support modifies immune function in patients sustaining severe head injury. *J Parenter Enteral Nutr.* 1995;19:387–392.
36. Spain D, DeWeese C, Reynolds M, et al. Transpyloric passage of feeding tubes in patients with head injuries does not decrease complications. *J Trauma.* 1995;39:1100–1102.
37. Minard G, Kudsk K, Melton S, et al. Early versus delayed feeding with an immune-enhancing diet in patients with severe head injuries. *J Parenter Enteral Nutr.* 1998;24:145–149.
38. Rapp R, Young B, Twyman D, et al. The favorable effect of early parenteral feeding on survival in head-injured patients. *J Neurosurg.* 1983;58:906–912.
39. Young B, Ott L, Haack D, et al. Effect of total parenteral nutrition upon intracranial pressure in severe head injury. *J Neurosurg.* 1987;67:76–80.
40. Ott L, Annis K, Hatton J, et al. Postpyloric enteral feeding costs for patients with severe head injury: blind placement, endoscopy, and PEG/J versus TPN. *J Neurotrauma.* 1999; 16:233–242.
41. Harbrecht B, Moraca R, Saul M, et al. Percutaneous endoscopic gastrostomy reduces total hospital costs in head-injured patients. *Am J Surg.* 1998;176:311–314.
42. Zaloga GP. Bedside method for placing small bowel feeding tubes in critically ill patients. *Chest.* 1991;100:1643–1646.
43. Thurlow PM. Bedside enteral feeding tube placement into duodenum and jejunum. *J Parenter Enteral Nutr.* 1986;10: 104–105.
44. Gabriel SA, Ackermann RJ, Castresana MR. A new technique for placement of nasoenteral feeding tubes using external magnetic guidance. *Crit Care Med.* 1997;25:641–645.
45. Davis TJ, Sun D, Dalton ML. A modified technique for bedside placement of nasoduodenal feeding tubes. *J Am Coll Surgeons.* 1994;178:407–409.
46. Salasidis R, Fleiszer T, Johnston R. Air insufflation technique of enteral tube insertion: a randomized, controlled trial. *Crit Care Med.* 1998;26:1036–1039.
47. Cresci G, Grace M, Park M, et al. Accurate and timely blind bedside placement of post-pyloric feeding tubes using an electromagnetic navigation device. *Nutr Clin Prac.* 1999;14:101.
48. Lord LM, Weiser-Maimone A, Pulhamus M, et al. Comparison of weighted vs. unweighted enteral feeding tubes for efficacy of transpyloric intubation. *J Parenter Enteral Nutr.* 1993;17:271–273.
49. Kittinger JW, Sandler RS, Heizer WD. Efficacy of metoclopramide as an adjunct to duodenal placement of small-bore feeding tubes: a randomized, placebo-controlled double-blind study. *J Parenter Enteral Nutr.* 1987;11:33–37.
50. Minard G. Enteral access. *Nutr Clin Prac.* 1994;9:172–182.
51. D'Amelio L, Hammond J, Spain D, et al. Tracheostomy and percutaneous endoscopic gastrostomy in the management of the head injured trauma patient. *Am Surg.* 1994; 60:180.
52. Klodell C, Carroll M, Carrillo E, et al. Routine intragastric feeding following traumatic brain injury is safe and well tolerated. *Am J Surg.* 2000;179:168–171.
53. Altmayer T, O'Dell M, Jones M, et al. Cisapride as a treatment for gastroparesis in traumatic brain injury. *Arch Phys Med Rehabil.* 1996;77:1093–1094.
54. Helling T, Evans L, Fowler D, et al. Infectious complications in patients with severe head injury. *J Trauma.* 1988; 28:1575–1577.

55. Spray S, Zuidema G, Cameron J. Aspiration pneumonia: Incidence of aspiration with endotracheal tubes. *Am J Surg.* 1976;131:701–703.

56. Hoyt D, Ozkan N, Hansbrough J, et al. Head injury: an immunologic deficit in T-cell activation. *J Trauma.* 1990; 30:759–767.

57. Quattrocchi K, Frank E, Miller C, et al. Impairment of helper T-cell function and lymphokine-activated killer cytotoxicity following severe head injury. *J Neurosurg.* 1991; 75:766–773.

58. Miller C, Quattrocchi K, Frank E, et al. Humoral and cellular immunity following severe head injury: review and current investigations. *Neurol Res.* 1991;13:117–124.

59. Imhoff M, Gahr R, Hoffmann P. Delayed cutaneous hypersensitivity after multiple injury and severe burn. *Ann Ital Chir.* 1990;61:525.

60. Quattrocchi K, Frank E, Miller C, et al. Suppression of cellular immune activity following severe head injury. *J Neutotrauma.* 1990;7:77.

61. Sacks G, Brown R, Teague D, et al. Early nutrition support modifies immune function in patients sustaining severe head injury. *J Parenter Enteral Nutr.* 1995;19:387–392.

62. Bengmark S. Immunonutrition—concluding remarks. *Nutrition.* 1999;15:57–61.

63. Zaloga G. Immune-enhancing enteral diets: where's the beef? *Crit Care Med.* 1998;26:1143–1146.

64. Barton R. Immune-enhancing enteral formulas: are they beneficial in critically ill patients? *Nutr Clin Prac.* 1997;12: 51–62.

65. Martindale RG, Cresci GA. The use of immune enhancing diet in head injury. *J Parent Enteral Nutr.* 2001;25 (Suppl):S27–S29.

66. Atanasov A. Pediatric trauma in Plovdiv: First international symposium on cardiovascular diseases and pediatric trauma. Sofia, Bulgaria. 1995:159.

67. Lazarov S. Metabolic changes in children with severe traumatic injuries. *Folia Medica.* 1999;41:23–29.

68. Winthrop A, Wesson D, Pencharz P, et al. Injury severity, whole body protein turnover, and energy expenditure in pediatric trauma. *J Pediatr Surg.* 1987;22:534–537.

69. Littlewood R, Wotten M, Trocki O, et al. Reduced body cell mass following severe head injury in children: implications for rehabilitation. *Pediatric Rehabilitation.* 1999;3:95–99.

70. Twyman D. Nutritional management of the critically ill neurologic patient. *Critical Care Clinics.* 1997;13:39–49.

CHAPTER

23 Nutritional Therapy in Acute Pancreatitis

Stephen A. McClave, M.D., Gerald W. Dryden, M.D., James K. Lukan, M.D.

Introduction	269
Importance of Pancreatic Rest	269
Reduced Pancreatic Stimulation with Jejunal Feeding	270
Importance of Maintaining Gut Integrity	271
Identifying Patients in Need of Aggressive Enteral Nutritional Support	273
Monitoring Patients on Early Enteral Feeding	274
Conclusions	275
Case Study	275
References	276

Introduction

Multiple factors contribute to the toxicity and overall disease severity of acute pancreatitis. Modulation of these factors through nutritional support is essential to the proper management of patients with this disorder. Certainly, it is important to reduce stimulation of the pancreas in an effort to allow resolution of inflammation within the gland. Although vital, this principle does not preclude use of the gut. An equally important factor affecting ultimate patient outcome may be the utilization of the gastrointestinal (GI) tract and maintenance of gut integrity. While the initial stress response on admission is dictated by the severity of pancreatitis and the presence or absence of necrosis within the gland, long-term complications and the speed with which the patient recovers from the systemic inflammatory response of pancreatitis may in part be related to the timing, route, and volume of enteral nutritional support.

On initial assessment, the clinician's efforts should be directed at identifying those patients with severe pancreatitis who would most benefit from establishing early enteral access and initiating a sufficient volume of enteral feeding. Monitoring the pancreatitis patient on jejunal feeding requires vigilance and the ability to clearly identify the point at which the patient is ready to advance to oral diet. Nutritional support in the patient with acute pancreatitis must be considered not only in the context of sustenance, but also as a critical therapeutic intervention with the potential risks and benefits of any pharmacologic agent.

Importance of Pancreatic Rest

That pancreatic rest and a reduction of exocrine secretion may allow a more expedient resolution of pancreatitic inflammation is an important clinical precept in the management of patients with acute pancreatitis. Fortunately, the most common deleterious effect of early advancement to oral diet is an uncomplicated exacerbation of symptoms, which in one multi-center trial occurred in 21% of patients recovering from acute pancreatitis.[1] Of greater concern is a true exacerbation of pancreatitis, which occurs in less than one-fifth of those patients who demonstrate an exacerbation of symptoms (or in 4.3% of patients overall).[1] Relapse in response to early advancement to oral diet does affect patient outcome with regard to length of hospitalization. Length of hospitalization after advancement to oral diet was prolonged from 7 days in those patients who advanced successfully, to 18 days in those patients who suffered relapse.[1] Total length of hospitalization was nearly doubled from 18 to 33 days ($p<0.002$) when relapse occurred in response to early advancement to oral diet.[1] The development of late complications of major peri-pancreatic infection in response to early dietary advancement described in early retrospective studies[2] has not been demonstrated in more recent prospective studies.

The understanding of what constitutes pancreatic rest has improved over the past decade. Reduction of the enzymatic protein portion of pancreatic exocrine secretion appears to be the most important factor in resolving the inflammatory response. While fluid volume and bicarbonate output from the pancreas are often simultaneously stimulated with increases in protein enzyme output, the three aspects of pancreatic secretion are not necessarily linked through the same stimulatory factors. Management strategies that reduce protein enzyme output with continued output of volume and bicarbonate may be sufficient to rest the pancreas and allow resolution of inflammation.[3] A reduction of protein enzyme output to basal unstimulated levels may not be required to rest the pancreas, as a reduction to subclinical levels may be sufficient to promote convalescence. This strategy may be guided by resolution of symptoms. Very little secretion in the pancreas may occur at the height of acute inflammation.[4] But most important, pancreatic rest may be achieved by early enteral feeding infused low in the gastrointestinal tract at the level of the jejunum with formulas that minimize pancreatic stimulation.

Reduced Pancreatic Stimulation with Jejunal Feeding

The safety of early enteral feeding and the ability to reduce pancreatic stimulation with jejunal infusion of nutrients was clearly demonstrated in the first prospective randomized trial of enteral versus parenteral feeding in acute pancreatitis.[5] As shown in Table 23.1, patients placed on early jejunal feeding within 48 hours of admission for acute pancreatitis demonstrated that there was no prolongation of the time to normalization of amylase, advancement to oral diet, length of time spent in the intensive care unit, or overall length of hospital stay.[5] Use of the enteral route did not increase nosocomial infections or affect overall mortality.[5]

The ability of early enteral feedings to rest the pancreas relates to the fact that there are various levels of stimulation throughout the GI tract.[6] These levels of pancreatic stimulation include the cephalic, gastric, and intestinal phases.[6] The cephalic phase begins as the sight, taste, and smell of food stimulate the pancreas via vagal innervation. Subsequent passage of food into the stomach likewise stimulates the pancreas via vagal innervation in the gastric phase. In addition, acid secretion in response to food and mechanical distension of the stomach contribute to pancreatic stimulation. The increase in acid stimulates gastrin output, which also directly stimulates the pancreas. The intestinal phase begins as food passes out of the stomach into the duodenal bulb, again affecting vagal stimulation of the pancreas. The major contribution to pancreatic secretion in the intestinal phase comes from release of cholecystokinin in response to luminal fat and protein, and secretin from acidic chyme entering the duodenum. The lower these nutrients are infused in the GI tract, the less likely they are to stimulate pancreatic secretion. Feeding low beyond the ligament of Trietz may not only bypass the stimulatory factors, but ironically may stimulate a number of inhibitory polypeptides. Pancreatic inhibitory polypeptide, polypeptide YY, somatostatin, luminal proteases, and even bile acids all inhibit or reduce pancreatic secretion and may be released in response to jejunal feeding.

Animal and human studies in acute pancreatitis have demonstrated the differential response of pancreatic secretion to nutrient stimulus delivered to individual levels of the GI tract. In a classic dog study,[7] Ragins et al. showed that feeding into the stomach stimulated fluid, bicarbonate, and enzyme secretion from the pancreas. Infusion into the duodenum stimulated fluid output only, with no increase in bicarbonate or enzyme output. Feeding into the jejunum resulted in no increase in volume, bicarbonate, or enzyme output.[7] Three patients who were part of a prospective randomized trial and were placed on jejunal feeds, normalized their amylase and resolved their abdominal pain over 5 days of jejunal feeding.[5] They all experienced relapse when advanced to oral clear liquid diets. One patient, whose tube was pulled, had to be made NPO for 5 more days before successfully advancing to oral diet. The other two patients were placed back on jejunal feeds.[5] Subsequently, their hyperamylasemia

TABLE 23.1

Safety of Early Jejunal Feeding in Acute Pancreatitis (means +/− SEM; *p<0.005)[5]

	TPN (n=16)	ETF (n=16)
Days to normal amylase	6.8 +/− 1.5	4.8 +/− 0.6
Days to oral diet	7.1 +/− 1.1	5.6 +/− 0.8
LOH (days)	11.9 +/− 2.6	9.7 +/− 1.3
Length ICU (days)	2.8 +/− 1.3	1.3 +/− 0.9
Nosocomial infection (%)	12.5 +/− 8.5	12.5 +/− 8.5
Mortality	0.0%	0.0%
Cost nutrition per patient	$3294 +/− 551.9	$761 +/− 50.3*

and pain resolved. Up to two additional attempts at oral feeding were required before the patients could be successfully advanced to a clear liquid diet. During each exacerbation, reinstating jejunal feeds resulted in resolution of symptoms and normalization of amylase.[5] A fourth patient randomized to jejunal feeds in the same study experienced clinical resolution of pancreatitis after 6 days of jejunal feeding.[5] When the tube was displaced into the stomach on the sixth day, the patient sustained a dramatic increase in the systemic inflammatory response syndrome exhibited by a rising temperature and white blood cell count. While the patient appeared clinically septic, cultures from the urine, blood, and sputum failed to show a putative pathogenic organism. Repositioning the tube and reinstating jejunal feeds led to resolution of the inflammatory response and the patient successfully advanced to oral diet 10 days later.[5] Clearly, low jejunal feeding in all of these patients allowed resolution of the inflammatory response and symptomatic convalescence, while feeding higher into the GI tract led to clinical relapses.

Specific characteristics and degree of digestive complexity of individual nutrients have a differential effect on pancreatic secretion.[6,8] Of the three major macronutrients, intraluminal fat is the most potent stimulus of the pancreas and intraluminal carbohydrate is the least. Long chain fatty acids appear to stimulate the pancreas more than medium chain triglycerides.[6,8] Intact protein stimulates the pancreas more than individual amino acids, and although this is controversial, small peptides may be the form of protein that has the least stimulatory effect. Agents with high osmolarity may stimulate the pancreas more than agents with low osmolarity.[8]

Studies in patients with pancreatitis have confirmed these differential effects of the individual components of luminal nutrients. In a unique post-operative patient with an isolated duodenal fistula and a surgically-placed jejunal feeding tube, pancreatic output in response to various formulas was evaluated.[9] Infused at the same level of the jejunum, elemental nearly fat-free formulas (Vivonex® [Novartis, Minneapolis, MN] and Criticare® [Mead Johnson, Evansville, IN]) showed no significant increase in volume, bicarbonate, amylase, or lipase output from the pancreas. Osmolite® (Ross Laboratories, Columbus, OH), with intact protein and long chain fatty acids, led to a statistically significant five-fold increase in lipase output (without change in volume, bicarbonate or amylase output).[9] In a separate study, patients recovering from alcoholic pancreatitis who were intolerant of a standard oral diet demonstrated normalization of amylase and resolution of abdominal pain when an elemental fat-free formula (Precision-LR) was given orally.[8]

With a basic understanding of these concepts, the clinician may envision a scale over which the degree of pancreatic stimulation is determined by the inherent nature and method of delivery by which nutrients are administered. At one end of the scale is oral feeding, which invokes the greatest degree of pancreatic secretion. Delivery of nutrients to progressively lower levels of the GI tract (from the stomach to the duodenum to jejunum) is associated with diminishing degree of stimulation. At the other end of the scale, parenteral infusion, in the absence of hypercalcemia or hypertriglyceridemia, has the least stimulatory effect and the lowest likelihood for relapse.[6] Similarly, with regard to components of the individual nutrients, fat would be at the end of the scale causing the greatest stimulation of the pancreas. Protein, and then carbohydrate, would be at the opposite end of the scale leading to lesser degrees of stimulation. The degree of disease severity (as determined by the presence or absence as well as the degree of pancreatic necrosis)[10] determines the maximal number of stimulatory factors that may be tolerated without relapse. Severe pancreatitis with significant pancreatitic necrosis may require feeding into the jejunum with a formula comprising either elemental amino acids or small peptides and minimal amounts of long chain fat, in order to reduce pancreatic stimulation below subclinical levels. On the other hand, in mild pancreatitis, the same formula may be given orally without exacerbating symptoms or inflammation.

Importance of Maintaining Gut Integrity

While the tenant of pancreatic rest is of central importance in managing patients with acute pancreatitis, maintaining gut integrity is equally important. The GI tract is the largest immune organ in the body, containing 65% of immune tissue overall and up to 80% of the immunoglobulin-producing tissue of the body.[11,12] As a result, utilization of the GI tract modulates overall systemic immunity and leads to a dramatic favorable impact on patient outcome.

In the fed state, the normal villi, rich blood supply, and intercellular tight junctions contribute to the overall integrity of the GI tract. Propulsive contractions keep the concentration of bacteria at normal levels and the secretion of bile salts and secretory IgA in response to luminal nutrients coat the bacteria and prevent adherence to the gut wall and subsequent translocation.[13,14] The healthy gut acts as an important antigen-processing organ, in which bacterial antigen is presented across the M-cells, stimulating the release and maturation of a population of pluripotential stem cells.[15,16] These cells will migrate out from the Peyer's patches, through the mesenteric lymph nodes and thoracic duct, into the systemic circulation as a mature line of B and T cell lymphocytes. A portion of these cells returns to the GI tract as gut-associated lymphoid tissue (GALT).[14–16] Lymphoid follicles are composed mostly of helper T-cells, which induce the production of secretory IgA by the plasma cells. Diffuse lymphoid tissue contained within the intestinal villi have a wider variety of cells, including helper T-cells, cytotoxic T-cells, B-cells, and plasma cells.[14–16] A separate population of cells generated in the maturation of the pluripotential stem cells migrates out as mucosal-associated lymphoid tissue (MALT) to distant sites such as the lungs, genitourinary, breast, and lacrimal glands.[13–16] Instead of seeing an increase in aspiration pneumonia in response to enteral feeding of critically ill patients, clinicians may instead see a reduced incidence of pneumonia[17] due to maintenance of MALT in the lung by the trophic effects of luminal nutrients on the intestinal immune components.[14–16]

In a situation of even brief disuse, gut integrity may deteriorate. In contrast to the fed state, fasting leads to villous atrophy, diminished blood flow, and loss of interepithelial tight junctions. This opens paracellular channels, allowing translocation of bacteria.[13] Reduced contractility promotes bacterial overgrowth.[13] Without nutrient-induced stimulation of secretory IgA and bile salts, bacteria are able to adhere to the luminal wall, promoting even greater translocation of bacteria and their secretory products (i.e., endotoxin).[13] The mass of GALT may diminish, as does the antigen-processing and buildup of MALT at distant sites.

The most important aspect of gut disuse may be the diminished blood supply to the gut, which leads to ischemia/reperfusion injury.[18] The generation of superoxide radicals in response to ischemia/reperfusion may promote the gut as a priming bed for macrophages.[18,19] Macrophages, primed and activated at the level of the gut, may migrate out to distant sites such as the liver, lung, and kidney. There, they may diapedese into these tissues, introducing oxidative species.[19] Activated macrophages are the key step linking issues of gut deterioration with more systemic factors that adversely affect patient outcome.[19,20] Activated macrophages initiate the arachidonic acid cascade. Generation of Prostaglandin E_2 suppresses delayed hypersensitivity reaction, generates superoxide radicals, and leads to an overall pattern of sepsis. Generation of Leukotriene B_4 leads to chemotaxis and edema and the Systemic Inflammatory Response Syndrome (SIRS). Thromboxane A_2, another product of this cascade, leads to vasoconstriction and thrombosis. This event, in turn, promotes physiologic shunts and multiple organ failure.[19,21]

Although simplified, the concepts presented point to the pivotal importance enteral nutrition plays in determining whether the gut promotes inflammation or enhances appropriate immune function in the setting of pancreatitis. Gut disuse, with or without parenteral feeding, leads to a process in which there is macrophage/neutrophil activation and a non-specific pattern of exaggerated systemic inflammatory response with multiple organ failure.[18–21] On the other hand, utilizing the gut and infusing luminal nutrients instead leads to a different process characterized by the orderly generation of GALT/MALT, and the incidence of nosocomial infection and organ failure is reduced.[14–16]

Data in patients with acute pancreatitis indicate that these factors are important in the disease process of pancreatitis and, to a large extent, determine degree of disease severity and ultimate patient outcome. A prospective study evaluating the effects of enteral feeding versus TPN and gut disuse in patients with pancreatitis compared these patients against a control group without pancreatitis.[22] A segment of jejunum was resected at surgery to evaluate the effect of enteral feeding on mucosal integrity and architecture.[22] The control group maintained on enteral feeding had essentially normal villi. Pancreatitis was associated with villous atrophy in the experimental arm, but the effect was minimized in the enteral nutrition group. Those patients with pancreatitis placed on TPN and gut disuse had the greatest villous atrophy. Longer periods of gut disuse completely transformed the mucosal architecture, resulting in a flattened, featureless surface.[22]

With loss of integrity, there is evidence in pancreatitis patients that the gut becomes "leaky." In a prospective randomized trial, Windsor showed that patients with pancreatitis maintained on enteral tube feeding had no change in IgM antibodies to endotoxin over a week of enteral feeding.[23] In contrast, controls placed on TPN and gut disuse demonstrated a statistically significant increase in IgM antibodies to endotoxin of 24.8% in response to a week of parenteral feeding ($p<0.05$).[23] Evidence that loss of integrity and a leaky gut led to an increased generation of superoxide radicals was shown in the same study by the fact that total antioxidant capacity (as measured by an enhancement chemiluminescence assay) was shown to be reduced by 27.7% in the group placed on TPN and gut disuse.[23] In contrast, study patients on enteral feeding showed a statistically significant increase in antioxidant capacity by 32.6% over a similar week of enteral feeding ($p<0.05$).[23]

The more important contribution from the leaky gut with compromised integrity relates to its effect on the overall stress response and disease severity caused by pancreatitis. In a prospective randomized trial, normal healthy volunteers randomized to TPN and gut disuse for 7 days demonstrated an exaggerated stress response to a standard intravenous challenge of E. Coli endotoxin, as evidenced by higher glucagon, epinephrine, tumor necrosis factor, and C-reactive protein levels compared to a study group receiving a week of enteral feeding.[24] Protein efflux across the lower extremity was greater in the group placed on TPN and gut disuse, indicating greater muscle catabolism.[24] In pancreatitis patients, significant increases in stress-induced hyperglycemia were seen in a control group placed on TPN and gut disuse.[5] No such increases in serum glucose levels were seen in the study group placed on enteral feeding.[5] In the same study, both enteral and parenteral groups at initiation of the study had similar mean Ranson Criteria, Marshal multi-organ failure scores, and APACHE III scores.[5] The curves for the serial mean values of these scoring systems separated during the course of hospitalization, as the group on enteral feeding tended to normalize and reduce their scores more readily than the group placed on TPN and gut disuse (only the third Ranson criteria, obtained on a mean 6.3 days following admission, was significantly lower in the enteral group compared to the parenteral group, $p=0.002$).[5] In a separate study, C-Reactive Protein levels in a group of pancreatitis patients randomized to TPN and gut disuse did not change over a week of parenteral feeding.[23] In contrast, C-Reactive Protein levels decreased significantly from 156 to 84 gm/dL in a study group placed on enteral feeding ($p<0.05$).[23] In the same study, APACHE II scores decreased significantly over a week of feeding within the enteral group, with no significant change in the group placed on TPN and gut disuse.[23] At the end of 1 week of nutritional therapy, 9 out of 11 patients in the enteral group had resolved the SIRS, contrasted with the group placed on TPN and gut disuse in which only 2 out of 12 patients resolved the SIRS over their first week of therapy ($p<0.05$).[23]

Most important, the issues of enteral access and maintenance of gut integrity in acute pancreatitis ultimately affect patient outcome. In a prospective randomized trial, patients with severe acute pancreatitis and necrosis on computerized tomography scans who were placed on enteral feeding developed significantly fewer septic complications compared to a similar group of patients placed on TPN and gut disuse (incidence of septic complications 28% versus 50% respectively, $p<0.03$).[25] Additionally, the number of infections in those patients who developed septic complications was reduced significantly as well, from 1.35 in the group randomized to TPN/gut disuse to 0.56 in the group on enteral feeding ($p<0.03$).[25] In fact, overall complications were reduced significantly, from 75% in the group placed on TPN/gut disuse to 44% in the early enteral group ($p<0.05$).[25]

Identifying Patients in Need of Aggressive Enteral Nutritional Support

Determining which patients need aggressive nutritional enteral support can be difficult for the clinician. Surprisingly, clinical assessment and physical examination on admission have been shown to be inferior to APACHE II scores in differentiating patients with severe pancreatitis with a higher likelihood of morbidity and mortality[26,27] from those with mild to moderate pancreatitis and a low likelihood of complications. In two studies, the sensitivity of clinical assessment in identifying patients with severe pancreatitis was only 34%–44%, whereas sensitivity for APACHE II score of >9 was 63%–82%.[26,27] While APACHE II score was superior to clinical assessment in predicting severe attacks on admission, overall accuracy for clinical assessment was higher on admission because most mild attacks were correctly predicted (see Table 23.2).[26,27] At 48 hours, sensitivity of both the APACHE II score >9 and Ranson Criteria >2 was greater (75%–82%) in identifying patients with severe pancreatitis than clinical assessment (44%–66%).[27] Overall accuracy for clinical assessment at 48 hours was 87%–89%, which was slightly higher than the two scoring systems at 69%–88%.[26,27] Further assurance that patients with severe pancreatitis have been correctly identified is indi-

TABLE 23.2

Identifying Patients with Severe Pancreatitis Who May Benefit from Aggressive Enteral Nutrition Support[26,27]

	Admission		48–72 Hours	
	Sensitivity	Accuracy	Sensitivity	Accuracy
Clinical Assessment	34-44%	83-84%	44-66%	87-89%
APACHE II Score >9	63%	77%	75-82%	76-88%
Ranson Criteria >2	N/A	N/A	75%	69%

cated by sequential APACHE II score profiles. Patients with severe pancreatitis demonstrated a median increase of 3.0 points, while patients with mild pancreatitis showed a decrease by 1.0 point ($p<0.0001$) over the first 48 hours of hospitalization.[27] Those patients with APACHE II scores >9 and Ranson Criteria >2 account for 20% of hospital admissions, tend to have pancreatic necrosis on CT scan, have a 19% mortality rate and a 38% incidence of complications, and are unlikely to achieve an oral intake successfully within 7 days of admission.[10,27–29] In contrast, those patients with APACHE II scores ≤9 and Ranson Criteria ≤2 account for 80% of hospital admissions, tend not to have necrosis on CT scan, have a 0% mortality rate, 6% complication rate, and a 81% incidence of reaching an oral diet successfully within 7 days of admission.[10,27–29] Using these parameters, the astute clinician can predict the patients likely to develop severe pancreatitis, who need aggressive enteral nutrition support and placement of early enteral access.

The presence of complications of acute pancreatitis such as pancreatitic ascites, fistulas, or pseudocysts does not preclude efforts at enteral feeding. In mostly retrospective case series, patients with these complications of acute pancreatitis have been shown to tolerate enteral feeding.[8,30,31] Typically, patients in these series languished in the hospital following the period of peak inflammation, continued to be intolerant of a standard oral diet, but tolerated elemental formulas given orally or by nasoenteric feeding tube. Development of diarrhea was only a minor complication and invariably ascites, fistulas and pseudocysts resolved over weeks of enteral feeding.[8,30,31]

Likewise, the need for surgery for hemorrhagic or infectious complications of acute pancreatitis again does not preclude enteral feeding, and in fact provides a unique opportunity for surgical placement of enteral access. In two case series, patients operated on for complications of acute pancreatitis tolerated jejunal feeds without incidence once surgical feeding tubes were placed successfully.[32–33] In two prospective trials, patients undergoing surgery for complications of pancreatitis were randomized post-op to either enteral or parenteral feeding. No differences were seen in pancreatic volume, bicarbonate, or enzyme output, and overall patient outcome were similar in both groups.[34,35]

Monitoring Patients on Early Enteral Feeding

Close vigilance of the pancreatitis patient on enteral feeding is important to ensure tolerance and to prevent complications from enteral nutrition support. Tolerance to enteral feeding in the pancreatitis patient is multifactorial, and relates to issues involving stimulation of the pancreas, intestinal contractility, position of feeding tube and level into which nutrients are infused, and overall absorptive capacity.

Initially, the feeding tube should be placed at or below the ligament of Treitz. Position throughout feeding may be confirmed by residual volumes less than 10cc[5], and/or periodic abdominal radiographs. While individual fluctuations in amylase and lipase may be seen during enteral feeding, the overall pattern should be a gradual decrease toward normalization (which should accompany gradual resolution of abdominal pain, nausea, and vomiting). Dramatic increases in fever, white blood cell count, abdominal pain, amylase, lipase, or residual volumes may indicate displacement of the tube back into the duodenum or stomach.[5] Patients with severe nausea and vomiting on admission may benefit from placement of a feeding tube with aspirate/feeding capabilities, in order to simultaneously decompress the stomach while delivering feeds into the jejunum. Feeding should be advanced only when glucose levels are maintained less than 200 g/dL and triglyceride levels less than 400 mg/dL. Early experience in one prospective randomized trial (in which 38% of patients had severe pancreatitis) showed that some degree of ileus was seen in 5 out of 16 patients on enteral feeding.[23] Surprisingly, enteral feedings did not have to be stopped in these patients, and only a decrease in a rate for 2 to 4 days was required before full feedings could be resumed.[23] Greater difficulty with tolerance was seen in a prospective study in 69 patients with pancreatitis (mean APACHE II score = 18, range 4–40) in which enteral feeding or a combination of enteral and parenteral feeding was successful in only 53% of patients.[36] Duration of ileus prior to attempts at enteral feeding may be a factor in predicting tolerance.[37] Ninety-two percent of patients in one prospective study who showed signs of resolving ileus by 48 hours tolerated attempts at enteral feeding, whereas only 50% of patients who sustained signs of ileus for up to 5 days tolerated attempts to advance to enteral feeding.[37]

Those patients in whom enteral access cannot be achieved, or those patients who demonstrate clear exacerbation of symptoms in response to jejunal feeding, should be considered for total parenteral nutrition (TPN). While the optimum timing of TPN is not clear, initiation should be delayed until after the fifth day of hospitalization to avoid exacerbation of the stress response and prolongation of length of hospitalization.[24,29] Fat should make up less than 15%–30% of overall calories to reduce the likelihood for immunosuppression, and the TPN should be advanced toward goal only as serum glucose and triglyceride levels can be well controlled (serum glucose <200 mg/dL and triglyceride <400 mg/dL).

The most difficult decision point is determining when the patient is ready to be advanced to an oral diet. In general, the patient with acute pancreatitis should be considered for advancement to clear liquid diet the point when there are minimal or no abdominal pain, resolution of nausea and vomiting, and decreasing amylase and lipase levels toward normal for at least 48 hours. In a prospective study, Levy et al. identified three factors associated with increased risk for relapse with the advancement to oral diet.[1] Duration of pain greater than 6 days, serum lipase three times normal, or presence of pancreatic necrosis on CT scan (Balthazar score ≥D) were all associated with a higher risk of relapse (35% to 39% incidence).[1] Those patients in whom these criteria were absent were found to be at low risk for relapse (12%–16% incidence).[1] Patients should demonstrate tolerance to clear liquids before further advancement in diet. The jejunal feeding tube should be kept in place for 24 to 48 hours while successful advancement in diet is confirmed. Patients who fail advancement to clear liquids may be placed immediately back on jejunal feeds.[5]

Patients on enteral jejunal feeds should have goal calories clearly identified by predictive equations or indirect calorimetry. Intake and output data should be monitored to ensure that the patient receives a sufficient volume to achieve the therapeutic endpoint of enteral feeding (i.e., gut integrity and attenuation of stress response). In an animal model and in patients undergoing bone marrow transplantation, at least 50% of goal calories were required to maintain gut integrity and eliminate bacterial translocation.[38,39] In patients with head injury and multiple trauma, aggressive strategies for infusing enteral feeds resulted in provision of 59.2% of goal calories, which led to significant reductions in incidence of infection, overall complications, and length of stay compared to the control group, who received only 36.8% of goal feeds.[40] In a prospective randomized trial in patients with acute pancreatitis, the study group placed on enteral tube feeding received only 21% of goal feeds over 4 days, and as a result showed no significant differences in outcome compared to a control group that was kept NPO.[41] Thus "trophic" or "trickle" feeds may be insufficient in patients with acute pancreatitis, and a volume sufficient to provide 50%–60% of goal calories may be required to maintain gut integrity, attenuate the stress response, and reduce overall disease severity.

Conclusions

The timing, route, constituents, and volume of early nutritional support affects the severity, morbidity, and ultimate outcome in patients with acute pancreatitis. Selecting appropriate patients with severe pancreatitis, achievement of enteral access, and vigilant monitoring of the patient on jejunal feeds are all critical for a successful outcome. Feeding low in the GI tract at the level of the jejunum appears to reduce pancreatic secretion to a subclinical level in order to allow resolution of the inflammatory response and convalescence of symptoms. Good clinical judgment is required to identify the optimal point at which patients may be advanced to oral diet. Early enteral feeding is most likely to benefit the patient with severe pancreatitis and pancreatic necrosis on CT scan, even when the clinical course is complicated by the development of fistulas, ascites, pseudocysts, or the need for surgical debridement.

Case Study

A 72-year-old obese African American male with known non-insulin dependent diabetes melitis (NIDDM), hypertension, and chronic renal insufficiency, was admitted with left upper quadrant abdominal pain, nausea, vomiting and fever for 72 hours prior to admission. Initial labs showed an elevated amylase and lipase, and a diagnosis of acute pancreatitis was made. Over the first 48 hours of admission, respiratory insufficiency with hypoxemia progressed, chest x-rays showed early adult respiratory distress syndrome, and the patient was placed on mechanical ventilation.

Physical examination at the time of the nutrition support team consultation showed a 72-year-old elderly obese African American male, alert, responsive and nasotracheally intubated. His height was 6 feet 0 inches, actual body weight 250 pounds, and ideal body weight 178 pounds. Vital signs included a fever of 103°F, blood pressure 190/80, heart rate 142, and respiratory rate 28. Coarse airway sounds with rales greatest on the right were noted. Cardiac exam was significant for distant heart sounds, but no obvious murmurs or gallops. Abdomen was distended, obese, with hypoactive bowel sounds and mild diffuse tenderness, but no masses or rebound tenderness. Extremities showed 1+ bilateral edema and stools were hemoccult negative.

Medications included Tylenol Elixir® (McNeil Consumer Healthcare, Fort Washington, PA), prophylactic Imipenem, Demerol, and Phenergan. Laboratories at the time of consultation included the following:

Na 156 mmol/L	Cl 110 mmol/L	BUN 55 mg/dL	WBC 19,000
K 5.6 mmol/L	CO_2 19 mmol/L	Creat 5.2 mg/dL	Hgb 11.2 Hct 33.8
Glucose 266 mg/dL	Albumin 2.6 g/dL	LDH 380 mg/dL	SGOT 305 mg/dL

Upon initial consultation, the nutrition team determined that the patient's APACHE II score was 22 and that he had 5 positive Ranson Criteria. A Computerized Tomography (CT) scan was obtained, which showed pancreatic necrosis in the head of the pancreas gland. The patient was felt to have severe pancreatitis and thought to be a candidate for aggressive, early enteral feeding. A nasoenteric tube was placed endoscopically and positioned approximately 20 cm below the ligament of Treitz. Feedings were started with a small peptide formula in which the majority of fat was composed of medium chain triglycerides. The rate was advanced over the first 48 hours to goal feeding. Over the first 6 days of hospitalization, the patient appeared to tolerate feedings well, with no nausea, vomiting, further distension, or diarrhea. Maximal daily temperature decreased gradually to 100.0°F, and white blood cell count decreased to 15,000. Residual volumes checked every 4 hours remained less than 10 cc.

On the seventh day of hospitalization, the patient developed sudden onset of "sepsis" with an elevated white count to 30,000, fever increasing to 104°F, and increasing tachycardia. Blood cultures, urine cultures, and cultures of the intravenous catheter tip were all negative. Cultures of the sputum showed only normal flora. Chest x-ray showed worsening ARDS, but the abdominal film confirmed that the feeding tube had slipped back into the stomach. The nurse's notes revealed that 12 hours before, residual volumes had increased to 30, 50, 80, and 120 cc. The patient was felt to be having increasing Systemic Inflammatory Response Syndrome (SIRS) in response to enteral feeding at the level of the stomach, leading to pancreatic stimulation and an exacerbation of the pancreatitis.

No new antibiotics were started (Imipenem had been stopped after the fifth day), and the tube was placed back down into the jejunum endoscopically. On the next day the white blood cell count had already begun decreasing to 28,000 and then 22,000, as did the fever from 104°F to 100°F. White blood cell count continued to decrease over the next 5 days, eventually down to 15,000. On day 16, the patient was successfully advanced to clear liquid diet and was ultimately discharged on day 18.

References

1. Levy P, Heresbach D, Pariente EA, et al. Frequency and risk factors of recurrent pain during refeeding in patients with acute pancreatitis: a multivariate multi-centre prospective study of 116 patients. *Gut.* 1997:40:262–266.
2. Ranson JHC, Spencer FC. Prevention, diagnosis and treatment of pancreatic abscess. *Surgery.* 1977; 82:99–106.
3. Cassim MM, Allardyce DB. Pancreatic secretion in response to jejunal feeding of elemental diet. *Ann Surg.* 1974;180:228–231.
4. Koretz RL. Nutritional support in pancreatitis: feeding an organ that has eaten itself. *Semin Gastrointest Dis.* 1993;4: 99–113.
5. McClave SA, Greene LM, Snider HL, et al. Comparison of the safety of early enteral versus parenteral nutrition in mild acute pancreatitis. *J Parenter Enteral Nutr.* 1997;21: 14–20.
6. Corcoy R, Ma Sanchez J, Domingo P, Net A. Nutrition in the patient with severe acute pancreatitis. *Nutrition.* 1998;4:269–275.
7. Ragins H, Levenson SM, Singer R, et al. Intrajejunal administration of an elemental diet at neutral pH avoids pancreatic stimulation. *Am J Surg.* 1973;126:606–614.
8. Parekh D, Lawson HH, Segal I. The role of total enteral nutrition in pancreatic disease. *S Afr J Surg.* 1993;31:57–61.
9. Grant JP, Davey-McCrae J, Snyder PJ. Effect of enteral nutrition on human pancreatic secretions. *J Parenter Enteral Nutr.* 1987;11:302–304.
10. Banks PA. Pancreatitis for the endoscopist-terminology, prediction of complications and management. ASGE Postgraduate Course, *Digestive Disease Week*, San Francisco, CA:May 1996:23–24.
11. Bengmark S. Gut microenvironment and immune function. *Curr Opinion Clin Nutrit Metab Care.* 1999;2:1–3.
12. Brandtzaeg P, Halstersen TS, Kett K, Krajci P, Kvale D, Rognum TO, et al. Immunobiology and immunopathology of the human gut mucosa: humoral immunity and intraepithelial lymphocytes. *Gastroenterology.* 1989;97: 1562–1584.
13. DeWitt RC, Kudsk KA. The gut's role in metabolism, mucosal barrier function, and gut immunology. *Inf Dis Clin North Amer.* 1999;13:465–481.
14. Kagnoff MF. Immunology of the intestinal tract. *Gastroenterology.* 1993;105:1275–1280.
15. Targan SR, Kagnoff MF, Brogan MD, et al. Immunologic mechanisms in intestinal diseases. *Ann Int Med.* 1987;106: 853–870.
16. Dobbins WO. Gut immunophysiology: a gastroenterologist's view with emphasis on pathophysiology. *Amer J Physiol.* 1982;242:G1–G8.

17. Kudsk KA, Croce MA, Fabian TC, et al. Enteral versus parenteral feeding—effects on septic morbidity after blunt and penetrating abdominal trauma. *Ann Surg.* 1992;215: 503–511.
18. Frost P, Bihari D. The route of nutritional support in the critically ill: physiological and economical considerations. *Nutrition.* 1997;13:58S-63S.
19. Moore EE, Moore FA. The role of the gut in provoking the systemic inflammatory response. *J Crit Care Nutr.* 1994;2:9–15.
20. Fink MP. Why the GI tract is pivotal in trauma, sepsis, and MOF. *J Crit Illness.* 1991;6:253–269.
21. Moore FA, Feliciano DV, Andrassy RJ, et al. Early enteral feeding, compared with parenteral, reduces postoperative septic complications. *Ann Surg.* 1992;216:172–183.
22. Groos S, Hunefeld G, Luciano L. Parenteral versus enteral nutrition: morphological changes in human adult intestinal mucosa. *J Submic Cytol Pathol.* 1996;28:61–74.
23. Windsor ACJ, Kanwar S, Li AGK, et al. Compared with parenteral nutrition, enteral feeding attenuates the acute phase response and improves disease severity in acute pancreatitis. *Gut.* 1998;42:431–435.
24. Fong, Y, Marano MA, Barber A, et al. Total parenteral nutrition and bowel rest modify the metabolic response to endotoxin in humans. *Ann Surg.* 1989;210:449–457.
25. Kalfarentzos F, Kehagias J, Mead N, et al. Enteral nutrition is superior to parenteral nutrition in severe acute pancreatitis: results of a randomized prospective trial. *Br J Surg.* 1997;84:1665–1669.
26. Wilson C, Heath DI, Imrie CW. Prediction of outcome in acute pancreatitis: A comparative study of APACHE II, clinical assessment and multiple factor scoring system. *Br J Surg.* 1990;77:1260–1264.
27. Larvin M, McMahon MJ. APACHE-II score for assessment and monitoring of acute pancreatitis. *Lancet.* 1989; 2:201–205.
28. Corfield AP, Cooper MJ, Williamson RCN, et al. Prediction of severity in acute pancreatitis: prospective comparison of three prognostic indices. *Lancet.* 1985;ii:403–407.
29. Sax HC, Warner BW, Talamini MA, et al. Early total parenteral nutrition in acute pancreatitis: lack of beneficial effects. *Am J Surg.* 1987:153:117–124.
30. Voitk A, Brown RA, Echave V, et al. Use of an elemental diet in the treatment of complicated pancreatitis. *Am J Surg.* 1973;125:223–227.
31. Bury KD, Stephens RV, Randall HT. Use of chemically defined, liquid elemental diet for nutritional management of fistulas of the alimentary tract. *Am J Surg.* 1971; 121: 174–183.
32. Lawson DW, Daggett WM, Civetta JM, et al. Surgical treatment of acute necrotizing pancreatitis. *Ann Surg.* 1970;172:605–615.
33. Kudsk KA, Campbell SM, O'Brien T, Fuller R. Postoperative jejunal feedings following complicated pancreatitis. *Nutr Clin Pract.* 1990;5:14–17.
34. Hernandez-Aranda JC, Gallo-Chico B, Ramirez-Barba EJ. Nutritional support in severe acute pancreatitis. *Nutricion Hospitalaria.* 1996;11:160–166.
35. Bodoky G, Harsanyi L, Pap A, Tihanyi T, Flautner L. Effect of enteral nutrition on exocrine pancreatic function. *Am J Surg.* 1991;161:144–148.
36. Schneider H, Boyle N, McCluckie A, Beal R, and Atkinson S. Acute severe pancreatitis and multiple organ failure: Total parenteral nutrition is still required in a proportion of patients. *Brit J Surg.* 2000;362–373.
37. Cravo M, Camilo ME, Marques A, Pinto Correia J. Early tube feeding in acute pancreatitis: A prospective study. *Clin Nutr.* 1989;8(suppl):14.
38. Nelson JL, Foley-Nelson TL, Gianotti L, et al. Caloric intake and bacterial translocation following burn trauma in guinea pigs. *Nutrition.* In press.
39. Mark DeMeo (personal communication).
40. Taylor SJ, Fettes SB, Jewkes C, et al. Prospective, randomized, controlled trial to determine the effect of early enhanced enteral nutrition on clinical outcome in mechanically ventilated patients suffering head injury. *Crit Care Med.* 1999;27:2525–2531.
41. Powell JJ, Murchison JT, Fearon KCH, et al. Randomized controlled trial of the effect of early enteral nutrition on markers of the inflammatory response in predicted severe acute pancreatitis. *Brit J Surg.* 2000;87:1375–1381.

CHAPTER 24

Nutritional Considerations for Dealing with Intestinal Diseases in the Intensive Care Unit

Walter L. Pipkin, M.D., Thomas R. Gadacz, M.D., F.A.C.S.

INTRODUCTION 279
PRINCIPLES OF THERAPY 279
ROUTES OF NUTRITIONAL SUPPORT 280
GUT SPECIFIC SUBSTRATES 280
DISEASE SPECIFIC THERAPY 281
Short Bowel Syndrome 281
Enterocutaneous Fistula 282
Inflammatory Bowel Disease 283
Low Flow States 284
CONCLUSIONS 284
REFERENCES 284

Introduction

The gastrointestinal tract has been regarded as both the "canary" of the body as well as the "motor" of multisystem organ failure.[1,2] The gut may in fact be the sentinel organ (canary) affected by subtle alterations in oxygen delivery and therefore potentially initiating the detrimental cascade (motor) leading to multiple organ failure. Patients admitted to the ICU with underlying gastrointestinal tract disorders often have multifactorial nutritional problems and are at high risk for adverse outcomes. The nutritional treatment plan must take into consideration the underlying illness, the intestinal disorder or extent of dysfunction, and available routes of nutritional support.

This chapter focuses on nutritional support of intensive care unit patients with underlying gastrointestinal disorders. The chapter discusses the options of enteral versus parenteral nutrition in critically ill patients, the macro and micronutrients that augment intestinal function and aid in mucosal protection, and the nutritional recommendations for selected intestinal disease processes. Nutritional support in disorders such as short gut syndrome, enterocutaneous fistulas, inflammatory bowel disease, and states of hemodynamic instability and marginal visceral blood flow is briefly reviewed.

Principles of Therapy

Enteral verses total parenteral nutrition (TPN) has been a much debated topic in the surgical literature. Despite persuasive data for the use of enteral nutrition whenever possible, there are indications for parenteral nutrition in the ICU. This is especially true for patients with complex gastrointestinal disorders. The indications for TPN also coexist with the contraindications for enteral nutrition. Patients with severe short gut syndrome with inadequate absorptive small bowel surface will require indefinite TPN. Many of these patients will not tolerate even small amounts of enteral feeds without significant GI side effects such as incapacitating dumping, or accelerated volume and electrolyte loss. Patients with a bowel obstruction (mechanical or functional) may also require short-term TPN until the problem is surgically corrected or resolves. Some patients with enterocutaneous fistulas will also require complete or partial parental nutritional support. Nutritional considerations in these complex conditions are discussed later in the chapter.

The multitude of benefits of enteral nutrition are covered elsewhere in this text. Suffice it to say that enteral nutrition has been reported to benefit essentially all organ systems. Early enteral feeding preserves the gut barrier function. Feeding the gut has also been shown to decrease the incidence of infectious complications in post-injury patients.[3,4] Gosche et al. showed that low levels of enteral nutrition restore luminal blood flow during sepsis.[5] Similarly, a lack of enteral feeding and dependence on TPN attenuate immune response. For example, a hypermetabolic response to lipopolysaccharide (LPS) challenge was noted in mice fed with only TPN.[6] Lack of enteral feeding also alters intestinal cytokines.[7] These alterations in cytokines have been shown to significantly affect neutrophil function and increase the mortality from gut ischemia in mice.[8] Additional important components of enteral nutrition are the maintenance of normal colonic flora and improvement of post-surgical glucose control.

Routes of Nutritional Support

Parental nutritional support requires placement of a central venous catheter. The subclavian and jugular veins are preferred. Femoral access is less ideal because of difficulty cleaning the groin area and the risk of deep venous thrombosis. The technique of line insertion, maintenance of catheter patency, prevention of infection, and monitoring for complications are reviewed in a preceding chapter.

Enteral nutrition can be provided by a nasogastric or nasoenteric tube positioned in the small intestine beyond the ligament of Treitz. Feedings through a nasogastric tube are commonly not tolerated in these critically ill patients and pose a significant risk of aspiration. Patients who have demonstrated inadequate gastric motility and have failed gastric feeding will require a nasoenteric tube. Another option is a percutaneous endoscopic gastrostomy (PEG). A PEG can be used to decompress the stomach and when desired, a second tube can be placed through the gastrostomy and positioned beyond the ligament of Treitz. Several manufacturers have marketed a dual lumen tube designed for this purpose. The distal or small bowel tube is used for enteral feedings with proximal gastric decompression. Gastrostomy tubes for decompression and jejunostomy tubes for enteral feeding can be placed laparoscopically or by open operation. Patients with fistulas pose significant challenges. In some cases a proximal tube can be used to help collect the fistula output and another tube, positioned into the distal bowel, is used for enteral feedings.

Gut Specific Substrates

It is clearly established that enteral feeding is superior to TPN when clinically feasible. Various macronutrients also have a specific role in augmenting enteric formulas. These macronutrients confer benefit not only to intestinal mucosa but also to systemic disease processes. Glutamine, arginine, fiber, and probiotics are examples of such substrates.

Many researchers have investigated the use of glutamine as an enteral additive. Glutamine is a nonessential amino acid that may become "conditionally essential" during stress.[9] Recent studies have shown that glutamine is utilized as a major fuel by enterocytes, colonocytes, and lymphoid tissue. A recent review on glutamine and the gastrointestinal tract by Zeigler et al. concluded that glutamine has specific beneficial effects in the GI tract: (1) Skeletal muscle exports large amounts of glutamine following sepsis, injury, or catabolic stress, and glutamine uptake and use by the gut increase during stress. (2) Glutamine supplementation enhances gut mucosal growth, facilitates repair, decreases infectious complications, and improves nitrogen balance. (3) Glutamine supplementation improves functional and clinical outcomes in catabolic patients compared to matched controls receiving little or no glutamine.[10] Determining the beneficial effects of the routine use of glutamine supplementation in postoperative or ICU patients needs additional clinical trials with well-defined outcomes.

Arginine is a nonessential amino acid in the unstressed state. With metabolic stress arginine, like glutamine, becomes conditionally essential. With increased utilization and need for arginine during these stressful conditions, it is not surprising that studies have shown arginine supplementation in the ICU patient is beneficial. Barbul et al. found that supplemental dietary arginine augments wound healing, immune response, and positive nitrogen balance.[11] There is further interest in arginine as a substrate for nitric oxide synthase. In several studies, nitric oxide (NO) has been shown to be a gastrointestinal mucosa protectant. Takeuchi et al. showed that inhibition of NO formation resulted in an increase in the mucosal damage to acid-induced gastric lesions.[12] Further studies are underway to enhance our current understanding and potential use of arginine in the ICU setting. More detailed explanation of both arginine and glutamine is given in Chapter 32.

Another nutrient that contributes to intestinal integrity is dietary fiber and the fermentable byproduct of soluble fiber, short chain fatty acids. There are two types of fiber—soluble and insoluble fiber. They can have opposing effects within the bowel. Both water soluble and insoluble fibers have been shown to stimulate small and large bowel mucosal growth and cellular proliferation.[13,14] Water soluble fibers like pectin can delay gastric emptying and prolong intestinal transit time.[15] The addition of pectin and other soluble fibers can be excellent supplementation to the diet of ICU patients with severe diarrhea. Fermentable fibers are metabolized by bacteria in the colon, resulting in the production of short chain fatty acids (acetate, propionate, and butyrate).[16] Short chain fatty acids (SCFA) are absorbed by the colonocyte and transported into the portal vein with systemic distribution as an energy source. These absorbed SCFA also enhance sodium and water absorption, increase intestinal transit time, and stimulate mucosal proliferation.[17] The efficacy of dietary fibers may be limited when conditions/interventions alter colonic flora and transit times. This is discussed during the disease-specific sections.

A recent area of interest in gastrointestinal research is the use of probiotics. In critically ill patients, there commonly are alterations in commensal intestinal flora. This is felt to be secondary to medications such as antibiotics, antimotility agents, bowel preps, histamine blockers, proton pump inhibitors, and narcotics. This change in flora is associated with a rise in the population of enteropathogenic bacteria and an increase in the mucosal permeability.[18] Probiotics involve placing live microbes into the gastrointestinal tract to confer benefit to the host organism.[19] The maintenance of the more normal lumen flora may prevent enteropathogenic species from adhering and invading mucosal cells and initiating the inflammatory and immune response.[20] Although probiotics are not currently the standard of care, several ongoing studies may alter our current practice of ICU antibiotic use and potential use of these live microbes. The concept of probiotics is extensively discussed in Chapter 34.

Disease Specific Therapy

Short Bowel Syndrome

Short bowel syndrome is secondary to either an anatomic or functional loss of mucosal absorptive surface resulting in diarrhea, steatorrhea, malabsorption, and/or maldigestion. Intestinal resection accounts for the majority of the cases, although mucosal diseases such as Crohn's disease and gluten-sensitive enteropathy can result in functional short bowel syndrome. The normal small bowel length is 300–500 cm. Ranges of severity exist, but symptoms generally begin with less than 50% of small bowel remaining. The factors that determine severity depends on the amount of bowel resected or diseased, the section of small bowel resected (jejunum or ileum), and the loss of the ileocecal valve. Patients will tolerate resection of the jejunum much better than the ileum. The ileum has a greater capacity for adaption and is able to absorb the larger load of nutrients and electrolytes. With loss of the ileum, the jejunum continues to allow efflux of chyme to the colon with little adaptation. There is a loss of bile salts and an eventual malabsorption of fats, resulting in steatorrhea. The ileum is also the site of vitamin B_{12} absorption when complexed with intrinsic factor. With ileal resection, vitamin B_{12} supplementation is required and can be given by intramuscular injection or intranasally.

Regardless of the cause, when a patient with short bowel syndrome is admitted to the intensive care unit, control of sepsis and hemodynamic stability is the first priority. High-volume fluid losses and electrolyte abnormalities should be monitored and replaced. Electrolyte imbalance can promote cardiac dysarrhythmias and commonly will inhibit bowel motility. See Table 24.1 for estimates of electrolyte composition from gastrointestinal fluid sources. When the patient has been stabilized, parenteral nutrition should be started to minimize further loss of lean body tissue.[21]

Once the electrolytes have been corrected and motility has returned, enteral nutrition should be initiated. Without ongoing peritonitis or sepsis, motility can be expected in two to three days. These early attempts of enteral nutrition are important since enteral nutrition is trophic to the gut mucosa. Early feeding should be limited because initiation of enteral nutrition can result in an increase in volume and electrolyte losses. To minimize osmotic loss, enteral formula should begin at a low rate as an elemental, semi-elemental, or peptide-based isotonic formula. TPN is given as needed to provide the necessary caloric and nitrogen requirements. As enteral feeds are tolerated and slowly advanced, TPN should be gradually reduced. Monitoring of effective absorption and utilization of nutrients is critical. Stool collection for deter-

TABLE 24.1

Fluid	Daily volume (mL)	(Na^+)	(K^+)	(CL^-)	(HCO_3^-)
Gastric	1000	60-80	15	100	0
Pancreatic	1000	140	5-10	60-90	40-100
Bile	1000	140	5-10	100	40
Small bowel	2000-5000	140	20	100	25-50
Large bowel	200-1500	75	30	30	0

mination of nitrogen and/or lipid content can be done but this is of limited clinical usefulness. It is much more practical to follow prealbumins as a nutritional assessment parameter. In addition to estimates of nutrient losses, special attention should be given to quantifying ostomy output/diarrhea. Although not the focus of this chapter, numerous novel approaches have been reviewed and published regarding nutritional support during the adaptive phase of care for short bowel syndrome.

Enterocutaneous Fistula

Nutritional management of patients with enterocutaneous fistulas (ECF) in the ICU setting can be extremely challenging depending upon the volume of output, location of the fistula, and the viability of the distal bowel. Abdominal operations account for greater than 80% of ECFs. Other predisposing conditions include Crohn's disease, neoplasia, infection, and radiation. Fistulas are classified by their location in the gastrointestinal tract and by their output. They are rather arbitrarily designated as either high output (>500 mL/d) or low output (<500 mL/d). Regardless of the cause or location of the fistula, many of these patients are metabolically unstable and are initially managed in an intensive care unit. The early management is similar to the care of the short bowel patient. First one must control the sepsis with broad-spectrum antibiotics, drainage of any abscesses, and aggressive resuscitation by restoring intravascular volume and electrolyte abnormalities. Table 24.1 again provides a reference for the volume of fluid and electrolyte composition of various gastrointestinal effluents. Following the urgent management of sepsis and volume resuscitation, skin protection and nutritional support are the next priority. Often the care of postoperative fistulas involves complex ostomy appliances using suction catheters and skin protective devices. An enterostomal nurse is critical to optimal skin care and ostomy management of these patients with often complex multifocal fistulous disease. If the ostomy output is poorly managed, this will significantly limit enteral nutritional support.

Early, aggressive nutritional support of these patients is vitally important to their ultimate outcome. ECF patients are commonly malnourished upon presentation to the ICU from poor volitional intake, excessive gastrointestinal secretions, and increased energy expenditure due to sepsis.[22] Prior to the implementation of TPN, there was a 64% mortality rate and only a 23% chance of spontaneous closure.[23] Since 1960, there has been a marked reduction in the mortality from ECFs that is multi-factorial but thought to be secondary to improvement in parasurgical care, including ventilator management, antibiotics, nutritional support, and improved ICU monitoring.[24]

Early in their ICU course, most ECF patients will require TPN as some component of calorie and electrolyte replacement. TPN should be started once the patient is adequately resuscitated and his or her abdominal sepsis controlled. This is usually begun on the third to fifth day of ICU management. Caloric requirement is approximately 25–35 kcal/kg/d and the protein requirement is 1.5 to 2.0 g/kg/d. The dextrose should be gradually advanced while monitoring serum glucose. The spontaneous closure rate varies from 30% to 70% depending on the location, comorbid factors, and nutritional state. Ninety percent of gastrointestinal fistulas that close spontaneously will do so within the first 30 days. With an uncomplicated, low-output distal fistula, a trial of parenteral nutrition only is advisable. If the patient has a more complex, high-output fistula with underlying gastrointestinal disease (radiation enteritis, inflammatory bowel disease, cancer) or foreign body such as mesh, the likelihood for spontaneous closure is less likely, and enteral nutrition can be advantageous. Enteral feeding has several advantages over TPN, including the ability to provide additional mucosal substrates like arginine, glutamine, omega fish oils, nucleosides, and nucleotides.[25,26] Location of the fistula will largely affect the route and success of nutritional support. If at least 100 cm of bowel exists between the ligament of Treitz and the fistula, nasoenteric feeds may be considered as the only nutrient source. Low residue/high protein formulas are initially recommended, which are slowly advanced to goal nutrition as tolerated. As with nutritional support in short bowel syndrome, there will be overlap with TPN while the tube feeds are being advanced to meet macro- and micronutrient goals.

ICU patients with high-output fistulas are more difficult to support but can be managed with partial or complete enteral nutrition. If the fistula is in the proximal bowel, enteral feedings can be delivered by placing a small-bore feeding tube into the distal limb. These are some of the most complex patients to manage from an infectious, metabolic, and nutritional standpoint and require a multidisciplinary team approach. Wound care and nutritional source/requirements will differ with the location of the fistula. Figure 24.1 provides relative site specific absorption of various nutrients, which should be considered when enteral feeding with ECFs.

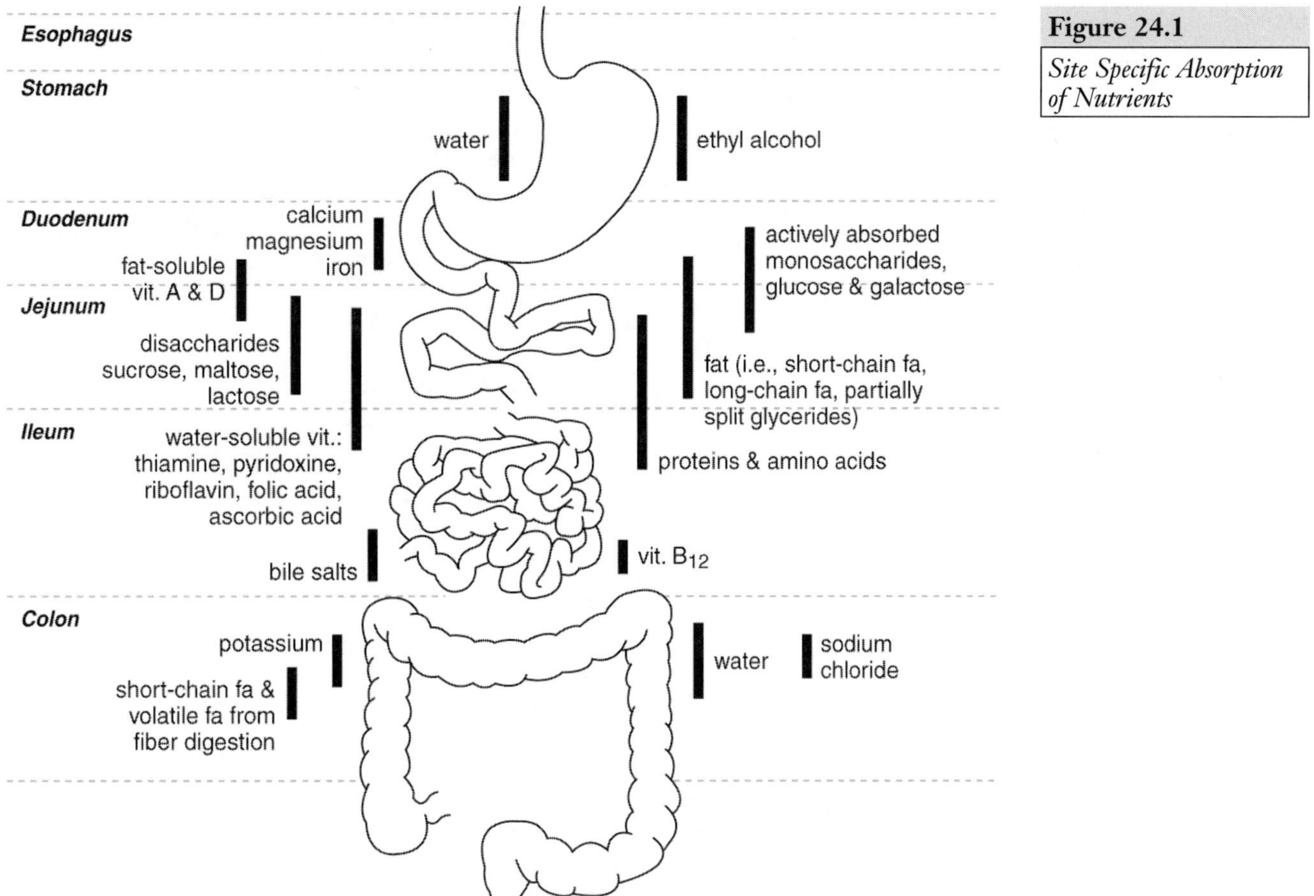

Figure 24.1

Site Specific Absorption of Nutrients

Inflammatory Bowel Disease

Patients with inflammatory bowel disease (IBD) often require multiple surgical interventions, which are commonly associated with intensive care unit stays. Indications for operations on these patients include obstruction, development of fistulas, abscess, perforation, hemorrhage, and failure of medical management. These patients may also develop short gut syndrome from the overall length of nonabsorptive mucosa or from multiple resections. Many of the nutritional considerations for these complications of IBD have been discussed in the previous sections.

Specific nutritional considerations also exist for patients with IBD. It is important not only to supply their nutritional needs but also to treat the underlying disease. Immune modulating drugs have long been employed in the treatment of these disorders by suppression of leukotriene and prostaglandin production. This alternative therapy has been termed immunonutrition.[27] Supplementation of fats in the diet with fish oils that contain omega-3 fatty acids inhibit the production of proinflammatory leukotriene B_4.[28] Studies have shown benefit in both Crohn's disease and ulcerative colitis.[29,30,31] Another study by Bousvaros et al. found a deficiency of fat soluble vitamins A and E in pediatric patients with active Crohn's and ulcerative colitis.[32] Because patients with inflammatory bowel disease often suffer from a short bowel syndrome from loss of absorptive surface, many investigators are studying modalities to augment mucosal growth. Glutamine is one of the micronutrients under investigation. Scheppach et al., as well as several other investigators, have shown that glutamine is trophic to gut mucosal cells.[33] Perhaps future investigations will focus less on inhibiting the inflammatory disease process and more on sustaining mucosal proliferation. It has been postulated that inflammatory bowel diseases are a pathologic immunologic response to luminal flora. The use of probiotics in patients with an intestinal pouch has been shown to decrease the incidence of pouchitis.[34] The intricate roles of nutrients and other substrates to provide nutritional support as well as to alter the disease process and promote mucosal function provide the possibility of better outcomes in these complicated patients. Although interesting, it will be some time yet before these novel IBD therapies are ready for trials in the population of ICU patients.

Low Flow States

In the past, critically ill patients with marginal visceral blood flow received only parental nutrition. Resurgence of interest in enteral feeding in this population has occurred secondary to continued reports of systemic as well as local benefits to the gastrointestinal mucosa with low levels of nutrient delivery. Disease processes commonly associated with altered visceral blood flow includes but is not limited to sepsis, hemorrhage, cardiac failure, an intra-aortic balloon pump, cardiac bypass, and ventilated patients with elevated positive end—expiratory pressure (PEEP).

The blood flow to the intestine consists of three parallel circulations: one each to the mucosa, the submucosa, and the muscularis. In the postprandial state, blood flow to the intestine increases two- to fourteenfold. The increase in flow to the mucosal circulation is modulated by digested nutrients initiating a local vasodilation. During a stressful event such as severe sepsis or hemorrhage, there is a 40% to 70% reduction in visceral blood flow, with shunting of blood to more central organs and muscle.[35] Decreased visceral flow has been postulated to increase gut permeability to bacteria and bacterial products initiating the development of multiple organ dysfunction.[36] Several studies have shown that this reduction in mucosal perfusion can be reversed with low levels of enteral feeds. In one of the first reports, Gosche et al., using an Escherichia coli sepsis model, showed that luminal nutrient delivery could restore intestinal flow.[5] Others have shown that enteral nutrient delivery could also restore visceral flow during active hemorrhage.[37] Several other models have now shown enhanced visceral perfusion and oxygenation in low flow states.

Another area of interest in multiple organ dysfunction syndrome has been termed gut priming. This involves the upregulation of adhesion molecules in the small intestinal vessels and the subsequent attraction of PMNs.[38] These primed neutrophils then circulate throughout the body and if a second inflammatory insult occurs, there is an exaggerated cytolytic response.[39] Because of promising evidence from in-vitro studies, it has been postulated that enteral nutrition may attenuate this inflammatory response. Moore et al. showed that enteral supplementation with arginine, omega-3 fatty acids, and nucleotides reduce the incidence of multiple organ dysfunction when compared to standard enteral controls.[40]

A clinical approach to these difficult patients would be to begin 10 to 20 mL/h of enteral feeds once the patient is adequately resuscitated. For the early aggressive feeding regimen to be successful requires close attention by ICU staff for the development of abdominal distension, changes in abdominal pain, feeding intolerance, or evidence of pneumatosis on X-ray. With any of these findings, feedings must be held. With appropriate resuscitation, feeding these patients may not be detrimental as was previously believed, but rather may prevent mucosal ischemia and its deleterious consequences.

Conclusions

Patients with underlying intestinal diseases admitted to the ICU are particularly difficult nutritional and metabolic problems. These patients have classically been kept NPO and/or received parenteral nutrition only. Enteral nutrition in many of these patients is crucial in improving their ultimate morbidity and mortality. We have discussed the early management of these patients, focusing on when and how to administer their nutrition. Many will initially require parenteral nutrition to meet metabolic needs and prevent loss of lean body tissue, but enteral nutrition can and should be attempted when feasible. The various macronutrients discussed are continuing to be investigated for their nutritional benefits as well as their possible therapeutic benefits to intestinal disease processes. Disease-specific formulas with appropriate macronutrients may prove to be the standard of care in the future.

References

1. Dantzker DR. The gastrointestinal tract—the canary of the body? *JAMA*. 1993;270:1247–1248.
2. Carrico CJ, Meaking JL, Marshall JC, et al. Multiple organ failure syndrome. The gastrointestinal tract: the "motor" of MOF. *Arch Surg*. 1986;121:196–208.
3. Moore FA, Moore EE, Jones TN, McCroskey BL, Peterson VM. TEN versus TPN following major abdominal trauma: reduced septic morbidity. *J Trauma*. 1989;29:16–23.
4. Kudsk KA, Croce MA, Fabian TC, et al. Enteral versus parenteral feeding: effects on septic morbidity following blunt and penetrating abdominal trauma. *Ann Surg*. 1992;215:503–513.
5. Gosche JR, Garrison RN, Harris PD, et al. Absorptive hyperemia restores intestinal blood flow during E. coli sepsis in rat. *Arch Surg*. 1990;125:1573–1576.
6. Fukatsu K, Zarzaur BL, Johnson CD, et al. Lack of enteral feeding increases expression of e-selectin after LPS challenge. *JSR*. 2001;97:41–48.
7. Wu Y, Kudsk KA, DeWitt RC, et al. Route and type of nutrition influence IgA-mediated intestinal cytokines. *Ann Surg*. 1999;229:662–668.

8. Fukatsu D, Zarzaur BL, Johnson CD, et al. Enteral nutrition prevents remote organ injury and mortality following a gut ischemic insult. *Ann Surg.* 2001 (in press).
9. Wilmore DW, Shabert JK. Role of glutamine in immunologic responses. *Nutrition.* 1998;14:618–626.
10. Ziegler TR, Bazargan N, Leader LM, et al. Glutamine and the gastrointestinal tract. *Curr Opin Clin Nutr Metab Care.* 2000;3:355–362.
11. Barbul A, Lazarou SA, Efron DT, et al. Arginine enhances wound healing and lymphocyte immune responses in humans. *Surgery.* 1990;108:331–337.
12. Takeuchi K, Kato S, Takehara K, et al. Role of nitric oxide in mucosal blood flow response and the healing of HCL-induced lesions in the rat stomach. *Digestion.* 1997;58: 19–27.
13. Sigleo S, Jackson MJ, Vahouny GV. Effects of dietary fiber constituents on intestinal morphology and nutrients transport. *Am J Physiol.* 1984;246:G34–G39.
14. Jacobs LR, Lupton JR. Effect of dietary fibers on rat large bowel mucosal growth and cell proliferation. *Am J Physiol.* 1984;246:G378–G385.
15. Spiller GA, Chernoff MC, Hill RA, et al. Effect of purified cellulose, pectin and a low-residue diet on fecal volatile fatty acids, transit time and fecal weight in humans. *Am J Clin Nutr.* 1980;33:754–759.
16. Wilmore, DW. Metabolic support of the gastrointestinal tract. *Cancer.* 1997;79:1794–1803.
17. Rombeau JL, Kripke SA. Metabolic and intestinal effects of short-chain fatty acids. *J Parenter Enteral Nutr.* 1990; 14(suppl):181–185.
18. Leveau P, Wang X, Soltesz V, et al. Alterations in intestinal permeability and microflora in experimental acute pancreatitis. *Int J Pancreatology.* 1996;20:119–125.
19. Ishibashi N, Yamazake S. Probiotics and safety. *Am J Clin Nutr.* 2001;73:465s-470s.
20. Vanderhoof JA, Young RJ. The role of probiotics in the treatment of intestinal infections and inflammation. *Current Opinion in Gastroenterology.* 2001;17:58–62.
21. Pritts T, Bower R. Short bowel syndrome. In: Cameron J, ed. *Current Surgical Therapy.* 7th ed. St. Louis: Mosby, Inc; 1998:161–166.
22. Rombeau, JL, Rolandelli RH. Enteral and parenteral nutrition in patients with enteric fistulas and short bowel syndrome. *Surg Clin N Amer.* 1987;67:551–559.
23. Edmunds G, Williams GM, Welch CE. External fistulas arising from the gastrointestinal tract. *Ann Surg.* 1960; 152:445.
24. Soeters PB, Ebied AM, Fischer JE. Review of 404 patients with gastrointestinal fistulas. *Ann Surg.* 1979;190:189–202.
25. Dudrick, SJ, Ashwin R, Mckelvey AA. Artificial nutritional support in patients with gastrointestinal fistulas. *World J Surg.* 1999;23:570–576.
26. Meguid MM, Campos AC. Nutritional management of patients with gastrointestinal fistulas. *Surg Clin N Amer.* 1996;76:1035.
27. Levy J. Immunonutrition: the pediatric experience. *Nutrition.* 1998;14:641–647.
28. Han P, Baldassano RN, Rombeau JL, et al. Nutrition and inflammatory bowel disease. *Gastroenterol Clin North Am.* 1999;28:423–443.
29. Griffiths AM. Inflammatory bowel disease. *Nutrition.* 1998;14:788–791.
30. Hawthorne AB, Daneshmend TK, Hawkey CJ. Treatment of ulcerative colitis with fish oil supplementation: a prospective 12 month randomized controlled trial. *Gut.* 1992; 33:922–928.
31. Belluzzi A, Brignola C, Campieri M, et al. Effect of an enteric-coated fish oil preparation on relapses in Crohn's disease. *N Engl J Med.* 1996;334:1557–1560.
32. Bousvaros A, Zurakowski D, Duggan C, et al. Vitamins A and E serum levels in children and young adults with inflammatory bowel disease: effect of disease activity. *J Pediatr Gastroenterol Nutr.* 1998;26:129–134.
33. Scheppach W, Loges C, Bartram P, et al. Effect of free glutamine and alanyl-glutamine dipeptide on musosal proliferation of the human ileum and colon. *Gastroenterology.* 1994;107:429–434.
34. Gioncheti P, Rizzello G, Venturi A, et al. Maintenance therapy of chronic pouchitis: A randomized, placebo-controlled, double blind trial with a new probiotic preparation. *Gastroenterology.* 1998;114:A4037.
35. Fink MP. Adequacy of gut oxygenation in endotoxemia and sepsis. *Crit Care Med.* 1993;21:54–58.
36. Deitch EA. Multiple organ failure: Pathophysiology and potential future therapy. *Ann Surg.* 1992;216:117–134.
37. Flynn WJ, Gosche JR, Garrison RN. Intestinal blood flow is restored with glutamine or glucose infusion after hemorrhage. *J Surg Res.* 1992;52:499–504.
38. Patrick DA, Moore EE, Moore FA, et al. Reduced PAF-acetyl-hydrolase activity is associated with postinjury multiple organ failure. *Shock.* 1997;7:170–174.
39. Botha AJ, Moore FA, Moore EE, et al. Early neutrophil sequestration after injury: a pathogenic mechanism for multiple organ failure. *J Trauma.* 1995;39:411–417.
40. Moore FA, Moore EE, Kudsk KA, et al. Clinical benefits of an immune-enhancing diet for early postinjury enteral feeding. *J Trauma.* 1994;37:607–615.

CHAPTER 25

Nutrition Support and Pregnancy

Thomas R. Howdieshell, M.D., F.A.C.S., F.C.C.P.,
Gail A. Cresci, M.S., R.D., L.D., C.N.S.D.,
Robert G. Martindale, M.D., Ph.D., F.A.C.S.

Body Composition Changes During Pregnancy 287
Anatomic and Physiologic Changes 287
Hormonal Changes 288
Metabolic Changes 288
Maternal Weight Gain 288
Placental Transfer of Nutrients 289
Nutritional Assessment 290
Nutrient Requirements 290
Nutritional Support 292
Total Enteral Nutrition 292
Total Parenteral Nutrition 292
Nutrition Intervention in the Critically Ill Pregnant Woman 293
Nutrition Assessment 293
Enteral Nutrition 293
Parenteral Nutrition 294
Case Study 294
References 295

Body Composition Changes During Pregnancy

Anatomic and Physiologic Changes

Pregnancy is a physiologic process associated with major alterations affecting nearly every maternal organ system and metabolic pathway. Most blood and urine measurements including nutrient assessment are significantly altered from nonpregnant values as a result of these changes. Values change as the pregnancy advances from the first to third trimester and on to delivery, and then return toward normal during the postpartum period. The major physiologic forces driving these changes include the 50% expansion of plasma volume and the 20% increase in hemoglobin mass, the former peaking in the middle of the third trimester, whereas the latter continues on to term; and the ever-increasing levels of estrogen, progesterone, and other placental-related hormones.[1]

The 30%–40% expansion of overall blood volume during the last trimesters (with the plasma component expanding 50%) reaches a peak between weeks 32 and 34 of gestation. The red cell mass also increases approximately 20% and peaks at the time of delivery. The physiologic dilution accompanying the expansion of blood volume results in a 12%–15% decrease in hemoglobin and hematocrit per deciliter of blood. Despite these changes, the mean corpuscular volume (MCV) and mean corpuscular hemoglobin concentration (MCHC) remain relatively unchanged in the nonanemic patient.[1]

Other adaptations include progressive increases in cardiac output peaking at 28 weeks, accumulation of body water, and changes in renal, respiratory, gastrointestinal, and genitourinary functions. The glomerular filtration rate (GFR) increases to accommodate the increase in maternal blood volume that must be filtered and to eliminate fetal waste products. As a result of this increase in GFR, small quantities of glucose, amino acids, and water-soluble vitamins may appear in the urine.[2] Although minor losses may be acceptable, a woman who excretes large amounts of protein may be experiencing a more serious problem termed pregnancy-induced hypertension, which requires strict medical monitoring.

Hormonal Changes

Numerous steroid hormones, peptide hormones, and prostaglandins influence the course of pregnancy. Some of them, such as the placental hormones human placental lactogen and human growth hormone, are produced only during pregnancy. Others, including insulin, glucagon, and thyroxin, are present in altered concentrations compared to the nonpregnant state, and have profound influences on gestational metabolism.[3]

Progesterone and estrogen have a particularly strong influence on pregnancy. The action of progesterone promotes development of the endometrium and relaxes the smooth muscle cells of the uterus. This relaxation serves both to help the uterus expand as the fetus grows and to prevent any premature contractions of the uterus. The same effect also influences other smooth muscle cells such as those in the gastrointestinal tract. The resultant slowing of the GI tract during pregnancy may increase the absorption of several nutrients, most notably iron and calcium. Annoying consequences of this decreased gut motility include constipation, heartburn, and delayed gastric emptying. In late pregnancy, these problems may be exacerbated by the weight of the uterus and fetus compressing contents of the abdominal cavity.[3]

Progesterone also causes increased renal sodium excretion during pregnancy. The body compensates for this sodium-losing mechanism by increasing aldosterone secretion from the adrenal gland and renin from the kidney. Sodium restriction during pregnancy, once thought to prevent hypertensive disorders of pregnancy, is actually harmful because it reduces plasma volume and cardiac output.[2] Estrogen promotes the growth of the uterus and breast during pregnancy and renders the connective tissues in the pelvic region more flexible in preparation for birth.[3]

Metabolic Changes

There are profound changes in maternal metabolism during pregnancy, and successful adaptation to these changes is necessary for a favorable pregnancy outcome. The basal metabolic rate (BMR) rises during pregnancy by as much as 15%–20% by term. This increase is caused by the increased oxygen needs of the fetus and maternal support tissues. There are alterations in maternal metabolism of protein, carbohydrate, and fat. The fetus prefers to use glucose as its primary energy source. Changes occur in maternal metabolism to accommodate this need of the fetus. The mother uses fat as her primary fuel source, thus permitting glucose to be available to the fetus. Increased macronutrient and micronutrient intake by the mother during pregnancy will ensure that these increased metabolic needs are met.[4]

Additional key metabolic alterations include increases in the plasma levels of T3 and T4. Therefore, a physiologic state of mild hyperthyroidism exists. Increases in plasma insulin levels result in variations in metabolism of glucose and the occurrence of gestational diabetes.[3] No other stress test can match this pronounced challenge of pregnancy for the identification of subsequent onset of adult diabetes. Calcium, iron, and zinc are required in proportionally greater quantity early because of the requirements of the placental transport enzymes and later due to the size of the fetal skeleton and blood-forming tissue.

The pregnant woman becomes anabolic for protein, with significant nitrogen retention, particularly during the first 24 weeks of gestation. Enhanced alterations in the lipid metabolic pathways occur, with doubling of the serum levels of triglycerides and cholesterol, as well as almost all of the blood clotting factors.[4] By converting blood values to levels per unit of hematocrit, partial adjustment can be made for expansion of maternal blood volume for a measure of absolute nutrient change in gestation.

Maternal Weight Gain

Maternal weight gain during pregnancy is an essential component of the normal growth and development of the mother and her fetus. During normal pregnancy, the components of weight gain consist of the fetus, placenta, amniotic fluid, enlarged uterine and breast tissue, and expanded maternal blood volume. Together, they comprise the obligatory weight gain associated with pregnancy.[5] In addition are highly variable accumulations of tissue fluid, adipose tissue, and protein stores. In studies from industrialized countries, obligatory weight gain amounts to approximately 7.5 kg. Among developing countries, obligatory maternal weight gain is approximately 20% less (6 kg), with lesser accumulation of adipose tissue and protein stores.[6]

In its 1990 report on maternal weight gain, the National Research Council recommended that all pregnant women have a BMI calculation at the time of entry into prenatal care (Table 25.1). If a woman has a BMI of less than 20, her weight gain target should be 0.5 kg of weight gain per week during the second and third trimester, in comparison to the woman whose BMI is greater than 26, with a weight gain target of only 0.3 kg/wk.[7] Excessive maternal weight gain has been associated with increased rates of labor problems,

TABLE 25.1

Recommended Total Weight Gain Ranges for Pregnant Women, by Prepregnancy Body Mass Index (BMI)

Weight-for-Height Category	Recommended Total Gain kg	lb
Low (BMI of <19.8)	12.5–18	28–40
Normal (BMI of 19.8–26.0)	11.5–16	25–35
High* (BMI of >26–29)	7–11.5	15–25

Young adolescent and African-American women should strive for gains at the upper end of the recommended range. Short women (<157 cm or 62 in) should strive for gains at the lower end of the range.

*The recommended target weight gain for obese women (BMI of >29.0) is at least 6 kg (13 lb).

caesarean section, fetal macrosomia, late delivery dates, and meconium staining of the fetus.

Placental Transfer of Nutrients

All nourishment is provided by the mother across the placental barrier during intrauterine life, and if the infant is breast-fed, by the mother and her mammary transfer system during extrauterine life. Both supply systems depend on an adequate maternal nutrient intake. These nutrient delivery systems are impeded if the mother is unable to ingest, absorb, metabolize, utilize, and transport nutrients to the placenta or breast. Maternal complications such as chronic cardiovascular and renal disease, diabetes, and pregnancy-induced toxemia compromise the maternal capacity to deliver nutrients as well as oxygen across the placenta to her fetus. Normal fetal growth reaches 30 grams per day during the last 16 weeks of gestation, 50% more than at any time during the neonatal period.[8]

The birth weight of the offspring depends on two maternal weight-related factors: How much weight did the mother put on during her pregnancy? What was her initial height/weight relationship or body mass index (BMI) when she began her pregnancy?[7]

Placental transfer of nutrients depends on their concentration in the maternal plasma and the adequacy of uterine blood flow perfusing the placenta. The transfer of nutrients increases up to six-fold as pregnancy advances. Most of the electrolytes, gases, and fat-soluble vitamins cross the placenta by simple diffusion. Carbohydrates cross by facilitated diffusion, and active transport is required for amino acids, water-soluble vitamins, and minerals such as calcium and iron.[9,10]

As a result of these three pathways, we find gradients in concentration of nutrients on the maternal and fetal side of the placenta, creating a maternal/fetal nutrient ratio. Certain molecules are lower in concentration in the fetus and higher in the mother, other items have equal concentration on both sides of the placental barrier, and additional molecules are lower in the mother and higher in the fetus. Levels of the water-soluble vitamins and some of the essential metals tend to be lower in the mother than in the fetus in the unsupplemented pregnant woman. Levels of the fat-soluble vitamins, in contrast, are higher in the mother than in the fetus, maintaining the diffusion gradient. Maternal supplementation of some of the water-soluble vitamins such as folic acid, pyridoxine, and vitamin B_{12} may alter but not eliminate these maternal/fetal ratios.[8]

The need of expanded blood volume during gestation is not entirely clear, but it is conceivable that it may be necessary to compensate for the hemodynamic changes caused by the increase in the uterine blood flow. In the rat, as well as in humans and other species, uterine blood flow increases several-fold during the course of pregnancy.[11] In order to maintain this high rate of blood flow to the uterus without reducing the rate of blood flow to other organs, expansion of blood volume and a proportional increase in cardiac output seem the most appropriate compensatory mechanisms. Consequently, if blood volume expansion early in pregnancy is inadequate, uterine blood flow may also be inadequate to sustain optimal fetal growth. It has been reported that maternal plasma volume expansion correlates with the birth weight of the infant.[12]

Malnutrition may influence maternal-fetal exchange of nutrients by altering placental development. Undernourished women and women living in poverty conditions in developing countries have a lower mean placental weight than well-nourished women or women from higher income groups.[13] Placentas from malnourished women have moderate reductions in DNA content and protein/DNA ratio.[14] The peripheral villous mass, trophoblastic mass, peripheral villous surface area, and peripheral villous capillary surface area were found to be reduced in poor Guatemalan women compared with middle-class American women.[15] A decreased number of villi in placentas of malnourished women has also been reported by additional studies.[13,14] The reduced villous surface area suggests a reduced area for maternal-fetal exchange, a finding that has obvious functional implications on maternal-fetal transfer.

A study done in low-income Indian women revealed that urinary excretion of estriol was reduced during the third trimester of pregnancy and that estriol excretion increased after the women received food supplements. In a similar population, reduced urinary excretion of pregnanediol and plasma levels of progesterone have also been described.[16] Thus, maternal malnutrition apparently reduces the ability of the feto-placental unit to synthesize steroid hormones.

A reduced maternal-fetal transfer of nutrients may be caused by a variety of placental and preplacental factors. For substances transported by simple or facilitated diffusion, placental blood flow, the size of the exchange area, and the thickness of the placental membrane probably play a decisive role in determining the rate of transfer.[17] For substances transported by active mechanisms, in addition to the previous factors, the metabolic activity of the trophoblast probably plays an important role in determining rate of transfer. In vitro studies of rat placenta have demonstrated that malnutrition does not interfere with the rate of uptake of radiolabeled alpha-amino isobutyric acid by placental slices.[17] Thus, preplacental factors such as placental blood flow are important determinates of the reduced rate of transfer of substances associated with maternal malnutrition.

Nutritional Assessment

An accurate nutritional assessment should include determination of the mother's weight history, gestational weight gain to date, and BMI. Short-term periods of starvation or semi-starvation in a previously well-nourished woman are well tolerated by the fetus and the mother in early pregnancy. Nutritional deficits in the last half of the pregnancy will have a greater effect on birth weight. Women at risk for marginal nutrient intake include teenagers, multipara, and mothers with inflammatory bowel disease, diabetes mellitus, hyperemesis gravidarum, pancreatitis, and low prepregnancy weight.[18]

It has been convenient to presume that the average prepregnant and pregnant woman in America has a more than adequate nutrient intake of calories, proteins, minerals, and vitamins. The results of a 1990 survey by the United States Department of Agriculture provide cause to question that conclusion. This survey showed that 50% to 60% of the female population failed to ingest 70% of the recommended nutrient intake.[19] When the patient's dietary intake is poor in green leafy vegetables, fruits, and dairy products, and is consistently less than 50% of the recommended dietary allowance (RDA), we should anticipate finding early clinical manifestations of nutritional disorders. These may not be the picture of classic nutritional deficiency, but rather the early manifestation of abnormalities such as evidence of protein and/or energy malnutrition (including muscle wasting, abnormal skin and hair texture, cheilosis, and angular stomatitis), lesions of the gums associated with low vitamin C, and hyperkeratosis of the skin over the arms associated with vitamin A deficits.[18] The pregnant woman needs more than a supplemental mineral/vitamin pill; she needs nutritional counseling. The responsibility of physicians and other members of the healthcare team should be to prove that their patients have an adequate nutrient intake. The biochemical assessment of nutritional status is designed to help in that determination.

Due to the multiple physiologic changes observed in normal pregnancy, the use of laboratory values in assessing the nutritional status of a pregnant patient should be carefully reviewed. Serum albumin levels decline rapidly during the first trimester, with an average decline of 1 gram per deciliter. Serum transferrin or TIBC levels increase during pregnancy and with iron deficiency, but decrease in the presence of chronic infection, stress, and protein malnutrition. Therefore, their interpretation in the pregnant patient should be addressed with caution. Iron deficiency, which is common in pregnancy, should be determined based on percent TIBC saturation, with less than 20% indicating a deficiency. Hemoglobin level declines in the first and second trimesters, and rises again in the third trimester. Accepted levels are 11.0, 10.5, and 11.0 g/dL in the first, second, and third trimesters, respectively. Characteristic blood glucose levels in pregnancy include fasting hypoglycemia and postprandial hyperglycemia. Hyperlipidemia is not uncommon during pregnancy. Triglycercides may increase 250% to 400% above normal. Cholesterol may increase on average by 25% but may increase up to 140% to 180%.[18]

Nutrient Requirements

Since the 1970s, the usual reference standard for the pregnant woman has been based on Hytten's calculation that a pregnancy requires an additional 80,000 kcal. This figure of 80,000 is based on a pregnancy in which the mother gained 12.5 kg and gave birth to an infant weighing 3.3 kg.[20] The increase accommodates the rise in maternal BMR during pregnancy as well as the synthesis and support of the maternal and fetal tissues. The current recommendation is that a woman consume an extra 300 kcal per day during the second and third trimesters of pregnancy.[21,22] Although she is eating for two, the expectant mother need not and should not double her food intake. However, it is important to recognize that energy needs differ from one woman to another. It is therefore not appropriate to make a single recommendation for all pregnant women. The best method of assessing individual energy status is by evaluating the rate of weight gain. In the first trimester, weight gain is expected to be between 0.9 and 2.2 kg. In the second and third trimesters, the average weight gain is 0.34 to 0.5 kg/wk.[23] During pregnancy, the body adapts to available energy stores, sparing energy for fetal growth when supplies are limited, adjusting basal metabolism and fat deposition if they are abundant.

Roughly 925 grams of protein are deposited in a normal-weight fetus and in the maternal accessory tissues. Thus, the 1989 RDA recommendations are for 10 grams of protein a day over the nonpregnant state. Additional protein for stress and/or extraordinary losses should be based on the disease state and metabolic demands. However, total protein intake should not exceed 1.5 g/kg in the normal pregnancy and 2.0 g/kg in the severely stressed pregnant woman. In a large population study, high protein intake in normal pregnancies was implicated in long-term detrimental effects on development.[24]

There are also alterations in vitamin, mineral, and trace element concentrations during pregnancy. Concentrations of water-soluble vitamins, including vitamins C and B_{12}, may decline independent of supplementation during pregnancy. Urinary excretion of water-soluble vitamins varies throughout pregnancy. For example, thiamine excretion decreases in the second and third trimesters, while riboflavin, niacin, and vitamin B_6 excretion increases in the second trimester.[25] Fat-soluble vitamin levels increase in pregnancy secondary to increased lipid levels. RDA recommendations are increased during pregnancy for most vitamins and minerals, except for vitamin A and vitamin D. As little as 10,000 IU of vitamin A per day and excessive vitamin D during pregnancy can each cause birth defects.[26]

During normal pregnancy, the average woman needs to absorb approximately 3 milligrams per day of elemental iron. Because only 10% to 30% of the dietary intake of iron is absorbed, the amount of ingested iron must be substantially increased. The average American diet provides 12–14 mg of iron/d. To ensure that sufficient iron is absorbed to satisfy the demands of pregnancy, a total intake of 30 milligrams per day of iron is required in most cases. Most prenatal vitamin and mineral supplements provide this recommended level of iron in the form of ferrous salts.[25,27]

Iron deficiency anemia is one of the most common complications of pregnancy. The iron requirement increases secondary to the expansion of the maternal red cell volume. Iron deficiency anemia can mean impaired oxygen delivered to the fetus, which may have severe consequences. In addition, during the last trimester, the fetus stores iron in its liver to use during the first four months of life.[27]

Current recommended calcium intake in pregnancy and lactation is 1200 milligrams per day. Hormonal factors in pregnancy cause the promotion of progressive calcium retention. Fetal use of calcium will peek during the third trimester with the formation of teeth and skeletal growth.[28] Studies have suggested that calcium supplementation in pregnancy has been associated with a reduction in pregnancy-induced hypertension as well as a reduced risk of preterm delivery in populations at risk for low calcium intake.[29] The role of maternal calcium intake on breast milk calcium and infant bone growth is not well understood, and additional research is needed before general advice is given to women to increase their calcium intake during pregnancy and lactation.[30]

Substantial research has demonstrated that folate is important for the prevention of neural tube defects such as spina bifida and anencephaly, one of the most common congenital malformations in the United States. Approximately 2500 to 3000 infants are born with neural tube defects each year in the United States, with an equal number likely lost to pregnancy termination and unknown numbers of spontaneous abortions. The U.S. Public Health Service and the American Academy of Pediatrics now recommend that all women of childbearing age who are capable of becoming pregnant receive a daily intake of 400 μg of synthetic folic acid (from vitamin supplements and fortified grains in other foods). During pregnancy, the RDA recommends increases to 600 μg dietary folate equivalents per day.[31,32]

Concentrations of numerous trace elements decline during pregnancy. Zinc blood levels begin to decline in the first trimester and continue throughout gestation to 20% to 35% below prepregnancy values, independent of supplementation. Therefore, the gestation age should be considered when zinc concentration status is evaluated. Current recommendations are to maintain plasma zinc concentrations at greater than 50 milligrams per deciliter. Copper levels increase during pregnancy in conjunction with increasing levels of ceruloplasmin. Serum levels below nonpregnant norms may indicate copper deficiency.[27] Plasma inorganic iodide concentration and thyroid clearance rates, considered diagnostic of iodine deficiency in nonpregnant women, are normal during pregnancy. Low levels of T3 and T4 may assist in the diagnosis of iodine deficiency since they are normally elevated in pregnancy.[3]

Nutritional Support

Total Enteral Nutrition

There have been numerous case reports using enteral feeding to support patients during pregnancy. In general, the indications for enteral nutrition in pregnancy are similar to those of all malnourished patients and include, but are not limited to neurological disease (cerebral hemorrhage, tumor), hypermetabolism due to trauma, GI diseases (pancreatitis, inflammatory bowel disease), and psychiatric disease (hyperemesis gravidarum, anorexia nervosa).[33,34] As long as the patient's gastrointestinal tract is functioning and intake is inadequate to meet maternal and fetal needs, enteral nutrition should be considered. Because the complications associated with enteral nutrition are less than those with parenteral nutrition, enteral nutrition should be utilized whenever possible.

Hyperemesis gravidarum (HEG) is characterized by severe nausea and vomiting, with onset between the fourth and tenth week of gestation and symptoms persisting beyond the fourteenth week of pregnancy. It is associated with dehydration, electrolyte imbalance, ketonuria, and weight loss of greater than 5% of body weight, usually requiring hospitalization. In most cases, the symptoms resolve by the twentieth week of gestation. The reported incidence of HEG is 0.3% to 1% of all pregnancies.[35] Various mechanisms for HEG have been proposed, including displacement of the gastrointestinal tract, hyperthyroidism, hyperparathyroidism, hypofunction of the pituitary gland and adrenal cortex, abnormal levels of human chorionic gonadotropin and estrogen, gastric dysmotility, abnormalities of the corpus luteum, and psychosomatic factors—although none of these have been proven.[36,37]

HEG patients are at risk of developing malnutrition with adverse effects on the fetus. In severe cases, serious complications such as Wernicke's encephalopathy and intrauterine growth retardation have been reported.[38] The mean intake of most nutrients has been shown to fall below 50% of the recommended daily allowance.[39] Nutrition support is therefore the cornerstone of management of HEG. Traditional measures include hospitalization for correction of fluid and electrolyte imbalance, temporarily withholding oral feedings, judicious use of antiemetic drugs, and psychological support. Most patients respond to these conservative measures, and a regular diet is reintroduced gradually. However, in some patients oral intake remains inadequate and enteral nutrition becomes necessary.[40]

Gulley et al.[41] described the use of continuous infusion of enteral feedings via a small-bore feeding tube in 30 patients with HEG. All the patients reported better control of nausea with nasoduodenal tube feedings than with traditional measures. The better response could be related to the fact that the enteral feedings bypassed the visual, oral, and psychological response to food, which stimulated salivary and gastric secretions, triggering nausea and vomiting.

An isoosmolar formula infused at 20 mL to 50 mL per hour can be initiated while the patient remains NPO. If, after 12 hours, tolerance has been established, the formula can be gradually increased until the estimated nutritional needs are met. Oral intake should be advanced slowly, with careful attention paid to tolerance when the patient is being weaned off of the tube feeding.[41]

In the Gulley et al.[41] study, aspiration was not determined to be a complication of the therapy. However, nasopharyngeal irritation and tube displacement were noted. Specific complications related to enteral feeding in the pregnant patient include gastric retention, diarrhea, and hyperglycemia.

Total Parenteral Nutrition

In the presence of an intact gastrointestinal tract, enteral hyperalimentation is preferable. However, in instances in which this mode of nutrition is not possible, total parenteral nutrition (TPN) can provide an adequate source of protein, glucose, lipids, electrolytes, and trace elements.[39]

The hesitation in the use of total parenteral nutrition in pregnancy appears to originate from the paucity of obstetrical patients requiring this intervention, indicating that most cases of severe medical illness necessitating TPN preclude pregnancy. In addition, many facilities are not staffed with nutritionists and dieticians who readily understand the nutritional demands of pregnancy and how these demands can be met through TPN.

To add to these limitations, Levine[42] reported an increased incidence of premature labor and fatty infiltration of the placenta in pregnant animals given parenteral fat emulsions to provide 50% or more of the total daily caloric intake. This statement is based on the presence of arachidonic acid and other precursor fatty acids (i.e., linoleic acid) found in most lipid emulsions used in TPN solutions.[43] The conversion of arachidonic acid to prostaglandins is felt to increase the risk of preterm labor. This phenomenon is usually seen with the use of experimental doses of fat emulsion, not with the usual therapeutic regimens. Preterm labor was most notably associated with the use of the compound Lipomul, which is no longer used in the United States.[44,45]

The indications for TPN in pregnancy are well documented.[46,47] Total parenteral nutrition is indicated for any pregnancy in which the mother is unable to tolerate oral intake to the extent of causing maternal malnutrition.[48–50] Specifically, it is instituted for several obstetrical and nonobstetrical conditions including:

1. Hyperemesis gravidarum not responsive to conservative therapy including intravenous fluid, antiemetics, sedatives, and enteral tube feeding
2. Maternal weight loss exceeding 1 kg per week times 4 consecutive weeks
3. Total weight loss of 6 kg or failure to gain weight
4. Prepregnancy malnutrition (patient below the 10th percentile of her ideal body weight)
5. Presence of a debilitating disease that increases nutritional demands and/or precludes enteral feedings (diabetic gastroenteropathy, small bowel obstruction, inflammatory bowel disease, unremitting pancreatitis)
6. Persistent ketosis, hypocholesterolemia, hypoalbuminemia (less than 2.0 grams per deciliter), macrocytic/microcytic anemia, negative nitrogen balance
7. Multiple gestations

Nutrition Intervention in the Critically Ill Pregnant Woman

Nutrition Assessment

The critically ill pregnant patient not only has increased metabolic needs due to pregnancy but also metabolic stress. Nutrient requirements are likely altered due to the nature of the injury and medical intervention. In order to accurately assess energy requirements, the use of indirect calorimetry is ideal. However, many institutions do not have this technology available so predictive equations are used. Traditional methods that estimate needs for hypermetabolic condition (see Chapter 4) may be used with 200–300 kcal/day added to support pregnancy. The patient's pre-pregnancy weight or ideal body weight should be used in these equations for energy requirement estimation. Caloric delivery should then be adjusted as needed based on frequent monitoring of maternal metabolic parameters, weight gain, and fetal growth using ultrasonography exams.[53]

Enteral Nutrition

Access

Although enteral nutrition is the preferred route of nutrient delivery in pregnancy, oftentimes successful and optimal enteral nutrient provision is difficult to achieve. In the critically ill pregnant patient, nasoenteric feeding tube placement is less invasive than other routes of enteral access (see Chapter 13). Achievement of post-pyloric feeding access is generally recommended for the pregnant critically ill patient over nasogastric feeds secondary to the increased risk of aspiration, particularly in someone unable to protect their airway (e.g., absent gag reflex). During pregnancy, decreased gastroesophageal sphincter tone and delayed gastric emptying commonly occur. A nasogastric tube prevents the gastroesophageal sphincter from closing, thus increasing the risk of gastric reflux into the esophagus.[53] There is limited data regarding the provision of enteral nutrition via percutaneous endoscopic gastrostomy (PEG) tube in pregnant women. PEG has several advantages over nasoenteric access. PEG feeding does not require radiologic confirmation for placement, and it may also reduce the potential for gastroesophageal reflux, esophagitis, sinusitis, and aspiration pneumonia.[54] However, placing a PEG tube in a pregnant woman is relatively contraindicated, and its success lies within the expertise of the endoscopist.

Formulations

Most enteral formulations have adequate macronutrient contents for metabolic support of the critically ill pregnant woman. Exceptions may include some specialized formulations with altered fat contents being either deficient in total fat, omega-3, omega-6 fatty acids, or all the above. The micronutrient content of formulations should be evaluated closely to assure they adequately supply pregnancy requirements (Table 25.2). If not, then supplementation of the deficient nutrients should be provided. As constipation is a common side effect of pregnancy, the use of fiber-containing formulas in addition to adequate free water provision may be beneficial. Prophylactic treatment with bulk-forming laxatives may also be necessary for optimal bowel motility.

TABLE 25.2

Daily Requirements in Normal Pregnancy[53]	
Vitamins	**Daily Reference Intakes (DRI)**
A	800 μg retinol equivalent
D	200 IU (5 μg cholecalciferol)
E (di-α-tocopheryl acetate)	10 mg α-tocopherol equivalents
Ascorbic acid	70 mg
Thiamin (B_1)	1.4 mg
Riboflavin (B_2)	1.4 mg
Pyridoxine (B_6)	1.9 mg
Niacin	18 mg
Pantothenic acid	6 mg
Biotin	30 μg
Folic acid	600 μg
B_{12}	2.6 μg
K	65 μg
Minerals and Trace Elements	**DRI (Enteral)**
Calcium 18 yr 19-30 yr 31-50 yr	 1300 mg 1000 mg 1000 mg
Phosphorus 18 yr 19-30 yr 31-50 yr	 1250 mg 700 mg 700 mg
Magnesium 18 yr 19-30 yr 31-50 yr	 360 mg 310 mg 320 mg
Zinc	15 mg
Copper	1.5-3.0 mg
Manganese	2.0-5.0 mg
Iodine	175 μg
Selenium	65 μg
Iron	30 mg
Chromium	0.05-0.2 mg

PARENTERAL NUTRITION

Catheter selection for parenteral nutrient delivery is based upon several factors, including anticipated duration of need for nutrition support (see Chapter 12). A peripherally inserted central catheter (PICC) is ideal for short-term (<30 days) duration. It has been suggested that placement of the PICC line in the right arm may be desirable with pregnancy, since in latter pregnancy patients are advised to rest in the left lateral decubitus position.[53] Provision of peripheral parenteral nutrition is not generally indicated in the critically ill catabolic patient. It is reserved for those anticipated to require intravenous nutrition for 5 to 7 days as with hyperemesis gravidarum, or as an adjunct to tube feeding.

Venous thromboembolism is estimated to be five times as likely to occur in pregnant women.[55,56] Prophylactic anticoagulant therapy for pregnant women receiving long-term TPN should be considered.

FORMULATIONS

Provision of parenteral macronutrients for the critically ill pregnant patient is similar to that for nonpregnant patients. The percent of total calories from carbohydrate usually should range from 40%–60%, from fat 20%–30%, and protein 15%–20%.[53] Standard parenteral amino acid solutions provide the appropriate balance of amino acids to support pregnancy when total estimated protein needs are met. Standard parenteral lipids contain adequate amounts of linoleic and linolenic acid for pregnancy if the above-stated amounts are provided. Standard multivitamins and trace element preparations may be lacking in various nutrients for pregnancy (e.g., folic acid, vitamin K, iron, iodine, selenium). Preparations should be analyzed and individual nutrients may need to be supplemented.[53]

Case Study

A 25-year-old female, 28 weeks pregnant, was admitted with a history of nausea, vomiting, and inability to tolerate even liquids that had persisted for weeks. She had lost 4 kg of weight over the previous 3 weeks. The patient's past medical history was significant for a previous laparotomy with small bowel resection and anastomosis following a motor vehicle accident. Abdominal x-rays upon admission revealed dilated loops of small bowel, air-fluid levels, and scattered colon gas suggestive of partial small bowel obstruction. A nasogastric tube and PICC were inserted for gastric decompression and initiation of parenteral nutrition.

A common method of calculating daily TPN caloric requirements utilizes the basal energy expenditure (BEE). For pregnancy, this equation is adjusted.[41,51,52]

$$\text{BEE (pregnant female)} = 655 + (9.6 \times \text{weight (kg)})^* + [(1.8 \times \text{height (cm)} - 4.7 \times \text{age})]$$

This value is then multiplied by a stress factor of 1.25 to account for the nutritional demands of pregnancy and partial bowel obstruction. Therefore, the total caloric requirement for 24 hours for this patient is:

$$\text{BEE} \times 1.25 \text{ kcal} + 300 \text{ kcal (pregnancy)}$$

This value for the average pregnant patient (5 feet 2 inches, 130 lb) is approximately 2000 kcal. For a standard 2 liter TPN solution, the number of kcal supplied by protein is calculated initially. Using a 6% amino acid solution (standard in most institutions), the proportion of protein calories is:

$$2000 \text{ mL} \times 0.06 \text{ (6\% amino acid solution)} = 120 \text{ g of protein}$$

$$120 \text{ g} + 10 \text{ g protein (pregnancy)} \times 4 \text{ kcal/g} = 520 \text{ kcal}$$

Therefore, the nonprotein caloric requirement for this patient is:

$$2000 \text{ kcal} - 520 \text{ kcal} = 1480 \text{ nonprotein calories}$$

No more than 30% to 35% of these calories should be supplied by fat. Therefore:

$$1480 \times 0.35 = 518 \text{ kcal of fat is given.}$$

Using a standard 20% Intralipid solution (2 kcal/mL), approximately 260 mL of Intralipid should be supplied over 24 hours. The remainder of the total caloric requirement is supplied by carbohydrates.

$$2000 \text{ kcal} - (520 + 518) = 962 \text{ kcal}$$

$$962 \text{ kcal} \div 3.4 \text{ kcal/g} = 283 \text{ g of carbohydrates}$$

To supply approximately 300 g of carbohydrate in a 2 liter solution, a 15% dextrose solution can be used.

$$2000 \text{ mL} \times 0.15 = 300 \text{ g}$$

Therefore, the TPN solution will consist of a D15, 6% amino acid solution to run at 83 mL/h with 260 mL of 20% Intralipid to infuse over 24 hours.

*If the patient is obese but less than 130% of her ideal body weight (IBW), the patient's actual weight should be used. If the patient is 130% or greater of her IBW, then the weight is calculated by (actual body weight − IBW) × 0.25 + IBW.

References

1. Whitehead RG. Pregnancy and lactation. In: Shils ME, Young VR, eds. *Modern Nutrition in Health and Disease*. 7th ed. Philadelphia: Lea and Febiger; 1988:931–943.
2. Van Der Post JA, Van Buul BJ, Hart AA, et al. Vasopressin and oxytocin levels during normal pregnancy: Effects of chronic dietary sodium restriction. *J Endocrin*. 1997;152: 345–357.
3. Lockitch G. Clinical biochemistry of pregnancy. *Crit Rev Clin Lab Sciences*. 1997;34:67–88.
4. Olson CM. Promoting positive nutritional practices during pregnancy and lactation. *Am J Clin Nutr*. 1994;59: 525–531.
5. Abrams BF, Laros RK, Prepregnancy weight, weight gain, and birth weight. *Am J Obstet Gynecol*. 1986;154:503–509.
6. Brown, JE, Jacobson HN, Askue LH. Influence of pregnancy weight gain on the size of infants born to underweight women. *Obstet Gynecol*. 1981;57:13–27.
7. Institute of Medicine, National Academy of Sciences. *Nutrition During Pregnancy: Weight Gain and Nutrient Supplements*. Washington, DC: National Academy Press; 1990.
8. Young, M. Placental factors and fetal nutrition. *Am J Clin Nutr*. 1981;34:738–743.
9. Young M. Transfer of amino acids. In: Chamberlain GP, Wilkinson AW, eds. *Placental Transfer*. London: Pitman Medical; 1979:142–160.
10. Blechner JN, Stenger VG, Prystowsky H. Uterine blood flow in women at term. *Am J Obstet Gynecol*. 1974;120: 633–652.
11. Bruce NW. The distribution of blood flow to the reproductive organs of rats near term. *J Reprod Fertil*. 1976;45: 359–371.
12. Croall J, Sheriff S, Mathews J. Non-pregnant maternal plasma volume and fetal growth retardation. *Br J Obstet Gynecol*. 1978;85:90–110.
13. Murthy LS, Agarwal KN, Khanna S. Placental morphometric and morphologic alterations in maternal undernutrition. *Am J Obstet Gynecol*. 1976;124:641–655.
14. Lechtig A, Yarbrough C, Delgado H, et al. Effect of moderate maternal malnutrition on the placenta. *Am J Obstet Gynecol*. 1975;123:191–209.
15. Laga EM, Driscoll SG, Munro HN. Comparison of placentas from two socio-economic groups. *Pediatrics*. 1972; 50:24–31.
16. Iyengar L. Urinary estrogen excretion in undernourished pregnant Indian women. *Am J Obstet Gynecol*. 1968;102: 834–850.
17. Rosso P. Nutrition and maternal-fetal exchange. *Am J Clin Nutr*. 1981;34:744–755.
18. MacBurney M. Pregnancy. In: Gottschlich M, Matarese L, Shronts E, eds. *Nutrition Support Dietetics Core Curriculum*. Silver Spring, MD: American Society for Parenteral and Enteral Nutrition; 1993:10–90.
19. United States Department of Agriculture. *Nationwide Food Consumption Survey. Report No. 85-1*. Hyattsville, MD: Nutrition Monitoring Division, Human Nutrition Information Service, U.S. Department of Agriculture; 1990.
20. Hytten, FE. Clinical physiology in obstetrics. In: Hytten, FE, Leitch I, eds. *The Physiology of Human Pregnancy*. 2nd ed. Oxford: Blackwell Scientific; 1971:20–60.
21. Brown JE, Kahn EB. Maternal nutrition and the outcome of pregnancy. *Clinics in Perinatology*. 1997;24:433–450.
22. Prentice AM, Spaaji CK, Goldberg GR, et al. Energy requirements of pregnant and lactating women. *Eur J Clin Nutr*. 1996;50:82.

23. King JC, Butte NF, Bronstein MN. Energy metabolism during pregnancy: Influence of maternal energy status. *Am J Clin Nutr*. 1994;59:439–445.

24. Martaugh MA, Weingart S. Individual nutrient effects on length of gestation and pregnancy outcome. *Sem Perinatal.* 1997;19:197–210.

25. Food and Nutrition Board. *Dietary Reference Intakes for Thiamine, Riboflavin, Niacin, Vitamin B6, Folate, Vitamin B12, Pantothenic Acid, Biotin, and Choline*. Washington, DC: National Academy of Sciences; 1998.

26. Rothman KJ, Moore LL, Singer MR, et al. Teratogenicity of high vitamin A intake. *N Engl J Med.* 1995;333:1369–1380.

27. National Research Council, National Academy of Sciences, Committee on Dietary Allowances, Food and Nutrition Board. *Recommended Dietary Allowances (RDA)*. 10th ed. Washington, DC: National Academy Press; 1989:60–62.

28. Prentice A. Maternal calcium requirements during pregnancy and lactation. *Am J Clin Nutr*. 1994;59:477–483.

29. Belizan JM, Villar J, Repke J. The relationship between calcium intake and pregnancy-induced hypertension: up-to-date evidence. *Am J Obstet Gynecol.* 1988;158:898–902.

30. Ritchie LD, Fung EB, Halloran BP, et al. A longitudinal study of calcium homeostasis during human pregnancy and lactation and after resumption of menses. *Am J Clin Nutr.* 1998;67:693–710.

31. Centers for Disease Control: *Recommendations for the Use of Folic Acid to Reduce the Number of Cases of Spina Bifida and Neural Tube Defects.* MMWR 41 (RR-14);1992:1–25.

32. Rush D. Periconceptional folate and neural tube defect. *Am J Clin Nutr*. 1994;59:511–516.

33. Brown RO, Vehe KL, Kaufman PA, et al. Long-term enteral nutrition support in a pregnant patient following head trauma. *Nutr Clin Pract.* 1989;4:101–104.

34. Nelson JH, McLean WT. Management of Landry-Guillain-Barré syndrome in pregnancy. *Ostet Gynecol.* 1985;65:25–29.

35. Kallen B. Hyperemesis during pregnancy and delivery outcome: A registry study. *Eur J Obstet Gynecol Reprod Biol.* 1987;26:291–301.

36. Chin RH, Lao TH. Thyroxine concentration and outcome of hyperemesis pregnancies. *Br J Obstet Gynecol.* 1988;95:507–509.

37. Koch KL, Stern RM, Vasey M, et al. Gastric dysrhythmias and nausea of pregnancy. *Dig Dis Sci.* 1990;35:961–968.

38. Lavin PM, Smith D, Kori SH, et al. Wernicke's encephalopathy: a predictable complication of hyperemesis gravidarum. *Obstet Gynecol.* 1983;62 (Suppl):153–155.

39. Van Stuijvenberg M, Schabort I, Labadavious R, et al. The nutritional status and treatment of patients with hyperemesis gravidarum. *Am J Obstet Gynecol.* 1995;172:1585–1591.

40. Barclay BA. Experience with enteral nutrition in the treatment of hyperemesis gravidarum. *Nutr Clin Pract.* 1990;5:153–155.

41. Gulley RM, Vander Pleog N, Gulley JM. Treatment of hyperemesis gravidarum with nasogastric feeding. *Nutr Clin Pract.* 1993;8:33–35.

42. Levine MG, Esser D. Total parenteral nutrition for the treatment of hyperemesis gravidarum: maternal nutritional effects and fetal outcome. *Obstet Gynecol.* 1988;72:102–107.

43. Greenspoon JS, Safarek RH, Hayashi JT, et al. Parenteral nutrition during pregnancy: lack of association with idiopathic preterm labor. *J Reprod Med.* 1994;39:87–91.

44. Driscoll DF, Baptista RJ, Bistrian BR, et al. Base solution limitations and patient-specific TPN admixtures. *Nutr Clin Pract.* 1987;2:160–163.

45. Amato P, Quercia RA. A historical perspective and review of the safety of lipid emulsion in pregnancy. *Nutr Clin Pract.* 1991;6:189–192.

46. Kirby DF, Fiorenza V, Craig R. Intravenous nutritional support during pregnancy. *J Parten Enteral Nutr.* 1988;12:72–80.

47. Herbert WP, Seeds JW, Bowes WA, et al. Fetal growth response to total parenteral nutrition in pregnancy. *J Reprod Med.* 1986;31:263–266.

48. Sandrock M, Amon E. Parenteral feeding and nutrition. In: Gleicher N, ed. *Principles and Practice of Medical Therapy in Pregnancy*. 2nd ed. Norwalk: Appleton and Lange; 1992:1297–1307.

49. Caruso A, Decarolis S, Ferrazzani S, et al. Pregnancy outcome and total parenteral nutrition in malnourished pregnant women. *Fetal Diagn Ther.* 1998;13:136–140.

50. Russo-Stieglitz KE, Levine AB, Wagner BA, et al. Pregnancy outcome in patients requiring parenteral nutrition. *J Matern Fetal Med.* 1999;8:164–167.

51. Driscoll DF, Blackburn GL. Total parenteral nutrition, a review of its current status in hospitalized patients and the need for patient-specific feeding. *Drugs.* 1990;40:346–363.

52. Greenspoon JS, Rosen DJ, Avet M. Use of the peripherally inserted central catheter for parenteral nutrition during pregnancy. *Obstet Gynecol.* 1993;81:831–834.

53. Hillhouse JH, Neiger R. Pregnancy and lactation. In: Gottschlich MM, Fuhrman MP, Hammond KA, et al., eds. *The Science and Practice of Nutrition Support.* 2nd edition. Dubuque, IA: Kendall Hunt; 2001:301–319.

54. Koh ML, Lipkin EW. Nutrition support of a pregnant comatose patient via percutaneous endoscopic gastrostomy. *J Parenter Enteral Nutr*. 1993;17:384–387.

55. Fabri PJ, Mirtallo JM, Ruberg RI, et al. Incidence and prevention of thrombosis of the subclavian vein during total parenteral nutrition. *Surg Gynecol Obstet.* 1982;115:238–242.

56. National Institutes of Health Consensus Development Conference. Prevention of venous thrombosis and pulmonary embolism. *JAMA.* 1986;256:744–748.

CHAPTER

26 Nutritional Considerations in the Intensive Care Unit: Neonatal Issues

Anjali Parish, M.D., Jatinder Bhatia, M.D.

INTRODUCTION 297
HISTORY OF TOTAL PARENTERAL NUTRITION IN INFANTS 297
NEED FOR TOTAL PARENTERAL NUTRITION 298
INTRAVENOUS FLUID AND ELECTROLYTE CONSIDERATIONS 298
Immediate Newborn Period 298
Glucose Homeostasis 300
Late Onset Hyponatremia in the Premature Infant 300
NUTRITIONAL GOALS FOR NICU PATIENTS 300
PARENTERAL NUTRITIONAL THERAPY 301
Energy Delivery 301
Protein Intake 302
Fat Intake 302
Vitamin, Mineral, and Trace Element Supplementation 302
Intravascular Access 303
Complications of TPN 303
ENTERAL NUTRITION 303
Initiating Enteral Feedings 304
Advancing Enteral Feedings 304
Which Formula to Use 305
How to Feed 305
OTHER NUTRITIONAL CONSIDERATIONS 305
Anemia of Prematurity 305
Breast Feeding after Discharge 305
Nutrition and Developmental Outcome of Premature Infants 306
CONCLUSIONS 306
REFERENCES 306

Introduction

Neonatal intensive care units care for a very diverse patient population, varying by weight, age, and medical problems. Problems in term infants may include congenital heart disease, sepsis, persistent pulmonary hypertension, or surgical lesions such as gastroschisis and congenital diaphragmatic hernia. Premature infants can have a variety of problems as well, such as respiratory distress syndrome and patent ductus arteriosus. As expected, this wide variation in medical diagnoses can lead to significant differences in nutritional needs among patients.

Since the introduction of surfactant in the 1990s, the United States has seen an improved survival rate of very low birthweight infants.[1] With this increasing survival, however, new challenges have arisen. Among them is keeping up with the nutritional demands of a rapidly growing, immature body. This field has evolved over the past few decades with advances in both parenteral and enteral nutritional therapy.

History of Total Parenteral Nutrition in Infants

The first published report of total parenteral nutrition (TPN) in an infant appeared in 1944. A five-month-old male infant with Hirschsprung's disease and failure to thrive was given complete intravenous feedings with fat, protein, and carbohydrate for 5 days while undergoing bowel rest. The patient had a return of his subcutaneous fat and improvement in energy level during this time until oral feedings could be restarted. The patient did suffer from phlebitis in the left leg where the first needle was placed for use to administer the fluids, but otherwise he had no known complications.[2] Without this use of TPN, the authors felt their patient would have died.

The hyperosmolarity of the original parenteral nutrition fluids required that venous sites be changed frequently and prevented fluids from being run on a continual basis, limiting the total nutrition delivered. In 1968, Stanley Dudrick and his colleagues published a report of long-term TPN delivered through central venous catheters that were placed percutaneously into the external jugular or subclavian vein and threaded into the superior vena cava.[3] By practicing sterile dressing changes every 3 days, catheters were maintained for an average of 19.7 days without concomitant sepsis.[4] Today, similar methods for central catheter placement and maintenance are still used.

A major benefit of TPN is the ability to provide amino acids to maintain positive nitrogen balance in patients who cannot tolerate enteral feedings. Amino acid solutions have evolved from casein or fibrin hydrolysates to crystalline L-amino acid solutions.[5] Amino acid solutions specific for different pathophysiologic processes are currently available as well. A major obstacle in the development of such solutions is a lack of a gold standard for comparison. Comparing amino acid concentrations of patients on TPN to those enterally fed may not be sufficient,[5] and specific amino acid needs for different disease states remain to be defined.

Initially, TPN depended on high concentrations of dextrose to deliver adequate calories. Dextrose concentrations as high as 20 grams per 100mL fluid were required to maintain an energy intake of 90–100 kcal/kg/d. Complications from such high dextrose delivery included hyperglycemia and glucosuria.[6] Ethyl alcohol was used in an attempt to decrease the dextrose load while still maintaining adequate calories. Problems with hypothermia, bradycardia, and apnea, as well as concerns for hepatic toxicity, led clinicians to abandon this technique.[6] The introduction of intravenous lipid preparations in the late 1960s provided a way to deliver adequate calories without the use of hyperosmolar dextrose solutions.[6]

Need for Total Parenteral Nutrition

Much of the original work for TPN in infants was done in patients with surgical problems. Patients who had gastrointestinal obstructions would often die after their surgeries not because of the actual procedure but because of malnutrition and its related consequences. Surgeons were among the first to recognize a need to supply patients with adequate nutrition during complete bowel rest. Today, TPN remains the cornerstone of therapy for infants undergoing abdominal surgery for congenital malformations like gastroschisis, omphalocele, and gastrointestinal obstructions. Through TPN, patients can be maintained in positive nitrogen balance, aiding in wound healing and immune system function, while waiting for adequate return of bowel function postoperatively.

The use of TPN in premature infants has also revolutionized their care. Prior to TPN, infants were effectively starved until full enteral feedings could be established.[7] Although many clinicians recognized the need for adequate nutrition in these small patients, many patients could not tolerate more than minimal amounts of enteral feedings. With total or supplemental parenteral nutrition, patients continue to grow and mature while enteral feedings are advanced as each individual patient tolerates.

Intravenous Fluid and Electrolyte Considerations

Immediate Newborn Period

The premature infant presents a unique challenge in the management of intravenous fluids during the first few days of life. Maintenance fluids are usually based upon urine output plus estimated insensible water loss (IWL) plus any known ongoing losses from other sites (i.e., gastrointestinal losses). Multiple studies have shown the younger the gestational age of an infant at birth, the higher the IWL through the skin.[8–10] Other factors that may increase IWL include placement under a radiant warmer, phototherapy for hyperbilirubinemia, and open skin sites such as gastroschisis or omphalocele. Such factors can increase IWL by greater than 100%. (Table 26.1)

Techniques to reduce IWL in the premature infant have also been studied. The plastic heat shield can reduce IWL by as much as 25%.[8] Topical agents such as paraffin[11] and possibly aquaphor[12] help reduce IWL in the premature infant as well. The blanket created from plastic wrap reduces IWL more than the rigid plastic body hood[13] and is just as effective as topical agents as well as being more cost efficient.[14] Whichever technique is employed, the goal is to effectively reduce IWL and prevent increases in body metabolism in order to conserve energy for growth.

Management of electrolytes in the extremely low birth weight infant (<1000 grams) is a considerable challenge. As insensible water loss continues, patients are at risk for hypernatremia. However, vigorous intravenous fluid therapy can increase the risk for patent

TABLE 26.1

Insensible Water Loss
Factors That Increase IWL
Prematurity
Radiant Warmer Heat
Phototherapy
Skin Defects
Omphalocele
Gastroschisis
Myelomeningocele
Tachypnea
Non-Humidified Oxygen
Factors That Decrease IWL
Mature Skin
Heat Shields
Plastic Wrap Blanket
Rigid Plastic Body Hood
Topical Skin Agents
Paraffin
Aquaphor
Covering Skin Defects
Humidified Oxygen

ductus arteriosus,[15,16] necrotizing enterocolitis[17] and bronchopulmonary dysplasia.[18–21] Maintenance fluids in infants are calculated by adding urine output plus estimated insensible water loss.[15] Insensible water loss estimates should be increased by at least 50% if the infant is under a radiant warmer or under phototherapy. Intravenous fluids should also be increased if the infant has excessive urine output or other areas of ongoing losses such as through nasogastric tube output. By using sodium restricted fluids, Costarino et al.[22] have shown reduced total intravenous fluid requirements and a decrease in incidence of bronchopulmonary dysplasia in very low birth weight infants. Regardless of initial intravenous fluids and rates, serial serum sodiums should be checked and adjustments made for hypernatremia (serum Na>150 mEq/L) and hyponatremia (serum Na<130 mEq/L) as needed.

Extremely low birth weight infants are also at risk for hyperkalemia despite adequate urine output. Nonoliguric hyperkalemia can result from an increase in exogenous potassium load (intravenous fluids, medications, transfusions) or from endogenous sources (hemolysis, hemorrhage, tissue necrosis),[23] but many times further investigation reveals none of these causes as the etiology for hyperkalemia. This hyperkalemia may be due to a shift in potassium from the intracellular space to the extracellular space due to decreased activity of Na+/K(+)-ATPase exchange pump in red blood cells of premature infants.[24,25] Management of hyperkalemia in the first few days of life includes use of fluids devoid of potassium, intravenous insulin, and rectal kayexalate.

Neonatal hypocalcemia is a particular problem in premature infants, asphyxiated infants, and infants of diabetic mothers. In the past, hypocalcemia was based on total serum calcium concentrations, but measurement of the biologically active ionized calcium is more accurate and is currently recommended for clinical use. In capillary blood samples taken from term infants, mean ionized calcium levels on the first day of life have been reported to be 1.24 ± 0.11 mmol/L by Wandrup et al.[26] and 1.21 ± 0.08 mmol/L by Nelson et al.[27] For healthy premature infants in the same studies, mean ionized calcium levels were 1.21 ± 0.16 and 1.11 ± 0.15 mmol/L respectively. The lower values found by Nelson et al.[26] may have been due to sample dilution with sodium heparinate. When whole arterial blood ionized calcium measurements were compared to capillary blood measurements, no clinically significant differences were found.[28]

Infants with asphyxia, polycythemia, or infants of diabetic mothers should have ionized calcium levels checked after birth and should receive calcium supplementation if necessary. Severely asphyxiated infants have a higher risk for hypocalcemia than less affected infants and are at risk for persistence of hypocalcemia after the first 24 hours of life.[29] Infants with polycythemia have higher serum phosphate levels than controls, and this hyperphosphatemia is one proposed mechanism behind the hypocalcemia seen in these infants.[30] Infants of diabetic mothers can have a variety of metabolic derangements, including neonatal hypocalcemia that are causes for high morbidity and mortality risks for these infants.[31,32] Therefore, screening for hypocalcemia should always be part of the initial evaluation in any infant with the above risk factors.

Hypocalcemia in the premature infant during the first 3 days of life is under much debate. Initially, premature infants were felt to have impaired parathyroid hormone (PTH) responses to hypocalcemia. However, several studies have now shown that premature infants are able to mount appropriate increases in PTH in the presence of hypocalcemia.[33–35] The same studies also show the premature infant is able to appropriately lower PTH levels during calcium supplementation. Nonetheless, it is often routine to supplement infants <1800 grams with calcium gluconate since these infants are born relatively osteopenic. Newer research is focusing on possible peripheral resistance to PTH as an etiology for hypocalcemia in premature infants.

Glucose Homeostasis

Prematurity, asphyxia, and maternal history of diabetes are also risk factors for hypoglycemia in the newborn period. Hypoglycemia cannot be reliably diagnosed by physical exam alone, because many infants are asymptomatic. Therefore, many institutions check glucose levels in each infant on arrival to the nursery. Prolonged symptomatic as well as asymptomatic hypoglycemia is associated with poorer long-term neurological outcome.[36] Though the lower limit for normal blood glucose in the neonatal period has been widely debated, a general consensus now exists that any glucose level less than 2.6 mmol/L (~45mg/dL) should be treated.[36–38] Infants in the intensive care unit require treatment via the intravenous (IV) route. For severe hypoglycemia (glucose <30 mg/dL) an intravenous minibolus followed by continuous glucose infusion should be used.[38,39] For milder hypoglycemia (glucose 30–45 mg/dL) a glucose infusion without a bolus may suffice.[38] (See Table 26.2). Regardless of treatment chosen, serial glucose checks should be done at least every 30 minutes until infusion rates have been adjusted to stabilize levels within the desired range.

Hyperglycemia (glucose >150 mg/dL) usually occurs as a result of intravenous glucose administration or use of certain drugs such as dexamethasone. First line of treatment is typically to decrease the rate of glucose being administered. However, the brain relies on glucose as its primary source of energy and requires a glucose delivery rate of at least 4–6 mg/kg/min. Furthermore, most premature infants are unable to produce alternative substrates (lactate and ketones) when their available glucose is decreased.[38] Insulin infusions have been shown to treat hyperglycemia without the need to reduce glucose administration.[40] Treatment for hyperglycemia still varies greatly between clinicians, and osmotic diuresis due to glucosuria resulting in dehydration is the most frequent complication.

TABLE 26.2

Treatment of Hypoglycemia
Definition of Hypoglycemia
Mild: Serum Glucose 40-50 mg/dL
Moderate: Serum Glucose 30-40 mg/dL
Severe: <30 mg/dL
Immediate Treatment
Mild: Begin dextrose infusion at 6-8 mg/kg/min and recheck serum glucose 20-30 minutes after infusion started.
Moderate: Begin dextrose infusion at 6-8 mg/kg/min and recheck serum glucose 20-30 minutes after infusion started.
OR
Give minibolus of dextrose (2-3 mL/kg of D10W) followed by dextrose infusion at 6-8 mg/kg/min and recheck serum glucose 20-30 minutes after minibolus is given.
Severe: Give minibolus of dextrose (2-3 mL/kg of D10W) followed by dextrose infusion at 6-8 mg/kg/min and recheck serum glucose 20-30 minutes after minibolus is given.
Continued Care
If patient remains hypoglycemic, dextrose delivery rate should be increased and minibolus repeated every 20-30 minutes until serum glucose stabilizes above 50 mg/dL.

Late Onset Hyponatremia in the Premature Infant

Late hyponatremia (serum sodium level < 130 mEq/L) occurs frequently after 1 week of age in infants born at less than 36 weeks gestational age and is different from hyponatremia in the first few days of life due to volume overload. Part of the reason for this hyponatremia may be a decrease in renal response to plasma aldosterone. Premature infants have plasma aldosterone levels similar to those of term infants; however, urinary excretion of aldosterone only rises with increasing gestational age.[41–43] As urinary excretion of aldosterone increases, sodium retention improves, and a positive sodium balance ensues. It is speculated that this increase in renal excretion of aldosterone by 36 weeks gestational age is one reason why term infants do not experience the hyponatremia preterm infants do.

Treatment of late onset hyponatremia varies. Evidence exists that sodium supplementation enhances weight gain for infants less than 35 weeks gestational age with 3–5 mEq/kg/d to maintain serum sodiums greater than 130 mEq/L during the first two weeks of life.[44] Furthermore, this weight gain is not due to expansion of the extracellular volume space and subsequent edema.[44,45] Given the fact that premature infants would have had positive sodium balance *in utero* during the last trimester of pregnancy and that bone mineralization also requires adequate sodium, sodium supplementation during the first 2 weeks of life should be considered for premature hyponatremic patients.

Nutritional Goals for NICU Patients

The average weight of a healthy term infant is 3.5 kg. Term infants are expected to lose up to 10% of their birth weight in the first week of life and to regain this weight by the end of their second week. Energy requirements for term infants have been estimated from 100–116 kcal/kg/d from 0–3 months and decline to about 100 kcal/kg/d by the end of the first year.[46] These estimates are based on the median intake of healthy infants, and adjustments need to be made for infants with complicating disease processes. Furthermore, parenteral energy requirements are less than enteral energy requirements.

The main goal for every neonatal patient is to maintain adequate growth along his or her individual growth curve. Premature infants are unique in requiring catch-up growth in addition to daily growth along their curves. Catch-up growth refers to the difference in weight, head circumference, and length between a fetus *in utero* compared to his or her prematurely born counterpart at the same post-conceptional age. In many instances premature infants are 2 standard deviations or more below the growth of their post-conceptual age-matched counterparts.[47] Partial catch-up growth can be achieved by manipulating the dietary intake of premature infants; however, the best way to achieve this goal has yet to be determined.[48] Healthy premature infants are predicted to gain 10–15 g/kg/d in body weight, which would require roughly 110–130 kcal/kg/d in energy.[49] Premature infants with complicating illnesses such as respiratory distress syndrome or necrotizing enterocolitis will require even more calories to grow.

Parenteral Nutritional Therapy

Parenteral nutrition should be used when full enteral feedings are not possible. Intravenous nutrition supplies energy through three major forms: carbohydrate as dextrose, protein as crystalline amino acids, and fat as a lipid emulsion. Vitamins, minerals, and trace elements can also be provided intravenously along with needed electrolytes, as previously discussed. Parenteral nutrition may require daily changes as a patient's growth and metabolic demands fluctuate, and frequent laboratory monitoring is required while intravenous nutrition is being initiated. See Table 26.3 for a suggested monitoring schedule. For those patients able to tolerate some enteral feedings, parenteral nutrition can be used to supplement total nutrient intake to maintain growth while enteral feedings are advanced.

Energy Delivery

In general for TPN, 30% to 40% of caloric requirement is provided through lipid emulsion, up to 15% by amino acids, and the remainder by carbohydrate. Studies estimate an average of 4.5 kcal of metabolizable energy (ME) is required for 1 gram of weight gain in low birthweight infants.[50] Adequate non-protein calories must be provided in order to achieve positive

TABLE 26.3

Suggested Monitoring Due to Parenteral Nutrition (PN)

Component	Initial	Later
Weight	Daily	Daily
Length	Weekly	Weekly
Head circumference	Weekly	Weekly
Na, K, Cl, CO_2	Daily until stable	Weekly
Glucose	Daily	PRN
Triglycerides	With every lipid change	Weekly or biweekly
Ca, PO_4	Daily until stable	Weekly or biweekly
Alkaline phosphatase	Day one of PN	Weekly or biweekly
Bilirubin		Weekly or biweekly
Mg	Day one of PN	Weekly or biweekly
Ammonia	PRN	PRN
Gamma GT	Day one of PN	Weekly or biweekly
ALT/AST	Day one of PN	Weekly or biweekly
Complete blood count	Day one of PN	Weekly or PRN

Adapted with permission from *CRC Handbook of Nutrition and Food* (in Press). Copyright CRC Press, Boca Raton, Florida.

nitrogen balance when amino acids are given. Carbohydrate delivery may be limited by the age and size of the patient as well as by the type of access used to deliver parenteral nutrition. In general, peripheral IV access should not be used to deliver fluids that contain more than 12.5 g of dextrose per 100mL. Furthermore, each patient's tolerance of parenteral nutrition will be different.

Protein Intake

Initiation of parenteral protein in infants not enterally fed should begin within the first 3 days of life. Studies have shown glucose infusions alone are not adequate to prevent protein catabolism,[51] and infants can lose up to 3% of their bodies' protein each day.[52] As little as 1 g/kg/d of protein delivery is needed to maintain positive nitrogen balance in extremely low birth weight infants,[52,53] and regimens of up to 2 g/kg/d of protein have been shown to be well tolerated in extremely low birth weight infants in the first 3 days of life.[53,54] Further studies are needed to determine the long-term effects and benefits of prevention of protein loss in the first few days of life.

In the first year of life, infants require 13.4 kcal of ME to deposit 1 gram of protein.[50] Protein deposition also depends on the amount of nitrogen available in the presence of adequate nonprotein calories. At nonprotein energy intakes of greater than 70 kcal/kg/d, the major determinant of nitrogen retention is nitrogen intake; however, nitrogen intakes of greater than 560 mg/kg/d (3.5 g/kg/d of protein) do not increase nitrogen retention even if calories are increased as well.[55] Therefore, the goal for protein intake during TPN is 3.0–3.5 g/kg/d, and protein balance is best predicted by protein intake.[56]

Fat Intake

The total amount of ME required to deposit 1 gram of fat is 10.8 kcal, and fat deposition is more energy efficient than protein deposition.[50] Furthermore, calories to produce fat can be provided from any source, leaving intravenous lipids as a means to boost total caloric intake and not to produce fat. Intravenous lipids are made in 10% and 20% emulsions. Each emulsion contains 1.2 g/dL of phospholipid emulsifier and 2.25 g/dL of glycerol. The 10% emulsion contains 10 g/dL of triglycerides, and the 20% emulsion contains 20 g/dL of triglycerides. When compared to the 10% emulsion, the 20% lipid emulsion is better tolerated by premature infants because of its lesser phospholipid delivery.[57] In most nurseries 10% lipid emulsion is no longer used. A serum triglyceride level should be checked following increases in lipid delivery.

Lipid infusions should be adjusted to maintain serum triglyceride levels less than 200 mg/dL. Most infants >28 weeks gestation can adequately clear 2 g/kg/d of lipids, while those >32 weeks can clear 3 g/kg/d.[58] Furthermore, lipid clearance is inversely related to the hourly rate of lipid infusion, and clearance is maximized when infusions are given over a 24-hour period.[59] Many centers choose to use a 20-hour lipid infusion period if 24-hour volumes are too small to run by infusion pumps. Lipid infusions should be started within the first 72 hours of life when possible with as little as 0.5–1.0 g/kg/d in order to prevent essential fatty acid deficiency.[60,61] A suggested parenteral nutrition regimen is depicted in Table 26.4.

Vitamin, Mineral, and Trace Element Supplementation

Only one intravenous multivitamin preparation for premature infants is currently available (M.V.I. Pediatric, Astra Pharmaceuticals, Westborough, MA). The recommended full daily dose is 5 ml for infants weighing over 3 kg, 65% of full dose (3.25 mL) for infants 1 to 3 kg, and 30% of full dose (1.5 mL) for infants weighing less than 1 kg (M.V.I. Pediatric, Astra Pharmaceuticals, Westborough, MA, 2000). Infants with loss of bowel due to surgical issues may require further zinc and vitamin B_{12} supplementation as well.[62] Cal-

TABLE 26.4

Suggested Nutrition Regimen in Infants <1000 g

	600–800 g	801–1000 g
Radiant Warmer		
IVF, mL/kg/d	100–120	80–100
Dextrose %	5[1]	10[1]
AA, g/kg/d	1.0[2]	1.0[3]
Lipids[3]	0.5	0.5
Incubator		
IVF, mL/kg/d	80–100	80
Dextrose %	7.5–10[1]	10[1]
AA, g/kg/d	1.5[2]	1.5
Lipids	0.5	0.5

No Na, K, Cl unless Na <130 mEq/L or K <3.5 mEq/L

AA (amino acid—Pediatric formulation)

[1] = Infants less than 1000 g may be intolerant to higher concentrations of glucose and may need adjustment based on serum glucose. Advancing glucose delivery is also dictated by tolerance.

[2] = Beginning on DOL 2, increase by 0.5 g/kg/d to max of 2–3/5 g/kg/d.

[3] = Start in conjunction to AA, 0.5 g/kg/d, increase by 0.5 g/kg/d to a max of 2–3 g/kg/d; monitor triglycerides at every increase and at max.

cium, phosphorus, and iron requirements deserve special attention and will be discussed separately.

Intravascular Access

Intravascular (IV) access is divided into either peripheral or central venous access. Peripheral access is obtained by placement of small plastic cannulas in superficial veins. These small cannulas have a median lifespan of only 30 hours[63] and are not preferred for the administration of hyperosmolar solutions. Most low-birth weight infants are going to require parenteral nutrition for weeks, and replacing peripheral cannulas every day is not feasible. Percutaneously inserted central venous catheters are now the access of choice to administer long-term parenteral nutrition. The average lifespan for these catheters in infants less than 1,000 grams was 34 ± 18 days when properly secured and dressed.[64] Complications of percutaneously inserted catheters include infection with prolonged use, thrombosis especially in smaller lines with low flow rates and without heparinized fluids, infiltration to skin sites as well as into the pleural or pericardial space with improperly placed lines,[65] and diaphragmatic palsy.[66] Frequent observation of skin sites, radiologic confirmation of appropriate placement of catheter tips, and frequent sterile dressing changes can help minimize these complications.

Complications of TPN

TPN-acquired cholestasis appears multifactorial in etiology. The first sign may occur by 2 weeks after starting TPN and is usually a rise in the conjugated bilirubin level to greater than 2.0 mg/dL. An earlier indicator of developing cholestasis is elevated gamma glutamyl transpeptidase levels.[67] Risk factors associated with developing cholestasis include recurrent sepsis, prolonged absence of enteral feedings, oxidation of TPN by light[68] and intestinal stasis with intraluminal bacterial overgrowth.[69] Cholestasis can progress to hepatic cirrhosis and liver failure; however, improvements in TPN and treatments for cholestasis are leading to a decline in mortality from this complication.[69]

Metabolic bone disease is a major complication in the premature infant requiring long-term parenteral nutrition. The most common presentations of metabolic bone disease are seen incidentally on radiologic studies and include fractures and progression of osteopenia. The leading cause of osteopenia in the premature infant is calcium and phosphorus deficiency.[47] Fetuses accumulate their largest quantities of calcium and phosphorus in the last trimester of pregnancy,[47] and whole-body mineral and calcium content is directly related to birth weight.[70] Calcium and phosphorus needs for the premature infant approach 200 mg/kg/d of calcium and 100 mg/kg/d of phosphorus.[71] Quantities of calcium and phosphorus in TPN preparations can be increased by the addition of cysteine hydrochloride to acidify the solutions; however, increasing delivery alone does not completely resolve the problem.[72] Aluminum toxicity, vitamin D metabolism, and nonphysiologic delivery of nutrients through continuous TPN solutions may also play a role.[72]

Sepsis in infants receiving long-term TPN is a frequent cause of morbidity and mortality in these patients. Several factors contribute to these recurrences including contamination of the TPN solutions.[73] Infected intracardiac thromboses in premature infants has also been reported.[74] Several methods to reduce episodes of TPN-related sepsis now exist, such as frequent sterile dressing changes and use of antibiotic-impregnated catheters, but none have completely eliminated this problem.

Other complications of TPN include hyperchloremia with metabolic acidosis and acquired neutrophil dysfunction. The use of acetate salts in addition to chloride salts has helped reduce the occurrence of hyperchloremia and metabolic acidosis in patients receiving TPN with supplemental sodium for various reasons.[75] The neutrophils of infants receiving TPN for greater than 10 days have significantly less intracellular killing of bacteria *in vitro* than the neutrophils from healthy infants and adults, and this acquired neutrophil dysfunction may be contributing to the higher risk for sepsis in infants on long-term TPN.[76] Most TPN-related complications improve as enteral feedings are advanced and TPN can be weaned (see Table 26.5).

Enteral Nutrition

Over the last few decades several benefits of early enteral feedings for premature infants have been elucidated. Advancing feedings and overcoming feeding intolerance in these small infants is still a major challenge. Definitions of feeding intolerance vary among clinicians and depend heavily on personal experiences. Term infants do not have the same issues as premature infants, but rather can suffer from a variety of very different conditions that may prevent enteral feedings. These infants each have a unique challenge to the advancement of feedings.

TABLE 26.5

Complications of Parenteral Nutrition

Mechanical
- Extravasation into surrounding tissue
- Embolization
- Thrombosis
- Displacement of catheter from intravascular space

Infections
- Bacterial sepsis
- Fungal sepsis
  - Candida species
  - Malaissiez furfur

Metabolic
- Errors of omission/commission
  - Hypo/hypernatremia
  - Hypo/hyperchloremia
  - Hypo/hyperkalemia
  - Hypo/hyperglycemia
  - Hypo/hypercalcemia
  - Hypophosphatemia
  - Essential fatty acid deficiency
- Hepatic dysfunction
- Metabolic bone disease

INITIATING ENTERAL FEEDINGS

Several studies have now shown that enteral feedings can be safely initiated in stable premature infants as early as the first 48 to 72 hours of life, even if they are on mechanical ventilation.[77,78] Feedings should be delayed in any infant with hypotension or hypoxia for at least 12 to 24 hours after these problems have resolved. Initial feedings can be started with any standard premature infant formula at no more than 20 to 30 mL/kg/d. Advancement of feedings depends on each patient's tolerance and clinical status and clinician preference. See Table 26.6 for one suggested feeding schedule. Small-volume feedings, which were started at 48 hours of life and held at 15–20 mL/kg/d for the next 7 days until advanced, improved feeding tolerance and shortened the time to achievement of full enteral feedings in premature infants when compared to controls who were not fed enterally for the first 9 days of life.[79] Furthermore, the infants who received early enteral feedings had lower peak indirect bilirubin levels and less complications of TPN, such as cholestatic jaundice and metabolic bone disease.[79] Intestinal motor function also matures more quickly in infants who have received early enteral feedings,[80] and this maturation depends on nutrients in the enteral feedings, not just volume being presented into the stomach.[81]

The major complication of initiating enteral feedings is development of necrotizing enterocolitis (NEC).

TABLE 26.6

Enteral Feeding Schedule

Weight (grams)	Beginning Rate	Daily Increase*
<750	0.5 mL/h	0.5 mL
750–1000	1.0 mL/h	1.0 mL
1001–1250	3.0 mL/h	1.0 mL
1251–1500	5-8 mL every 3 hours	1-2 mL
1501–1800	5-10 mL every 3 hours	3 mL
1801–2000	8-10 mL every 3 hours	5-8 mL
>2000	10-30 mL every 3 hours	5-10 mL

*For continuous feeding as indicated; for bolus feeding or PO, increase is per feed.

It is generally agreed that abdominal symptoms (such as distention, hematochezia, and bilious gastric residuals) with radiologic changes consistent with pneumotosis intestinalis constitute NEC. The most important aspect of treatment is discontinuation of enteral feedings for at least 7 days. However, several studies have shown that early enteral feedings do not increase a patient's risk for NEC.[82–84] The cause of NEC is multifactorial, and one aspect is the exposure of an immature gastrointestinal tract to nutrients. However, with careful evaluation of symptoms when they present, minimal enteral feedings can be started early to the benefit of the patient.

Infants with hypotension secondary to any etiology are also at risk for necrotizing enterocolitis. During hypotensive episodes, the body restricts blood flow to the splanchnic region in order to preserve flow to the brain, heart, and adrenal glands. This restriction in splanchnic blood flow can lead to mesenteric ischemia, which predisposes the bowel to necrotizing enterocolitis. Infants born with birth depression, sepsis, acute hypovolemia, symptomatic hypermagnesemia, or congenital heart defects are all at risk for hypotension, and feedings should be held until hypotension is completely resolved.

ADVANCING ENTERAL FEEDINGS

Advancement of feedings is done differently by every clinician. Most physicians advance feedings slowly in infants who weigh less than 1500 grams and do not reach full enteral nutrition until 2 to 3 weeks of age. Larger infants may be advanced more quickly, especially if they are feeding by mouth and not by tube. Signs of feeding intolerance include abdominal distention, increasing gastric residuals and emesis. If abdominal gas patterns remain normal on plain radiographs, feedings can usually be continued if the volume of feeding is reduced (see Table 26.6).

Which Formula to Use

Breast milk is still the first choice for all infants when available. Mature human milk fed to premature infants needs to be supplemented with a fortifier in order to deliver adequate calories, protein, and other nutrients to the babies. If breast milk is not available, premature infant formulas containing at least 24 cal/oz should be used for infants weighing less than 1800 grams, and premature infant formulas with at least 22 cal/oz should be used once an infant passes 1800 grams until he or she is at least 4 months corrected gestational age. When premature infants are at least 4 months corrected gestational age and are demonstrating adequate growth along their individual growth curves, term formulas fortified with iron may be used as the primary source of nutrition. Any infant with potential for absorption problems, such as short bowel syndrome or gastroschisis, should have enteral feedings initiated with an elemental formula.

How to Feed

Infants less than 34 weeks gestational age cannot orally feed and require gavage feedings. Two methods of gavage feeding are used, gastric and transpyloric. Studies have not conclusively shown transpyloric feedings to be advantageous over gastric feedings, and they require radiographs to confirm placement.[85,86] On the other hand, transpyloric feedings can be a safe alternative in infants not tolerating gastric feedings, and some authors have found caloric intake may be advanced more quickly by the transpyloric route.[87] Nasogastric (NG) tube placement can cause airway obstruction in the neonate who is an obligate nose breather, and NG tubes can lead to impaired pulmonary mechanics in infants recovering from respiratory distress syndrome.[88] However, if long-term placement is anticipated, NG tubes are easier to secure than orogastric tubes and require less frequent replacement.

Initiation of oral feedings should not begin until at least 34 weeks corrected gestational age. Even at this age, some infants may experience significant desaturations during oral feedings, which resolve by restarting gavage feedings.[89] Gavage feedings may be given on a continuous or intermittent bolus schedule. Studies have shown hormonal release patterns of infants are different between the two feeding patterns, but the clinical significance has yet to be established.[90] Also, infants receiving continuous feedings expend less energy for thermogenesis than those infants receiving bolus feedings.[91] The ability to tolerate bolus feedings depends on an infant's gastric emptying time. Factors that improve gastric emptying are feeding with breast milk[92] and positioning the infant in the prone or right lateral decubitus position.[93] In general, infants less than 1000 grams are continuously fed while the larger infants are tried on bolus feedings first.

Other Nutritional Considerations

Anemia of Prematurity

Constituting less than 0.01% of body weight, iron is considered a trace element. The growing fetus accumulates iron at a rate of 1.6–2.0 mg/kg/d in the third trimester[72] to reach a total body iron content of 75 mg/kg at term.[49] When born prematurely, an infant loses this period of iron accumulation, resulting in lower iron stores. Furthermore, the more ill the infant, the more blood lost through laboratory sampling and procedures, further depleting total body iron content. Iron supplementation should begin as early as 2 weeks of age[49] at no less than 2 mg/kg/d. Requirements will increase for patients with chronic illness and for those undergoing treatment with erythropoietin for anemia of prematurity.

Data are clear that premature infants do increase red cell production when given recombinant erythropoietin subcutaneously and supplemental iron in their diets.[94] Further studies are showing that the response to erythopoietin is improved if intravenous iron is given as opposed to just oral iron supplementation.[95–97] Although side effects from treatment with recombinant erythropoietin have not been reported, the question has been raised of a possible increase in retinopathy of prematurity in infants treated with recombinant erythropoietin and iron.[98] Whether all premature infants should receive recombinant erythropoietin is still under study; however, iron supplementation is appropriate for every infant born preterm.

Breast Feeding after Discharge

Much attention has been turned towards the adequacy of human milk as the sole dietary source for the premature infant. Most centers will supplement human milk with fortifiers while premature infants are in the hospital. The debate is whether this supplementation should continue after discharge home and how. A multi-center trial in Great Britain showed infants fed preterm formula regained birth weight more quickly than those exclusively fed human milk.[99] Breast-fed infants who received preterm formula supplementation also gained weight more quickly than exclusively breast-fed infants, but not at the same rate as formula-fed babies.[99] Long-term implications of these growth differences are currently under study.

Breast milk does contain properties not available in commercial formulas, which have positive effects on premature infants. Most notably, it seems to have a neuro-developmental stimulatory effect. Early research found that preterm babies who were exclusively provided breast milk had an average IQ score 10% higher than those fed preterm formula, even after adjustment for social and educational factors.[100] Therefore, by supplementing breast milk, one can enhance growth as well as provide the many advantages of mother's milk to the premature infant. Breast milk remains best for any baby (with rare exceptions); supplemented breast milk is even better for today's premature baby.

Nutrition and Developmental Outcome of Premature Infants

Current dietary supplementations for the premature infant have arisen out of desire to help prevent long-term morbidity associated with preterm birth. Otherwise healthy premature infants still have increased risks for lower developmental IQ than their term counterparts. Researchers have turned their attention toward reducing these risks through dietary manipulations. Although most work is ongoing, good evidence now exists that even short-term dietary improvements can have positive effects.

Of particular interest is neuro-developmental outcome for the otherwise healthy preterm infant. A preliminary study that showed premature infants (at 18 months post term age) fed specialized preterm formula had higher developmental and social quotient scores than those fed standard term formula.[101] Short term beneficial effects have also been reported.[102] Furthermore, they had a lower incidence of moderate developmental impairment.[101] Unpublished data from this same study suggest that this effect of diet on developmental performance persists at 7.5 to 8 years of age.[47] These infants were fed preterm formula for only 4 weeks postnatally, and studies involving longer supplementation periods are ongoing.

Conclusions

Nutritional considerations in the neonatal intensive care unit center around sick premature and term infants and their many problems. Most ongoing research is focused on improving current parenteral nutrition regimens and finding ways to initiate enteral feedings as soon as possible. The pathogenesis of necrotizing enterocolitis is still poorly understood, and NEC is still the major cause of nutritionally related morbidity for premature infants. As survival from lung disease continues to improve, future research must focus on ways to reduce growth delay in premature infants in hopes of improving cognitive outcome.

References

1. Paranka MS, Yoder BA, Brehm W. Improved outcome of extremely premature infants in the 1990s. *Military Medicine.* 1999;164:568–571.
2. Helfrick FW, Abelson NM. Intravenous feeding of a complete diet in a child. *J Pediatr.* 1944;24:400–403.
3. Dudrick SJ, Wilmore DW, Vars HM, et al. Long-term total parenteral nutrition with growth, development, and positive nitrogen balance. *Surgery.* 1968;64:134–142.
4. Wilmore DW, Dudrick SJ. Prevention of cannular sepsis—preliminary report. *N Eng J Med.* 1967;277:433.
5. Winters RW, Heird WC, Dell RB. History of parenteral nutrition in pediatrics with emphasis on amino acids. *Federation Proceedings.* 1984;43:1407–1411.
6. Heird WC, Driscoll Jr JM, Schullinger JN, et al. Intravenous alimentation in pediatric patients. *J Pediatr.* 1972;80: 351–372.
7. Smallpiece V, Davies PA. Immediate feeding of premature infants with undiluted breast-milk. *Lancet.* 1964;2:1349–1352.
8. Fanaroff AA, Wald M, Gruber HS, et al. Insensible water loss in low birth weight infants. *Pediatrics.* 1972;50:236–245.
9. Rutter N, Hull D. Water loss from the skin of term and preterm babies. *Arch Dis Child.* 1979;54:858–868.
10. Hammarlund K, Sedin G, Stromberg B. Transepidermal water loss in newborn infants. *Acta Paediatr Scand.* 1983; 72:721–728.
11. Rutter N, Hull D. Reduction of skin water loss in the newborn. I. Effect of applying topical agents. *Arch Dis Child.* 1981;56:669–672.
12. Pabst RC, Starr KP, Qaiyumi S, et al. The effect of application of aquaphor on skin condition, fluid requirements, and bacterial colonization in very low birth weight infants. *J Perinatolo.* 1999;19:278–283.
13. Baumgart S, Fox WW, Polin RA. Physiologic implications of two different heat shields for infants under radiant warmers. *J Pediatr.* 1982;100:787–790.
14. Brice JEH, Rutter N, Hull D. Reduction of skin water loss in the newborn. II. Clinical trial of two methods in very low birthweight babies. *Arch Dis Child.* 1981;56:673–675.
15. Baumgart S, Costarino AT. Water and electrolyte metabolism of the micropremie. *Clin Perinatolo.* 2000;27:131–146.

16. Bell EF, Warburton D, Stonestreet BS, et al. Effect of fluid administration on the development of symptomatic patent ductus arteriosus and congestive heart failure in premature infants. *N Eng J Med.* 1980;302:598–604.

17. Bell EF, Warburton D, Stonestreet BS, et al. High-volume fluid intake predisposes premature infants to necrotising enterocolitis. *Lancet* 1979;90.

18. Brown ER, Start A, Sosenko I, et al. Bronchopulmonary dysplasia: possible relationship to pulmonary edema. *J Pediatr.* 1978;92:982–984.

19. Spitzer AR, Fox WW, Delivoria-Papadopoulos M. Maximum diuresis—a factor in predicting recovery from respiratory distress syndrome and the development of bronchopulmonary dysplasia. *J Pediatr.* 1981;98:476–479.

20. Palta MP, Gabbert D, Weinstein MR, et al. Multivariate assessment of traditional risk factors for chronic lung disease in very low birth weight neonates. *J Pediatr.* 1991; 119:285–292.

21. Van Marter LJ, Pagano M, Allred EN, et al. Rate of bronchopulmonary dysplasia as a function of neonatal intensive care practices. *J Pediatr.* 1992;120:938–946.

22. Costarino AT, Gruskay JA, Corcoran L, et al. Sodium restriction versus daily maintenance replacement in very low birth weight premature neonates: a randomized, blind therapeutic trial. *J Pediatr.* 1992;120:99–106.

23. Gruskay J, Costarino AT, Polin RA, et al. Nonoliguric hyperkalemia in the premature infant weighing less than 1000 grams. *J Pediatr.* 1988;113:381–386.

24. Stefano JL, Norman ME, Morales MC, et al. Decreased erythrocyte Na+, K(+)-ATPase activity associated with cellular potassium loss in extremely low birth weight infants with nonoliguric hyperkalemia. *J Pediatr.* 1993;122: 276–284.

25. Sato K, Kondo T, Iwao H, et al. Sodium and potassium in red blood cells of premature infants during the first few days: risk of hyperkalaemia. *Acta Pediatr Scand.* 1991;80: 899–904.

26. Wandrup J, Kroner J, Pryds O, et al. Age-related reference values for ionized calcium in the first week of life in premature and full-term neonates. *Scand J Clin Lab Invest.* 1988;48:255–260.

27. Nelson N, Finnstrom O, Larsson L. Plasma ionized calcium, phosphate and magnesium in preterm and small for gestational age infants. *Acta Pediatr Scand.* 1989;78:351–357.

28. Husain SM, Veligati N, Sims DG, et al. Measurement of ionised calcium concentration in neonates. *Arch Dis Child.* 1993;69:77–78.

29. Ilves P, Kiisk M, Soopold T, et al. Serum total magnesium and ionized calcium concentrations in asphyxiated term infants with hypoxic-ischaemic encephalopathy. *Acta Paediatr.* 2000;89:680–685.

30. Merlob P, Amir J. Pathogenesis of hypocalcemia in neonatal polycythemia. *Medical Hypotheses.* 1989;30:49–50.

31. Hod M, Merlob P, Friedman S, et al. Gestational diabetes mellitus: A survey of perinatal complications in the 1980s. *Diabetes.* 1991;40(Suppl 2)74–78.

32. Mimouni F, Tsang RC, Hertzberg VS, et al. Polycythemia, hypomagnesemia, and hypocalcemia in infants of diabetic mothers. *AJDC.* 1986;140:798–800.

33. Cooper LJ, Anast CS. Circulating immunoreactive parathyroid hormone levels in premature infants and the response to calcium therapy. *Acta Pediatr Scand.* 1985;74: 669–673.

34. Rubin PL, Posillico JT, Anast CS, et al. Circulating levels of biologically active and immunoreactive intact parathyroid hormone in human newborns. *Pediatr Res.* 1991;29: 201–207.

35. Dilena BA, White GH. The responses of plasma ionised calcium and intact parathyrin to calcium supplementation in preterm infants. *Acta Pediatrica Scandinavica.* 1991;80: 1098–1100.

36. Lucas A, Morley R, Cole TJ. Adverse neurodevelopmental outcome of moderate neonatal hypoglycemia. *Br Med J.* 1988;297:1304–1308.

37. Hawdon JM, Ward Platt MP, Aynsley-Green A. Prevention and management of neonatal hypoglycemia. *Arch Dis Child.* 1994;70:F60–F65.

38. Farrag HM, Cowett RM. Glucose homeostasis in the micropremie. *Clin Perinatolo.* 2000;27:1–22.

39. Lillen LD, Pildes RS, Srinivasan G, et al. Treatment of neonatal hypoglycemia with minibolus and intravenous glucose infusion. *J Pediatr.* 1980;97:295–298.

40. Collins Jr JW, Hoppe M, Brown K, et al. A controlled trial of insulin infusion and parenteral nutrition in extremely low birth weight infants with glucose intolerance. *J Pediatr.* 1991;118:921–927.

41. Honour JW, Shackleton CHL, Valman HB. Sodium homeostasis in preterm infants. *Lancet.* 1974;1147.

42. Sulyok E, Nemeth M, Tenyi I, et al. Relationship between maturity, electrolyte balance and the function of the renin-angiotensin-aldosterone system in newborn infants. *Biolog Neonate.* 1979;35:60–65.

43. Sulyok E, Kovacs L, Lichardus B, et al. Late hyponatremia in premature infants: role of aldosterone and arginine vasopressin. *J Pediatr.* 1985;106:990–994.

44. Al-Dahhan J, Haycock GB, Nichol B, et al. Sodium homeostasis in term and preterm neonates III: Effect of salt supplementation. *Arch Dis Child.* 1984;59:945–950.

45. Roy RN, Chance GW, Radde IC, et al. Late hyponatremia in very low birthweight infants (<1.3 kilograms). *Pediatr Res.* 1976;10:526–531.

46. Bhatia J, Bucher C, Bunyapen C. Feeding the term infant. CRC Press (In Press)

47. Tsang R, Namgung R. Newborn bone development. *Report of the 106th Ross Conference on Pediatric Research.* 1996: 21.

48. Kashyap S, Schulze K, Ramakrishnan R, et al. Evaluation of a mathematical model for predicting the relationship between protein and energy intakes of low-birth-weight infants and the rate and composition of weight gain. *Pediatr Res.* 1994;35:704–712.

49. Bhatia J, Bucher C, Bunyapen C. Feeding the premature infant. CRC Press (In Press).

50. Roberts SB, Young VR. Energy costs of fat and protein deposition in the human infant. *Am J Clin Nutr.* 1988;48: 951–955.

51. Anderson TL, Muttart CR, Bieber MA, et al. A controlled trial of glucose versus glucose and amino acids in premature infants. *J Pediatr.* 1979;94:947–951.

52. Saini J, Macmahon P, Morgan JB, et al. Early parenteral feeding of amino acids. *Arch Dis Child.* 1989;64:1362–1366.

53. van Lingen RA, van Goudoever JB, Luijendijk IHT, et al. Effects of early amino acid administration during total parenteral nutrition on protein metabolism in pre-term infants. *Clin Sci.* 1992;82:199–203.

54. Rivera A Jr., Bell EF, Stegink LD, et al. Plasma amino acid profiles during the first three days of life in infants with respiratory distress syndrome: effect of parenteral amino acid supplementation. *J Pediatr.* 1989;115:465–468.

55. Zlotkin SH, Bryan MH, Anderson GH. Intravenous nitrogen and energy intakes required to duplicate in utero nitrogen accretion in prematurely born human infants. *J Pediatr.* 1981;99:115–120.

56. Thureen PJ, Anderson AH, Baron KA, et al. Protein balance in the first week of life in ventilated neonates receiving parenteral nutrition. *Am J Clin Nutr.* 1998;68:1128–1135.

57. Haumont D, Deckelbaum RJ, Richelle M, et al. Plasma lipid and plasma lipoprotein concentrations in low birth weight infants given parenteral nutrition with twenty or ten percent lipid emulsion. *J Pediatr.* 1989;115:787–793

58. Innis SM. Fat. In: Tsang RC, Lucas A, Uauy R, eds. *Nutritional Needs of the Premature Infant.* Baltimore: Williams and Wilkins; 1993:65

59. Brans YW, Andrew DS, Carrillo DW, et al. Tolerance of fat emulsions in very-low-birth-weight neonates. *Am J Dis Child.* 1988;142:145–152.

60. Thureen PJ, Hay Jr WW. Intravenous nutrition and postnatal growth of the micropremie. *Clin Perinatolo.* 2000;27: 197–219.

61. Foote KD, MacKinnon MJ, Innis SM. Effect of early introduction of formula vs fat-free parenteral nutrition on essential fatty acid status of preterm infants. *Am J Clin Nutr.* 1991;54:93–97.

62. Meadows N. Monitoring and complications of parenteral nutrition. *Nutrition.* 1998;14:806–808.

63. Johnson RV, Donn SM. Life span of intravenous cannulas in a neonatal intensive care unit. *Am J Dis Child.* 1988; 142:968–971.

64. Durand M, Ramanathan R, Martinelli B, et al. Prospective evaluation of percutaneous central venous silastic catheters in newborn infants with birth weights of 510 to 3920 grams. *Pediatrics.* 1986;78:245–250.

65. Hogan MJ. Neonatal vascular catheters and their complications. *Radiol Clin North Amer.* 1999;37:1109–1125.

66. Williams JH, Hunter JE, Kanto Jr WP, et al. Hemidiaphragmatic paralysis as a complication of central venous catheterization in a neonate. *J Perinatolo.* 1995;15:386–388.

67. Black DD, Suttle EA, Whitington, et al. The effect of short-term total parenteral nutrition on hepatic function in the human neonate: a prospective randomized study demonstrating alteration of hepatic canalicular function. *J Pediatr.* 1981;99:445–449.

68. Bhatia J, Moslen MT, Haque AK, et al. Total parenteral nutrition—associated alterations in hepatobiliary function and histology in rats: is light exposure a clue? *Pediatr Res.* 1993;33:487–492.

69. Kubota A, Yonekura T, Hoki M, et al. Total parenteral nutrition—associated intrahepatic cholestasis in infants: 25 years' experience. *J Ped Surg.* 2000;35:1049–1051.

70. Rigo J, De Curtis M, Picaud JC, et al. Whole body calcium content in term and preterm neonates. *Eur J Pediatr.* 1998;157:259–260.

71. Greer, F. Vitamin and mineral requirements for very-low-birth-weight infants fed human milk. *Report of the 108th Ross Conference on Pediatric Research.* 1999;60.

72. Klein GL. Metabolic bone disease of total parenteral nutrition. *Nutrition.* 1998;14:149–152.

73. Tresoldi AT, Padoveze MC, Trabasso P, et al. Enterobacter cloacae sepsis outbreak in a newborn unit caused by contaminated total parenteral nutrition solution. *Am J of Infect Control.* 2000;28:258–261.

74. De Schepper J, Hachimi-Idrissi S, Cham B, et al. Diagnosis and management of catheter-related infected intracardiac thrombosis in premature infants. *Am J Perinatolo.* 1993;10:39–42.

75. Peters O, Ryan S, Matthew L, et al. Randomised controlled trial of acetate in preterm neonates receiving parenteral nutrition. *Arch Dis Child.* 1997;77:F12–F15.

76. Okada Y, Klein NJ, Pierro A, et al. Neutrophil dysfunction: The cellular mechanism of impaired immunity during total parenteral nutrition in infancy. *J Ped Surg.* 1999; 34:242–245.

77. Heicher D, Philip AGS. Orogastric supplementation in small premature infants requiring mechanical respiration. *Am J Dis Child.* 1976;130:282–286.

78. Slagle TA, Gross SJ. Effect of early low-volume enteral substrate on subsequent feeding tolerance in very low birth weight infants. *J Pediatr.* 1988;113:526–531.

79. Dunn L, Hulman S, Weiner J, et al. Beneficial effects of early hypocaloric enteral feeding on neonatal gastrointestinal function: Preliminary report of a randomized trial. *J Pediatr.* 1988;112:622–629.

80. Berseth CL. Effect of early feeding on maturation of the preterm infant's small intestine. *J Pediatr.* 1992;120:947–953.

81. Berseth CI, Nordyke C. Enteral nutrients promote postnatal maturation of intestinal motor activity in preterm infants. *Am J Phys.* 1993;264:G1046–G1051.

82. Book LS, Herbst JJ, Lung AL. Comparison of fast- and slow-feeding rate schedules to the development of necrotizing enterocolitis. *J Pediatr.* 1976;89:463–466.

83. La Gamma EF, Ostertag SG, Birenbaum H. Failure of delayed oral feedings to prevent necrotizing enterocolitis. *Am J Dis Child.* 1985;139:385–389.

84. Ostertag SG, LaGamma EF, Reisen CE, et al. Early enteral feeding does not affect the incidence of necrotizing enterocolitis. *Pediatrics.* 1986;77:275–280.

85. Laing IA, Lang MA, Callaghan O, et al. Nasogastric compared with nasoduodenal feeding in low birthweight infants. *Arch Dis Child.* 1986;61:138–141.

86. Pereira GR, Lemons JA. Controlled study of transpyloric and intermittent gavage feeding in the small preterm infant. *Pediatrics.* 1981;67:68–72.

87. Van Caillie M, Powell GK. Nasoduodenal versus nasogastric feeding in the very low birthweight infant. *Pediatrics.* 1975;56:1065–1072.

88. Sasidharan P, Rejjal A, Krishnaswamy R. NG Tube feeding is not recommended in infants recovering from RDS. *Pediatr Res.* 1990;27:224A.

89. Poets CF, Langner MU, Bohnhorst B. Effects of bottle feeding and two different methods of gavage feeding on oxygenation and breathing patterns in preterm infants. *Acta Paediatrica.* 1997;86:419–423.

90. Aynsley-Green A, Adrian TE, Bloom SR. Feeding and the development of enteroinsular hormone secretion in the preterm infant: Effects of continuous gastric infusions of human milk compared with intermittent boluses. *Acta Paediatr Scand.* 1982;71:379–383.

91. Grant J , Denne SC. Effect of intermittent versus continuous enteral feeding on energy expenditure in premature infants. *J Pediatr.* 1991;118:928–932.

92. Cavell B. Gastric emptying in preterm infants. *Acta Paediatr Scand.* 1979;68:725–730.

93. Yu VYH. Effect of body position on gastric emptying in the neonate. *Arch Dis Child.* 1975;50:500–504.

94. Bechensteen AG, Haga P, Halvorsen S, et al. Erythropoietin, protein, and iron supplementation and the prevention of anemia of prematurity. *Arch Dis Child.* 1993;69:19–23.

95. Meyer MP, Haworth C, Meyer JH, et al. A comparison of oral and intravenous iron supplementation in preterm infants receiving recombinant erythropoietin. *J Pediatr.* 1996;129:258–263.

96. Carnielli VP, Da Riol R, Montini G. Iron supplementation enhances response to high doses of recombinant human erythropoietin in preterm infants. *Arch Dis Child. Fetal Neonatal Edition* 1998;79:F44–F48.

97. Pollak A, Hayde M, Hayn M, et al. Effect of intravenous iron supplementation on erythropoiesis in erythropoietin-treated premature infants. *Pediatrics.* 2001;107:78–85.

98. Romagnoli C, Zecca E, Gallini F, et al. Do recombinant human erythropoietin and iron supplementation increase the risk of retinopathy of prematurity? *Eur J Pediatr.* 2000; 159:627–628.

99. Lucas A, Gore SM, Cole TJ, et al. Multicentre trial on feeding low birthweight infants: effects of diet on early growth. *Arch Dis Child.* 1984;59:722.

100. Lucas A, Morley R, Cole TJ, et al. Breast milk and subsequent intelligence quotient in children born preterm. *Lancet.* 1992;339:261–264.

101. Lucas A, Morley R, Cole TJ, et al. Early diet in preterm babies and developmental status at 18 months. *Lancet.* 1990;335:1477–1481.

102. Bhatia J, Rassin DK, Cerreto MC, et al. Effect of protein/energy ratio on growth and behavior of premature infants: preliminary findings. *J Pediatr.* 1991;119:103–110.

CHAPTER

27 Nutrition Support in the Pediatric Intensive Care Unit

Diane L. Olson, R.D., C.N.S.D., C.S.P., L.D.,
W. Frederick Schwenk II, M.D., C.N.S.P.

Introduction	311
Nutrition Assessment	311
Nutrition Requirements	312
Energy	312
Protein	314
Electrolytes, Vitamins, and Minerals	315
Nutrition Support	315
Oral Feeding	315
Enteral Nutrition	315
Parenteral Nutrition	320
Special Pediatric Disease States	321
Neurologic Impairment	321
Inborn Errors of Metabolism	321
Conclusions	321
Case Study	321
References	322

Introduction

Nutrition support in the pediatric intensive care unit (PICU) has many similarities with such therapy in adults. Most aspects of the nutrition assessment do not depend upon age. Children seem to have the same metabolic responses to illness that adults do, and the components of both enteral and parenteral nutrition are similar in adults and children.

However, this chapter will highlight important differences between children and adults with respect to nutrition support in the pediatric intensive care unit. Children have increased energy requirements and decreased energy reserves compared to adults. As a general rule, an inverse relationship exists between age and the risk of developing malnutrition.[1] Because malnutrition has been associated with an increased risk of infection and mortality in critically ill children, many professionals caring for patients in a pediatric intensive care unit advocate early administration of nutrition support to these patients.[2–4]

Another major differences between children and adults with respect to nutrition support is that far fewer clinical studies have examined the role of nutrition support in children compared to adults. One factor causing this discrepancy is that energy expenditure is difficult to measure in children. In addition, most pediatric institutional review boards are reluctant to approve studies in healthy children, since children are unable to give informed consent. Without normal controls, metabolic measurements in critically ill children are difficult to interpret. Notwithstanding the limitations, many of the studies showing benefit of nutrition support in the intensive care unit have been done in infants.[5]

Another difference between pediatric-aged and adult patients is the scope of the disease states that might be represented. Pediatric care-givers may more likely encounter patients with neurologic impairment, as well as with inborn errors of metabolism. These special diagnoses will be discussed briefly within this chapter.

Nutrition Assessment

The elements that are part of a nutritional assessment of a patient in a pediatric intensive care unit are similar to those used in adults. They include anthropometric, clinical, laboratory, and review of previous, current and required intake.[6] Careful nutrition and metabolic assessment should help in providing optimal nutrition support with a minimal number of complications.

The most important anthropometric data in a child or teenager are accurate measurements of weight and length or height.[7] In children less than 2 years of age, weight is measured without the clothes or diaper, while length is measured using a length board with fixed headboard and a moveable right-angle footboard. Accurate measurement of length requires two individuals, one to hold the head in position and the other to move the footboard and make the measurement. Measurement of length should be accurate to within 0.5 cm. In children less than 3 years of age, measurement of head circumference is also important.

For children over 2 years of age, measurement of weight is made with the child wearing light clothing. Height is ideally determined by using a stadiometer, where the child stands against a fixed scale at right angles to the floor. Such measurements are usually accurate to within 1–2 mm. However, in the intensive care unit setting, accurate height measurements are often impossible to obtain, in which case the care-giver needs to use recent height measurements made outside the hospital if they are available. Length measurements made on a hospital bed using a measuring tape are rarely accurate.

New reference growth charts for children in the United States have been available since the year 2000.[8] These data are derived from measurements made in a cross-section of children in the United States. For children less than 3 years of age, normal weight-for-length data are provided, while for older children, body mass index (BMI) for age is shown. Both weight for length and BMI charts are available for children 2 to 3 years of age. These latter two charts can be used to identify children at particular nutritional risk—those who fall below the 3% in their weight relative to their length or who have a BMI less than the 3% for age. Children who have crossed percentiles on these latter two curves are also more likely to have nutrition deficiencies.

No specific laboratory tests can be used to assess the nutritional status of infants and children. One problem is that for many laboratories, normal values for infants and children have not been established. In such cases, it may be necessary to rely upon published normal data,[9–12] recognizing the limitations of these values. In addition, in smaller children, there may be limitations on the amount of blood that can be safely obtained by venipuncture. Specific laboratory tests must be chosen after considering the child's underlying diagnosis and risk for nutritional deficiencies.

Any nutritional assessment must also include accurate dietary information. Attention must be given to the child's development—specifically, whether the child is able to eat independently.[7] Calorie counts are frequently useful in hospitalized patients to assess adequacy of intake.

Nutrition Requirements

Energy

No consensus exists as to how best to estimate the energy requirements of a critically ill child. The recommended allowances for children from the National Research Council assume that the child is healthy, active, and growing. None of these apply to a child in an intensive care unit. Use of these allowances for critically ill children overestimates the energy requirements of most children in a pediatric intensive care unit.[12]

While burns and sepsis may cause hypermetabolism in a critically ill child, uncomplicated operative procedures in infants and children have not been shown to cause hypermetabolism.[13–15] The explanation for this lack of hypermetabolism is not known. One hypothesis is that in such patients, there is secretion of cytokines and counter-regulatory hormones that diverts the energy that would normally be used for protein synthesis for growth into protein synthesis for repair of tissue damage.[3,14,15]

Most practitioners assume that similar complications seen in adults with overfeeding and underfeeding also apply to children. Overfeeding is thought to increase the likelihood of hepatic dysfunction and respiratory compromise, as well as increase the risk of mortality. As reported in adults, it is assumed that overfeeding can lead to hypermetabolism and that overfeeding cannot by itself reverse tissue catabolism.[16] In contrast, underfeeding is assumed to alter immune function and have negative effects on the cardiovascular system and gastrointestinal tract.[17]

A number of ways of predicting energy requirements in a critically ill child have been proposed.[3,18–22] Unfortunately, no clinical studies have compared outcomes using the various caloric estimation formulas in critically ill children. Results of a survey of practitioners in 64 pediatric intensive care units across the United States confirm this lack of consensus (Figure 27.1).

Most approaches to predicting energy requirements begin with an estimation of resting energy expenditure (REE) or basal metabolic rate (BMR). These values usually differ by no more than 10%. Tables 27.1 and 27.2 show how to predict REE and BMR, respectively, in critically ill children using equations or data from WHO/FAO/UNU.[19]

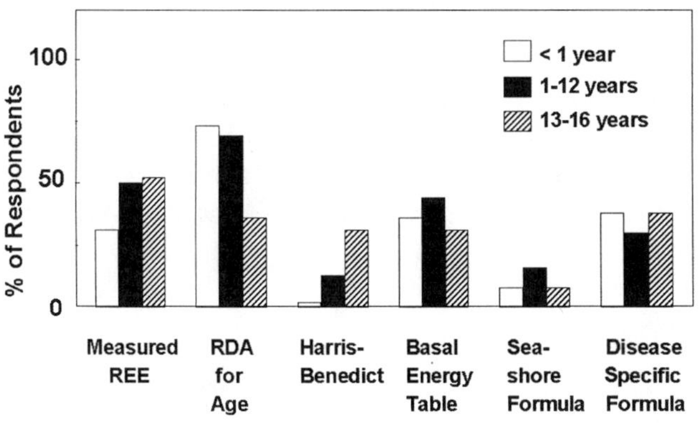

Figure 27.1

Methods Used to Determine Energy Requirements in Infants and Children in Pediatric Intensive Care Units. (N = 64). Data from a survey conducted by D.O. in 1992.

TABLE 27.1

Equations from WHO/FAO/UNU for Predicting Resting Energy Expenditure from Age, Sex, and Body Weight[a]

Sex and Age Range (years)	Equation to Derive REE in kcal/d
Boys	
0–3	(60.9 × wt) - 54
3–10	(22.7 × wt) + 495
10–18	(17.5 × wt) + 651
Girls	
0–3	(61.0 × wt) - 51
3–10	(22.5 × wt) + 499
10–18	(12.2 × wt) + 746

[a]weight of person in kilograms

Reprinted with permission from National Academy of Sciences. *Recommended Dietary Allowance.* 10th ed. Washington, DC: National Academy Press; 1989.

TABLE 27.2

Basal Metabolic Rates from WHO/FAO/UNU According to Weight and Sex

Body Weight (kg)	Metabolic rate (kcal/24 h) Boys	Metabolic rate (kcal/24 h) Girls	Body Weight (kg)	Metabolic rate (kcal/24 h) Boys	Metabolic rate (kcal/24 h) Girls
3.0	120	144	36.0	1268	1148
4.0	191	191	38.0	1316	1172
5.0	239	239	40.0	1340	1172
6.0	287	311	42.0	1363	1196
7.0	357	383	44.0	1387	1220
8.0	431	431	46.0	1435	1220
9.0	478	502	48.0	1459	1244
10.0	550	550	50.0	1483	1268
11.0	622	622	52.0	1507	1268
12.0	670	670	54.0	1531	1292
13.0	718	718	56.0	1579	1316
14.0	765	765	58.0	1603	1316
15.0	813	813	60.0	1627	1340
16.0	861	837	62.0	1650	1363
17.0	885	861	64.0	1674	1387
18.0	909	885	66.0	1698	1411
19.0	933	909	68.0	1722	1435
20.0	957	933	70.0	1746	1459
22.0	1005	957	72.0	1746	1459
24.0	1058	981	74.0	1770	1483
26.0	1100	1005	76.0	1794	1507
28.0	1124	1055	78.0	1818	1507
30.0	1172	1076	80.0	1842	1532
32.0	1196	1100	82.0	1866	1555
34.0	1244	1124	84.0	1890	1579

Reprinted with permission from Kleiber M. American Society for Nutritional Sciences. *Journal of Nutrition.* 1972;102:307.

An alternative approach is to calculate BMR from an empirical equation developed by J. Seashore.[22] This equation can be used for children who are between the 10th and 90th percentiles for weight. If a patient's weight falls above the 90th percentile or below the 10th percentile, weight-age rather than chronological age can be used in the formula. (Weight-age is the age for which the patient's present weight would be at the 50th percentile.) Figure 27.2 shows how accurately the Seashore equation predicts BMR over a wide range of ages and weights. Table 27.3 shows the guidelines for using Seashore's equation for the estimation of BMR to estimate total daily energy requirements. It should be noted that this method is appropriate for children up to age 15. Beyond age 15, the Harris-Benedict equations may be more appropriate.

To calculate total energy requirements of a patient in a pediatric intensive care unit, other factors may need to be considered beyond the BMR or REE. Energy needs may be increased by 13% for each degree of temperature elevation over 37°C.[22] The specific dynamic action of the food may account for an additional 5%–10% of BMR.[12,19] A similar percent of additional calories may be important in very young children to account for growth.[18] In contrast to children outside of an intensive care unit, activity is likely to be minimal and have little effect on energy expenditure.

A few recent studies have measured energy expenditure in children in an intensive care unit.[23–28] Results from these studies show a wide variability in energy expenditure, particularly in children receiving ventilation. The techniques described above are not always useful in accurately assessing energy requirements. However, in order to carry out indirect calorimetry in ventilated patients, a cuffed endotracheal tube must be utilized, and children are usually intubated using non-cuffed tubes. In addition, at the present time most pediatric intensive care units do not have the ability to measure energy expenditure utilizing indirect calorimetry. While theoretically such measurements may be of benefit, implementation of indirect calorimetry in pediatric-aged patients awaits better outcome data. Indirect calorimetry may be particularly useful in children who are difficult to wean from a ventilator, have a severe closed head injury, or have multiple trauma or burns.[12,17,21]

Protein

Infants and children in pediatric intensive care units have a net negative nitrogen balance, since the level of

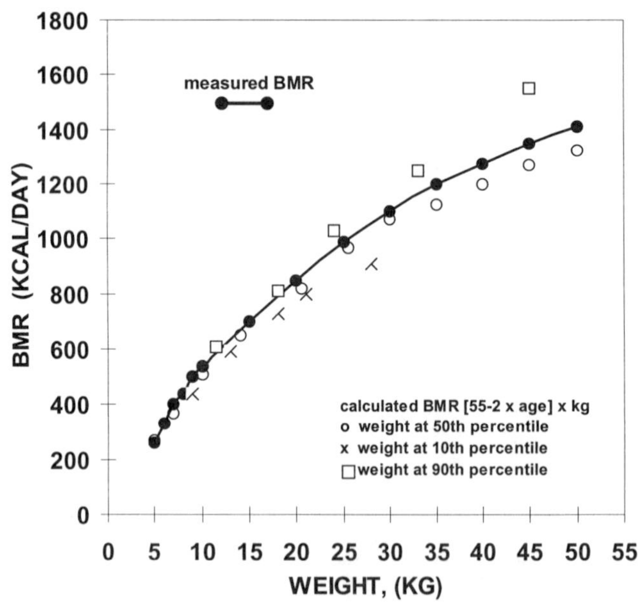

Figure 27.2

Basal Metabolic Rate in Children Measured and Predicted Using the Seashore Equation

TABLE 27.3

Estimations of Energy Requirements Using the Seashore Formula	
Basal = (55 - 2 × age) × kg =	______
Maintenance, 20% × basal =	______
Activity, 0–25% × basal =	______
Sepsis, 13%/1°C × basal =	______
Burns, 50–100% × basal =	______
Total =	______

Adapted with permission from Seashore JH: Nutritional support of children in the intensive care unit. *Yale J Biol Med.* 1984;57:111–134.

catabolism does not equal the rate of protein synthesis. Exogenously administered protein, along with adequate calories, can help to ameliorate this net protein loss. However, giving too much protein can increase the risk of metabolic acidosis and azotemia.[2] If adequate non-protein calories are not administered along with the protein, the amino acids may be used for gluconeogenesis rather than protein synthesis.[21] Consequently, the minimum ratio of administered non-protein calories to amino nitrogen is felt to be at least 240:1 during acute illness.[12]

Overall, expressed in grams per kilogram body weight per day, protein requirements for children decrease with size. Critically ill infants and children up to 2 years of age may require as much as 2.5 to 3 g/kg body weight/d, 2 to 11 year old children may require 2 g of protein/kg while children over 12 years of age require 1.5 to 2 g of protein/kg.[21] Protein requirements may be increased when the protein is administered parenterally, since elemental amino acids are not used as efficiently. Protein requirements are also increased when the patient has a severe burn, significant blood loss, large amounts of chest tube drainage, and/or major organ trauma.[2] Guidelines for parenteral and protein requirements are noted in Table 27.4.

Electrolytes, Vitamins, and Minerals

Few studies have documented electrolyte, vitamin, and mineral requirements during acute illness in infants and children. For this reason, vitamins and minerals are usually administered at rates to meet the Dietary Reference Intakes (DRIs) for age. These requirements are listed in Tables 27.5 and 27.6.

In comparison to adults and expressed per kilogram body weight, infants and children have increased requirements of iron, calcium, phosphorus, and vitamin D. Iron, calcium, and phosphorus needs are also increased in adolescent patients. Additional supplementation of selected nutrients may be required if a deficiency is noted or there are continuing losses of specific nutrients occur, such as in burns, renal disease, or diarrhea. Potentially, children who are particularly malnourished may develop hypophosphatemia during refeeding.[31]

TABLE 27.4

Daily Protein Requirements (grams/kg) for Parenteral Nutrition for Pediatric Patients*	
Infants	2.0–2.5
Children	1.5–2.0
Adolescents	0.8–2.0

*Assumes normal age-related organ function

Reprinted with permission from National Advisory Group: Safe practices for parenteral nutrition formulations. *J Parenter Enteral Nutr.* 1998;22:49–66.

Nutrition Support

After assessing the baseline nutrition status and requirements of an infant or child in the intensive care setting, decisions must be made about the most appropriate way to deliver nutrition support and the most appropriate food or formula to use. A useful decision-making flow chart is outlined in Figure 27.3.[33]

The optimal time to administer nutrition support to these young patients is unclear. Because of decreased nutrient stores, many authors suggest beginning nutrition support in a pediatric intensive care unit within a few days in infants, within 5 days in older children, and within 7 days in adolescents.[2,3]

Oral Feeding

The least invasive way of administering nutrition support to the infant or child in an intensive care unit is to provide oral feedings. This also has the advantage of using the gastrointestinal tract. A contraindication to oral feedings would be a high risk for aspiration.

In general, small frequent feeds are usually better tolerated than three large meals. High protein and/or high kilocalorie supplements may be added to the feedings for the infant or child who is unable or unwilling to increase their volume of intake. Close monitoring of how much and what is being ingested can help to determine whether the patient is meeting nutrition goals.

Enteral Nutrition

The optimal way to provide nutrition support in a pediatric intensive care unit is through tube feedings. Such therapy is appropriate for patients who are, or are likely to become, malnourished and who cannot maintain their nutrition orally. Children with neurologic disorders, inborn errors of metabolism such as glycogen storage disease type 1, cystic fibrosis, inflammatory bowel disease, cancer, bronchopulmonary dysplasia, human immunodeficiency virus, cerebral palsy, and congenital heart disease all may benefit from such treatment.[6]

The most common and least invasive way of administering such nutrition is through the use of an oral or nasogastric feeding tube.[37] However, this may not be appropriate in patients who have intractable vomit-

TABLE 27.5

Daily Vitamin Requirements for Infants and Children

Life stage group	Vitamin A (μg/d)[a]	Vitamin C (mg/d)	Vitamin D (μg/d)[b,c]	Vitamin E (mg/d)[d]	Vitamin K (μg/d)	Thiamin (mg/d)	Riboflavin (mg/d)	Niacin (mg/d)[e]	Vitamin B_6 (mg/d)	Folate (μg/d)[f]	Vitamin B_{12} (μg/d)	Pantothenic Acid (mg/d)	Biotin (μg/d)	Choline[g] (mg/d)
Infants														
0–6 mo	400*	40*	5*	4*	2.0*	0.2*	0.3*	2*	0.1*	65*	0.4*	1.7*	5*	125*
7–12 mo	500*	50*	5*	5*	2.5*	0.3*	0.4*	4*	0.3*	80*	0.5*	1.8*	6*	150*
Children														
1–3 y	300	15	5*	6	30*	0.5	0.5	6	0.5	150	0.9	2*	8*	200*
4–8 y	400	25	5*	7	55*	0.6	0.6	8	0.6	200	1.2	3*	12*	250*
Boys														
9–13 y	600	45	5*	11	60*	0.9	0.9	12	1.0	300	1.8	4*	20*	375*
14–18 y	900	75	5*	15	75*	1.2	1.3	16	1.3	400	2.4	5*	25*	550*
Girls														
9–13 y	600	45	5*	11	60*	0.9	0.9	12	1.0	300	1.8	4*	20*	375*
14–18 y	700	65	5*	15	75*	1.0	1.0	14	1.2	400	2.4	5*	25*	400*

*RDAs and AIs may both be used as goals for individual intake. RDAs are set to meet the needs of almost all (97% to 98%) individuals in a group. For healthy breast-fed infants, the AI is the mean intake. The AI for other life-stage and gender groups is believed to cover needs of all individuals in the group, but lack of data or uncertainty in the data prevent being able to specify with confidence the percentage of individuals covered by this intake.

[a]As retinol activity equivalents (RAEs). 1 RAE=1 μg retinol, 12 μg β-carotene, 24 μg α-carotene, or 24 μg β-cryptoxanthin in foods. To calculate RAEs from REs or provitamin A carotenoids in foods, divide the REs by 2. For preformed vitamin A in foods or supplements and for provitamin A carotenoids in supplements, 1 RE=1 RAE.

[b]Cholecalciferol. 1 μg cholecalciferol=40 IU vitamin D.

[c]In the absence of adequate exposure to sunlight.

[d]As α-tocopherol. α-Tocopherol includes RRR-α-tocopherol, the only form of α-tocopherol that occurs naturally in foods, and the 2R-stereoisomeric forms of α-tocopherol (RRR-, RSR-, RRS-, and RSS-α-tocopherol) that occur in fortified foods and supplements. It does not include the 2S-stereoismeric forms of α-tocopherol (SRR-, SSR-, SRS-, and SSS-α-tocopherol), also found in fortified foods and supplements.

[e]As niacin equivalents (NE). 1 mg of niacin=50 mg of tryptophan; 0–6 months=preformed niacin (not NE).

[f]As dietary folate equivalents (DFE). 1 DFE=1 μg food folate=0.6 μg of folic acid from fortified food or as a supplement consumed with food=0.5 μg of a supplement taken on an empty stomach.

[g]Although AIs have been set for choline, few data assess whether a dietary supply of choline is needed at all stages of the life style, and it may be that the choline requirement can be met by endogenous synthesis at some of these stages.

In view of evidence linking folate intake with neural tube defects in the fetus, it is recommended that all women capable of becoming pregnant consume 400 μg from supplements or fortified foods in addition to intake of food folate from a varied diet. It is assumed that women will continue consuming 400 μg from supplements or fortified food until their pregnancy is confirmed and they enter prenatal care, which ordinarily occurs after the end of the periconceptional period—the critical time for formation of the neural tube;

Reprinted with permission from Trumbo P, Yates AA, Schlicker S, et al. Dietary reference intakes: vitamin A, vitamin K, arsenic, boron, chromium, copper, iodine, iron, manganese, molybdenum, nickel, silicon, vanadium, and zinc. *Journal of the American Dietetic Association.* 2001;101:294–301.

TABLE 27.6

Daily Mineral and Trace Element Requirements for Infants and Children

Life stage group	Calcium (mg/d)	Chromium (μg/d)	Copper (μg/d)	Fluoride (μg/d)	Iodine (μg/d)	Iron (mg/d)	Magnesium (mg/d)	Manganese (mg/d)	Molyb-denum (μg/d)	Phosphorus (mg/d)	Selenium (μg/d)	Zinc (mg/d)
Infants												
0–6 mo	210*	0.2*	200*	0.01*	110*	0.27*	30*	0.003*	2*	100*	15*	2*
7–12 mo	270*	5.5*	220*	0.5*	130*	**11**	75*	0.6*	3*	275*	20*	**3**
Children												
1–3 y	500*	11*	**340**	0.7*	**90**	**7**	**80**	1.2*	**17**	**460**	**20**	**3**
4–8 y	800*	15*	**440**	1*	**90**	**10**	**130**	1.5*	**22**	**500**	**30**	**5**
Males												
9–13 y	1,300*	25*	**700**	2*	**120**	**8**	**240**	1.9*	**34**	**1,250**	**40**	**8**
14–18 y	1,300*	35*	**890**	3*	**150**	**11**	**410**	2.2*	**43**	**1,250**	**55**	**11**
Females												
9–13 y	1,300*	21*	**700**	2*	**120**	**8**	**240**	1.6*	**34**	**1,250**	**40**	**8**
14–18 y	1,300*	24*	**890**	3*	**150**	**15**	**360**	1.6*	**43**	**1,250**	**55**	**9**

NOTE: This table presents Recommended Dietary Allowances (RDAs) in **bold type** and Adequate Intakes (AIs) in ordinary type followed by an asterisk (*). RDAs and AIs may both be used as goals for individual intake. RDAs are set to meet the needs of almost all (97 to 98 percent) individuals in a group. For healthy breastfed infants, the AI is the mean intake. The AI for other life stage and gender groups is believed to cover needs of all individuals in the group, but lack of data or uncertainty in the data prevent being able to specify with confidence the percentage of individuals covered by this intake.

SOURCES: Dietary Reference Intakes for Calcium, Phosphorus, Magnesium, Vitamin D, and Fluoride (1997); Dietary Reference Intakes for Thiamin, Riboflavin, Niacin, Vitamin B_6, Folate, Vitamin B_{12}, Pan-Chromium, Copper, Iodine, Iron, Manganese, Molybdenum, Nickel, Silicon, Vanadium, and Zinc (2001). These reports may be accessed via www.nap.edu. Copyright 2001 by the National Academy of Science. Courtesy of the National Academy Press, Washington, D.C.

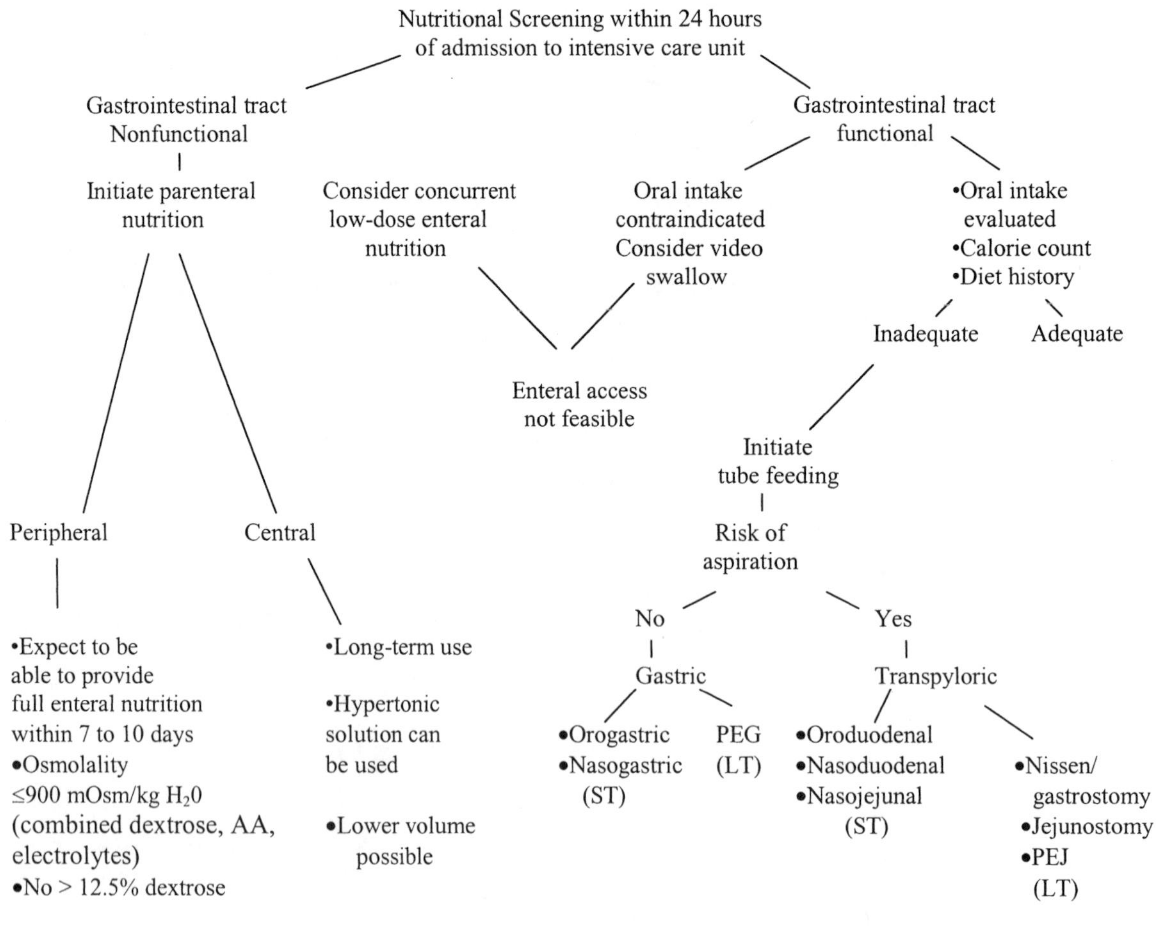

ST = short term; anticipated tube feedings for <6 weeks
LT = long term; anticipated tube feedings for >6-8 weeks
Oral stimulation is an important adjunct to any form of long term nutritional support, especially in infants <6 months old
PEG = percutaneous endoscopic gastrostomy
PEJ = percutaneous endoscopic jejunostomy
(Adapted from Huddleston KC, Ferraro-McDuffie A, Wolff-Small T. Nutritional support of the critically ill child. *Crit Care Nurs Clin North Am.* 1993;5:71 with permission of WB Saunders.)

Figure 27.3

Decision-Making Flow Chart for Deciding upon Nutrition Support in an Infant or Child

ing, delayed gastric emptying, esophageal reflux, or an endotracheal tube.[37] Children who are intubated may be at particular risk for aspiration, since pediatric endotracheal tubes typically do not have cuffs. An alternative to giving enteral nutrition into the stomach is to place the tube transpylorically. This can be done using fluoroscopy, endoscopy, surgery, or even using pH guided placement.[37,38]

Enteral feeding has several advantages over parenteral feeding. Besides decreased cost and ease of administration, enteral feeding is associated with decreased hepatobiliary complications and physiological maintenance of structural and functional gastrointestinal integrity.[6,39,40] Enteral nutrition in the pediatric intensive care unit also appears to be well tolerated.[41,42] Common complications of enteral feeding include vomiting, diarrhea, and abdominal distention.

In the pediatric intensive care unit, enteral feedings are usually initiated as a continuous infusion using a pump with an initial rate of 1–2 mL per kilogram body weight per hour. If the feeding is well tolerated, the rate of infusion can be increased every 6 to 8 hours. If the feeding is into the stomach, a gastric residual in excess of the previous hour's feeding is considered significant, and the feedings typically are held for an hour. Recurrent gastric residuals or high residuals would be an indication for the use of a prokinetic agent or an alternate feeding route (such as transpyloric feedings). In children who have fasted for several days, enteral feedings are usually initiated more slowly.

Table 27.7 lists criteria that may be useful in selecting an appropriate formula to use for enteral feedings. Breast milk is an appropriate choice for feeding infants. Specialized formulas exist not only for infants, but for children ages 1 to 10. Infant formulas are usually 20 kcal/oz, while formulas used for older children are 30 kcal/oz. Infant and pediatric enteral formulations usually have a higher ratio of energy to protein and increased amounts of calcium, phosphorus, and vitamin D.

The electrolyte, vitamin, and mineral content of an enteral feeding needs to be determined to make

TABLE 27.7

Characteristics of Selected Enteral Formulas

Formula Classification	Product Characteristics	Possible Indications for Use	Infant Formula (Manufacturer)	Pediatric Formula (Manufacturer)
Standard milk-based (SMB)	Intact protein Contains lactose Long-chain triglycerides Low residue Low osmolality	Normally functioning gastrointestinal tract Lactose tolerant	Human milk Similac (a) Enfamil (b) Carnation Good Start (whey hydrolysate) (c)	Compleat Pediatric ‡ (e)
Standard milk-based altered	Intact protein Electrolyte manipulation (low iron) SMB lactose free Added rice starch	Renal Lactose intolerant Mild reflux	Similac PM 60:40† (a) Lactofree (b) Similac Lactose Free (a) Enfamil AR (b)	Pediasure Enteral (a) ‡ Resource Just for Kids§ ‡ (e)
Standard soy-based lactose free	Intact protein Low residue Low osmolality	Primary lactose deficiency Secondary lactose deficiency Galactosemia	Isomil (a) Prosobee (b) Carnation Alsoy (c)	None
Standard fiber-containing	Intact protein Lactose free 4.3–6.3 g fiber per 1,000 mL Low to moderate osmolality	Constipation Diarrhea Normal digestive and absorptive capacity	None	Compleat Pediatric ‡ (e) Kindercal§ ‡ (b) Pediasure‡ with fiber enteral (a)
Lactose free/modified fat	Intact protein Fat content is 88% medium chain triglycerides and 12% long-chain triglycerides	Chylothorax Intestinal lymphangiectasia Severe steatorrhea Cholestasis Liver disease	Portagen‡ • (b)	Portagen • ‡ (b)
Semi-elemental	Hydrolyzed protein (peptides and amino acids) Lactose free Low to moderate osmolality Partial medium-chain triglyceride content	Steatorrhea Intestinal resection Cystic fibrosis Chronic liver disease Inflammatory bowel disease Diarrhea associated with hypoalbuminemia Allergy to cow's milk and soy proteins Not needed for jejunal feedings in patients with normal gastrointestinal function	Pregestimil ‡ • (b) Alimentum ‡ (a) Nutamigen ¶ (b)	
Elemental	Protein in form of free amino acids or peptides Lactose free May have high osmolality Carbohydrate in form of glucose oligosaccharides	Intestinal fistula Glycogen storage disease Short gut syndrome HIV+ inflammatory bowel disease	Neocate (d)	Ele Care ‡ (a) Neocate One+ ‡ (d) Vivonex Pediatric ‡ (e) Peptamen Junior ‡ (c)
Transitional	Increased nutrients 22 calories per ounce from ex-premies	Expremature babies for up to the first year of life	NeoSure ‡ (a) EnfaCare ‡ (b)	

†Low in phosphorus; only available in low iron form
‡ Contains medium-chain triglycerides as part of its total fat
• Standard preparation from powder at a 20 kcal/oz dilution for infants and a 30 kcal/oz dilution for children. Essential fatty acid deficiency may occur with long-term use in infants with chronic liver disease
¶Does not contain medium-chain triglycerides
(a) Ross Laboratories, Columbus, OH; (b) Mead Johnson, Evansville, IN; (c) Nestle Nutrition, Deerfield, IL; (d) Scientific Hospital Supplies, Gaithersburg, MD; (e) Novartis, Minneapolis, MN.

Adapted from and reprinted with permission from Samour PQ, Helm KK, Long CE, eds. *The Handbook of Pediatric Nutrition.* 2nd ed. 1999:517–519, Aspen Publishers Inc.

sure that adequate amounts are being provided. In addition, the daily intake of calories, protein, and fluid should be monitored. Laboratory parameters that may be useful to follow include electrolytes, blood urea nitrogen (BUN), and glucose.[44]

Parenteral Nutrition

Parenteral nutrition is indicated in pediatric-aged patients in an intensive care unit when they are malnourished or are at risk for developing malnutrition, and they are unable to take nutrition by mouth or through an enteral feeding device.[45] These patients would typically include patients who have had gastrointestinal surgery and/or who have short bowel syndrome, inflammatory bowel disease, intractable chylothorax, intractable diarrhea of infancy, or intensive cancer treatment, when the medical treatment contraindicates placement of a feeding tube.[45,46] The most common complications of the use of parenteral nutrition are infections and technical problems with the catheter.[47]

To administer parenteral nutrition, a venous access device is needed. A catheter placed in a peripheral vein may be used if the parenteral support is likely to be 2 weeks or less or if central venous access is not possible.[45] Peripherally given nutrition support limits the osmolarity of the parenteral solution. In addition, in order to achieve adequate calories, it is often necessary to give a larger amount of intravenous lipid, as well as fluid.[6] When nutrition support is given centrally, a number of venous access devices are possible, including a tunneled or non-tunneled, cuffed central venous catheter, an implanted catheter, or a peripherally inserted central catheter (PICC).

The major difference between adult and pediatric parenteral nutrition support is that protein, lipid, and electrolytes are often prescribed on a per kilogram body weight per day basis[44] for infants and children. These are slightly less than the protein needs of the critically ill child referred to on page 315. Protein, electrolyte, and trace element requirements are listed in Tables 27.4, 27.8, and 27.9. Lipid intakes usually range from 1.5 to 3.0 grams of lipid per kilogram body weight per day. If a patient is receiving propofol, the fat emulsion base in which the propofol is administered should be taken into consideration when determining the amount of lipid to administer with the parenteral nutrition.[48]

It should be noted that calcium and phosphorus requirements are increased on a per kilogram body weight basis in infancy. However, there are limits as to how much calcium and phosphorus can be added to a parenteral nutrition solution due to the possibility of calcium phosphate precipitation.[44,49]

TABLE 27.8

Daily Parenteral Electrolyte and Mineral Requirements for Infants and Children

Electrolyte	Infants/Children	Adolescents
Sodium	2-6 mEq/kg	Individualized
Chloride	2-5 mEq/kg	Individualized
Potassium	2-3 mEq/kg	Individualized
Calcium	1-2.5 mEq/kg	10-20 mEq
Phosphorus	0.5-1 mmol/kg	10-40 mmol
Magnesium	0.3-0.5 mEq/kg	10-30mEq

Reprinted with permission from National Advisory Group: Safe practices for parenteral nutrition formulations. *J Parenter Enteral Nutr.* 1998;22:49-66.

TABLE 27.9

Daily Parenteral Trace Element Requirements for Infants and Children*‡

Trace Elements	Term neonates (ug/kg)	< 5 years old (ug/kg)	Older children and adolescents
Zinc	300	100	2-5 mg
Copper	20	20	200-500 μg
Manganese	1	2-10	50-150 μg
Chromium	0.2	0.14-0.2	5-15 μg
Selenium	2-3**	2-3**	30-40 μg
Iodide	1†	1†	—

*Assumes normal age-related organ function
**Limit = 40 μg/kg per day
†Percutaneous absorption from protein-bound iodine may be adequate
‡Recommended intakes of trace elements cannot be achieved through the use of a single pediatric multitrace product. Only through the use of individualized trace element products can recommended intakes of trace elements be achieved.

Reprinted with permission from National Advisory Group: Safe practices for parenteral nutrition formulations. *J Parenter Enteral Nutr.* 1998;22:49-66.

Two other differences between pediatric and adult parenteral nutrition are that the pediatric trace element formulations typically do not contain selenium and that the pediatric multivitamin preparations do contain vitamin K.[30,50] If a child is to be on parenteral nutrition for more than a month, a dose of selenium of 2 μg per kilogram body weight per day up to a maximum dose of 30–40 μg is recommended.[30,50]

Besides selenium deficiency in the unsupplemented child on parenteral nutrition, another long-term complication seen primarily in infants and children is aluminum toxicity. Aluminum is a commercial contaminant of phosphorus, trace elements, calcium, and vitamins.[51] Excess aluminum has been reported to cause osteopenia, fractures, osteomalacia, anemia, and encephalopathy in children.[52] Children on long-term parenteral nutrition who have any of these symptoms should have aluminum concentrations measured.

In the pediatric intensive care unit, parenteral nutrition is usually given as a continuous infusion.[53] A continuous infusion makes it easier to manage the electrolyte, acid-base, and fluid disturbances that are often seen in this patient population. In addition, due to the secretion of counter-regulatory hormones, these children are often insulin resistant, so a continuous rather than a more concentrated infusion of glucose is easier for them to tolerate without developing hyperglycemia.

There are no standard monitoring schemes for children who are on parenteral nutrition. However, electrolytes and glucose are usually monitored daily. Infants and young children are particularly vulnerable to cholestatic liver disease; liver function needs to be followed carefully in these patients.[54] As soon as a patient is able to tolerate enteral nutrition, a transition from parenteral nutrition is made.

Special Pediatric Disease States

Neurologic Impairment

Children with severe neurologic impairment frequently are found in a pediatric intensive care unit. These children often have nutritional problems due to developmental delays in feeding skills, gastroesophageal reflux, oral motor dysfunction, ingestion of foreign bodies, and/or behavioral issues.[55,56] Energy requirements in these children are variable. When estimating energy requirements, calculations based on height or height-age, rather than age or weight, are probably more accurate.[7]

Inborn Errors of Metabolism

Another population of patients who are more often seen in a pediatric intensive care unit are children with inborn errors of metabolism. In order to understand the optimal way to provide nutrition support, an understanding of the metabolic processes involved is needed.[57] Many of these children require specialized formulas in order to optimize their metabolic control.[58,59] When they are acutely ill, high rates of glucose may be helpful to increase insulin concentrations and suppress catabolism.

Conclusions

In contrast to adults, optimal nutrition support for patients in a pediatric intensive care unit may be more urgent due to the increased energy and protein requirements in children compared to adults. While the basic principles of nutrition support in children and adults may be similar, a number of differences including nutrition assessment, nutrition formulations, and nutrition complications have been outlined in this chapter.

Case Study

LA is a 3-year-old boy who presented to the emergency room with vomiting and abdominal pain. He was found to have a mid-gut volvulus and malrotation. At the time of surgery, much of the small intestine had to be removed, although at least 10 centimeters of small intestine was left including the ileocecal valve. The patient now has an iliostomy. Prior to the surgery, the patient's weight and height were 15 kg and 95 cm, respectively. This plotted at the 50% for height, 50–75% for weight and 50–75% for BMI on the standard National Center for Health Statistics growth chart.

While this patient seemed to be well nourished prior to surgery, he will need nutrition support following surgery. Because of the surgical resection of his small intestine, he is unlikely to be able to absorb enough calories enterally in order to maintain his nutrition. This patient would be considered to have "short gut syndrome," and therefore would be a candidate for parenteral nutrition. He is also likely to require parenteral nutrition support for a prolonged period of time, so that placement of a more permanent central line rather than a PICC line would be appropriate.

Parenteral nutrition should be initiated as soon as the patient's fluid and electrolyte status stabilizes. His maintenance energy requirements would be about 860 kcal/d using Table 27.1 or 882 kcal/d using the Seashore equation (basal + 20%). His maintenance fluid requirements would be around 1500 mL.[56] IV lipid emulsion should make up about 30% of his total calories, or between 1.5 and 2.0 g/kg body weight/d. About 2.0 g of protein/kg body weight/d should be administered. Assuming a total volume of 1350 mL of parenteral nutrition (1500 mL – 150 mL of 20% lipid), the final dextrose concentration would be about 10%. The electrolyte and mineral content of the parenteral nutrition solution could be determined using Table 27.8. In addition, the patient's formulation would require the addition of trace elements and vitamins to meet his daily requirements. This patient would be at risk for both dehydration and electrolyte and mineral disturbances due to his ostomy.

As soon as possible, a continuous enteral infusion should be started. The presence of nutrients within the gut may enhance growth of the remaining short bowel greatly enhancing this child's likelihood of long-term survival. There is no agreement on the type of enteral feeding to use when treating short bowel syndrome in infants. Breast milk, hydrolyzed protein formulas and amino acid based formulas have been utilized. Due to carbohydrate malabsorption, a hydrolysate formula with a lower percentage of carbohydrate and higher percentage of fat may be better absorbed.[61] Both the rate of the enteral infusion and amount of carbohydrate in the formula could be slowly increased as tolerated. The overall prognosis of this child is guarded, since he is at risk for developing liver disease as a result of long-term parenteral nutrition.

References

1. Pollack MM, Wiley JS, Holbrook PR. Early nutritional depletion in critically ill children. *Crit Care Med.* 1981;9: 580–583.
2. Norris MKG, Steinhorn DM. Nutrition management during critical illness in infants and children. *AACN Clinical Issues.* 1994;5:485–492.
3. Ford EG. Nutrition support of pediatric patients. *Nutr Clin Prac.* 1996;11:183–191.
4. Cunningham, JJ. Body composition and nutrition support in pediatrics: what to defend and how soon to begin. *Nutr Clin Prac.* 1995;10:177–182.
5. Lloyd DA. Energy requirements of surgical newborn infants receiving parenteral nutrition. *Nutrition.* 1998;14: 101–104.
6. ASPEN Guidelines for the use of parenteral and enteral nutrition in adult and pediatric patients. 2002 (in press)
7. Olson DL. Pediatric nutritional assessment. In: Nelson JK, Moxness KE, Jensen MD, et al., Eds. *Mayo Clinic Diet Manual.* 7th ed. St. Louis: Mosby; 1994:419–426.
8. National Center for Health Statistics, Centers for Disease Control and Prevention, U.S. Department of Health and Human Services, http://www.cdc.gov/growthcharts/
9. Burritt MF, Slockbower JM, Forsman RW et al. Pediatric reference intervals for 19 biologic variables in healthy children. *Mayo Clin Proc.* 1990;65:329–336.
10. Barone MA. In: McMillan JA, et al (eds). *Oski's Pediatrics Principles and Practice.* 3rd ed. Philadelphia: Lippincott, Williams & Wilkins; 1999:2216–2225.
11. Behrman RE, Kliegman RM, Jensen HB. *Nelson Textbook of Pediatrics.* 16th ed. Philadelphia: WB Saunders; 2000: 2184–2223.
12. Torres JR A, Wiggins PA. Nutrition in the pediatric intensive care unit patient. In: Tobias JD, ed. *Pediatric Critical Care: The Essentials.* Armonk, NY: Futura Publishing Co.; 1999.
13. Groner JI, Brown MF, Stallings VA, et al. Resting energy expenditure in children following major operative procedures. *J Pediatr Surg.* 1989;24:825–828.
14. Powis MR, Smith K, Rennie M, et al. Effect of major abdominal operations on energy and protein metabolism in infants and children. *J Pediatr Surg.* 1998;33:449–453.
15. Shanbhogue RLK, Lloyd DA. Absence of hypermetabolism after operations in the newborn infant. *J Parenter Enteral Nutr.* 1992;16:333–336.
16. Chwals WJ. Overfeeding the critically ill child: fact or fantasy? *New Horizons.* 1994;2:147–155.
17. Joosten KFM, Verhoeven JJ, Hazelzet JA. Energy expenditure and substrate utilization in mechanically ventilated children. *Nutrition.* 1999:15:444–448.
18. Torres Jr A, Wiggins PA. Nutrition support in a pediatric intensive care unit. *Nutr Clin Prac.* 1999;14:64–68.
19. Baugh N, Recupero MA, Kerner Jr JA. Nutritional requirements in pediatric patients. In: *A.S.P.E.N. Nutrition Support Practice Manual.* Christensen ML, section editor. Silver Spring, MD: American Society for Parenteral and Enteral Nutrition;1998:24-1–24-13.
20. Marian M. Pediatric nutrition support. *Nutr Clin Prac.* 1993;8:199–209.
21. ASPEN. Guidelines for the use of parenteral and enteral nutrition in adult and pediatric patients. Critical Care. 2002 (in press)
22. Seashore JH: Nutritional support of children in the intensive care unit. *Yale J Biol Med.* 1984;57:111–134.
23. Tilden SJ, Watkins S, Tong TK, et al. Measured energy expenditure in pediatric intensive care patients. *AJDC.* 1989;143:490–492.
24. Steinhorn DM, Green TP. Severity of illness correlates with alterations in energy metabolism in the pediatric intensive care unit. *Crit Care Med.* 1991;19:1503–1509.
25. Coss-Bu JA, Jefferson LS, Walding D, et al. Resting energy expenditure and nitrogen balance in critically ill pediatric patients on mechanical ventilation. *Nutrition.* 1998; 14:649–652.
26. Verhoeven JJ, Hazelzet JA, van der Voort E, et al. Comparison of measured and predicted energy expenditure in mechanically ventilated children. *Intensive Care Med.* 1998; 24:464–468.
27. Coss-Bu JA, Jefferson LS, Walding D, et al. Resting energy expenditure in children in a pediatric intensive care unit: comparison of Harris-Benedict and Talbot predictions with indirect calorimetry values. *Am J Clin Nutr.* 1998;67:74–80.
28. White MS, Shepherd RW, McEniery JA. Energy expenditure measurements in ventilated critically ill children: within- and between-day variability. *J Parenter Enteral Nutr.* 1999;23:300–304.

29. Yates AA, Schlicker SA, Suttor CW. Dietary reference intakes: the new basis for recommendations for calcium and related nutrients, B vitamins and choline. *J Am Diet Assoc.* 1998;98:699–706.

30. National Advisory Group. Safe practices for parenteral nutrition formulations. *J Parenter Enteral Nutr.* 1998;22: 49–66.

31. Worley G, Claerhout SJ, Combs SP. Hypophosphatemia in malnourished children during refeeding. *Clin Pediatr.* 1998;37:347–352.

32. Trumbo P, Yates AA, Schlicker S, et al. Dietary reference intakes: vitamin A, vitamin K, arsenic, boron, chromium, copper, iodine, iron, manganese, molybdenum, nickel, silicon, vanadium, and zinc. *J Am Diet Assoc.* 2001;101:294–301.

33. Huddleston KC, Ferraro-McDuffie A, Wolff-Small T. Nutritional support of the critically ill child. *Crit Care Nurs Clin North Am.* 1993;5:65–78.

34. Brant CQ, Stanich P, Ferrari AP Jr. Improvement of children's nutritional status after enteral feeding by PEG: An interim report. *Gastrointest Endosc.* 1999;50:183–188.

35. Miller TL, Awnetwant EL, Evans S, et al. Gastrostomy tube supplementation for HIV-infected children. *Pediatrics.* 1995;96:696–702.

36. Pietsch JB, Ford C, Whitlock JA. Nasogastric tube feedings in children with high-risk cancer: a pilot study. *J Pediatr Hematol Onc.* 1999;21:111–114.

37. ASPEN. Guidelines for the use of parenteral and enteral nutrition in adult and pediatric patients. Enteral Access Devices. 2002 (in press)

38. Dimand RJ, Veereman-Wauters G, Braner DAV. Bedside placement of pH-guided transpyloric small bowel feeding tubes in critically ill infants and small children. *J Parenter Enteral Nutr.* 1997;21:112–114.

39. Lo CW, Walter WA. Changes in the gastrointestinal tract during enteral or parenteral feeding. *Nutr Rev.* 1989;47: 193–198.

40. Brown HD, Levine ML, Lipkin M. Inhibition of intestinal epithelial cell renewal and migration inducted by starvation. *Am J Physiol.* 1963;205:868.

41. Chellis MJ, Sanders SV, Webster H, et al. Early enteral feeding in the pediatric intensive care unit. *J Parenter Enteral Nutr.* 1996;20:71–73.

42. Panadero E, Lopez-Herce J, Caro L, et al. Transpyloric enteral feeding in critically ill children. *J Pediatric Gastroenterology and Nutrition* 1998;26:43–48.

43. Samour PQ, Helm KK, Long CE, eds. *The Handbook of Pediatric Nutrition.* 2nd ed. Gaithersburg, MD: Aspen Publishers Inc. 1999;517–519.

44. Baker MR, Olson DL. Nutrition support in pediatrics. In: Nelson JK, Moxness KE, Jensen MD, et al., eds. *Mayo Clinic Diet Manual.* 7th ed. St. Louis: Mosby; 1994:599–613.

45. ASPEN. Guidelines for the use of parenteral and enteral nutrition in adult and pediatric patients. Types and routes (access) of administration of parenteral nutrition. 2002 (in press)

46. Baker SS. Indications for parenteral nutrition. In: Baker RD, Baker SS, Davis AM, eds. *Pediatric Parenteral Nutrition.* New York: Chapman & Hall; 1997:18–30.

47. Davis A. Initiation, monitoring and complications of pediatric parenteral nutrition. In: Baker RD, Baker SS, Davis AM, eds. *Pediatric Parenteral Nutrition.* New York: Chapman & Hall; 1997:212–237.

48. Roth MC, Martin AB, Katz JA. Nutritional implications of prolonged propofol use. *Am J Health-Syst Pharm.* 1997;54: 694–695.

49. Lifshin LS, Baumgartner TG. Pharmacy of parenteral nutrition. In: Baker RD, Baker SS, Davis AM, eds. *Pediatric Parenteral Nutrition.* New York: Chapman & Hall; 1997: 238–253.

50. Greene HL, Hambridge KM, Schanler R. Guidelines for the use of vitamins, trace elements, calcium, magnesium, and phosphorus in infants and children receiving total parenteral nutrition. *Am J Clin Nutr.* 1988;48:1324–1342.

51. Popinska K, Kierkus J, Lyszkowska M, et al. Aluminum contamination of parenteral nutrition additives, amino acid solutions and lipid emulsion. *Nutrition.* 1999;15:683–686.

52. American Academy of Pediatrics. Aluminum toxicity in children. *Pediatrics* 1996;97:413–416.

53. Friel C, Bistrian B. Cycled total parenteral nutrition: is it more effective? *Am J Clin Nutr.* 1997;65:1078–1079.

54. Hofmann AF. Defective biliary secretion during total parenteral nutrition: probable mechanisms and possible solutions. *J Pediatr Gastroenterol.* 1995;20:376–390.

55. ASPEN. Guidelines for the use of parenteral and enteral nutrition in adult and pediatric patients. Neurologic impairment. 2002 (in press)

56. Pipes PL, Pritkin R. Nutrition and special health needs. In: Trahms CM, Pipes PL, eds. *Nutrition in Infancy and Childhood.* Columbus, Ohio: WBC/McGraw-Hill, 1997: 337–405.

57. ASPEN. Guidelines for the use of parenteral and enteral nutrition in adult and pediatric patients. Inborn errors of metabolism.

58. Elsas II LJ, Acosta PB. Metabolic support of inherited metabolic disease. In: Shils ME, Olson JA, Shike M, et al., (eds) *Modern Nutrition in Health and Disease*, Vol 2. 9th ed. Baltimore: Williams & Wilkins; 1999:1003–1056.

59. Acosta PB. Nutrition support of inborn errors of metabolism. In: Queen PM, Helm KH, Lang CE, eds. *Handbook of Pediatric Nutrition.* 2nd ed. Gaithersburg, MD: Aspen Publishers, Inc.; 1999:243–292.

60. Davis A. Indications and techniques for enteral feeds. In: Baker SB, Baker RD, Davis AM, eds. *Pediatric Enteral Nutrition.* New York: Chapman & Hall; 1994:76.

61. ASPEN. Guidelines for the use of parenteral and enteral nutrition in adult and pediatric patients. Short bowel syndrome. 2002 (in press)

CHAPTER

28

Nutritional Support for the Obese Patient

Scott A. Shikora, M.D., F.A.C.S., Michael J. Naylor, M.D.

INTRODUCTION 325

DEFINING OBESITY 325

PREVALENCE OF OBESITY 326

CO-MORBIDITIES OF OBESITY 326

THE HAZARDS OF STANDARD NUTRITIONAL APPROACHES 327
- Fluid Load 327
- Glucose Load 327
- Lipid Load 328

HYPOCALORIC FEEDING 328
- Benefits of Hypocaloric Feeding 328
- Fat Oxidation 328
- Maximizing Protein Sparing 329
- Adverse Effects of Hypocaloric Feeding 329
- Enteral Hypocaloric Feeding 329

ESTIMATING CALORIC REQUIREMENTS 329
- Energy Equations 329
- Indirect Calorimetry 330

DOES HYPOCALORIC FEEDING WORK? 331

ACCESS ISSUES 331
- Central Venous Access 331
- Enteral Access 332

CONCLUSIONS 333

REFERENCES 333

Introduction

Most critical care clinicians are painfully aware the severely obese patients present unique challenges not encountered when caring for less obese patients. For this patient population, many aspects of treatment that are usually considered routine become complicated.[1] These differences can be attributed to both the diseases suffered by many severely obese patients, as well as the physical difficulties encountered when caring for the overweight. Not surprising, these issues spill over into the field of nutritional support. As with the less obese, when critically ill, the severely obese are likely to require (and entitled to receive) early, aggressive, involutional feeding. However, this lifesaving intervention introduces additional difficulties unique to this population. Calculating macronutrient, micronutrient, and fluid requirements, and obtaining and maintaining reliable access can be extremely difficult. In addition, although there is little published information regarding their unique nutritional needs, there is concern that standard formulations and techniques may not be appropriate and may even be harmful.

Unique approaches to nutritional intervention may better serve this population. This chapter will discuss the issues regarding nutrition support of the critically ill, severely obese patient, including the hazards of standard nutritional approaches, the difficulties of estimating requirements, the problems with establishing and maintaining access, and the hypothetical benefits of a hypocaloric feeding regimen.

Defining Obesity

Obesity simply stated is a condition of excess adiposity. It encompasses a wide range of adiposity from very mildly overweight to extremely obese. Unfortunately, most of the simple measures for determining whether a patient is obese poorly correlate with the degree of adiposity. For example, the simplest method for determining whether a patient is obese is to use the patient's body weight. Although higher body weights usually correlate with obesity, body weight does not account for body size. Obviously, if two patients have the same body weight but different heights, the smaller patient may be obese, while the taller may not.

Weight-for-height tables derived from actuarial data have been used as standards for ideal or desirable weight. Actual weight-for-height is compared to these tables to estimate the degree of obesity. Again, higher weights-for-height would be a likely indicator of obesity. Unfortunately, the ideal weights are somewhat arbitrary, and use of these tables does not take into account the wide variation in body composition. Two patients may have the same weight and height; however, one may be extremely muscular while the other is not.

Body mass index (BMI) is another popular method to analyze weight-for-height:

$$\text{BMI} = \text{weight (kg)/height (m}^2\text{)}$$

BMI is easy to calculate and generally correlates well with body fat. Unfortunately, it also suffers from the same inaccuracies as the standard tables. It does not take into account the extremes of muscularity and adiposity. Despite the known limitations, most clinicians still use BMI or comparisons to the ideal body weight tables to judge the degree of obesity.[2]

The BMI or percent over ideal body weight at which obesity is defined is somewhat controversial and subject to change. The U.S. National Health and Nutrition Examination Surveys (NHANES)[3] originally defined overweight for women as a BMI $\geq$27.3 kg/m^2 and for men as a BMI $\geq$27.8 kg/m^2. Recently, these levels have been lowered to 25 kg/m^2 for both men and women. Currently overweight is defined as a BMI of 25–29.9 kg/m^2 and obesity defined as a BMI of 30 kg/m^2 or greater.[4] Morbid or extreme obesity is generally defined as a BMI of 40 kg/m^2 or greater. Obesity is also defined as body weight 20% greater than the ideal standard and morbid as 100% or greater than ideal.

More accurate measures of body composition include bioelectrical impedance analysis, dual-energy x-ray absorptiometry (DEXA), CT scanning, and others. However, these modalities are often very expensive and are usually available only at specialized centers.

Prevalence of Obesity

Despite the increased awareness of the hazards of being overweight and the growth of the weight loss industry, obesity continues to increase in prevalence in the United States.[3] In 1985, it was estimated that 25% of Americans were considered overweight (BMI 25–29 kg/m^2) and approximately 14% were obese (BMI $\geq$30 kg/m^2).[5] In 1991, the percentage of Americans classified as overweight had climbed to over 30%.[3] In 1994, while the percentage of Americans who were overweight remained at just over 30%, the number classified as obese dramatically increased to over 22% of the population. Therefore, by 1994, more than half of all Americans were either overweight or obese. Even more significant was the finding that as many as 6 million Americans were extremely obese (BMI $\geq$40 kg/m^2).[6] Unfortunately, these numbers are thought to be even higher in the new millennium. The causes for this increase are many and include dietary factors such as the abundance of energy-dense foods and a decrease in energy expenditure as the population becomes more sedentary.

The high prevalence of obesity in society, and the predictions that this will continue to increase, guarantee that all critical care clinicians will be treating severely obese patients at some time in their practice, and therefore must understand the unique factors involved in the care of this population.

Co-Morbidities of Obesity

Obesity is now a major health concern for society. In terms of cost, it has been estimated in 1986 that severe obesity costs society approximately 39.3 billion dollars or 5.5% of the entire health expenditure.[7] These figures are expected to increase as both the cost of health care and the prevalence of obesity escalate. In 1995, the direct cost associated with obesity was estimated to be $51.6 billion and represented 5.7% of the total health care expenditure.[8]

Several diseases are associated with severe obesity (Table 28.1). In addition, the risk of illness or even death from the co-morbid conditions increases exponentially as weight increases.[9]

These conditions also adversely affect recovery from both surgical and non-surgical procedures. Therefore, the severely obese would be more likely than the non-obese to suffer complications requiring

TABLE 28.1

The Obesity-Associated Medical Conditions	
Coronary artery disease	Hypertension
Cardiomyopathy	Cerebrovascular disease
Diabetes mellitus	Endocrine abnormalities
Infertility	Hepatobiliary disease
Malignancies	Depression
Degenerative joint disease	Chronic back pain
Respiratory abnormalities	Gallstones
Hepatic steatosis	Gastroesophageal reflux
Sudden death	

critical care and might be expected to respond less well to critical care therapies.

The Hazards of Standard Nutritional Approaches

The discipline of nutrition support as evolved to the point that it is no longer controversial to state that all critically ill patients regardless of their adiposity, (or lack thereof) deserve aggressive nutritional support as part of their overall treatment plan. The consequences of starvation and malnutrition in the hospitalized patient have been reported elsewhere and are not directly relevant to the topic at hand. However, it is important to emphasize that even the severely obese can develop the adverse sequelae of protein deficiency with critical illness.

Standard nutritional support, whether parenteral or enteral, typically involves the infusion of a concentrated formulation comprised of protein, carbohydrate, and lipid. Most patients will be prescribed approximately 1.0–2.0 g of protein/kg of actual body weight/d. Carbohydrate is usually given as dextrose and can range from as little as 150 grams to as much as 700 grams daily. Lipid calories are often provided to a level of 30%–40% of the total calories. Total calorie infusion for most patients falls within the range of 20–35 kcal/kg of actual body weight per day.[10] Standard nutritional formulas may be potentially harmful for the severely overweight.

Fluid Load

The stress response of severe illness promotes the retention of salt and water. Involutional feeding requires a volume load to serve as a vehicle for delivering the nutrients. Restricting volume may lead to the delivery of inadequate nutrition. This is particularly true with the use of the enteral route, as formulas are usually isoosmolar or mildly hyperosmolar. This fluid load can rapidly expand blood volume. The close association of obesity with heart disease places the critically ill overweight patient at risk for myocardial infarction, pulmonary edema, and congestive heart failure.

Glucose Load

The concentrated glucose solution provided by feeding may have a number of adverse effects for the severely obese (Figure 28.1). Concentrated dextrose can cause hyperglycemia in both glucose-intolerant and "normal" stressed patients. Elevated blood glucose levels have been implicated in poor wound healing[11] and immune dysfunction, leading to an increased susceptibility to infections.[12–15] Extremely overweight patients are three times more likely to be diabetic than nonobese patients.[5] Excessive glucose infusion is particularly dangerous. The administration of excess parenteral glucose can enhance lipogenesis, causing hepatic steatosis, and subsequent hepatic dysfunction.[16] In addition, excess glucose can also increase the production of CO_2, which increases respiratory work. For the

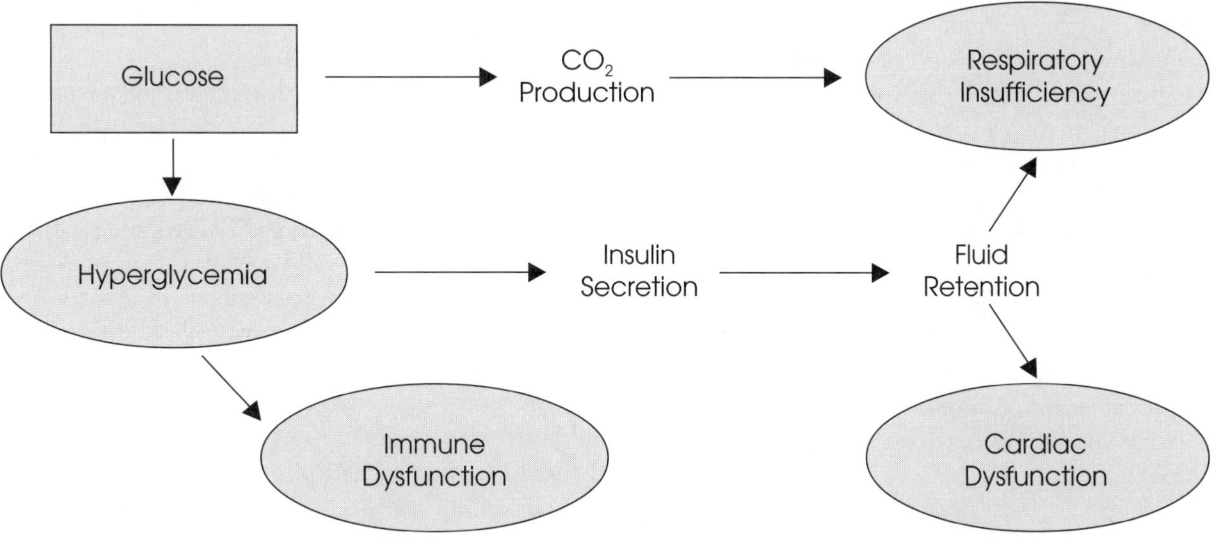

Figure 28.1
The Hazards of Glucose

obese with underlying respiratory compromise, consistently elevated CO_2 levels may lead to respiratory failure.[17,18] The infusion of a concentrated glucose load will also increase the secretion of insulin. Insulin is a potent antinatriuretic hormone leading to further salt and water retention, which can exacerbate the fluid-overloaded state and place the patient at risk for cardiac failure, infarction, and/or pulmonary edema.

Lipid Load

Unlike dextrose, lipids are generally safe for obese patients. However, fats provide significant calories. Since obesity is a state of both fat and energy excess, in the short run, there may be little benefit to infusing lipid. In addition, estimating calorie requirements in the severely obese patient is difficult and often inaccurate. Therefore, the standard use of energy-dense lipids to meet estimated needs may lead to overfeeding in this population. This will be discussed in more detail later in the chapter.

Hypocaloric Feeding

Since standard nutritional practices may be harmful for the obese patient, a nutritional formulation that restricts calories and, in particular calories from glucose, is attractive. This approach, often referred to as *hypocaloric* feeding, is based on the theory that an energy deficit caused by restricting calorie administration below actual requirements can be safely compensated for by the mobilization of endogenous fat. In addition, by providing adequate protein, nitrogen homeostasis is maintained.

Hypocaloric nutritional intervention for the critically ill obese was developed from the experience with a safe, effective, and widely used outpatient diet for weight loss known as the *Protein Sparing Modified Fast (PSMF)*.[19] Briefly, this diet provided patients with adequate protein while intentionally underfeeding energy. By meeting protein requirements and limiting glucose calories, it enabled safe weight loss while patients remained in nitrogen balance. Typically, a PSMF diet provides approximately 1.5–2.0 g of protein/kg of ideal or adjusted body weight. Calories are limited to approximately 60% of the resting energy expenditure (REE) mainly as dextrose. Fats are usually not prohibited.

Benefits of Hypocaloric Feeding

A protein-sparing, hypocaloric formulation may have potential short-term benefits for use in the critically ill obese[20–22] (Table 28.2). Although dextrose is the sole source for non-protein calories, elevated blood sugars are rarely seen. Since the likelihood of hyperglycemia is reduced, many dextrose associated complications are avoided. Therefore, one would anticipate improved wound healing, fewer wound infections, enhanced immune function, the promotion of diuresis, and decreased carbon dioxide production. By promoting diuresis and avoiding increased carbon dioxide production, respiratory work may be decreased, thus decreasing the need for mechanical ventilatory support. Despite the deliberate restriction in energy provision, protein anabolism and successful wound healing have been reported in critically ill obese patients placed on this feeding regimen.[21,22] Additionally, although insulin secretion is decreased, the need for exogenous insulin administration is markedly decreased or even avoided altogether, even in diabetic patients.

TABLE 28.2

Theoretical Advantages of Hypocaloric Feeding
Avoidance of glucose-related complications
Avoidance of hyperglycemia
Decrease in endogenous insulin secretion
Marked decrease of or avoidance of need for exogenous insulin, even in diabetic patients
Improved ventilatory mechanics
Improved diuresis
Decreased CO_2 production
Enhanced protein anabolism
Promotion of positive nitrogen balance
Enhanced wound healing
Improved immune function

Fat Oxidation

Although a hypocaloric feeding regimen has many theoretical benefits for the severely obese patient, its success is based predominantly on the premise that the critically ill patient can oxidize stored fat for needed calories and spare protein stores. This concept has not to date been conclusively validated. In the non-stressed patient, decreased insulin secretion and insufficient calorie administration would favor fat oxidation. However, critical illness may alter normal metabolic pathways. Currently, only two studies have considered this issue. Jeevanandam and colleagues demonstrated poor fat oxidation in a population of fasted obese critically ill patients.[23] In contrast, using indirect calorimetry to analyze substrate utilization, Dickerson and colleagues estimated fat oxidation at 68% of nonprotein energy expenditure in a similar population of stressed postoperative obese patients who were receiving hypocaloric parenteral nutrition.[21] They also reported that their patients achieved protein anabolism, increases in serum proteins, and complete wound healing. Since this study did not compare a hypocaloric regimen with a standard, it could not prove superiority. It does however, demonstrate that this approach seems safe.

Maximizing Protein Sparing

Since the major benefits of hypocaloric feeding are secondary to the reduced glucose infusion, it would be attractive to postulate that completely eliminating non-protein calories from the infusion would have an even greater impact. However the contrary seems true. The infusion of a dextrose-free amino acid solution was shown to decrease net nitrogen loss but not prevent it.[24] The addition of a non-protein calorie source such as glucose appears necessary to improve the protein sparing.[25] This is thought to be due, in part, to the need for protein catabolism to fuel gluconeogenesis in a glucose deficient state. After rapid depletion of the glycogen stores, the body relies on gluconeogenesis to provide glucose to the glucose-dependent tissues such as the immune system, the healing wound, and the peripheral nervous system.[26–28]

The amount of glucose necessary to achieve maximal protein sparing is unknown. Nitrogen preservation increases with higher energy administration, but the effect is blunted as energy delivery increases above 60% of REE.[29] Therefore, it may be postulated that to maximize the protein-sparing effect yet still limit caloric intake, the total energy provided should exceed about 50% of the energy expenditure to be effective. A severely energy-restricted diet, i.e., providing less than 50% of the energy expenditure, would compromise protein sparing, while a less restricted diet would risk the complications of a higher dextrose infusion.

Adverse Effects of Hypocaloric Feeding

To date, no reports in the literature have found any adverse effects with hypocaloric feeding. This author's experience agrees with that of others, in that it seems to be safe and has few contraindications. Despite the limited use (or absolute avoidance) of lipid, an essential fatty acid deficiency is unlikely to develop. Linoleic acid, the most important essential fatty acid, accounts for approximately 10% of the stored lipid. Mobilization of fat releases more than the 2–3.5 g of linoleic acid required daily.[30] Even if lipolysis and fat oxidation are less efficient in the stressed obese patient, most patients would only require this form of nutritional support for a relatively limited period of time. If a patient requires longer support, an intralipid infusion can be given once weekly to prevent an essential fatty acid deficiency.

Enteral Hypocaloric Feeding

Although the hypocaloric protein-sparing approach was originally conceived for parenteral nutritional support, it can be applied to enteral feeding as well. To produce this type of formula regimen, one can either construct an enteral formulation out of modular protein and dextrose components, or utilize a commercially prepared product. In the later case, several high protein, low-fat formulas are available. Furthermore, standard products can also be used and are usually more cost-effective.

The daily administration of a standard solution can be based on the provision of 60% of the calculated energy requirements. Additional protein can be added to meet 100% of the protein needs. Although these formulas tend to provide approximately 30% of the total calories as lipid, with a hypocaloric regimen, the lipid contribution will be minimized and of no consequence.

When using the enteral route, one must be mindful of meeting vitamin and mineral requirements. Most standard commercially available enteral products contain sufficient vitamins and minerals to meet the FDA guidelines when 2000 kcals are administered daily. Since hypocaloric feeding generally will provide less than 2000 kcals, additional micronutrients may be required.

Estimating Caloric Requirements

Energy Equations

Not much information is available on energy expenditure in the obese. The estimation of energy expenditure can be difficult in this population of patients. Body composition is quite different from the non-obese, in which most energy expenditure equations have been derived (Table 28.3). As compared to the non-obese, the majority of overweight patients have both an increased fat mass and increased lean body mass.[31] However, the proportion of lean body mass to fat mass can vary greatly.

Obesity is characterized by the accumulation of excess adipose tissue within the body. Adipose tissue can be divided into two major components: extracellular and intracellular. The extracellular space contains fluid, electrolytes, protein, and blood vessels.

TABLE 28.3

Body Composition Changes Associated with Obesity
Increased adipose tissue
Increased lean body mass
Increased total body water
Increased extracellular fluid (ECF)
Increased intracellular fluid (ICF)
Increased ECF:ICF
Increased protein content
Increased mineral weight

The major cellular component is the adipocyte. The intracellular components include fluid, protein and triglycerides.

Adipose tissue on average is approximately 80% lipid, 15% water and 5% protein.[32] In individuals of normal weight, extracellular fluid (ECF) is about 40%–50% of total body water. Adipose tissue has an elevated ECF to intracellular fluid (ICF) ratio on the order of 3 or 4:1.[32] It would then follow that the obese have a higher proportion of fat free mass as ECF.[32]

The expanded fat free mass of obesity is in part due to excess fat free adipose tissue (i.e. adipocyte elements). Organ enlargement, increased skeletal muscle mass, and increased skeletal weight are also seen. The result is that obese patients have more total body water, protein content, and mineral weight than the non-obese.[32]

Other obesity-associated factors may also affect body composition. Obesity in adults is often associated with hypertension, edema, and congestive heart failure, all of which may be secondary to overexpansion of the ECF. It has been shown that total body water, ECF, ICF and the ratio of ECF/ICF are significantly increased in obese women compared to normal weight subjects.[33]

Therefore these derangements in body composition, and the great variability from patient to patient, make using ideal body weight in standard energy expenditure equations inaccurate. Given the larger lean body mass, using ideal body weight will generally underestimate caloric requirements. However, using actual body weight may massively overestimate energy expenditure, as fat is less metabolically active than fat free tissue and body fluid is inactive. Many practitioners, including this author, use a contrived weight estimate called the adjusted body weight.[34] It is calculated by using the following equation:

$$\text{Adjusted BW} = .25\ [\text{Actual BW} - \text{Ideal BW}] + \text{Ideal BW}$$

This equation assumes that the obese possess a lean body mass that is approximately 25% greater than the non-obese. Unfortunately, there is no scientific basis for this equation; neither does it take into account the great variability in body composition in the obese.

Numerous formulas are available to estimate energy requirements for patients. All suffer from inaccuracies that have been described elsewhere.[35–37] Most rely on weight as a gross estimate of lean body mass. Some differentiate men from women and the young from the old. Most have been criticized for lack of accuracy for the critically ill. To the knowledge of this author, only one equation, the Ireton-Jones Equation, even considers obesity as an independent variable.[38] However, the formula only considers whether obesity is present or absent. It does not take into account whether the obesity is mild, moderate or severe. Since body composition, lean body mass, and fat mass vary greatly from patient to patient, it is unlikely that a formula such as the Ireton-Jones Equation can accurately estimate energy expenditure for a wide range of obesity.[39]

Indirect Calorimetry

Respiratory indirect calorimetry is considered the gold standard for accurately measuring energy expenditure. It does not rely on body weight, sex, age, or any other patient characteristics. Simply stated, a portable gas analyzer (CART) measures oxygen consumption and carbon dioxide production. It then converts this data into REE by utilizing the modified Weir equation.[40]

$$\text{REE}=1.44\ [3.9(O_2\ \text{consumption})+1.1(CO_2\ \text{production})]$$

This formula determines energy expenditure based solely on metabolic activity. It has been shown to be "extremely accurate." Obviously, the referenced studies were performed by investigators experienced with the correct operation of the device. However, the accuracy of the metabolic CART is based upon the ability to properly use it. Improper use may greatly compromise the results. Although the proper technique is not difficult to learn, it does require training. However, there may be significant variability in the experience and training of clinicians with the device. Furthermore, to date, no studies that have specifically analyzed the accuracy of indirect calorimetry in the obese. However, since it only relies on gas exchange, there is no reason to doubt its potential accuracy in this unique patient population. Unfortunately, many institutions do not possess this technology.

An alternative to respiratory indirect calorimetry, is circulatory indirect calorimetry. This technique does not require a metabolic CART. Instead, it utilizes the thermodilution method, which requires a pulmonary artery catheter, commonly found in use in most intensive care units.[41] Cardiac output (CO), arterial oxygen, and mixed venous oxygen saturations are measured and then applied to the Modified Fick equation:

$$REE = CO(L/min) \times hemoglobin(g/dL) \times [SaO_2(\%) - Sa\dot{V}O_2(\%)] \times 95.18$$

Although this technique is easy, rapid and readily available, one study demonstrated that it suffered from unacceptable variability compared to respiratory indirect calorimetry.[42] This prospective trial was done with critically ill patients and not limited to obese patients; however, there is no reason to suspect that a trial exclusively involving obese patients, would demonstrate different results.

Does Hypocaloric Feeding Work?

Although the concept of a specialized approach for nourishing the severely ill obese patient has been considered for a number of years, few studies in the literature evaluate this technique, and even fewer prospective randomized trials compare it to standard feeding regimens (Table 28.4).

In a nonrandomized trial, Dickerson et al.[21] placed 13 obese patients requiring parenteral nutrition for post-operative complications on a hypocaloric regimen. The researchers reported net protein anabolism, complete tissue healing, and lack of major complications. Borge and colleagues,[22] in a randomized, prospective trial of non-critically ill patients, compared a hypocaloric parenteral formulation with a standard approach. In both groups, positive nitrogen balances were achieved. However, these researchers did not report the incidence of complications or the effect on outcome. In a second prospective, randomized trial by the same group of investigators, Choban and colleagues[43] studied both critically ill and non-critically ill obese patients. Positive nitrogen balances were again achieved in both groups. Glucose control was better in the hypocaloric group, but did not reach statistical significance. This may reflect the small study size. Complication rates were equivalent, and no untoward effects were noted in the group given the lower energy formulations. Importantly, they were able to obtain these results without the need for indirect calorimetry. Unfortunately, effects on outcome were not reported.

Access Issues

Although little is written in the literature describing the possible difficulties of establishing feeding access in the severely obese, most clinicians are familiar with them. Obese patients are probably more prone to access-related complications as a result of their body habitus and concomitant medical conditions (Table 28.5).

Central Venous Access

Most clinicians who place central venous access are quite aware of the difficulties obtaining access in the severely obese. Their increased body size obscures the normal anatomical landmarks, which greatly increases the likelihood of unsuccessful venous cannulation and complications such as pneumothorax, hemothorax, hemorrhage, and infection. Ultrasonography and even fluoroscopy may be necessary to "find the vein." To further complicate the situation, many severely obese patients are unable to tolerate lying flat or being placed in the reverse Trendelenberg position (angling the bed with the legs up and head down). This maneuver is extremely important for venous cannulation.

TABLE 28.4

Published Studies Utilizing Hypocaloric Feeding in the Obese

	Study Type	Patients	Results
Dickerson[21]	Prospective	13 postoperative Patients with complications	Protein anabolism Wound healing
Burge[22]	PRDBT	16 hospitalized patients No critically ill patients	Positive N2 balance Outcome not studied
Choban[43]	PRDBT	30 hospitalized patients Including critically ill	Positive N2 balance Outcome not studied

PRDBT = Prospective, randomized, double-blind trial

TABLE 28.5

Access Problems in the Obese Patient
Central Venous Access
Normal anatomical landmarks are obscured
Patients may be unable to tolerate reverse Trendelenberg positioning
Needles may not be long enough to reach the vein
Complications: hemothorax, pneumothorax, infection, hemorrhage, arrhythmias, hypoxia, respiratory failure
Enteral Access
Soft tissue adiposity complicates nasal placement
Patient weight may preclude use of fluoroscopy
Patients may not tolerate lying flat for the duration of the procedure
Gastroesophageal reflux may lead to aspiration
Sedatives may be contraindicated secondary to respiratory concerns
Abdominal wall transillumination for endoscopy may be impossible
Increased intraabdominal pressure may lead to gastric wall necrosis
Patients are high risk for surgical tube placement
Complications:
Nasal placement: epistaxis, esophageal perforation, tube misplacement, aspiration, respiratory failure
Endoscopic placement: respiratory failure, infection, tube misplacement, gastric wall necrosis, aspiration
Surgical placement: increased likelihood of all of the usual risks associated with surgery and anesthesia, infection, wound dehiscence, respiratory compromise

Currently, there is no data comparing central venous placement in the internal jugular vein vs. the subclavian. Both approaches can be quite challenging. Short, wide necks and large chest walls may compromise the ability to identify the typical anatomical landmarks. Standard prepackaged catheter kits may not have sufficiently long needles. Each patient should be carefully scrutinized prior to determining which site to attempt. Both anatomical issues and access needs should be considered.

In general terms, the best recommendations for venous access placement are to have the most experienced clinician attempt to place the line with good illumination and adequate assistance. Should the patient need to go to surgery, the operating room is an excellent place for central venous catheter placement or exchange.

ENTERAL ACCESS

Enteral access can also be challenging.[44] Blind nasal-enteric placement is made more difficult by the increased adiposity of the soft tissues of the palate and pharynx. This can lead to an increase in the complications from tube misplacement including epistaxis, esophageal perforation or hemorrhage, inadvertent placement into the trachea or bronchus, and pneumothorax. Fluoroscopic tube placement may be impossible for patients weighing over 400 lb, as many fluoroscopy tables are not designed for patients who weigh more than 350 lb. In addition, underlying conditions such as pulmonary insufficiency or severe degenerative joint disease may prevent the patient from being able to lie still in the supine position for the duration of the procedure. Respiratory difficulties may be compounded by the occlusion of a nostril with the tube. Gastroesophageal reflux is thought to occur more commonly in the severely obese, placing them at higher risk for aspiration pneumonia both during tube placement and while feeding.[45]

Endoscopic tube placement in this population is also risky. Lying supine and the need for sedation can compromise respiration. With most endoscopic techniques, illumination of the abdominal wall is necessary to insure that the stomach is adjacent to the abdominal wall without other viscera in between. Inability to transilluminate the skin secondary to the large layer of subcutaneous fat may increase the risk of colon injury. Once the tube is placed, increased intraabdominal pressure, common in these patients, can cause tension on the tube that can lead to gastric wall necrosis, leakage with peritonitis, necrotizing fasciitis, or superficial infections.

Surgical tube placement carries all of the potential problems associated with surgery. These include complications associated with medical diseases (cardiac, pulmonary, thromboembolic, etc), and those associated with the actual surgery. The operative incision is more prone to infection and healing complications. The incisional discomfort will limit ambulation, cause respiratory splinting, and require treatment with analgesics. All of these issues could increase the risk of respiratory insufficiency, pneumonia, and thromboembolic events.

While laparoscopic surgery minimizes problems associated with an "incision," it is not immune to other complications. Patients still require general anesthesia for laparoscopy. The carbon dioxide gas used to create the pneumoperitoneum may lead to carbon dioxide retention in patients with pulmonary insufficiency. Standard trocars and laparoscopic instruments may be too short to be used for patients with massive abdominal walls. The increased intraabdominal pressure created by the pneumoperitoneum (necessary to elevate the anterior abdominal wall to create a work space), and the heavy abdominal wall can cause derangements in venous blood return to the heart.

Conclusions

Critically ill severely obese patients can be extremely difficult to provide care for. This group is more prone to become severely ill and therefore to require involutional nutritional support. Unfortunately, the standard nutritional regimens intended to support these patients may be harmful. Many of the potential risks of traditional feeding regimens are secondary to the dependence on the infusion of large quantities of glucose. The protein-sparing, hypocaloric approach is a unique feeding regimen that restricts glucose infusion and is offered as a safe alternative.

Many issues remain to be resolved with hypocaloric feeding. While this approach seems to be safe, is it effective? Currently none of the relatively few investigations that have analyzed the hypocaloric feeding regimen have reported improved outcome. Additionally, all of the published studies have utilized a parenteral approach whereas, currently, most patients requiring nutritional support are fed enterally. Since enteral nutrition seems to offer advantages over parenteral for most patients, an enterally delivered hypocaloric regime might also be worthy of study. Like many areas in nutrition support, large prospective, randomized trials are still necessary to analyze whether this unique approach truly offers benefits.

References

1. Shikora SA, Johannigman JA. The Obese Surgical Patient. In Civetta JM, Taylor RW, Kirby RR, eds. *Critical Care*. 3rd ed. Philadelphia, PA: Lippincott Company; 1996: 1277–1286.
2. Ireton-Jones CS, Francis C. Obesity: Nutrition support practice and application to critical care. *Nutr Clin Pract*. 1995;10:144–149.
3. Kuczmarski RJ, Flegal KM, Campbell SM, et al. Increasing prevalence of overweight among US adults: The National Health and Nutrition Examination Surveys, 1960 to 1991. *JAMA*. 1994;272:205–211.
4. NHLBI Obesity Education Initiative Expert Panel on the Identification, Evaluation, and Treatment of Overweight and Obesity in Adults. *Clinical Guidelines on the Identification, Evaluation, and Treatment of Overweight and Obesity in Adults*. National Institutes of Health, June 1998.
5. Van Itallie TB. Health implications of overweight and obesity in the United States. *Ann Intern Med*. 1985;103(6 pt 2):983–988.
6. Flegal KM, Carroll MD, Kuczmarski RJ, et al. Overweight and obesity in the United States: prevalence and trends 1960–1994. *Int J Obes*. 1998,22:39–47.
7. Colditz GA. Economic costs of obesity. *Am J Clin Nutr*. 1992;55:503S–507S.
8. Wolf AM, Colditz GA. Current estimates of the economic cost of obesity in the United States. *Obesity Research*. 1998;6:97–106.
9. Lew EA, Garfinkel L. Variations in mortality by weight among 750,000 men and women. *J Chron Dis*. 1979;32: 563–576.
10. Hunter DC, Jaksic T, Lewis D, et al. Resting energy expenditure in the critically ill: Estimations versus measurement. *Br J Surg*. 1988,75:875–878.
11. McMurray JF. Wound healing with diabetes mellitus. Better glucose control for better wound healing in diabetes. *Surg Clin North Am*. 1984;64:769–778.
12. Bagdade JD, Stewart M, Walters E. Impaired granulocyte adherence. A reversible defect in host defense in patients with poorly controlled diabetes. *Diabetes*. 1978;27:677–681.
13. Jones RL, Peterson CM. Hematologic alterations in diabetes mellitus. *Am J Med*. 1981;70:339–352.
14. Hostetter MK. Handicaps to host defense. Effects of hyperglycemia on C3 and Candida Albicans. *Diabetes*. 1990; 39:271–275.
15. Pomposelli JJ, Baxter JK 3rd, Babineau TJ, et al. Early postoperative glucose control predicts nosocomial infection rate in diabetic patients. *J Parenter Enteral Nutr*. 1998;22:77–81.
16. Baker AL, Rosenberg IH. Hepatic complications of total parenteral nutrition. *Am J Med*. 1987;82:489–497.
17. McMahon MM, Benotti PN, Bistrian BR. A clinical application of exercise physiology and nutritional support for the mechanically ventilated patient. *J Parenter Enteral Nutr*. 1990;14:538–542.
18. Askanazi J, Rosenbaum SH, Hyman AI, et al. Respiratory changes induced by the large glucose loads of total parenteral nutrition. *JAMA*. 1980;243:1444–1447.
19. Bistrian BR. Clinical use of a protein-sparing modified fast. *JAMA*. 1972;240:2299–2302.

20. Baxter JK, Bistrian BR. Moderate hypocaloric parenteral nutrition in the critically ill, obese patient. *Nutr Clin Pract.* 1989;4:133–135.
21. Dickerson RN, Rosato EF, Mullen JL. Net protein anabolism with hypocaloric parenteral nutrition in obese stressed patients. *Am J Clin Nutr*. 1986;44:747–755.
22. Burge JC, Goon A, Choban PS, et al. Efficacy of hypocaloric total parenteral nutrition in hospitalized obese patients: A prospective, double-blind randomized trial. *J Parenter Enteral Nutr.* 1994;18:203–207.
23. Jeevanandam M, Young DH, Schiller WR. Obesity and the metabolic response to severe multiple trauma in man. *J Clin Invest.* 1991;87:262–269.
24. Greenberg GR, Marliss EB, Anderson GH, et al. Protein sparing therapy in post-operative patients. *N Engl J Med.* 1976;294:1411–1416.
25. Young GA, Hill GL. A controlled study of protein-sparing therapy after excision of the rectum. *Ann Surg.* 1980;192: 183–191.
26. Blackburn GL. Nutrition in surgical patients. In Hardy JD, Kukora JS, Pass HI, eds. *Hardy's Textbook of Surgery.* 2nd ed. Philadelphia, PA: JB Lippincott; 1988: 86–104.
27. Hensle TW, Askanazi J. Metabolism and nutrition in the perioperative period. *J Urol.* 1988;139:229–239.
28. Douglas RG, Shaw JHF. Metabolic response to sepsis and trauma. *Br J Surg.* 1989;76:115–122.
29. Elwyn DH, Kinney JM, Askanazi J. Energy expenditure in surgical patients. *Surg Clin North Am.* 1981;61:545–556.
30. Mascioli EA, Smith MF, Trerice MS, et al. Effect of total parenteral nutrition with cycling on essential fatty acid deficiency. *J Parenter Enteral Nutr.* 1979;3:171–173.
31. Benedetti G, Mingrone G, Marcoccia S, et al. Body composition and energy expenditure after weight loss following bariatric surgery. *J Am Coll Nutr.* 2000;19:270–274.
32. Waki M, Kral JG, Mazariegos M, et al. Relative expansion of extracellular fluid in obese vs. nonobese women. *Am J Physiol.* 1991;261:E199–E203.
33. Heymsfield SB, Lichtman S, Baumgartner RN, et al. Assessment of body composition: An overview. In: Bjorntorp P, Brodoff BN, eds. *Obesity.* 1st ed. Philadelphia: JB Lippincott Co; 1992:37–54.
34. Wilkens, K. Adjustment for obesity. *ADA Renal Practice Group Newsletter*, Winter 1984.
35. Osborne BJ, Saba AK, Wood SJ, et al. Clinical comparison of three methods to determine resting energy expenditure. *Nutr Clin Pract.* 1994;9:241–246.
36. Daly JM, Heymsfield SB, Head CA, et al. Human energy expenditure: Overestimation by widely used prediction equations. *Am J Clin Nutr.* 1985;42:1170–1174.
37. Cortes B, Nelson LD. Errors in estimating energy expenditure in critically ill surgical patients. *Arch Surg.* 1989; 124:287–290.
38. Ireton-Jones CS, Turner WW, Liepa GU, et al. Equations for estimation of energy expenditures in patients with burns with special reference to ventilatory status. *J Burn Care Rehabil.* 1992;13:330–333.
39. Amato P, Keating KP, Quercia RA, et al. Formulaic methods of estimating calorie requirements in mechanically ventilated obese patients: A reappraisal. *Nutr Clin Pract.* 1995;10:229–232.
40. Weir JB de V. New methods for calculating metabolic rate with special reference to protein metabolism. *J Physiol.* 1941;109:1–9.
41. Ligett SB, St John RE, Lefrak SS. Determination of resting energy expenditure utilizing the thermodilution pulmonary artery catheter. *Chest.* 1987;4:562–566.
42. Ogawa AM, Shikora SA, Burke LM, et al. The thermodilution technique does not agree with indirect calorimetry for the critically ill patient. *J Parenter Enteral Nutr.* 1998; 22:347–351.
43. Choban PS, Burge JC, Scales D, et al. Hypoenergetic Nutrition Support in Hospitalized Obese Patients. A Simplified Method for Clinical Application. *Am J Clin Nutr.* 1997;66:546–550.
44. Shikora SA. Enteral feeding tube placement in obese patients: Considerations for nutrition support. *Nutr Clin Pract.* 1997;12:S9–S13.
45. Vaughan RW, Bauer S, Wise L. Volume and pH of gastric juice in obese patients. *Anesthesiology.* 1981;55:180.

CHAPTER

29 Nutrition in the Immunocompromised Intensive Care Unit Patient

Chris C. Carlson, M.D.

INTRODUCTION	335	CONCLUSIONS	339
ALGORITHM FOR PROVIDING NUTRITION	335	REFERENCES	339
IMMUNOCOMPROMISE	337		
Sepsis	337		
Cancer	338		
HIV/AIDS	339		

Introduction

Over the course of the last century, critical care medicine has evolved into an exacting science utilizing state-of-the-the art monitoring along with the newest biomodulating agents. Cellular and molecular processes of illness have been elucidated that allow the physician to "dial in" the metabolic, endocrine, and physiologic responses desired, greatly increasing patients' chances of surviving what were once thought fatal insults. No field has undergone more change nor had a greater increase in the depth of understanding than provision of nutrition. Where once it was believed that the gastrointestinal tract was nonfunctional in the critically ill, it is now understood that the gut-mucosa barrier and gut-associated lymphoid tissue (GALT) play a pivotal role in the onset, response, and resolution of critical illness. With these new discoveries has come the requirement for physicians to understand the complex changes that the gastrointestinal tract undergoes during severe illness and to what extent nutritional support benefits the patient.

Nutrition in the immunocompromised host while in the intensive care unit is a complex series of minute adjustments designed to improve the patient's chance to heal wounds and recover from the stressors of illness. Often the etiology of these stressors is multifactorial and effects are seen in multiple organ systems. The exact nutritional needs are also subject to change throughout the course of the patient's convalescence as the body responds and either adapts or fails. Frequently the already difficult job of providing proper balanced nutrition to patients is complicated by their immunocompromised state. Assessment of the body's nutritional status and a thorough understanding of the etiology of the immunocompromise become imperative in assuring recovery from the insults related to surgical disease, sepsis, trauma, cancer, adjuvant chemoradiation, and infection.

Algorithm for Providing Nutrition

Increases in catecholamines, cortisol, and acute phase proteins in ICU patients induce glycogenolysis, gluconeogenesis, lipolysis, and skeletal muscle proteolysis in an effort to provide high-energy substrates to the brain, heart, and red blood cells. This hypermetabolic response, however, can be detrimental as the loss of lean body mass secondary to muscle proteolysis has been shown to increase morbidity and mortality in the ICU patient. In the immunocompromised patient this becomes even more crucial, as the patient's ability to resist further insults is diminished.

Prior to initiating any nutritional support, an algorithm to define the most efficacious mode of delivery should be followed (Figure 29.1). One of the few requirements for the provision of nutrition is that the patient be hemodynamically stable, as gut mucosal

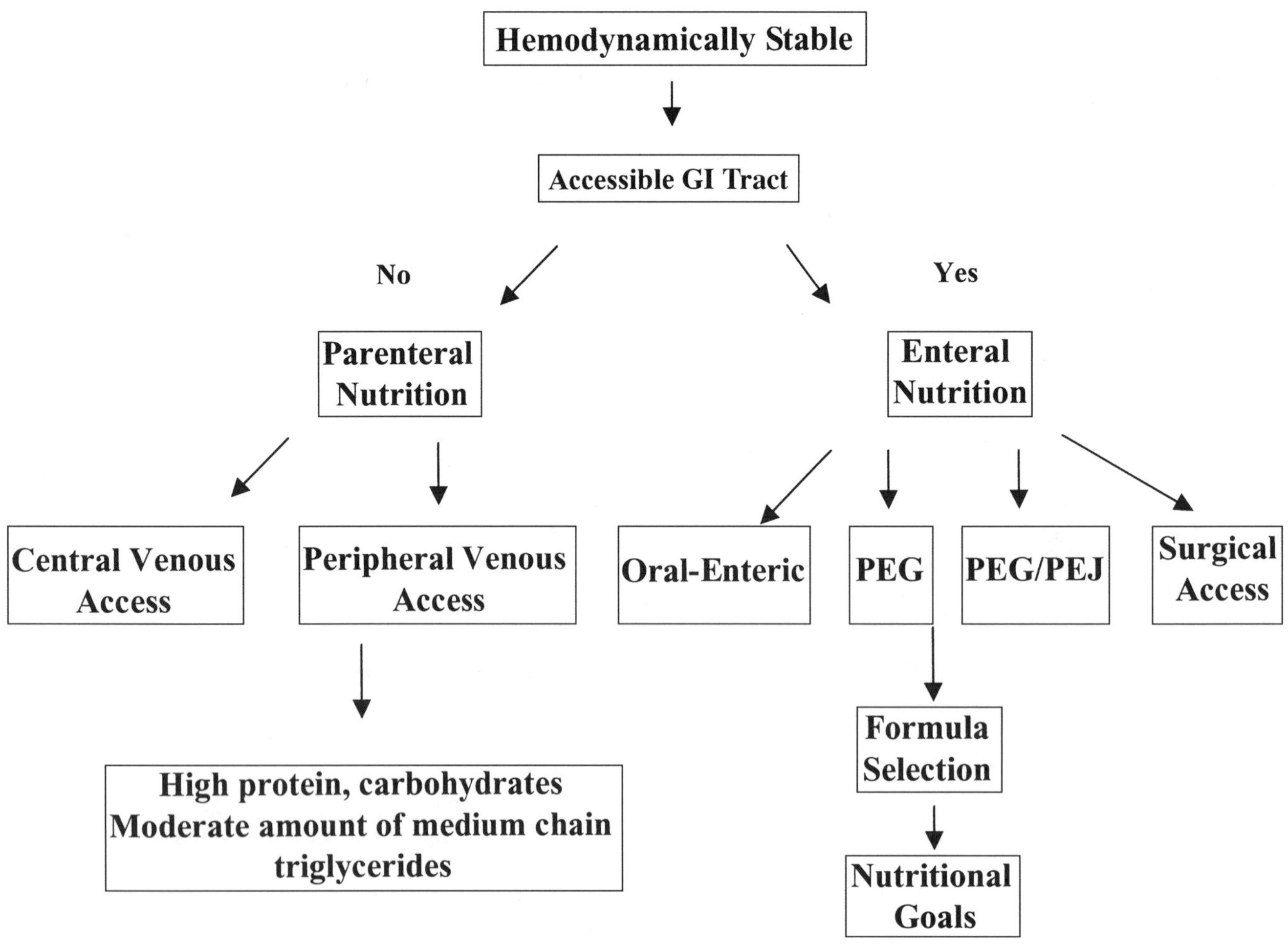

Figure 29.1

Nutrition Therapy in the Immunocompromised Host

blood flow is one of the first capillary beds shunted in the stress response and decreased gastrointestinal blood flow decreases absorption and potentially leads to gut ischemia. Studies in the burn literature, however, have even questioned whether holding feeds to await hemodynamic stability is an absolute necessity.[1,2] Arguments supporting the concept of trophic gastrointestinal tract feeds—defined as only small amounts of readily absorbable nutrients designed to maintain villous architecture—posit that even in the heightened stress response of the acutely ill patient, small amounts of enteral feeds pose no danger and could possibly speed the GI tract return to function as well as decrease the rate of bacterial translocation.[3] Small intestinal absorption of enteral feeds does not appear to be decreased by surgery or illness, and early problems with diarrhea and feeding intolerance appear to be related to feeding the stomach. Of benefit especially to the immunocompromised patient, enteral diets have been shown to decrease gut permeability as well as maintain mucosal immunity and gut-associated lymphoid tissue (GALT).[4]

The route of administration and accessibility of the GI tract must next be considered. Enteral administration of feeds via a nasogastric or nasoenteric tube is the optimal method of provision of nutrition but carries certain risks in the immunocompromised patient. Nasal tubes prevent proper sinus drainage and predispose to sinusitis, a potentially fatal complication in the patient with poor immune function.[5] One study performed in ICU patients with indwelling nasogastric or nasotracheal tubes showed an increase in the incidence of sinusitis from 1.8% to 43.1% with nasal tubes.[6] In addition, placement of a nasoenteric tube is often a laborious and time-consuming process, causing a delay in provision of nutrition while multiple attempts are made and x-rays taken.[7] Recently techniques for bedside placement of nasoenteric tubes have been perfected and success ranges from 70% to 90%.[8] Long-term access to the GI tract is not feasible with a nasogastric or enteric tube, and often requires surgical placement of feeding access for convenience and ease of administration. Percutaneous endoscopic gastrostomy (PEG), PEG with a jejunal extension, and percutaneous endoscopic jejunostomy (PEJ) are three modalities of providing access to the GI tract for long-term enteral feeding. These procedures require endoscopically guided placement of catheters in the gastrointestinal tract that exit the abdominal wall and allow enteral feeds to be placed directly into the gut without the patient discomfort or inconvenience of the nasally inserted tubes. Although an improvement compared to nasal tubes, the percutaneously placed tubes have their own share of problems, including accidental dislodgement, clogging of the tube, and peri-tube superficial infections. Thrombocytopenia and coagulopathy contribute to morbidity when surgical access is required for nutrition administration and can even preclude percutaneous placement. While few studies have investigated complications of percutaneous GI access in immunocompromised patients, the decreased risk of sinusitis and the ease of care of percutaneous enteral access should warrant their use in most routine cases. Neutropenia with absolute granulocyte counts of <1000 has been reported as a relative contraindication. Spillage of a small amount of gastric contents during the PEG procedure is not uncommon. Even minute amounts of spillage into the peritoneal cavity in the severely immunocompromised population can be life threatening. PEG placement may also be used in rare instances of severe intraabdominal malignancies or carcinomatosis causing obstruction as a method of gastric decompression and may preclude the need for long-term NG tube therapy, minimizing the sinusitis complications.

Parenteral administration of nutrition to the immunocompromised ICU patient can be accomplished via either peripheral or central access. Peripheral access prevents supplementation of greater than 10% dextrose concentrations because of its hypertonicity, but can often serve as a temporary bridge to more definitive nutrition access. Central venous access for parenteral nutrition, in addition to the understood chance of pneumothorax (less than 4%), subclavian artery injury, air embolism, thoracic duct injury, and catheter malposition, carries additional risk in the immunocompromised patient. Immunocompromised patients are especially susceptible to line sepsis,[9] which, coupled with their already decreased cellular and humoral immunity, can lead to overwhelming bacterial infection. Immunocompromise also mandates the placement of either a subclavian or internal jugular vein central line, as the risk of infection of femoral lines prohibits femoral access.[10]

Immunocompromise

Nutritional support of the immunocompromised patient poses a particular challenge to the clinician, requiring a more aggressive approach to the provision of nutrition and a more vigilant watch for associated complications. Compromise of the immune system occurs in the surgical and medical ICU patient for a host of reasons and etiologies. The stress of critical illness, combined with immunosuppressive medications, breaching of the skin barrier, and altered host flora, places a great burden on the host's ability to ward off infection. In addition, many of the disease processes faced by the ICU medical staff cause or are associated with decreased immune function, such as sepsis, diabetes, malnutrition, renal failure, AIDS, and neutropenia secondary to adjuvant chemotherapy in cancer. This chapter will focus briefly on providing nutrition for immunocompromised patients with the most commonly encountered etiologies of immunocompromise—sepsis, cancer, and AIDS.

Sepsis

Sepsis is defined as the systemic inflammatory response to a severe clinical insult that is characterized by two or more of the following: elevated heart rate, respiratory rate, temperature, white blood cell count, or percent of immature white blood cells. The metabolic demands of sepsis coupled with decreased ability of the immunocompromised to fight infection pose a challenge to the physician. The general hypermetabolism resulting from stress hormone and catecholamine release leads to a marked hyperglycemia. Combined with peripheral insulin resistance noted in critically ill patients, this can quickly lead to the metabolic sequelae of dehydration, such as non-ketotic hyperosmolar coma. The nutritional goals in the septic patient involve providing adequate calories to prevent peripheral muscle proteolysis as well as improving the body's ability to utilize the calories given.

Studies have demonstrated the profound suppression of cellular immunity with even modest elevations of serum glucose. Neutrophil chemotaxis, adherence to bacteria, phagocytosis, oxidative burst, and superoxide production are all reduced with even minor elevations in blood glucose.[11] Hyperglycemia of sepsis, however does not preclude giving patients adequate calories necessary for healing and for prevention of the catabolism associated with starvation. Strict glucose control utilizing an insulin drip and hourly serum blood glucose levels is often required as well as routine monitoring of urinary output for ketone bodies and acetone.

One of the most recent areas of interest relates the decrease in nosocomial pneumonia by maintenance of the gut-mucosal barrier with enteral feeding. Multiple studies have shown the benefits of enteral versus parenteral feeding on critically ill patients and the reduction of septic morbidity and mortality.[12–14] One theory states that the reduction in extraintestinal septic complications may be due to decreased translocation of bacteria and possibly toxins leading to infection elsewhere in the body.[15] A second theory proposes the gut to be the major source for the production of both intraintestinal and extraintestinal mucosal immunity and that enteral feedings preserve IgA-dependent immunity.[16]

In general, the septic immunocompromised patient requires the strictest attention to glucose control as well as early feeding to prevent catabolism. Enteral access is the most physiologically sound method and avoids the infectious complications associated with central venous access. Enteral nutrition may also have an advantageous effect by preventing the further translocation of microbes and prevention of further extraintestinal infections.

Cancer

Malnutrition and cachexia in the ICU patient further contribute to the immunocompromise associated with cancer and the side effects of chemotherapeutic agents. Approximately 60% to 80% of cancer patients experience weight loss, with 50% having lost weight at the time of diagnosis. The role of proper nutritional supplementation in the cancer patient is designed to lessen the effects of malnutrition as well as improve responses to treatment.

The etiology of cancer cachexia is believed to result from alterations in food intake, absorption, and nutrient use.[17] Decreased appetite secondary to tumor burden, and chemotherapeutics causing nausea, vomiting, mucositis, and food aversions all increase the difficulty in provision of nutrition. Arguments have even been posited for circulating factors produced by tumors playing an anorexigenic role. Tumor necrosis factor α is one such cytokine believed to play a role in the metabolic changes associated with cancer. These factors result in protein-calorie malnutrition that, when coupled with adjuvant chemotherapy and radiation treatment, can significantly increase morbidity and mortality. Malnutrition in the cancer patient has also been shown to suppress antibody-dependent and cellular immunity, with antibody-dependent immunity being affected much earlier and more severely.[18]

Host metabolism appears to undergo severe changes in the cancer patient that must be addressed when providing nutrition. Skeletal muscle protein synthesis decreases while proteolysis increases[19] and hepatic protein synthesis significantly increases.[20,21] Patients demonstrated hyperglycemia and peripheral glucose intolerance.[22] Hepatic glucose production is increased 25% to 40% in the face of starvation possibly secondary to increased tumor production of lactate,[19] serving as a substrate for gluconeogenesis. Cancer patients likewise show increased lipid mobilization,[23] increased free fatty acid oxidation,[24] and decreased serum lipid clearance secondary to suppression of lipoprotein lipase.[25]

Parenteral nutrition in the cancer patient has met with disappointing results, showing little benefit in restoration of lean body mass[26] and no improvement in outcome.[27] The American College of Physicians does not endorse the routine use of TPN in cancer patients because it does not appear to improve survival or response to therapy when reviewed globally.[28]

The benefits of enteral feeding in the immunocompromised cancer patient range from being less costly than TPN to being more easily maintained and more physiologic. Enteral feeds maintain the normal villous architecture and function of the gastrointestinal tract. They also result in increased total gut weight, mucosal thickness, protein and DNA content, and brush border enzyme activity.[29] As mentioned previously, enteral feeds maintain the integrity of the gut-mucosal barrier, helping to decrease intra- and extraintestinal infections in patients who are already immunocompromised from their disease as well as from the treatment. Enteral feeding has also been shown to maintain host immunologic function[30] as measured by challenge with endotoxin. The benefits of enteral feeds in host immune function are discussed in detail in Chapter 11.

Despite the fact that multiple studies have shown improvement in the metabolic and immunologic function of the cancer patient given enteral nutrition, few have shown a clinical benefit. The need for blinded prospective trials is obvious and will likely show improvement in survival and definitely in quality of life for cancer patients given enteral nutrition.

HIV/AIDS

As the incidence of AIDS increases in the United States, more and more physicians will be dealing with the complex medical problems afflicting these patients, and thus a significant proportion of ICU patients will be afflicted. In addition to the immune dysfunction caused by the viral illness, AIDS patients are victims of a severe wasting characterized by loss of both body fat and body cell mass.[31] This wasting is believed to be multifactorial, arising from mechanical problems of the GI tract, loss of appetite, diarrheal illnesses with resultant malabsorption, and alterations in metabolic rate and resting energy expenditure. Approximately 50% of patients with AIDS have GI tract involvement, with diarrhea present in 60%, dysphagia in 40%, and rectal pain in 20%.[32,33]

One of the earliest hallmarks of AIDS in the otherwise asymptomatic patient is malnutrition followed by cachexia. Thus, early recognition and treatment are advisable, as those patients presenting with involuntary loss of 10% or more of their reference weight require nutritional supplementation.

Parenteral nutrition has a role in the AIDS patient with a dysfunctional GI tract, as can occur with neoplasia, dysmotility syndromes associated with AIDS, or infectious disorders of the GI tract. In patients whose malnutrition was due to increased intake or malabsorption, one study has shown that TPN was capable of increasing body cell mass.[34] Others have shown that TPN at home can maintain a zero or positive nitrogen balance, normal visceral proteins, and may maintain or increase weight.[35,36]

In the AIDS patient with a functional GI tract, however, enteral nutrition is the preferred method of nutrition. Avoidance of line complications in a patient with dysfunctional cellular immunity, as occurs in AIDS, is desirable, although conflicting studies have shown no increase up to a 36% increased incidence of catheter sepsis in AIDS patients.[37,38] Feeding via a nasoenteric or gastric tube often is poorly tolerated secondary to oral candidiasis or esophagitis, thus PEG or PEG/PEJ placement is more feasible. Tailoring of enteral supplementation depends upon the patient's energy expenditure, ability to supplement with oral intake, and the presence and quality of malabsorption and/or diarrhea. For low-volume diarrhea, use of a low-fiber, lactose-free, or fat-free formula may be advisable. More severe diarrhea has been somewhat successfully treated with elemental formulas and peptide formulas.[39]

Nutritional supplementation in the AIDS patient is, to some extent, a controversial topic, and arguments have been made that it does not improve survival. Nutritional supplementation can, however, improve the clinical and functional status of the patient. Body cell mass depletion has also been shown to be linked to survival, suggesting that nutritional support may improve survival[40] in future studies.

Conclusions

Providing adequate nutrition to patients with a serious illness is an obvious key step in returning them to health. This is even more important in the immunocompromised patient, who often does not have the reserves to fight infections and is unable to tolerate further infectious insults. A detailed algorithm must be followed when choosing a method of delivery and the specific metabolic derangements addressed when considering nutrient provision in the immunocompromised. In general, avoidance of central venous access and the problems associated with indwelling catheters is advisable. Enteral feeds may not only maintain the gastrointestinal tract, thus allowing patients to return sooner to regular oral intake, but may also decrease infections elsewhere in the body and maintain surface mucosal immunity.

References

1. Hansbrough JF. Enteral nutritional support in burn patients. *Gastro Endo Clin N Amer.* 1998;8:645–647.
2. McDonald WS, Sharp CW, Deitch EA. Immediate enteral feeding in burn patients is safe and effective. *Ann Surg.* 1991;213:177–183.
3. Deitch EA. Bacterial translocation of the gut flora. *J Trauma.* 1990;30:S184–S189.
4. Dewitt RC, Kudsk KA. General nutritional therapeutic issues: enteral nutrition. *Gastro Clin.* 1998;27:2.
5. Aebert H, Hunefeld G, Regel G. Paranasal sinusitis and sepsis in ICU patients with nasotracheal intubation. *Int Care Med.* 1988;15:27–30.
6. Salord F, Gaussorgues P, Marti-Flick J, et al. Nosocomial maxillary sinusitis during mechanical ventilation: a prospective comparison of orotracheal versus the nasotracheal route for intubation. *Int Care Med.* 1990;390–393.
7. Garvin CG, Brown RO. Nutritional support in the intensive care unit: are patients receiving what is prescribed? *Crit Care Med.* 2001;29:204.
8. Hernandez-Socorro CR, Marin J, Ruiz-Santana S, et al. Bedside sonographic-guided versus blind nasoenteric feeding tube placement in critically ill patients. *Crit Care Med.* 1996;24:1690–1694.
9. Raad II, Bodey GP. Infectious complications of indwelling vascular catheters. *Clin Infect Dis.* 1992;15:197.

10. Hampton AA, Sheretz RJ. Vascular-access infections in hospitalized patients. *Surg Clin North Am.* 1988;68:57–71.
11. McManus LM, Bloodworth RC, Prihoda TJ, et al. Agonist-dependent failure of neutrophil function in diabetes correlates with extent of hyperglycemia. *J Leukocyte Biology.* 2001;70:395–404.
12. Kudsk KA, Croce MA, Fabian TC, et al. Enteral versus parenteral feeding. Effects on septic morbidity after blunt and penetrating abdominal trauma. *Ann Surg.* 1992;215: 503–515.
13. Moore FA, Moore EE, Jones TN, et al. TEN vs. TPN following major abdominal trauma: reduced septic morbidity. *J Trauma.* 1989;29:916–923.
14. Moore FA, Feliciano DV, Andrassy RJ, et al. Early enteral feeding, compared with parenteral, reduces postoperative septic complications. The results of a meta-analysis. *Ann Surg.* 1992;216:172–183.
15. Ziegler TR, Smith RJ, O'Dwyer ST, et al. Increased intestinal permeability associated with infection in burn patients. *Arch Surg.* 1988;123:1313–1319.
16. Kudsk KA, Li J, Renegar KB. Loss of upper respiratory tract immunity with parenteral feeding. *Ann Surg.* 1996; 223(6):629–635.
17. Harrison LE, Fong Y. Enteral nutrition in the cancer patient. In: Rombeau JL, Rolandelli RH, eds. *Clinical Nutrition: Enteral and Tube Feeding.* 3rd ed. Philadelphia: WB Saunders; 1997:300–323.
18. Emery PW, Edwards RHT, Rennie MJ, et al. Protein synthesis in muscle measured in vivo in cachectic patients with cancer. *Br Med J.* 1984;289:584.
19. Shaw JHF, Humberstone DM, Douglas RG, et al. Leucine kinetics in patients with benign disease, non-weight-losing cancer, and cancer cachexia: studies at the whole-body and tissue level and the response to nutritional support. *Surgery.* 1991;109:37.
20. Lundholm K, Ekman L, Karlberg I, et al. Protein synthesis in liver tissue under the influence of methyl-cholanthrene-induced sarcoma in mice. *Cancer Res.* 1979;39: 4657.
21. Yoshikawa T, Noguchi Y, Matsumoto A. Effects of tumor removal and body weight loss on insulin resistance in patients with cancer. *Surgery.* 1994;116:62.
22. Richtsmeier WJ, Dauchy R, Sauer LA. In vivo nutrient uptake by head and neck cancers. *Cancer Res.* 1987;47: 5230.
23. Beck SA, Tisdale MJ. Production of lipolytic and proteolytic factors by a murine tumor-producing cachexia in the host. *Cancer Res.* 1987;47:5919.
24. Eden E, Edstrom S, Bennegard K, et al. Glycerol dynamics in weight-losing cancer patients. *Surgery.* 1985;97:176.
25. Vlassara H, Spiegal RJ, Doval DS. Reduced plasma lipoprotein lipase activity in patients with malignancy associated weight loss. *Horm Metab Res.* 1986;18:698.
26. Cohn SH, Gartenhaus W, Varstky D, et al. Body composition and dietary intake in neoplastic disease. *Am J Clin Nutr.* 1981;34:1997.
27. Brennan MF. Total parenteral nutrition in the cancer patient. *N Engl J Med.* 1981;305:375.
28. McGeer AJ, Detsky AS, O'Rourke K. Parenteral nutrition in patients receiving cancer chemotherapy. *Ann Intern Med.* 1989;110:734.
29. Jackson WD, Grand RJ. The human intestinal response to enteral nutrients: a review. *J Amer Coll Nutr.* 1991;10:500.
30. Fong Y, Marano MA, Barber A, et al. Total parenteral nutrition and bowel rest modify the metabolic response to endotoxin in humans. *Ann Surg.* 1989;210:449.
31. Holt DR, Barbul A. Parenteral nutrition and acquired immunodeficiency syndrome. In: Rombeau JL, Caldwell MD, eds. *Parenteral Nutrition.* 2nd ed. Philadelphia: WB Saunders; 1993:748–755.
32. Santangelo WC, Krejs GJ. Southwestern internal medicine conference: gastrointestinal manifestations of the acquired immunodeficiency syndrome. *Am J Med Sci.* 1986; 292:328–334.
33. Gelb A, Miller S. AIDS and gastroenterology. *Am J Gastroenterol.* 1986;81:619–622.
34. Kotler DP, Tierney AR, Culpepper-Morgan JA, et al. Effect of home total parenteral nutrition upon body cell mass in AIDS (Abstract). V International Conference on AIDS. The Scientific and Social Challenge. Abstracts. International Development Research Center, Montreal; 1989:218.
35. Janson DD, Teasley KM. Parenteral nutrition in the management of gastrointestinal Kaposi's sarcoma in a patient with AIDS. *Clin Pharm.* 1988;7:535–544.
36. Singer P, Askanazi J, Roghkopf MM, et al. Home parenteral nutrition in AIDS (Abstract). V International Conference on AIDS. The Scientific and Social Challenge. Abstracts. International Development Research Center, Montreal; 1989:425.
37. Raviglione JH, Battan R, Pablos-Mendez A, et al. Infections associated with Hickman catheters in patients with acquired immunodeficiency syndrome. *Am J Med.* 1989; 86:780–786.
38. Prichard JG, Nelson MJ, Burns L, et al. Infections caused by central venous catheters in patients with acquired immunodeficiency syndrome. *South Med J.* 1988;81:1496–1497.
39. Resler SS. Nutrition care of AIDS patients. *J Am Diet Assoc.* 1988;88:828–832.
40. Kotler DP, Tierney AR, Wang J, et al. Magnitude of body cell mass depletion and the timing of death from wasting in AIDS. *Am J Clin Nutr.* 1989;50:444–447.

CHAPTER

30 Nutrition in Solid Organ Transplantation

Jeffrey A. Lowell, M.D., F.A.C.S., Mary Ellen Beindorff, R.D., L.D.

INTRODUCTION	341
TRANSPLANTATION OVERVIEW	341
INDICATIONS FOR TRANSPLANT	341
CONTRAINDICATIONS FOR TRANSPLANT	341
IMMUNOSUPPRESSION	341
PHASES OF TRANSPLANT	342
Pre-Transplant	342
Acute Post-Transplant	343
MONITORING AND FOLLOW-UP	345
CONCLUSIONS	346
REFERENCES	346

Introduction

Advances in surgical technique, immunosuppressive medications, and critical-care medicine have led to an increase in the utilization of organ transplantation for the treatment of organ function failure. Both patient and transplant organ survival have dramatically increased. However, these improvements would probably not be possible without the equally significant advances in the field of nutritional support. Transplantation patients are unique and have unique nutritional requirements. This chapter will review the issues pertaining to the safe and appropriate nutritional support for patients undergoing heart, lung, kidney, or liver transplant.

Transplantation Overview

Organ transplantation continues to grow as the number and type of transplants increase each year. Medical advances have led to better survival rates for recipients, and more patients are now being referred to transplant programs. The United Network of Organ Sharing (UNOS) reports the existence of 270 transplant centers in the United States, and although the number of solid organ transplants increases every year, it cannot keep pace with the number of people awaiting organs. As of January 2001, approximately 75,069 people were listed and awaiting transplant. Each year, these waiting lists continue to grow because the pool of cadaveric organ donors is limited.

Indications for Transplant

Transplant is indicated for individuals with end-stage organ failure. For patients waiting for liver, heart, or lung transplants, inability to obtain an organ will result in death. However, patients with kidney, pancreas, or intestinal failure can survive without a transplant since they can receive dialysis, insulin therapy, or parenteral nutrition. Unfortunately, these patients will probably have a poor quality of life and may die an untimely death from life-threatening complications.

Contraindications for Transplant

Relative contraindications for organ transplant include life-threatening medical conditions such as HIV infection, malignancy, sepsis, multi-organ failure, severe pulmonary hypertension, cardiopulmonary disease, active substance abuse, active psychiatric problems, age, a combination of chronic illnesses with poor prognosis, and a lack of social support post-transplant. In certain cases, financial support may also be a contraindication.[1]

Immunosuppression

The introduction of immunosuppressive drugs revolutionized the field of organ transplantation. Both patient and organ graft survival dramatically increased. Today, numerous immunosuppressive medications can be used in combination to prevent and treat rejection.

TABLE 30.1

Drug	Side Effect	Management
Cyclosporine	Hypertension	Sodium restriction
	Hyperkalemia	Potassium restriction
	Hyperglycemia	Decrease simple sugars
	Hyperuricemia	Increase fluid intake
	Hyperlipidemia	Limit fat and maintain ideal weight
	Hypomagnesemia	Increase magnesium intake
	Neurotoxicity	Correct electrolyte abnormalities
Tacrolimus	Hyperglycemia	Decrease simple sugars
	Hyperkalemia	Potassium restriction
	Nausea and vomiting	Adjust food as needed
		Monitor intake for adequacy
Prednisone	Hyperglycemia	Decrease simple sugars
	Hyperlipidemia	Limit fat and maintain ideal weight
	Increased appetite	Increase activity
		Monitor calorie intake
	Fluid retention	Limit sodium intake
	Calcium wasting	Supplement 1-1.5 g/d
Azathioprine	Nausea, vomiting	Adjust food as needed
	Sore throat, decreased taste	Monitor intake for adequacy
	Macrocytic anemia	Folate supplements
	Mouth sores	Soft, bland foods

Nutritional Effects of Common Immunosuppressive Drugs

Reprinted with permission from Lowell JA, Beindorff ME. Nutritional Assessment and Therapy in Abdominal Organ Transplantation. In: Shikora SA, Blackburn GL, eds. *Nutrition Support Theory and Therapeutics.* Gaithersburg, MD: Aspen Publishers; 1997:437.

Each of these medications has side effects that can affect the nutritional status of organ recipients (Table 30.1).

Phases of Transplant

There are three main phases of transplantation: pre-transplant, acute post-transplant, and chronic post-transplant. The pre-transplant period addressed here encompasses the acutely ill, end-stage organ failure patient. These patients are usually in the intensive care unit awaiting transplant, or death. The acute post-transplant period refers to the first 2 to 4 weeks after surgery. The chronic post-transplant period describes patients who are more than 6 weeks after surgery. Since the focus of this book is nutritional considerations in the intensive care unit, we will concentrate on the first two phases.

Pre-Transplant

The primary goal of the pre-transplant phase is to maximize the patient's nutritional status. Patients with adequate nutritional stores pre-transplant predictably fare better post-transplant with fewer complications and better recovery times than those with insufficient nutritional stores.[2,3] Many patients awaiting transplant are malnourished.[4,5] End-stage liver, heart, and lung patients are most commonly malnourished, as are longstanding dialysis patients. Numerous factors contribute to a poorly nourished pre-transplant patient, depending on which organ is failing (Table 30.2).

The main goals of nutritional therapy at this stage include limiting catabolism, providing adequate calories to meet energy needs, correcting electrolyte abnormalities, repleting macronutrients, and avoiding nutrition-associated complications. However, obtaining a functioning allograft is the most important need and should not be delayed to allow for additional nutritional replacement.

The nutritional assessment of a pre-transplant patient's nutritional status should utilize a combination of objective and subjective parameters. Body weight measurements are simple to perform and reproducible but are affected by body fluid derangements and are therefore often unreliable. Serum protein laboratory values and urinary collections are reproducible and low cost but may be affected by many non-nutritional factors (fluid status, liver and kidney function, etc.) and can also be unreliable. Other tests, such as indirect calorimetry and bioelectrical impedance, are often unavailable and more expensive to perform. The subjective global assessment (SGA) is a simple and inexpen-

TABLE 30.2

Factors Contributing to Nutrition Problems by Organ—Pre-Transplant		
Organ	**Complication**	**Treatment**
Liver	Ascites	Sodium restriction Diuretic therapy
	Hypernatremia	Fluid restriction
	Steatorrhea	Lower fat diet, supplement with water-soluble form of fat-soluble vitamins
	Encephalopathy	Treat with lactulose and/or neomycin Restrict protein to .6–.8 g/kg until encephalopathy resolves then increase protein as tolerated to 1.0–1.2 g/kg/d
	Pruritis	Treat with bile-sequestering agents
	Muscle-wasting	Provide adequate protein as tolerated
	Early satiety	Provide multiple small feedings
Kidney	Fluid overload	Sodium restriction and fluid restriction if necessary
	Iron deficiency	Iron supplementation orally or parenterally, epogen treatment
	Nausea/vomiting	Treat uremia
	Hyperkalemia	Limit potassium intake
	Hyperphosphatemia	Treat with phosphorus binders, limit phosphorus intake
	Osteopenia	Calcium supplementation, increased physical activity
Heart	Cardiac cachexia	Provide adequate calories and protein in small frequent feedings
	Fluid overload	Restrict sodium and fluid
	Hyperkalemia	Restrict potassium
	Hypokalemia	Supplement potassium
	Osteopenia	Supplement calcium and Vitamin D
Lung	Dyspnea	Small frequent feedings
	Malabsorption	Supplement fat-soluble vitamins in a water-soluble form Provide pancreatic enzymes to cystic fibrosis patients

sive technique often used to evaluate the nutritional status of pre-transplant patients. The SGA has been validated in liver-failure patients by Hasse et al.[2] and better accounts for weight changes due to fluid and gastrointestinal derangements. Pikul et al.[3] also reported using the SGA successfully to assess the degree of malnutrition in patients awaiting liver transplant. Specific energy, protein, fluid, and micronutrient recommendations for pre-transplant patients are found in Table 30.3.

ACUTE POST-TRANSPLANT

ENERGY

Transplant recipients generally have increased energy needs as a result of surgical stress, steroid administration, and poor nutritional status prior to transplant. Most patients are not hypermetabolic unless sepsis is present. Studies of energy requirements of post-transplant recipients using indirect calorimetry demonstrate that resting energy expenditure varies from 7% to 38% above predicted values.[6–8] In these studies, energy-expenditure measurements were obtained anywhere between the second and 28th day following the operation. Based on these investigations, post-operative transplant recipients should generally be provided 1.3 to 1.5 times the basal energy expenditure (BEE) or 30 to 35 kcal/kg.

PROTEIN

Protein requirements for acute post-transplant patients can be affected by steroid use, the stressed state, previous nutritional status, and protein losses from drains, stomas and/or wounds. Studies of urinary nitrogen excretion after transplant show increased nitrogen losses leading to persistently negative nitrogen balance even with increased protein intake. For these patients, 1.5 to 2.0 g/kg are most commonly used to provide adequate protein intake.[9–12]

TABLE 30.3

Detailed Nutrient Needs Specific to Organ Failing—Pre-Transplant		
Organ	**Nutrient**	**Needs**
Liver	Calories	1.2–1.3 × BEE
	Protein	1.0–2.0 g/kg
	Stage I encephalopathy	1.0–1.2 g/kg
	Stage II encephalopathy	.8–1.0 g/kg
	Stage III encephalopathy	.6–.8 g/kg
	Stage IV encephalopathy	.5–.6 g/kg
	Fluid	25–30 mL/kg/d unless Serum sodium <125 mEq/dL then restrict to 1–1.5 L/d
	Fat	30% of total calories, increase to provide adequate calories
		Restrict or include Medium Chain Triglyceride (MCT) sources if steatorrhea present
	Sodium	Restrict to 2000 mg/day
	Fat-soluble vitamins	Provide in a water-soluble form
	B-complex vitamins	Provide to patients with alcohol abuse history
	Calcium	Provide to patients with low intake or cholestatic disease
Kidney	Calories	1.2–1.3 × BEE
	Protein	Prerenal: .8 g/kg
		Hemodialysis: 1.0–1.5 g/kg
		CAPD: 1.3–1.5 g/kg
	Fat	30% of total calories, increase to provide adequate calories
	Fluid	25–30 mL/kg unless urine output minimal, then urine output + 1 L/d
	Sodium	Restrict to 2000–4000 mg/d
	B-complex vitamins	Provide supplement
	Iron	Provide oral supplement, add parenteral iron and/or epogen if necessary
	Vitamin C	Provide supplement
	Calcium	Usually provided as a phosphorus binder but if serum calcium levels increased may need to switch binders
	Potassium, magnesium, and phosphorus	Limit intake, use phosphorus or potassium binders if necessary
Heart	Calories	1.2–1.5 × BEE
	Protein	1.0–2.0 g/kg/d
	Fat	30% of total calories
	Fluid	1.0–1.5 L/d as necessary
	Sodium	2000 mg/d
	Potassium	Monitor closely, may need restriction or supplementation
	Calcium, magnesium, and phosphorus	Supplementation often necessary
Lung	Calories	1.2–1.5 × BEE
	Protein	1.0–2.0 g/kg/d
	Fat	30% of total calories, increase to provide adequate calories
	Fluid	25–30 mL/kg, restrict if necessary
	Fat-soluble vitamins	Provide in a water-soluble form
	Sodium	May need to supplement
	Calcium	Supplementation often necessary

Studies in animal models have shown some promising results in regard to the type of protein administered. Dietary supplementation with specific nutrients such as arginine and RNA, or the omission of nucleotides have been studied. However, no recommendations can be made for humans at this time.[13,14]

FLUID

Requirements for fluid are dependent on the patient's post-operative volume status. Decreased urine output and increased fluid administration contribute to fluid overload. Commonly patients are fluid overloaded prior to surgery and then receive excessive crystalloid fluids during the transplant itself. On the other hand, excessive fluid losses from diarrhea, chest tubes, nasogastric tubes, and any abdominal drain or ostomy will increase fluid needs. After the major fluid shifts have equilibrated, patients with good renal function will require approximately 2000 mL/d of fluid. Fluid-restricted patients often must be ardently encouraged to drink enough fluid to match their urine output.

ELECTROLYTES AND MICRONUTRIENTS

Immediately after surgery, transplant recipients require very careful attention to their intake of electrolytes and micronutrients. Phosphorus and magnesium, for instance, are two micronutrients that can deplete rapidly after transplantation secondary to medications such as glucocorticoids, Cyclosporine, or Tacrolimus, or from refeeding. Increased intake of oral phosphorus in the diet may not be adequate and oral supplementation may be necessary. Oral replacement of magnesium during this phase is often inadequate and parenteral magnesium is usually necessary for repletion. Diuretics can also deplete potassium and magnesium levels. Cyclosporine can cause increased magnesium loss and potassium retention. Tacrolimus can cause potassium retention as well. Both Cyclosporine and Tacrolimus can precipitate renal dysfunction, which may lead to hyperphosphatemia or hyperkalemia. Biliary obstruction and bile drainage can affect copper levels in liver-transplant recipients, but in practice copper levels are rarely monitored. Particularly in renal transplant patients, iron deficiency after transplant is common. An iron/total iron-binding capacity of less than 20% or transferrin saturation of less than 20 mg/dL is indicative of iron deficiency. Parenteral iron may be warranted to replete stores. In addition, excess blood loss will cause iron loss. Vitamin C and zinc requirements will be increased secondary to wound healing. Even though the efficacy of vitamin supplementation has not been documented, it is reasonable to start or continue with a multivitamin after transplant.

NUTRITION SUPPORT

Early post-operative transplant patients require adequate provision of appropriate macronutrients and micronutrients. Immediately after surgery, operative stress and catabolism, as well as high doses of steroids, will affect nutritional requirements. Depending on the degree of pre-operative malnutrition, adequate nutritional support should begin as soon as possible. Ideally, post-transplant, recipients will be extubated within 24 hours and advanced to clear liquid diets within a day or two. When there are no complications, patients often advance to a regular diet within 48 to 72 hours. However, when complications occur, patients usually will require nutritional support. For most patients, consideration should be given to feeding enterally. The benefits of enteral feeding will be described elsewhere in this book. However, these benefits are also beneficial for transplant patients.[7,15] The type of transplant, projected duration of need, and individual hospital ICU protocols will determine the type of tube to be placed. Although post-op transplant patients have been fed successfully via nasogastric tubes, nasointestinal tubes for post pyloric feeding are often preferred.[16] Once a small bowel feeding tube is in place, feedings can be started at a minimal rate and increased as tolerated to goal. Many transplant centers have tube-feeding protocols in place and may initiate feedings as early as 12 hours post-operatively or when the patient is hemodynamically stable. Intestinal absorption capability and other conditions should also be considered and may affect type, rate, and amount of formula given. These conditions have been summarized in Table 30.4.

When the patient is extubated and can start oral feeding, supplemental tube feeding should be continued until patient is able to orally take in at least 50% of energy and protein needs. Supplemental tube feeding can be given overnight to improve daytime appetite and decrease early satiety. Total parenteral nutrition (TPN) should be reserved for only those patients whose gastrointestinal tracts cannot be used for nutrition.

Monitoring and Follow-Up

All transplant recipients require close monitoring. If a patient is eating, a careful record of nutrient intake should be followed to assess adequacy. The addition of nutrition supplements or having patients eat several

TABLE 30.4

Post-Transplant Conditions and Type of Feeding Recommended	
Problem	**Tube Feeding Formulation**
Acute posttransplant, normal digestive tract	Polymeric, high nitrogen formula
Renal failure	Renal formula (feeding with restricted potassium, phosphorus and sodium, usually concentrated)
Diarrhea or constipation	Fiber-containing formula
Hyperglycemia	Polymeric, high nitrogen formula
Fluid overload	Concentrated, polymeric, high nitrogen formula
Malabsorption	Semi-elemental formula

small meals can help to maximize intake. Inadequate intake from lack of appetite, early satiety, nausea, or vomiting may require placement of a feeding tube. Complications post-transplant may include rejection, infection, hypertension, intestinal complications, or impaired mental status. These problems and even their treatments may cause interruption in adequate intake and necessitate placement of a feeding tube.

For patients on tube feedings, daily weights, intake and output records, and laboratory values (particularly glucose, sodium, potassium, carbon dioxide, phosphorus, magnesium, and calcium) should be closely monitored. Patients requiring TPN should be monitored by watching their weight, intake and output, and laboratory values (BUN, glucose, triglycerides, ammonia, sodium, potassium, phosphorus, magnesium, and calcium).

Conclusions

Solid organ transplantation patients are nutritionally and metabolically complicated. Many are significantly malnourished prior to transplant secondary to their underlying organ failure. The surgery and ensuing medications can also affect nutritional status. Therefore, providing post-transplant recipients with optimal nutrition support should improve patient survival and quality of life. Feeding patients adequately (particularly those malnourished pre-operatively) can decrease complications and possibly shorten length of hospital stays after surgery. However, safe and appropriate feeding requires that the clinicians and/or dietitians involved with these patients understand the unique aspects of their nutritional management.

References

1. Marsh JW, Miller SB, Carroll PB, et al. Medical evaluation and recipient selection for organ transplantation. In: *The Handbook of Transplantation Management*. Makowka L, ed. Austin, TX: R.G. Landes Co; 1991:1–43.
2. Hasse JM, Strong G, Gorman, MA, et al. Subjective global assessment—alternative nutritional assessment technique for liver transplant candidates. *Nutrition*. 1991;9:339–343.
3. Pikul J, Sharpe MD, Lowndes R, et al. Degree of preoperative malnutrition is predictive of postoperative morbidity and mortality in liver transplant recipients. *Transplantation*. 1994;57:469–472.
4. DiCecco SR, Wieners EJ, Wiesner RH, et al. Assessment of nutritional status of patients with end-stage liver disease undergoing liver transplantation. *Mayo Clin Proc*. 1989;64:95–102.
5. Porayko MK, DiCecco S, O'Keefe SJ. Impact of malnutrition and its therapy on liver transplant candidates. *Nutrition*. 1993;9:339–343.
6. Delafosse B, Faure JL, Bouffard Y, et al. Liver transplantation—energy expenditure, nitrogen loss and substrate oxidation rate in the first two postoperative days. *Transplant Proc*. 1989;21:2453–2454.
7. Hasse JM, Blue LS, Liepa GU, et al. Early enteral nutrition support in patients undergoing liver transplantation. *J Parenter Enteral Nutr*. 1995;19:437–443.
8. Plevak DJ, Dicecco SR, Wiesner RH, et al. Nutritional support for liver transplantation: identifying caloric and protein requirements. *Mayo Clin Proc*. 1994;69:225–230.
9. Hasse JM. Diet therapy for organ transplantation: a problem-based approach. *Nurs Clin North Am*. 1997;13:15–26.
10. Hasse J. Solid organ transplantation. In: Matarese LE, Gottschlich MM, eds. Contemporary Nutrition Support Practice. Philadelphia, PA: WB Saunders Co; 1998:547–560.
11. Shanbhogue RLK, Bristrian BR, Jenkins RL, et al. Increased protein catabolism without hypermetabolism after human orthotopic liver transplantation. *Surgery*. 1987;101:146–149.
12. Hasse JM. Nutrition Assessment and Support of Organ Transplant Recipients. *J Parenter Enteral Nutr*. 2001;25:120–131.
13. Van Buren CT, Kim E, Kulkarni AD, et al. Nucleotide-free diet and suppression of immune response. *Transplant Proc*. 1987;19(4 Suppl 5):57–59.
14. Alexander JW, Dreyer D, Greenberg N, et al. Oral L-arginine with and without canola oil modulates blood pressure and renal function in patients following kidney transplantation. *J Parenter Enteral Nutr*. 1999;23:S19.
15. Wicks C, Somasundaram S, Bjarnason I, et al. Comparison of enteral feeding and total parenteral nutrition after liver transplantation. *Lancet*. 1994;344:837–840.
16. Hasse JM, Blue LS, Liepa GU, et al. Early enteral nutrition support in patients undergoing liver transplantation. *J Parenter Enteral Nutr*. 1995;19:437–443.
17. Reilly J, Mehta R, Teperman L, et al. Nutritional support after liver transplantation: a randomized prospective study. *J Parenter Enteral Nutr*. 1990;14:386–391.

CHAPTER

31

Anabolic Agents in the Intensive Care Unit

Leah Gramlich, M.D., F.R.C.P.(C),
Demetrios J. Kutsogiannis, M.D., M.H.S., F.R.C.P.(C)

INTRODUCTION 347
THE METABOLIC RESPONSE TO CRITICAL ILLNESS 347
THE INFLAMMATORY RESPONSE IN CRITICAL ILLNESS 348
NUTRITIONAL MODULATION OF ANABOLISM AND CATABOLISM 349
Energy Metabolism 349
Protein Metabolism 349
Carbohydrate Metabolism 350
Lipid Metabolism 350
Micronutrients 350
ANABOLIC AGENTS IN CRITICAL ILLNESS 351
Insulin 351
Testosterone 351
Anabolic Steroids 351
GROWTH HORMONE AND INSULIN-LIKE GROWTH FACTOR-1 351
Neuroendocrine Alteration of GH Secretion in Critical Illness 351
Metabolic Effects of GH in Critical Illness 352
Clinical Studies Utilizing GH in the Critically Ill 352
CONCLUSIONS 354
REFERENCES 354

Introduction

Central to the role of regulating the catabolic response to critical illness are the hormones released by and other physiological effects mediated through the neuroendocrine axis and the sympathetic nervous system. The precise cellular mechanisms by which other mediators released in the stress response contribute to catabolism are less well understood. Cytokines released from inflammation, such as IL-1 and tumor necrosis factor (TNF-α), play a role in the injury response and catabolism either directly or through other immunologic changes seen in the severely ill patient. Collectively, these responses may have either anabolic or catabolic effects at the cellular level. This chapter will focus on anabolism and catabolism in critical illness and discuss the role of the systemic inflammatory response syndrome (SIRS), nutritional therapy, and catabolic and anabolic strategies in critical illness.

The Metabolic Response to Critical Illness

The immunologic, coagulation, and neuroendocrine responses to critical illness produce a diverse array of effects on tissue metabolism. The catabolism (breakdown of complex compounds, often with the liberation of energy) that accompanies the stress response to injury and infection represents a deviation from the normal physiologic function in an attempt to optimize healing and improve survival. The biologic imperative is to provide energy, primarily in the form of glucose and amino acids, for acute phase protein production, wound healing, and the augmentation of the immune response. This is accomplished by altering the normal proportion of metabolic substrates that are used as an energy source.

Nutrient utilization in critical illness is different from that found in the non-stressed starved state, where 90% of the calories are derived from fat with only 5%–8% of the calories coming from protein.[1] In patients with critical illness, fat is not readily available as an energy substrate and protein is not spared. While fatty acids can readily provide two carbon fragments used for general tissue fuel, they cannot be used to provide a net gain of carbohydrate intermediates, namely glycogen or circulating glucose, which are preferentially demanded in the catabolic state. As a result, protein degradation is relied on as an energy substrate. Body protein is a low-energy fuel and exists in the body with approximately three parts of water, hence the 4 kcal/g of dry protein becomes 1 kcal/g of hydrated lean tissue when body protein is degraded following injury. Consequently, the extreme weight loss of injury and sepsis is attributable to the body meeting its modest increases in energy demands with a relatively low energy fuel (protein) rather than having to meet very high energy demands with a normal proportion of substrates including carbohydrate, fat, and protein.[2]

With persistence of catabolism and net protein breakdown, the significant protein losses demonstrated in critical illness cannot be reconciled by any amount of intensive nutritional support that provides both energy and protein substrates. As a result, loss of lean body mass is ongoing in critical illness and contributes directly to mortality and morbidity particularly in the critically ill patient with losses in excess of 40% of lean body mass. Therefore, nutritional therapy in critical illness is primarily supportive, its goal being to obviate catabolism as opposed to promoting anabolism. Despite this limited role of nutritional calories to influence catabolism, other roles for nutritional therapy have been advocated including the immune modulating effects and special metabolic effects of certain substrates. Investigators have used ω-3 fatty acids and alternative protein substrates such as glutamine, arginine, and nucleotides to enhance immunity through nutrition.[3,4] Discussion has also considered the importance of feeding enterally as compared to parenterally and its ability to obviate SIRS.[5]

The Inflammatory Response in Critical Illness

Critical illness, resulting from sepsis, burn injury, trauma, or the post operative state is often manifest through the host's inflammatory response. This response depends on the balance between the pro-inflammatory response, namely the systemic inflammatory response syndrome (SIRS), and the anti-inflammatory response, namely the compensatory anti-inflammatory response syndrome (CARS). At the cellular level, the inflammatory response in critical illness is composed of a multitude of molecular interactions and cellular signaling systems that are complex and highly integrated. These molecular components include pro- and anti-inflammatory cytokines, chemokines, lipid mediators, nitric oxide, and the coagulation cascade. The neuroendocrine axis and sympathetic nervous system also play an important role and interact with the aforementioned molecular components.

Cytokines are proteins or glycoproteins that serve as chemical messengers that regulate tissue repair and the immune response. The most important cytokine mediators of both the innate and specific immune response include the pro-inflammatory cytokines; tumor necrosis factor alpha (TNF-α); interleukin-1 (IL-1) and interleukin-6 (IL-6); and the anti-inflammatory cytokines, interleukin-4 (IL-4) and interleukin-10 (IL-10).[6] Although increased plasma concentrations of TNF-α and IL-6 have been demonstrated to correlate with mortality in septic patients, monoclonal antibodies directed against human TNF-α have not provided a survival advantage in clinical trials.[7] Moreover, the anti-inflammatory effect mediated by IL-10 is associated with a higher severity of injury and a higher incidence of sepsis in trauma patients.[8,9] Hormones such as glucocorticoids stimulate neutrophil release from the bone marrow and inhibit gamma interferon (γ-IFN), interleukin-1 (IL-1), and interleukin-2 (IL-2) production.[10] Cortisol levels and the cortisol response to corticotropin have been demonstrated to be an independent predictor of mortality in patients with septic shock.[11]

Platelet function and the coagulation cascade are influenced by the effects of lipid mediators and cytokines. Inflammatory lipid mediators, including platelet activating factor and the eicosanoids, have many effects including that of regulating vasomotor tone and platelet aggregation.[12] TNF-α, IL-1β, and IL-6 activate coagulation and inhibit fibrinolysis resulting in microvascular thrombosis and multiple organ system failure (MOSF).[13,14,15] In a critically ill population, a greater consumption of coagulation factors and platelets and a greater increase in fibrinogen and thrombin-antithrombin complexes have been demonstrated in patients with septic shock than in those with sepsis alone.[16] Similarly, reduced levels of the natural anticoagulant protein C are present in septic patients and correlate with increased mortality. A recent randomized controlled trial demonstrated a survival advantage in septic patients who were administered activated protein C.[17]

The sum of these and other microbiological, immunological, hemodynamic, and biochemical events has been postulated to cause MOSF and may ultimately be mediated through the apoptotic process.[18] Apoptosis of cells is the morphologic feature that characterizes multi-organ system failure; however, it is still debatable whether this is a protective or harmful response. Morphologically, apoptosis is characterized by cellular dehydration, compaction of nuclear chromatin, and nuclear fragmentation.[19] Apoptosis is an active genetically regulated program for cellular self-destruction that may occur under physiological or pathological conditions. Increased release of cytokines, oxygen-free radicals, heat shock proteins, glucocorticoids, and bacterial products into the circulation increases apoptotic rates in cells.[19] Central to the role of apoptosis are a group of cysteine-aspartate proteases termed "caspases," particularly caspase-3, which are released in response to proapoptotic signals and result in the disassembly of the cells. In septic patients, caspase-3 mediated apoptosis results in significant lymphocyte apoptosis and may contribute to the impaired immune response that is seen in sepsis.[20] However, to date it is not certain whether apoptosis and lymphocyte apoptosis in particular could hamper T-cell function, thus predisposing septic patients to secondary infection, or whether it is beneficial to the host survival by down-regulating the inflammatory response seen in sepsis. ICU mortality is more commonly attributable to MOSF rather than to the initial pathologic insult. Ultimately, all of these cellular processes have an effect on tissue metabolism.

Nutritional Modulation of Anabolism and Catabolism

The progressive loss of lean body mass associated with catabolism in the setting of critical illness is itself associated with morbidity and mortality, independent of the initiating event.[21] Despite appropriate nutritional therapy in the severely catabolic patient, losses of 60–100 gm of protein per day are well recognized, suggesting that the neuroendocrine mediators involved in inflammation cannot be obviated by nutrition support alone.[1] There are three important variables in the interaction between nutrition and the inflammatory response: (1) nutritional status; (2) severity of the inflammatory response; and (3) duration of starvation and injury.[5] All of these variables will influence what is "optimal nutrition support" in a given patient.

Energy Metabolism

Many equations allow us to estimate energy requirements in patients who are critically ill. These include the Harris-Benedict equation, which estimates energy requirements as 25 kcal/kg. Studies using an indirect calorimeter to measure energy expenditure in patients with critical illness have suggested that our estimates may be inaccurate (>110% or <90% of measured energy expenditure) in up to 50% of patients.[22] Measurement of energy expenditure by indirect calorimetry in critically ill patients requiring nutrition support for over a week is highly recommended when available. At present most of the literature suggests that for the majority of hospitalized critically ill patients energy requirements range between 25 and 30 kcal/kg. Exceptions to this requirement are burn and trauma patients who may require 40–45 cal/kg/d or individuals who have a body mass index <20 kg/m^2.[23]

Protein Metabolism

Increased protein intake in the presence of adequate calories is a standard anti-catabolic/anabolic approach to critical illness.[1] Intake of 1.5–2 g/kg/d is considered optimal to attenuate catabolism by providing adequate substrate for protein synthesis. In the past, patients were fed up to 4 g/kg/d of protein, but more recent studies assessing protein synthesis and nitrogen retention suggest that higher levels of protein intake during the "stress response" are not utilized effectively.[1] Indeed, excess protein intake is deleterious since amino acids not used for protein synthesis need to be oxidized, resulting in a formation of increased urea and heat. This increased urea production can be problematic in the presence of renal dysfunction. The type of protein that patients receive may also be influential with respect to anabolic potential. Enterally delivered protein has been reported to be better utilized for synthesis than protein delivered parenterally.[24] One explanation for this is the fact that much of the protein delivered enterally is in the form of peptides derived from protein hydrolysate, and nitrogen retention from these administered peptides is noted to be significantly greater than that from whole protein or amino acids typically found in parenteral preparations.

Following acute injury there is increased efflux of amino acids, especially glutamine, alanine, and phenylalanine from muscle.[25] The increased amino acid and protein recycling is important in critically ill patients for maintenance of gut integrity, to provide substrates to facilitate wound healing, and to optimize immune status. Glutamine is the major fuel of at least two important cellular components involved in wound healing, including fibroblasts and stimulated lymphocytes,[25] and is the preferred fuel for rapidly dividing enterocytes. The availability of glutamine is recognized as a rate-limiting step in muscle protein synthesis, and the rate of protein turnover in muscle depends in part on the availability of glutamine. The catabolism and resultant loss of intramuscular glutamine present in patients who have undergone surgery is attenuated by providing nutritional support containing supplemental glutamine.[1]

Arginine is an integral substrate of the urea acid cycle and is not considered to be an essential amino acid. However, under periods of severe stress, arginine is thought to become an essential dietary nutrient. It is felt to be important in healing during deficiency states but may also promote wound healing when given as a supplement.[25] Arginine appears to achieve many of its demeliatory actions via the hypothalamopituitary axis. It is a secretagogue for insulin, glucagon, prolactin, and growth hormone.

Carbohydrate Metabolism

Carbohydrates are an important source of energy during nutritional support of the critically ill patient. Carbohydrates should be given to meet 50%–70% of the energy requirements of a given patient. In the setting of critical illness, hormonal and cytokine mediators of the inflammatory response also influence carbohydrate metabolism. However, at infusion rates of >4 mg/kg/min the ability to metabolize glucose is impaired. This is often manifest by increased serum glucose levels. Hyperglycemia may also be related to insulin resistance in the setting of increased levels of cortisol, growth hormone, and the catecholamines. Glucagon and the catecholamines are characterized as counter-regulatory anti-insulin or stress hormones. Cortisol stimulates gluconeogenesis and increases proteolysis and alanine synthesis as well as sensitizing adipocytes to the action of lipolytic hormones. Cortisol causes insulin resistance and facilitates the action of catecholamines. This helps maintain cardiovascular stability during stress. Cortisol has a synergistic effect with catecholamines and glucagon with the result of diverting glucose utilization from skeletal muscle to central organs such as the brain. As a group, the stress hormones cause hyperglycemia. Glucagon increases hepatocyte cycloadanine monophosphate concentrations and promotes gluconeogenesis, glycogenolysis, lipolysis, and ketogenesis in the liver. Catecholamines cause increased glycogenolysis, hepatogluconeogenesis, and gluconeogenic precursor mobilization and promote lipolysis. Glucagon and catecholamines have a synergistic effect with resulting gluconeogenesis. All of these changes lead to a common end point—increased glucose production at the expense of widespread catabolism.[25,26]

Lipid Metabolism

The stress response causes increased lipolytic activity resulting in increased serum concentrations of free fatty acids and glycerol and a decreased rate of ketogenesis. Since ketone bodies are one of the primary energy sources utilized to decrease protein catabolism, this response would indicate that critically ill patients may require increased amounts of carbohydrate and protein in their diet to prevent protein catabolism and achieve a positive nitrogen balance. The metabolism of fatty acids is significantly increased in critical illness with increased rate of production of physiologically active prostaglandins that have immunosuppressive activity.[25] One means of limiting the effect of metabolism to physiologically active prostaglandins (i.e., PGE-II) has been to replace the omega-6 fatty acids obtained from standard vegetable and animal oils with the omega-3 fatty acids from fish oil.[27]

Micronutrients

Micronutrients include electrolytes, minerals, vitamins, and trace elements. In the setting of catabolism it is vitally important to consider the refeeding syndrome, particularly in malnourished patients who become critically ill. To this end, judicious application of volume, sodium, and carbohydrate must be considered. Adequate repletion of phosphorus, magnesium, and potassium to facilitate lean body mass repletion are also vital.

In the United States, recommended daily allowances have been established by the Committee on Dietary Allowances of the Food & Nutrition Board.[28] However, these requirements were established for healthy populations, not for specific individuals. In the setting of critical illness, there are no specific recommended daily intakes of micronutrients and vitamins. However, there have been suggestions made by Debiasse[28] and others.[25] The vitamins can be categorized as being safe at levels of 50–100 times the recommended daily allowance, and these vitamins include vitamin B_1, niacin, vitamin B_2, pantothenic acid, biotin, folic acid, vitamin B_{12}, vitamin C, and vitamin E. Vitamins that are safe at 10 times the recommended daily allowance (RDA) include vitamin B_6, vitamin A, vitamin D, and vitamin K. In certain instances, vitamin supplementation should be limited, including considerations for pregnancy, renal failure, and anti-coagulation with vitamin K antagonists.

Anabolic Agents in Critical Illness

Insulin

Insulin has been shown to increase skeletal muscle protein synthesis and to decrease its degradation in numerous in vitro and in vivo studies when amino acids are provided intravenously.[29] In catabolic patients, a combined insulin and glucose infusion produces strikingly greater inhibition of protein breakdown than an infusion of glucose alone. Moreover, glucose alone is marginally more protein sparing than a regimen containing primarily fat.[30] It is of note that the availability of amino acid substrates is vital for the maximization of the anabolic effect of insulin. In the past the anabolic effects of insulin have been evaluated mainly through the use of an intravenous amino acid infusion model. In a more recent study, the anabolic effect of intravenous insulin on protein kinetics (3-Methylhistidine excretion rates) was not evident in patients who had enteral provision of nutrients.[29] This would suggest that the route of administration does affect insulin's anabolic effect.

Testosterone

Testosterone levels are decreased immediately after severe trauma or critical illness and throughout the recovery period from catabolism. Exogenously administered testosterone is rapidly metabolized resulting in a modest increase in anabolic activity as compared to that demonstrated with the use of other testosterone analogues. This limited beneficial effect has been more than offset by the androgenic side effects noted with the use of testosterone, including hirsuitism, mood change, and hypersexualism. Similarly, testosterone has been used to increase lean mass in debilitative patients but only with moderate success. Complications relate mainly to androgenic side effects, which include mood changes, hirsuitism, and gynecomastia.

Anabolic Steroids

Anabolic steroids are derivatives of testosterone that were developed in an attempt to dissociate the androgenic and anabolic effects of testosterone so that only the anabolic effects were maintained while the androgenic side effects were minimized. These agents can be given orally or parenterally.

Anabolic steroids have been used in the area of sports medicine but also in treatment of patients following major burns.[31,32] Clinical trials using oxandrolone have been conducted in patients with severe burns and have shown significant increases in weight gain as a result of increased muscle mass. This increase in lean mass is significantly higher than that seen with nutrition alone. Like other anabolic agents, optimal nutrition is necessary for maximal anabolic effect. The anabolic effects of synthetic anabolic steroids also appear to be dose-dependent. The main contraindications for oxandrolone are the presence of carcinoma of the male breast and prostate, as these tumors have androgenic receptors. More recently, Gervasio et al.[33] studied the effects of the administration of oxandrolone following multiple trauma in 62 patients requiring enteral nutrition. Oxandrolone at 20 mg/day did not have obvious beneficial effects on nutritional or clinical outcomes such as length of hospital or intensive care unit stay and frequency of pneumonia or sepsis. In the context of other large-scale studies looking at anabolic agents and critical illness this likely warrants further investigation.

Growth Hormone and Insulin-Like Growth Factor-1

Neuroendocrine Alteration of GH Secretion in Critical Illness

Critical illness imparts a myriad of effects involving the immunologic, hormonal, cytokine, and coagulation systems. Nutrition, hormones, and cytokines modulate the somatotropic axis in both health and disease. The hypothalamus responds to cytokine stimulation by increasing the thermoregulatory set-point and by elaboration of stress hormones such as catecholamines, cortisol, and glucagons.[25] The initial endocrine response to stress results in a peripheral inactivation of anabolic activity with a preservation of pituitary activity. The delay in the anabolic state is thought to be adaptive for the provision of metabolic substrate for the survival of the host. Initially pulsatile secretion of anterior pituitary hormones such as ACTH, TSH, LH, prolactin, and GH is preserved; however, this response is diminished in protracted critical illness. Furthermore, the impairment of this response in the chronic phase of critical illness appears to be a result of hypothalamic dysfunction as the pituitary response to releasing factors is preserved.[34] In the acute phase of critical illness both peak GH levels and GH pulse frequency are increased. This has been attributed to acquired peripheral resistance to GH resultant from the effects of cytokines such as IL-1, IL-6, and TNF-α, as well as from the downregulation of the GH receptor in the liver and skeletal muscle.[35] In contrast to the acute phase of critical illness, GH secretion in the chronic phase of critical illness is chaotic with a reduced pulsatile release and a concomitant reduction in circulating insulin-like growth factor-1 (IGF-1) concentrations. During this chronic phase, reduced serum levels of GH dependent IGF-1 and IGF binding proteins such as insulin-like factor binding protein-3 (IGFBP-3) are correlated with biochemical markers of impaired anabolism and muscle wasting.[34] It has been hypothesized that a low availability of somatostatin, growth hormone releasing hormone (GHRH), or thyrotropin releasing hormone (TRH)—one of the endogenous ligands of the growth hormone releasing peptide (GHRP) receptor—may be responsible for the reduced GH amplitude and burst frequency.[34] The GHRPs are a class of peptides acting on the pituitary and the hypothalamus to release GH through activation of a G protein coupled receptor.[36] In humans it has been demonstrated that infusion of GHRP-2 but not GHRH or TRH synchronizes the serum profiles of GH, TSH, and prolactin.[37] Moreover, the combined administration of GHRH and GHRP-2 appears to elicit a more pronounced increase in basal and pulsatile levels of GH than either alone.[34,36,37]

Metabolic Effects of GH in Critical Illness

During the normal response to stressful stimuli, skeletal muscle degradation produces amino-acid substrate for hepatic gluconeogenesis. There is an increased efflux of amino acids such as alanine, glutamine, and phenylalanine, from muscles following burn injury. This protein recycling is important to support collagen synthesis and immune function.[25] As a result of a defect in amino acid transport, this protein catabolism cannot be reversed by the provision of amino acids alone. However, the defect may be reversed by anabolic agents such as GH and IGF-I.[25] Growth hormone has direct and indirect anabolic effects, the latter of which are mediated by insulin-like growth factor-1 (IGF-1).[38] The direct effects of GH include protein synthesis in muscle, amino acid transport, lipolysis, and insulin antagonism.[38,39] These effects may benefit the ill fasting patient by averting protein synthesis while providing metabolic fuels in the form of fatty acids. However, in the late stages of critical illness, the use of fatty acids as metabolic substrate does not persist, and fat is stored in vital organs such as the liver, and therefore continue to lose skeletal muscle protein.[34]

The anabolic effect of GH is thought to be mediated through IGF-1, which is produced by many cell types but predominantly in the liver.[35] In critically ill adults, IGF-1 positively correlates with the basal component, the pulsatile component, and the total amount of nightly GH secretion.[36] IGFs are bound to specific binding proteins, the most abundant of which is insulin-like growth factor binding protein 3 (IGFBP-3). IGF-1 forms a ternary complex with IGFBP-3 and an acid labile subunit that restricts the circulatory efflux of the unit, increases its half-life, and represents a reservoir of IGF-1 activity.[35,40] IGF-1 enhances glucose uptake in muscle and has little effect on suppressing hepatic glucose production or adipocyte lipolysis as compared with insulin.[38] A decrease in IGF-1 synthesis and secretion is generally demonstrated after traumatic or burn injury and catabolic states, accompanied by an inconsistent reduction in IGFBP-3. Insulinopenia, acidosis, IL-1, and TNF-α all contribute to the reduction of IGF-1 in trauma, burns, and inflammation.[35] Moreover, during inflammatory processes, generated proteases cleave the IGF-1 ternary complex, which results in a reduction in the half-life and potency of the peptide.[41]

Clinical Studies Utilizing GH in the Critically Ill

The majority of the human studies of GH in the critically ill have utilized the recombinant form of GH (rhGH) or IGF-1 and have recruited small numbers of patients focusing primarily on hormonal, metabolic, and immunologic endpoints such as GH/IGF-1 concentrations, nitrogen balance, and CD4/CD8 ratios respectively. The most optimistic results of rhGH therapy have been demonstrated in burn injured patients.[42]

In general, a sustained rise in plasma concentrations of IGF-1,[40,43–48] insulin-like growth factor binding protein 3 (IGFBP-3),[40] and insulin[40,46,47,49] have been observed after the administration of exogenous GH.

The majority of studies evaluating nitrogen balance as an endpoint to rhGH therapy have demonstrated an improved nitrogen balance in critically ill patients. Net protein catabolism and urea production rate have been demonstrated to decrease in surgical patients with sepsis after treatment with rhGH;[44,50] the effect was more pronounced in those patients who were less catabolic.[50] The administration of rhGH significantly reduced nitrogen excretion, urea generation, and potassium and phosphorus excretion in a population of trauma patients[43] and improved the cumulative changes in nitrogen, potassium, and phosphate balance in patients with pancreatic and gastrointestinal dysfunction who required total parenteral nutrition (TPN).[51] In combination with TPN, rhGH improves nitrogen metabolism and increases plasma free amino acid levels in the immediate posttraumatic period.[52] The administration of 0.1 mg/kg/d of rhGH on days 2, 3, and 4 after admission for sepsis resulted in an improved nitrogen balance and a decrease in 3-methylhistidine excretion, indicating a reduction of muscle breakdown.[47] A related study in nonseptic patients also demonstrated improvement in nitrogen balance with rhGH therapy; however, there was no effect of rhGH on the excretion of 3-methylhistidine.[48] Postoperative muscle biopsies of patients undergoing elective cholecystectomy and on TPN have also demonstrated a preservation of total ribosome and polyribosome concentration in those treated with rhGH compared to those not receiving therapy.[49] The anabolic effects of rhGH may also be responsible for the changes in extracellular water seen in critically ill patients. Using the indicator dilution technique to measure extracellular and total body water, critically ill surgical patients at 3 to 4 weeks after their hospital admission given rhGH maintained extracellular and intracellular water, indicating a preservation of body cell mass compared with control patients who developed a marked expansion of extracellular water and a reduction in intracellular water and hence body cell mass.[53] This effect may be mediated by an improvement in the efficiency of the cellular pump mechanisms or enhancing the synthesis of cellular proteins. However, other investigators have not demonstrated a change in skeletal muscle extracellular water with rhGH therapy.[40] Similarly, albumin synthesis is known to be increased in critically ill patients; in a randomized trial of 22 critically ill patients no changes in the rate of albumin synthesis were observed between controls and those treated with GH.[54]

Perhaps the most optimistic results with the use of rhGH have been in populations of pediatric burn patients. The use of rhGH improved nitrogen balance and decreased the requirement for albumin replacement in pediatric burn patients[55] and also reduced first and second donor-site healing times and decreased hospital length of stay compared to placebo in children with burn injuries.[56] Attenuation of protein catabolism has also been shown in a group of severely burned children after the administration of IGF-1/IGF-3 complex.[42] In contrast to the wealth of evidence suggesting improved nitrogen balance with the use of rhGH, in a randomized trial of 14 trauma patients, rhGH did not increase either daily or cumulative nitrogen balance, nor did it affect plasma or muscle concentrations of total free amino acids or glutamine when compared to controls.[40] The resistance to nitrogen metabolism was thought to be secondary to impaired IGF-1 action at the cellular level due to a receptor or postreceptor defect. Likewise, despite convincing evidence for an improved cumulative nitrogen balance after the administration of rhGH in patients with respiratory failure, this response is not accompanied by an improvement in muscle strength or a shorter duration of mechanical ventilatory support possibly because of preferential redistribution of protein toward central organs as opposed to muscle.[46]

The use of rhGH also influences parameters of lipid and glucose metabolism. Several studies have demonstrated an increase in plasma free fatty acid (FFA) levels after administration of rhGH in pediatric burn patients,[45] patients with sepsis,[47] and in nonseptic patients.[48] The anabolic effect of GH may be mediated in part by the increased availability of FFA as a fuel. Hyperglycemia requiring insulin therapy has been noted as an adverse effect of rhGH in several trials.[43,48,49,51,57,58] In a randomized trial of 14 burn injured patients, those treated with rhGH had increased insulin and glucagon levels accompanied by increased insulin resistance.[45] Systemic calcium levels have also been noted to increase in rhGH treated patients.[57]

There appears to be an interaction between growth hormone and endogenous catecholamines as well as therapeutic cardiac inotropes such as dopamine. Administration of rhGH to high-risk burn patients was shown to increase norepinephrine levels by 45% and epinephrine levels by 162% compared with controls. The increase in catecholamine levels in response to rhGH was thought to be mediated by increased insulin levels.[45] Mean serum GH concentration, GH secretory amplitude, and the mass of GH secreted per burst are decreased during prolonged dopamine infusion in critically ill patients.[59] Patients suffering from severe head injury typically have a reduction in their circulating CD4 cell counts. In a randomized trial of 14 head injured patients the administration of early aggressive nutrition eliminated the otherwise depressed CD4/CD8 ratio; and in the group randomized to a 7-day course of IGF-1 treatment, CD4/CD8 ratios were significantly above those treated with nutrition alone at 7 days.[60]

Few studies have investigated the influence of rhGH on mortality in critically ill patients, the largest studies demonstrating a significant increase in mortality for those patients receiving rhGH. In a matched case control study of 54 adult burn injured patients, the administration of 0.06 to 0.15 mg/kg/d of rhGH was associated with an 11% mortality as compared with a 37% mortality seen in controls.[57] In several small studies of adult patients, rhGH was not associated with an increase in morbidity or mortality.[47,48,50,61] Similarly, one study of 40 pediatric burn patients did not have any mortality in either the rhGH or placebo treatment groups and the length of hospital stay was decreased in those children receiving rhGH.[56] However, in two large multicenter clinical trials of the therapeutic use of rhGH in an adult population of 247 patients in Finland and 285 patients in other European centers, there was a significant increase in the relative risk of death of 1.9 in the Finnish study and 2.4 in the European study.[58] Multiple organ failure, septic shock, and uncontrolled infection were reported more frequently in the rhGH treated groups in both studies, which suggests that rhGH may interact detrimentally on immunologic function in this population of patients. The discrepancy between the results of these two large randomized trials with previous studies in burn or trauma patients may be due to differences in patient populations and the time at which therapy was initiated. The studies by Takala et al.[58] excluded burn patients, and patients with trauma accounted for only 10% of the population. RhGH therapy was initiated 5 to 7 days after ICU admission in Takala's studies concurrent with the early phase of the augmented inflammatory response seen in critically ill patients as compared with later administration of rhGH in other studies. Consequently the early administration of rhGH may have accelerated cellular metabolic rate and increased catecholamine levels leading to a further energy deficit in these patients at a time when their cellular oxygen demands were the highest.[62] This theory is congruent with the evolving observation of GH resistance in the early phases of critical illness followed by a reduced pulsatile release of GH with low circulating levels of IGF-1 during the chronic phase.[34] Other patient and nutritional characteristics that complicate the use of GH and other anabolic agents and complicate the interpretation of clinical trials of rhGH have been outlined by Wilmore.[41] The most important of these are the nutritional status of the patient, the interaction between GH and the nutrients delivered, and the effect of inflammation on GH mediated protein synthesis. Moreover, an interaction exists between patient albumin levels and site of surgery, with those undergoing esophageal, pancreatic, or gastric surgery at greatest risk for postoperative morbidity and mortality. Consequently, care should be taken to enroll and stratify patients with these high risk characteristics appropriately prior to randomization into trials assessing nutritional or anabolic agents.[63]

Conclusions

Future considerations in the use of anabolic agents in the ICU must consider the nutritional status of the patient, the timing of the therapeutic intervention with respect to the onset of the inflammatory response, and the specific peptide within the GH axis to be used to promote anabolism. Preference may be given to GHRH related peptides or IGF-1 over rhGH. An infusion of GHRP-2 or GHRH plus GHRP-2 resulted in a 60%–100% rise in serum IGF-1 levels, which may be more pronounced than that generated by high doses of daily exogenous GH, hence providing a rationale for the use of these peptides in order to endogenously (vs. exogenously) stimulate IGF-1 production.[36] Alternatively, theoretical advantages of IGF-1, including the fact that IGF-1 enhances cellular proliferation and insulin sensitivity and attenuates intestinal atrophy and abnormal ion transport induced by TPN, may provide a rationale to use a combination of rhGH and IGF-1 as anabolic agents in critically ill patients.[39]

References

1. Chang DW, DeSanti L, Demling RH. Anticatabolic and anabolic strategies in critical illness: a review of current treatment modalities. *SHOCK.* 1998;10:155–160.
2. Kinney JM, Duke JH, Long CL, et al. Tissue fuel and weight loss after injury. *J Clin Path.* 1970;23[Suppl]:65–72.
3. Moore FA. Effects of immune-enhancing diets on infectious morbidity and multiple organ failure. *J Parenter Enteral Nutr.* 2001;25:S36–S43.
4. Oltermann MH, Rassas TN. Immunonutrition in a multidisciplinary ICU population: a review of the literature. *J Parenter Enteral Nutr.* 2001;25:S30–S35.
5. Bistrian BR. Influence of total parenteral nutrition on immune function. In: Faist E, Baue AE, Schildberg FW, eds. *The Immune Consequences of Trauma, Shock and Sepsis—Mechanisms and Therapeutic Approaches.* Volume 2/2. Pabst Science Publishers; 1996:881–885.
6. Oberholzer A, Oberholzer C, Moldawer LL. Cytokine signaling-regulation of the immune response in normal and critically ill states. *Crit Care Med.* 2000;28[Suppl.]:N3–N12.
7. Reinhart K, Wiegand-Lohnert C, Grimminger F, et al. Assessment of the safety and efficacy of the monoclonal anti-tumor necrosis factor antibody-fragment, mak 195f, in patients with sepsis and septic shock: a multicenter, randomized, placebo-controlled, dose-ranging study. *Crit Care Med.* 1996;24:733–742.

8. Neidhart R, Keel M, Steckholzer U, et al. Relationship of Interleukin-10 plasma levels to severity of injury and clinical outcome in injured patients. *J Trauma.* 1997; 42:863–870.
9. Sherry RM, Cue JI, Goddard JK, et al. Interleukin-10 is associated with the development of sepsis in trauma patients. *J Trauma.* 1996;40:613–616.
10. Weissman C. The metabolic response to stress: an overview and update. *Anaesthesiology.* 1990;73:308–327.
11. Annane D, Sebille V, Troche G. et al. A 3-level prognostic classification in septic shock based on cortisol levels and cortisol response to corticotropin. *JAMA.* 2000;283: 1038–1045.
12. Bulger, EM, Maier RV. Lipid mediators in the pathophysiology of critical illness. *Crit Care Med.* 2000;28[Suppl.]: N27–N36.
13. Esmon CT, Taylor FB Jr, Snow TR. Inflammation and coagulation: linked processes potentially regulated through a common pathway mediated by protein C. *Thromb Haemost.* 1991;66:160–165.
14. Stouthard JM, Levi M, Hack CE, et al. Interleukin-6 stimulates coagulation, not fibrinolysis, in humans. *Thromb Haemost.* 1996;76:738–742.
15. Bevilacqua MP, Pober JS, Majeau GR, et al. recombinant tumor necrosis induces procoagulant activity in cultured human vascular endothelium: characterization and comparison with the actions of interleukin 1. *Proc Natl Acad Sci USA.* 1986;12:4533–4537.
16. Mavrommatis AC, Theodoridis T, Orfanidou A, et al. Coagulation system and platelets are fully activated in uncomplicated sepsis. *Crit Care Med.* 2000;28:451–457.
17. Bernard GR, Vincent JL, Laterre PF, et al. Efficacy & safety of recombinant human activated protein C for severe sepsis. *New Engl J Med.* 2001. Mar 8;344:699–709.
18. Matushak GM. Multiple organ system failure: clinical expression, pathogenesis and therapy. In: Hall JB, Schmidt GA, Wood LDH, eds. *Principles of Critical Care*, 2nd Edition. New York: McGraw-Hill; 1998:221–248.
19. Papathanassoglou ED, Moynihan JA, Ackerman MH. Does programmed cell death (apoptosis) play a role in the development of organ dysfunction in critically ill patients. A review and theoretical framework. *Crit Care Med.* 2000;28:537–549.
20. Hotchkiss RS, Swanson PE, Freeman BD, et al. Apoptotic cell death in patients with sepsis, shock and multiple organ dysfunction. *Crit Care Med.* 1999;27:1230–1251.
21. Graves RJ. *Lectures on the Practice of Medicine*. Dublin: New Sydenham Society;1884.
22. McClave SA, Iowen CC, Kleber MJ, et al. Are patients fed appropriately according to their caloric requirements? *J Parenter Enteral Nutr.* 1998;22:375–387.
23. Ahmad A, Duerksen DR, Munroe S, et al. An evaluation of resting energy expenditure in hospitalized, severely underweight patients. *Nutrition.* 1999;15:384–388.
24. Chang DW, DeSanti L, Demling RH. Ref 41 A.S.P.E.N. Board of Directors: Guidelines for the use of parenteral and enteral nutrition in adult and pediatric patients. *J Parenter Enteral Nutr.* 1993;17:1–52.
25. Meyer NA, Muller MJ, Herndon DN. Nutrient support of the healing wound. *Soc of Crit Care Med.* 1994;2:202–214.
26. Shamoon H, Hendler R, Sherwin RS. Synergistic interactions of anti-insulin hormones in man. *J Clin Endocrinol Metab.* 1981;52:1235–1241.
27. Gottlisch M, Jenkins M, Warden G, et al. Differential effects of three enteral regimens on selective outcome variables and burn patients. *J Parenter Enteral Nutr.* 14:225–236.
28. Debiasse MA, Wilmore DW. What is optimal nutritional support? *Soc of Crit Care Med.* 1994;2:122–130.
29. Clements RH, Hayes CA, Gibbs ER, et al. Insulin's anabolic effect is influenced by route of administration of nutrients. *Arch Surg.* 1999;134:274–277.
30. Woolfson AMJ, Heatley RV, Allison SP. Insulin to inhibit protein catabolism after injury. *N Engl J Med.* 1979;300: 14–17.
31. Haupt HA, Rovere GD. Anabolic steroids: a review of the literature. *Amer J Sports Med.* 1984;12:469–484.
32. Demling RH, DeSanti L. Increased protein intake during the recovery phase after severe burns increases body weight gain and muscle function. *J Burn Care & Rehab* 1998;19:161–168.
33. Gervasio JM, Dickerson FN, Sweeringen J, et al. Oxandrolone in trauma patients. *Pharmacotherapy.* 2000;20: 1328–1334.
34. Van den Berghe G. Novel insights into the neuroendocrinology of critical illness. *Euro J Endocrinol.* 2000;143:1–13.
35. Frost RA, Lang CH. Growth factors in critical illness: regulation and therapeutic aspects. *Curr Opin Clin Nutr Metab Care.* 1998;1:195–204.
36. Van den Berghe G, DeZegher F, Veldhuis JD, et al. The somatotropic axis in critical illness: effect of continuous growth hormone (GH)-releasing hormone and GH-releasing peptide-2 infusion. *J Clin Endocrinol Metab.* 1997; 82:590–599.
37. Van den Berghe G, Wouters P, Bowers CY, et al. Growth hormone-releasing peptide-2 infusion synchronizes growth hormone, thyrotropin and prolactin release in prolonged critical illness. *Euro J Endocrinol.* 1990;140:17–22.
38. Ross RJM, Rodriguez-Arnao J, Bentham J, et al. The role of insulin, growth hormone and IGF-I as anabolic agents in the critically ill. *Intensive Care Med.* 1991;19:S54–S57.
39. Ney DM. Effects of insulin-like growth factor-1 and growth hormone in models of parenteral nutrition. *J Parenter Enteral Nutr.* 1999;23:S184–S189.
40. Roth E, Valentini L, Semsroth M, et al. Resistance of nitrogen metabolism to growth hormone treatment in the early phase after injury of patients with multiple injuries. *J Trauma: Injury, Infect & Crit Care.* 1995;38:136–141.
41. Wilmore DW. Impediments to the successful use of anabolic agents in clinical care. *J Parenter Enteral Nutr.* 1999; 23:S210–S213.
42. Ramzy PI, Wolf SE, Herndon DN. Current status of anabolic hormone administration in human burn injury. *J Parenter Enteral Nutr.* 1999;23:S190–S194.

43. Ziegler TR, Young LS, Ferrari-Baliviera E, et al. Use of human growth hormone combined with nutritional support in a critical care unit. *J Parenter Enteral Nutr.* 1990; 14:574–581.

44. Gottardis M, Benzer A, Koller W, et al. Improvement of septic syndrome after administration of recombinant human growth hormone (rhGH)? *J Trauma.* 1991;31:81–86.

45. Fleming RYD, Rutan RL, Jahoor F, et al. Effect of recombinant human growth hormone on catabolic hormones and free fatty acids following thermal injury. *J Trauma.* 1992;32:698–702.

46. Pichard C, Kyle U, Chevrole J, et al. Lack of effects of recombinant growth hormone on muscle function in patients requiring prolonged mechanical ventilation: a prospective, randomized, controlled study. *Crit Care Med.* 1996;24:403–413.

47. Voerman BJ, Strack van Schijndel RJM, Groeneveld ABJ, et al. Effects of recombinant human growth hormone in patients with severe sepsis. *Ann Surg.* 1992;216:648–655.

48. Voerman BJ, Strack van Schijndel RJM, Groeneveld ABJ, et al. Effects of human growth hormone in critically ill nonseptic patients: results from a prospective, randomized, placebo-controlled trial. *Crit Care Med.* 1995;23:665–673.

49. Hammarqvist F, Stromberg C, Von Der Decken A, et al. Biosynthetic human growth hormone preserves both muscle protein synthesis and the decrease in muscle-free glutamine and improves whole-body nitrogen economy after operation. *Ann Surg.* 1992;216:184–191.

50. Koea JB, Breier BH, Douglas RG, et al. Anabolic and cardiovascular effects of recombinant human growth hormone in surgical patients with sepsis. *Br J Surg.* 1996;83: 196–202.

51. Ziegler TR, Rombeau JL, Young LS, et al. Recombinant human growth hormone enhances the metabolic efficiency of parenteral nutrition: a double blind, randomized controlled study. *J Clin Endo Metab.* 1992;74:865–873.

52. Jeevanandam M, Ali MR, Holaday NJ, et al. Adjuvant recombinant human growth hormone normalizes plasma amino acids in parenterally fed trauma patients. *J Parenter Enteral Nutr.* 1995;19:137–144.

53. Gatzen C, Scheltinga MR, Kimbrough TD, et al. Growth hormone attenuates the abnormal distribution of body water in critically ill surgical patients. *Surgery.* 1992;112:181–187.

54. Barle H, Gamrin L, Essen P, et al. Growth hormone does not affect albumin synthesis in the critically ill. *Intensive Care Med.* 2001;27:836–843.

55. Ramirez RJ, Wolf SE, Barrow Re, et al. Growth hormone treatment in pediatric burns: a safe therapeutic approach. *Ann Surg.* 1998;228:439–448.

56. Herndon DN, Barrow RE, Kunkel KR, et al. Effects of recombinant human growth hormone on donor-site healing in severely burned children. *Ann Surg.* 1990;212:424–429.

57. Knox, J, Demling R, Wilmore D, et al. Increased survival after major thermal injury: the effect of growth hormone therapy in adults. *J Trauma: Injury, Infection & Crit Care.* 1995;39:526–530.

58. Takala J, Ruokonen E, Webster NR, et al. Increased mortality associated with growth hormone treatment in critically ill adults. *N Eng J Med.* 1999;341:785–792.

59. Van den Berghe G, De Zagher F, Lauwers P, et al. Growth hormone secretion in critical illness: effect of dopamine. *J Clin Endocrinol Metab.* 1994;79:1141–1146.

60. Kudsk, KA, Mowatt-Larssen C, Bukar J, et al. Effect of recombinant human insulin-like growth factor 1 and early total parenteral nutrition on immune depression following severe head injury. *Arch Surg.* 1994;129:66–71.

61. Voerman BJ, Strack van Schijndel RJ, de Boer H, et al. Effects of human growth hormone on fuel utilization and mineral balance in critically ill patients on full intravenous nutritional support. *J Crit Care.* 1994;9:143–150.

62. Demling R. Growth hormone therapy in critically ill patients. *N Engl J Med.* 1999; 341:837–838.

63. Kudsk KA. Discrepancies between nutrition outcome studies: is patient care the issue? *J Parenter Enteral Nutr.* 2001;25:S57–S60.

CHAPTER

32 Special Nutrient Formulas (Neutraceuticals)

Hank Schmidt, M.D., Robert G. Martindale, M.D., F.A.C.S.

INTRODUCTION	357	OMEGA-3 FATTY ACIDS	360
ARGININE	358	CLINICAL EVIDENCE	361
GLUTAMINE	359	REFERENCES	363
NUCLEOTIDES	360		

Introduction

The importance of nutritional support in surgical patients cannot be overstated, particularly in the realm of intensive care settings. In the past two decades we have come to understand the benefits of enteral feeding over total parenteral nutrition. Prevention of mucosal atrophy and stimulation of the gut-associated lymphoid tissue (GALT) by early enteral feeding in post-operative surgical patients has only recently become part of our standard of care. Feeding the gut is clearly a stimulant for the immune system and plays a key role in lower infection rates measured in patients receiving enteral as opposed to parenteral nutrition. This association between nutrition and infection has been known for centuries. The World Health Organization report in 1968 clearly defines this association and begins to set goals in clinical nutrition.[1] The understanding of the gastrointestinal tract as a major component of the human immune system and a key modulator of the organism's response to stress and injury has subsequently opened the door to an exciting new field of specialized enteral preparations sometimes referred to as neutraceuticals.

The recent expansion of our understanding of stress metabolism and the systemic inflammatory response has influenced critical care nutrition on two levels. First, as stated above, is the importance of provision of enteral macro-nutrients, namely a patient's requirement for protein, carbohydrate, and lipids. Secondly, research in neutraceuticals seems to have focused on various combinations of micro-nutrients and "conditionally" essential nutrients. Neutraceuticals are felt to function in cellular metabolic pathways where increased demands associated with stress response benefit from supplementation. These nutrients may be the key to fine-tuning enteral formulas for specific clinical scenarios.

For centuries, man has sought the therapeutic benefits of naturally occurring substances as components of the human diet, acknowledging the connection between health and nutrition. Herbal teas, roots, plants, and animal products are by no means limited to the history of medicine, as the market for alternative pharmaceuticals continues to expand.[2] With the explosion of knowledge and analytical techniques in biochemistry and molecular biology, investigators may now pinpoint the specific role of many of these elements in human metabolism. This same knowledge has also produced a far greater understanding of the systemic response to stress, affected by severe catabolism and loss of lean body mass.[3] Historically, nutritional support in critically ill patients has sought to provide adequate calories and protein to induce nitrogen balance, preventing peripheral muscle breakdown. However, we have learned that provision of adequate protein and calories does not prevent loss of lean body mass in the critically ill patient. With an enhanced appreciation for the connection between enteral feeding and immune response, our attention has turned to supplementation of caloric requirements with specific nutrients designed to affect critical metabolic pathways. One of the earliest clinical studies evaluating such selective supplementation randomized burn patients to receive a modular tube feeding recipe (MTF), or one of two other enteral nutritional regimens traditionally used in this population. The MTF consisted of a high-protein, low-fat formulation enriched in omega-3 fatty acids, arginine, cysteine, histidine, zinc, vitamin A, and ascorbic acid. Significant benefits were observed in MTF fed patients, who had lower infection rates (75% fewer) and shorter length of hospital stay (31%) on a percent burn basis. This study may also lend support to the immunosuppressive effects of omega-6 polyunsaturated fats, as 70% of total deaths occurred in the group supported with higher fat and linoleic acid content formulations.[4]

Since the first recognition of enteral nutrition as an immunomodulatory phenomenon, investigators have been challenged to find "the right mix" for any given patient or clinical scenario. This knowledge has also essentially created a market to drive pharmaceutical research in this direction. There are six products currently marketed as immunonutrition formulas. We are now faced with the challenge of optimizing specific preparations through in-depth analysis of micronutrients and their individual roles in human metabolism. A wealth of in vitro, in vivo, animal, and human data has been produced in the process of examining the physiology of dietary nucleic acids, arginine, glutamine, omega-3 fatty acids, and an array of other less studied nutrients. (See Table 32.1.)

Arginine

Arginine, like glutamine, is classified as a non-essential amino acid in unstressed conditions since the body synthesizes adequate arginine for normal maintenance of tissue metabolism, growth, and repair.[5] During major catabolic insults such as trauma or surgery, an increase in urinary nitrogen, excreted largely as urea, represents the end products of increased lean body tissue catabolism and reprioritized protein synthesis. As the activity of the urea cycle increases, so does the

TABLE 32.1

Immune-Modulated Enteral Formulas

Formula	Manufacturer	Major additives
Crucial®	Nestle	Marine oil; Arginine
Immuno-Aid®	BBraun	Arginine; Glutamine BCAA; Nucleic acids
Impact®	Novartis	Arginine; Structured lipid RNA
Intensical®	Meade/Johnson	Arginine; Canola oil; Fish oil
Optimental®	Ross	Arginine; Structured lipid; Fish oil; Canola oil

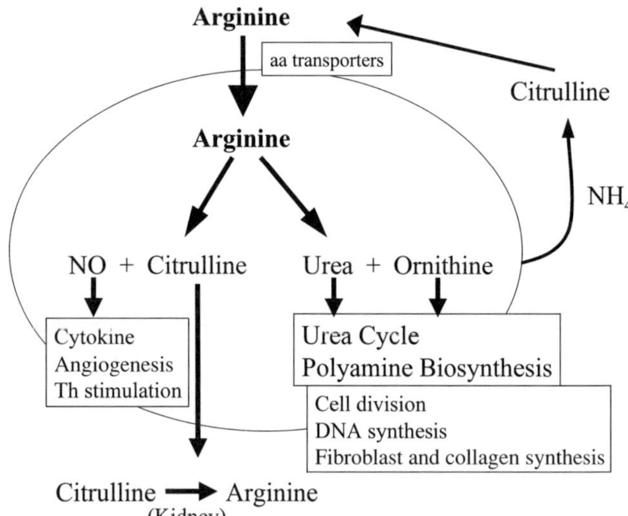

Figure 32.1

Arginine Metabolism

metabolic demand for arginine. Arginine during these stress situations becomes conditionally essential in that demand is greater than endogenous supply (Figure 32.1).

Numerous animal and human studies indicate that supplemental dietary arginine is beneficial for accelerated wound healing, enhanced immune response, and acceleration in attainment of positive nitrogen balance.[6] The exact mechanisms for these benefits are yet to be entirely understood but may in part be the result of arginine's role as a potent anabolic hormone secretagogue. Growth hormone, glucagons, prolactin, and insulin release are all increased with supplemental arginine. Arginine is also the substrate for production of nitric oxide and citrulline by nitric oxide synthase. Nitric oxide is a ubiquitous molecule with significant roles in the maintenance of vascular tone, coagulation cascade, immunity, stimulation of angiogenesis, modulation of the effects of endotoxin, and regulation of GI tract absorptive and barrier function.[7] Nitric oxide has also been implicated as a participant in numerous disease states as diverse as sepsis, hypertension, and cirrhosis. Arginine is also the substrate for the enzyme arginase with end products urea and ornithine. Through the production of ornithine and urea, arginine promotes proliferation of fibroblasts and collagen, both essential for later stages of wound healing. Arginine and its metabolite ornithine also serve as precursors for polyamine biosynthesis. Polyamines play a pivotal role in cell division and DNA synthesis.[8] By supplying the amidino group for creatine synthesis, arginine is important in maintaining the reserve of high energy phosphate required for ATP generation in muscle.

In animal models arginine supplementation has been associated with improved wound healing with increased wound tensile strength and collagen deposition. Using a wound healing model, Barbul et al.[6] observed enhanced collagen deposition in human volunteers with supplemental arginine. Arginine-supplemented rats have been shown to have improved thymic function as assessed by thymic weight, the total number of thymic lymphocytes, and the mitogenic reactivity of thymic lymphocytes to phytohemagglutinin and concanavalin A.[7] Animal studies using arginine supplementation have shown improved survival in burns, intraperitoneal bacterial challenge, cecal ligation and puncture, and tumor implantation models.[7]

The majority of human studies have included arginine in combination with other so called "immune modulating" elements, making it impossible to define the specific arginine influence. While supplemental arginine has been shown to improve survival in various animal models as well as a number of in vitro measures of immune function in animals and humans, the benefit of arginine supplementation alone needs further large scale studies to confirm its benefits in the clinical setting. Certainly the early data suggest that arginine upregulates immune function, modulates vascular flow patterns, and supports nitrogen balance.[9,10]

Glutamine

Glutamine is the most abundant amino acid in the body and makes up greater than 50% of the free amino acid pool.[11] Containing five carbons and two nitrogen moieties makes glutamine the major interorgan donor of nitrogen and carbon. Glutamine is now considered conditionally essential, meaning that during major catabolic insults, demand for glutamine is greater than supply. Glutamine can be synthesized in most tissues of the body, but skeletal muscle, by virtue of its mass, produces the majority of endogenous glutamine. Glutamine is the primary fuel for many rapidly dividing tissues such as the small bowel mucosa and proliferating lymphocytes.[12] Glutamine has numerous metabolic roles including maintenance of acid-base status, as a precursor of urinary ammonia, as the primary fuel source for enterocytes, as fuel source for lymphocytes and macrophages, and as a precursor for nucleotides, arginine, glutathione, and glucosamine.[13] Glutamine is also a major contributor to gluconeogenesis and is the primary substrate for renal gluconeogenesis in humans.[13] Recent reports also support a role for glutamine in decreasing peripheral insulin resistance in stress models.[13] A 50% reduction in free glutamine supply has been documented after both elective operations as well as major injury. During catabolic illness glutamine uptake by the small intestine and immunologically active cells may exceed glutamine synthetic rates and release from skeletal muscle, making glutamine a conditionally essential amino acid.[11,14]

There is a rapidly growing volume of human data regarding the use of glutamine supplementation both enterally and parenterally.[5] The majority, estimated at 70% to 80% of luminally supplied glutamine, is metabolized by the enterocyte, minimizing access to the systemic circulation. Clearly the target for enterally supplied glutamine is the splanchnic bed and gut associated lymphoid tissue (GALT). In animal models, supplemental glutamine has been shown to enhance intestinal adaptation after massive small bowel resection,[15] to attenuate intestinal and pancreatic atrophy,[5] and to prevent hepatic steatosis associated with parenteral and enteral feeding.[13] Glutamine appears to maintain gastrointestinal tract mucosal thickness, maintain DNA and protein content, reduce bacteremia and mortality after chemotherapy, and reduce bacteremia and mortality following sepsis or endotoxemia.[13]

In humans undergoing surgical stress, glutamine-supplemented parenteral nutrition appears to help maintain nitrogen balance and the intracellular glutamine pool in skeletal muscle.[16] A recent trauma study reported a greater than 50% decrease in pneumonia compared to an isonitrogenous, isocaloric control population.[17] A decrease in bacteremia and sepsis was also noted. In critically ill patients, glutamine supplementation may attenuate villous atrophy and the increased intestinal mucosal permeability associated with parenteral nutrition. Intravenous glutamine supplementation in a randomized, blinded trial of 84 critically ill patients showed significant improvement in long-term mortality.[18] In another study bone marrow transplant patients were randomized in a blinded fashion to glutamine or an isonitrogenous formula, resulting in fewer infections, improved nitrogen balance, and significantly shorter mean hospital length of stay.[19] Glutamine supplementation has also been shown to aid in protecting the GI tract against chemotherapy induced mucosal toxicity.[17] Oral glutamine supplementation reduced the severity and decreased the duration of stomatitis that occurred during chemotherapy in bone marrow transplant.[20] Glutamine supplementation at 30 g/d in esophageal cancer patients undergoing radiation was shown to preserve lymphocyte response and decrease gut permeability.[21]

While a large volume of animal and human data supports the concept that glutamine is beneficial in a variety of experimental models, the benefit of routine enteral glutamine supplementation in critically ill human patients remain somewhat controversial. Well-designed clinical trials with clearly defined endpoints and adequate statistical power are needed to assess whether the beneficial effects demonstrated in GI physiology, immune function and postoperative metabolism translate into a reduction in hospital stay and mortality rate in all ICU populations. It is clear that glutamine is a major contributor to homeostasis in the ICU population.

Nucleotides

Nucleotides are yet another important component in the concept of immune modulation. The average American diet contains 1–2 grams per day of nucleotides. Nucleotides are made up of the purine and pyrimidine backbone with a ribose and one to three phosphates. Human breast milk contains approximately 30% of its protein as nonprotein nitrogen while nucleotides make up 5% of the nonprotein nitrogen. In the production of commercial formula, the nucleotides are removed during processing for whey and casein concentrates. This has led to the speculation that critically ill patients fed enteral formulas may in fact have an inadequate supply of nucleotides. Several infant and animal models have shown that supplementation of nucleotides can decrease GI infections and increase natural killer (NK) cells, villous height, and mucosal enzyme activity.

Nucleotides are available to the host via de novo synthesis or from salvage pathways of DNA and RNA degradation. The synthesis requires substrates of glutamine, aspartate, glycine, and formate. Activity and contribution of the salvage pathways may vary among tissues and with phases of the cell cycle. Nucleotides serve an array of vital functions including signal transduction, regulation of enzyme activity, synthesis of macromolecular compounds such as glycogen and phospholipids, promotion of gut development and maintenance of mucosal integrity, tissue repair, and cell turnover. Ogoshi et al. have reported various combinations of nucleotides in specific ratios to be cytoprotective, increase hepatic regrowth after partial hepatectomy, increase oxidative phosphorylation, and decrease TPN-induced gut permeability in a rat model.[22]

Therefore, one may speculate that in critical illness, nucleotide requirements are elevated in the face of hypermetabolism and activated immune response. This scenario is confirmed by numerous animal studies demonstrating impaired mucosal function in nucleotide depleted diets that could be reversed by oral supply of these substrates.[23,24] In a model system for Crohn's disease involving indomethacin-induced enteritis in rats, supplementation of diets with 1% yeast RNA allowed a significant improvement in ulcer healing.[25] Studies using supplemental oral nucleotides are somewhat more controversial in that only 0.05% of each oral dose is measured in the circulation. This may in fact be a protective mechanism, preventing overstimulation of purinergic signal activation. The benefits of nucleotide supplementation appear consistent across tissues and species in relation to gut barrier and immune function. The exact mechanisms to explain these benefits are far from understood. Clearly it is not just immune stimulation or alteration in the inflammatory response. Nucleotide supplementation does appear safe at the levels currently supplied in commercial formulas.

Omega-3 Fatty Acids

Considerable effort has also been dedicated to investigation of the role of fatty acid metabolism in the inflammatory and immune response. The typical western diet now contains significantly more omega-6 than omega-3 fatty acids. In addition it is now apparent that lipid membranes are strongly influenced by dietary lipid profiles. Dietary changes in lipids have been shown to alter T-cell proliferation, cell-cell adhesive properties, plasma membrane fluidity, and cytokine response to various stimuli.[26]

It has also recently been shown that high levels of polyunsaturated fatty acids (PUFA), especially linoleic acid, have a suppressive effect on neutrophils, lymphocytes, monocytes, and macrophage function in both in-vitro and in-vivo studies. The more specific immunosuppressive influence includes inhibition of lymphocyte proliferation, decrease in neutrophil chemotaxis and migration, impairment of the reticuloendothelial system, and decrease in the bactericidal capacity. Exchange of subtypes of fatty acids limits production of arachadonic acid metabolites such as thromboxane A2, prostaglandin E2 and I2, as well as leukotriene B4, all mediators of the systemic inflammatory response and hypermetabolism in sepsis. Therefore, the effect of omega-3 fatty acids likely comes from profound alteration in the immunoregulatory process achieved by elaboration of various cytokines, interleukins, and interferons.[27] Early studies in the Eskimo population of

Greenland demonstrated that their diets enriched in omega-3 fatty acids conveyed lower risk of coronary artery disease, likely due to diminished platelet aggregation and thrombosis, both of which are directly influenced by platelet activating factor release stimulated by cytokines and other products of membrane phospholipid metabolism.[28] Omega-3 fatty acids have been reported to decrease cardiovascular disease, inflammatory diseases, autoimmune disease, and type I diabetes, and have been associated with a lower incidence of colon and breast cancer. A number of animal studies have confirmed the benefit of omega-3 fatty acids in terms of reduction of post-burn metabolic rate, mortality from infection, bacterial translocation rate, and response to LPS. With regard to critically ill patients, the relevance of dietary omega-3 fatty acids is clear in light of their attenuation of the inflammatory response, anti-thrombotic effects, prevention of overproduction of PGE-2 to stress stimuli, and depression of plasma triglyceride levels. In addition to the dietary influence in cell membrane changes, recent evidence now indicates that fatty acid ratio changes can have acute effects on platelet adhesiveness, neutrophil function, membrane stability, and alteration in microvascular perfusion. Reduced production of vasoactive mediators by elimination of omega-6 fatty acids likely limits splanchnic vasoconstriction thereby modulating gut ischemia during stress, minimizing bacterial translocation, and preserving GALT integrity. Clearly, numerous complex molecular mechanisms are involved that are beyond the scope of this chapter. In general it is felt that in the critical care setting, increasing omega-3 fatty acid levels compete with cyclo-oxygenase metabolism to limit the omega-6 production of PGE-2 and leukotrienes of the 4 series, all of which are pro-inflammatory and/or function to limit microvascular flow. Numerous animal studies and one very important clinical study in ARDS patients, using a formula enriched with omega-3 fatty acids, reported fewer ventilator days and shorter duration of ICU stay.[29]

Clinical Evidence

Since 1990 there have been 26 prospective randomized human trials investigating the effects of immunonutrition in hospitalized patients. Results of these studies vary; they have been extensively scrutinized for several variables, including lack of feeding comparisons, lack of homogenous study population comparisons, and methods of data analysis. Despite the variations in study design, the majority of the well-designed studies demonstrate a clear benefit in terms of reduced infection rates, decreased antibiotic use, and reduced ICU and hospital length of stay. These studies may be best approached by categorizing each into subgroups including general ICU, gastrointestinal surgery, trauma, burn, and sepsis/multi-organ system failure patients. Obviously some overlap exists in these patient populations; however, this classification is adequate for examination of trends in all series combined. Bower and colleagues examined a general intensive care unit population of 296 patients, randomized to enteral feedings supplemented with arginine, dietary nucleotides, and fish oil (Impact®, Novartis, Minneapolis, MN) or a control formula within 48 hours of study entry event.[30] Patients given the experimental formula had a substantial reduction in length of hospital stay and a significant reduction in frequency of acquired infections.

Five prospective randomized trials have been published limiting the study to include only trauma patients.[31–35] Of these studies, four demonstrated advantages to early immune-enhancing enteral feedings in terms of incidence of SIRS, resolution of hypermetabolism, infectious complications, length of hospital stay, incidence of intra-abdominal abscesses, and multi-system organ failure. The patient populations in these studies ranged from 32 to 98 subjects, and each protocol compared different formulations (Impact® [Novartis, Minneapolis, MN], Perative® [Ross Laboratories, Columbus, OH], or Immun-Aid® [BBraun, Irvine, CA]). The study by Mendez and colleagues failed to show significant improvements in outcome measures. This study reported an increase in ventilator days and more ARDS in the experimental group. Several concerns of study design have limited the acceptance of this study. Mendez et al.[32] had a 25% unexplained dropout rate, with the experimental group enduring significantly higher rates of ARDS at initiation of the study.

Supplemented enteral formulas allowed significantly fewer infectious complications and shorter length of stay in acutely burned patients as well.[4] Similar analyses have been carried out in "general surgery" patient populations, many of whom presented for resection of gastrointestinal cancer.[36–43] The vast majority of these studies revealed a lower rate of postoperative infections and shorter length of hospital stay in patients given supplemented enteral formulas. Other benefits included earlier liberation from mechanical ventilation, shorter length of ICU stay, improved phagocytic ability of monocytes, and decreased IL-6 plasma concentrations. Three studies in particular were able to predict a cost savings per patient in treating fewer complications when using supplemented enteral formulations. It is likely that this result may be extrapolated to other studies when shorter length of hospital stay and decreased cost incurred by infectious complications are weighed against provision of an immune-enhancing enteral feeding.

There are now three meta-analyses encompassing most major prospective randomized clinical trials on supplemented enteral feeding[9,44,45] (Table 32.2). Both studies published in 1999 demonstrated reduced infection rates and shorter duration of hospital stay in patients with critical illness who received enteral nutrition supplemented with key nutrients. The study by Heys et al.[9] found no change in overall mortality, however, in this patient population. In the meta-analysis by Beale et al.[44] of 1482 patients in 12 trials, patients administered the supplemented enteral formula also spent significantly fewer days supported with mechanical ventilation. The third meta-analysis by Heyland et al.[45] examined 2402 patients in 22 randomized trials involving enteral nutrient formulas supplemented with omega-3 fatty acids, arginine, and nucleotides. As in previous studies, immunonutrient formulas were associated with decreased infection rates and decreased length of stay. In a subset analysis, critically ill septic patients (as opposed to surgical patients) demonstrated a higher mortality rate when given supplemented formulas. Overall Impact® and Immun-Aid® produced lower mortality rates than in groups using other formulas. Therefore, the authors conclude that further study is necessary to identify subgroups of patients who will benefit from neutraceuticals.

We are now able to examine a significant number of patients enrolled in randomized studies on immune enhancing nutrition. From this data we are obligated to develop a new standard of care for use of neutraceuticals in critically ill patients. We may now be able to define which patients benefit from this intervention as opposed to which patients incur higher mortality, which formula should be given, when should it be used and for what duration. Some of these issues were recently addressed at the U.S. Summit on Immune-Enhancing Enteral Therapy (San Diego, CA; May, 2000)[46] in an attempt to clarify recommendations for use (Table 32.3). This group proposed a benefit for patients undergoing elective gastrointestinal surgery who are moderately to severely malnourished (albumin <3.5), as well as patients presenting with blunt and penetrating torso trauma (abdominal trauma index 20; injury severity score 18).[46] Therefore, immune enhancing diets (IED) should be of little benefit in well-nourished pre-operative patients with albumin >3.5. The consensus group added other populations who "should" benefit from IED, however the data at this time is insufficient to firmly justify IED use. This list includes major vascular surgery in patients with COPD, major head and neck resection with malnutrition preoperatively, severe head injury (GCS <8), major burn (>30% TBSA), and ventilator-dependent patients at high risk for subsequent infections. Likewise, populations expected *not* to benefit were also specified by the group, including patients resuming oral ad lib diet in 5 days, ICU patients requiring monitoring only, presence of bowel obstruction distal to the site of access, incomplete resuscitation, low perfusion states, and presence of major upper gastrointestinal hemorrhage. Another issue addressed was the time of initiation of IED. It appears that many patients benefit from this therapy even before the insult of injury or other stress. In any case nutrients should be supplemented immediately after resuscitation. The authors recommend a dose of approximately 1200 to 1500 mL per day or until 50% to 60% of nutrient goal is met.

In summary, we now have a wealth of animal and human data attempting to elucidate the appropriate mix of "immune modulating" nutrients, the adequate

TABLE 32.2

Immunonutrition

Author	Journal	Patients	Studies	Outcome
Heys	Ann Surg 1999	1009	11	Decreased infection rate Decreased hospital stay No change in mortality
Beale	CCM 1999	1482	12	Decreased infection Decreased ventilator days Decreased hospital stay
Heyland	JAMA	2419	22	Decreased infection Decreased hospital stay ? mortality

TABLE 32.3

Immunonutrition: Consensus Statement May, 2000

Expected benefit

- Major GI surgery
- Serious trauma (ISS >17, ATI >19)

Probable benefit

- Major vascular with COPD
- Major head and neck resection
- Severe closed head injury (Glascow <9)
- Major burn (>30% TBSA)
- Ventilator dependent with high risk for subsequent infection

level of nutrient required to show benefit, and most important, the clinical scenarios yielding the best outcome with use of immune modulating formulas. Some basic tenets should be observed prior to any attempt at nutritional immune modulation: patients must be adequately volume resuscitated; enteral nutrition is the preferred route of delivery; enteral feeding should be advanced only when tolerated; and basic calorie, protein, and micronutrient needs must be met and not exceeded.

What is more controversial, yet apparent from multiple clinical trials is that the concept of immunonutrition is now not only theoretical, but can yield clinical benefit. Subtle differences in patient selection, population studies, and nutrient mix can explain the outcome differences in the relevant studies. As mentioned above, the "exact" blend of nutrients is yet to be established. Additional research is needed in the arena of single nutrient supplementation to better define mechanisms in humans. We can state that nutritional modulation of the metabolic and immune response is possible, appears beneficial in specific patient populations, and is safe when used appropriately. Continued, rigorous, critical evaluations of the data are needed as more immunonutrients and "nutraceuticals" are reported for modulation of immune function. Increasing awareness of the potential beneficial pharmacologic effects of nutrients in promoting optimal ICU outcomes can only be helpful.

References

1. Scrimshaw NS, Taylor CE, Gordon JE. Interactions of Nutrition and Infection. Geneva, Switzerland: World Health Organization; 1968. Monograph series Number 57.
2. Gorski T. Defining and assessing alternative medicine practices. *JAMA*. 1996;276:195–196.
3. Wilmore DW. Homeostasis: Bodily changes in trauma and surgery In: Sabiston DL, ed. *Textbook of Surgery: The Biological Basis of Modern Surgical Practice*. Philadelphia: WB Saunders, 1997:55–67.
4. Gottschlich MM, Jenkins M, Warden GD, et al. Differential effects of three enteral dietary regimens on selected outcome variables in burn patients. *J Parenter Enteral Nutr*. 1990;14:225–236.
5. DeBandt JP, Cynober LA. Amino acids with anabolic properties. *Curr Opin Clin Nutr Metab Care*. 1998;1:263–272.
6. Barbul A, Lazarou SA, Efron DT, et al. Arginine enhances wound healing and lymphocyte immune responses in humans. *Surgery*. 1990;108:331–337.
7. Evoy D, Lieberman MD, Fahey TJ, et al. Immunonutrition: the role of arginine. *Nutrition*. 1998;14:611–617.
8. Cynober L, LeBoucher J, Vasson MP. Arginine metabolism in mammals. *J Nutr Biochem*. 1995;6:402–413.
9. Heys SD, Walker LG, Smith I, et al. Enteral nutrition supplementation with key nutrients in patients with critical illness and cancer. *Ann Surg*. 1999; 229:467–477.
10. Beale RJ, Bryg DJ, Bihari DJ. Immunonutrition in the critically ill. A systemic review of clinical outcome. *Critical Care Med*. 1999;27:2799–2805.
11. Wilmore DW, Shabert JK. Role of glutamine in immunologic responses. *Nutrition*. 1998;14:618–626.
12. Ziegler TR, Bazargan N, Leader LM, Martindale RG. Glutamine and the gastrointestinal tract. *Curr Opin Clin Nutr Metab Care*. 2000;3:355–362.
13. Griffiths RD. Glutamine: establishing clinical indication. *Curr Opin Clin Nutr Metab Care*. 1999;2:177–182.
14. Schloerb PR. Immune-enhancing diets: products components, and their rationales. *J Parenter Enteral Nutr*. 2001; 25:S3–S7.
15. Fukuchtl S, Bankhead R, Rolandelli RH. Parenteral nutrition in short bowel syndrome. In: Rombeau JL, Rolandelli RH, eds. *Parenteral Nutrition. 3rd Ed*. Philadelphia: WB Saunders; 2001:282–303.
16. Stehle P, Zander J, Mertes N, et al. Effects of parenteral glutamine peptide supplements on muscle glutamine loss and nitrogen balance after major surgery. *Lancet*. 1989; 1:231–233.
17. Houdijk APJ, Rijnsburger ER, Jansen J, et al. Randomized trial of glutamine-enriched enteral nutrition on infectious morbidity in patients with multiple trauma. *Lancet*. 1998; 352:772–776.
18. Van Der Hulst RRW, Van Krell BK, Von Meyenfeldt MF, et al. Glutamine and the preservation of gut integrity. *Lancet*. 1993;341:1363–1365.
19. Ziegler TR, Young LS, Benfell K, et al. Clinical and metabolic efficacy of glutamine supplemented parenteral nutrition after bone marrow transplantation. A randomized, double blind controlled study. *Ann Intern Med*. 1992;116: 821–828.
20. Anderson PM, Ramsay NK, Shu XO, et al. Effect of low-dose oral glutamine on painful stomatitis during bone marrow transplantation. *Bone Marrow Transplantation*. 1998;22:339–344.
21. Yoshida S, Matsui M, Shirouza Y, et al. Effect of glutamine supplements and radiochemotherapy on systemic immune and gut barrier function in patients with advanced esophageal cancer. *Ann Surg*. 1998;227:485–491.
22. Iwasa Y, Iwasa M, Ohmori Y, et al. The effect of the administration of nucleosides and nucleotides for parenteral use. *Nutrition*. 2000;16:598–602.
23. Cosgrove M. Perinatal and infant nutrition. Nucleotides. *Nutrition*. 1998;14:748–751.
24. Kulkarni AD, Rudolph F, Van BC. The role of dietary sources of nucleotides in immune function: a review. *J Nutrition*. 1994;124:1442S-1446S.
25. Sukumar P, Loo A, Magur E, et al. Dietary supplementation of nucleotides and arginine promotes healing of small bowel ulcers in experimental ulcerative ileitis. *Dig Dis Sci*. 1997;42:1530–1536.

26. Grimble RF. Dietary lipids and the inflammatory response. *Proceedings of the Nutrition Society.* 1998;57:535–542.

27. Suchner U, Kuhn KS, Furst P. The scientific basis of immunonutrition. From the Clinical Nutrition and Metabolism Group Symposium on 'Nutrition in the severely-injured patient.' *Proceedings of the Nutrition Society.* 2000; 59:553–563.

28. Dyerberg J, Bang HO. Lipid metabolism, atherogenesis, and haemostasis in Eskimos: the role of the prostaglandin-3 family. *Haemostasis.* 1979;8:227–233.

29. Gadek JE, Demichele SJ, Karlstad MD, et al. Effect of enteral feeding with eicosapentaenoic acid, gamma-linolenic acid, and antioxidants in patients with acute respiratory distress syndrome. Enteral Nutrition in ARDS Study Group. *Crit Care Med.* 1999;27:1409–1420.

30. Bower RH, Cerra FB, Bershadsky B, et al. Early enteral administration of a formula (Impact®) supplemented with arginine, nucleotides, and fish oil in intensive care unit patients: Results of a multicenter, prospective, randomized clinical trial. *Crit Care Med.* 1995;23:436–449.

31. Weimann A, Bastian L, Bischoff WE, et al. Influence of arginine, omega-3 fatty acids, and nucleotide-supplemented enteral support on Systemic Inflammatory Response Syndrome and Multiple Organ Failure in patients after severe trauma. *Nutrition.* 1998;14:165–172.

32. Mendez C, Jurkovich GJ, Garcia I, et al. Effects of an immune-enhancing diet in critically injured patients. *J Trauma Injury Infect Crit Care.* 1997; 42(5):933–941.

33. Kudsk D, Minard G, Croce M, et al. A randomized trial of isonitrogenous enteral diets after severe trauma. *Ann Surg.* 1996;224:531–543.

34. Moore FA, Moore EE, Kudsk KA, et al. Clinical benefits of an immune-enhancing diet for early postinjury enteral feeding. *J Trauma.* 1994;37:607–615.

35. Brown RO, Hunt H, Mowatt-Larssen CA, et al. Comparison of specialized and standard enteral formulas in trauma patients. *Pharmacotherapy.* 1994;14:314–320.

36. Gianotti L, Braga M, Vignali A, et al. Effect of route of delivery and formulation of postoperative nutritional support in patients undergoing major operations for malignant neoplasms. *Arch Surg.* 1997;132:1222–1229.

37. Senkal M, Mumme A, Eickhoff U, et al. Early postoperative enteral immunonutrition: clinical outcome and cost-comparison analysis in surgical patients. *Crit Care Med.* 1997;25:1489–1496.

38. Heslin MJ, Latkany L, Leung D, et al. A prospective, randomized trial of early enteral feeding after resection of upper gastrointestinal malignancy. *Ann Surg.* 1997;226: 567–580.

39. Daly JM, Weintraub FN, Shou J, et al. Enteral nutrition during multimodality therapy in upper gastrointestinal cancer patients. *Ann Surg.* 1995;221:327–338.

40. Braga M, Vignali A, Gianotti L, et al. Immune and nutritional effects of early enteral nutrition after major abdominal operations. *Eur J Surg.* 1996;162:105–112.

41. Daly JM, Lieberman MD, Goldfine J, et al. Enteral nutrition with supplemental arginine, RNA, and omega-3 fatty acids in patients after operation: Immunologic, metabolic, and clinical outcome. *Surgery.* 1992;112:56–67.

42. Braga M, Gianotti L, Radaelli G, et al. Perioperative immunonutrition in patients undergoing cancer surgery: results of a randomized double-blind phase 3 trial. *Arch Surg.* 1999;134:428–433.

43. Senkal M, Zumtobel V, Bauer K, et al. Outcome and cost-effectiveness of perioperative enteral immunonutrition in patients undergoing elective upper gastrointestinal tract surgery. *Arch Surg.* 1999;134:1309–1316.

44. Beale RJ, Bryg DJ, Bihari DJ. Immunonutrition in the critically ill: a systemic review of clinical outcome. *Crit Care Med.* 1999;27:2799–2805.

45. Heyland DK, Novak F, Drover JW, et al. Should immunonutrition become routine in the critically ill patient? A systematic review of the evidence. *JAMA.* 2001;286: 944–953.

46. Proceedings from summit on immune-enhancing enteral therapy. *J Parenter Enteral Nutri.* 2001;25(Supplement): S1–S63.

CHAPTER

33 Aggressive Perioperative and Intra Operative Enteral Nutrition, Strategy for the Future

Stig Bengmark, M.D., Ph.D.

A Rediscovered Concept 365
Early Enteral Nutrition Should Mean Early 366
Intestinal Starvation: A Key to Morbidity 367
Immunostimulatory Nutrition Is Complex 367
Supply of Antioxidants Essential 368
Modulation of the Acute Phase Response 369
The Acute Phase Response Is Instantaneous 369
A Narrow Therapeutic Window 369
Exaggerated Cytokine Response a Prognosticator 370
Need of Calories and Nitrogen Balance Overrated 371
Immune Control More Important 371
Preoperative Enteral Starvation to Be Reduced 372
Uninterrupted Jejunal Feeding 372
GI Secretions Important in Immune Defense 373
Secretion Inhibited by Drugs 374
Gastric Secretion Important in Infection Control 375
Nitric Oxide—The Key to GI Motility and Blood Flow 375
EN and LAB Might Modulate Rejection 376
Use of Special Immunomodulatory Nutrients 377
Conclusions 377
References 377

"Sometimes imagination is better than knowledge."
Albert Einstein

A Rediscovered Concept

As early as the 5th century BC, Hippocrates understood the need to protect the sick patient through proper nutrition.[1] He also recognized the association between illness and malfunction of the large intestine. During most of the history of surgery, of course, feeding patients by mouth was the only option. As a result, aggressive oral/enteral nutrition in connection with surgery is not a novel concept. Almost 100 years ago, for example, Andresen[2] reported successful postoperative enteral feeding immediately following gastrojejunostomy. During the first half of the 20th century, it was not unusual to offer food to surgical patients on their first postoperative day. In the 1940s and 1950s, Scandinavian surgeons routinely gave sandwiches of salted and fermented herring on the first day after procedures such as gastric resection. Many believed it was a formula for success.

During World War II, two groups led by renowned American surgeons Mulholland[3] and Rhoads[4] performed studies comparing oral gastric feeding—or feeding through jejunostomy—with parenteral nutrition. Both reported definite advantages of enteral nutrition (EN) over parenteral nutrition (PN). Neither group, however, regarded these findings as an incentive to use enteral nutrition more actively. Instead, they interpreted the results as an indication of the "primitive" state of parenteral formulas, and as an incentive to develop more effective parenteral procedures (formulas).

Both industry and scientists made enormous efforts during the following 30 years to develop the "perfect parenteral formula." When judging these efforts now, it should be remembered that very little was known about the sensitivity of various nutrients to processing and preservation, nor was much known about antioxidants and their clinical importance. Furthermore, neither the need to supply dietary fibers, nor the importance of flora had yet been widely recognized. The general belief was that, with time, chemically defined and residue-free (elemental) diets would be available for the nutritional support of critically ill patients.

Numerous experimental and clinical studies, conducted during the 1970s and 1980s, supported the superiority of EN over PN, but they passed unnoticed and had no discernable influence on general nutrition policy. Several key 1980 observations should have alerted medical professionals to the benefits of enteral nutrition. Among them:

1. Enteral nutrition significantly increases visceral (splanchnic and mucosal) circulation.[5]
2. The intestinal mucosa is unable to nourish itself from the blood—it needs direct nutrition from the gut lumen.[6]
3. Enteral nutrition leads to an early positive nitrogen balance.[7]
4. Enteral nutrition rich in protein increases survival.[8]

Past studies have shown that both small bowel motility and absorption function normally in the immediate postoperative period—for review see Ryan Jr., et al.[9] This information led to early attempts to provide enteral nutrition with residue-free solutions immediately after partial colectomy. The EN-treated patients lost 2.4% of body weight compared to 6.1% in the PN group ($p<0.005$) and required intravenous (IV) catheter for only 1.8 days compared to 6.6 days in the IV-treated group ($p<0.005$).[9] Another study compared patients undergoing extensive esophageal, gastroduodenal, biliary, and pancreatic procedures. The patients receiving immediate enteral nutrition demonstrated a mean cumulative, 10-day nitrogen balance of $+11.7 \pm 5.4$ g compared to -44.7 ± 6.5 g for the patients with parenteral nutition.[7]

Nevertheless, the medical world remained more or less unresponsive to proposals for increased use of EN in surgical care. It continued to be driven by the idea that one day the perfect TPN solution would be reality—superior to natural food and to foods supplied via the normal oral route. Several controlled studies in the 1980s showed definite advantages of EN over PN. However, it was not until Moore, et al.[10] published their meta-analysis in 1991—a study based on eight prospective randomized trials—that more serious attention was given to EN as a promising alternative in postoperative nutrition. This meta-analysis demonstrated a significant decrease in postoperative sepsis rate when EN was provided in the early postoperative period—an average 18% of infections compared to 35% in the patients fed parenterally. Even more impressive differences were demonstrated the following year, when Kudsk, et al.[11] reported a 76% lower sepsis rate in a prospective study of abdominal-trauma patients, when fed enterally compared to parenterally.

In recent years, the failure of antibiotics (including selective decontamination) to solve infection problems, increased awareness of the dangers of antibiotics, and the failure of total parenteral nutrition (TPN) to solve nutritional demands and prevent sepsis have turned the focus of interest to enteral nutrition. Above all, the documented capacity of EN to meet nutritional demands and reduce morbidity, in addition to ecological and immunological factors, makes EN today a promising alternative.[12,13] But, as will be emphasized below, only if we do it right.

Early Enteral Nutrition Should Mean Early

It is crucial to define what is called "early" as clearly as possible. In the literature, it is not unusual for enteral nutrition starting as late as 72 hours after first sign of disease (emergency medicine) or end of operation (surgery) to be called "early." It is my conviction that such a definition is far too liberal. One cannot exclude the possibility that we would observe significant differences in outcome by comparing those who receive their first EN within 24 hours, and those who wait until to the third day for enteral nutrition. Experimental and clinical observations support the assumption of a narrow therapeutic window for the early hours after injury—meaning that the ability to influence the course of disease diminishes as time passes.

It appears increasingly evident that the main reason for early enteral nutrition is not so much to provide calories as to modulate the gut immune system. It is important to remember that up to 75%–80% of the total immune system is in the gut, especially the colon (Figure 33.1a,b).[14] This observation should be an incentive to provide enteral nutrition solutions in the early postoperative phase that also contain nutritional fibers for the lower parts of the gut. In other words, a tool as simple as food can modulate the acute phase response (APR). The strong immunological effects

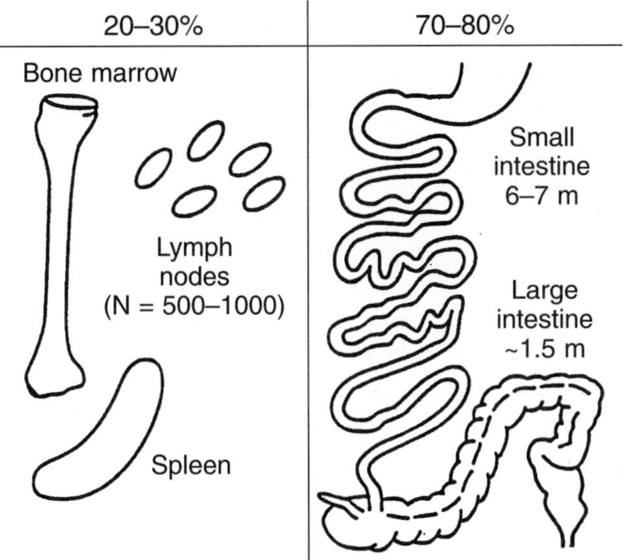

Figure 33.1

Distribution (percent) of Immunoglobulin-Producing Immunocytes. All classes are included, but the respiratory and upper alimentary tracts are not taken into account.

Adapted from Brandtzaeg P, Halstensen TS, Krajci P, et al. Immunobiology and immunopathology of human gut mucosa: humoral immunity and intraepithelial lymphocytes. *Gastroenterlogy*. 1989;97:1562–1584 with permission WB Saunders Company.

produced by enteral nutrition are also reasons why immunological parameters are increasingly introduced in clinical nutrition.

The largest proportions of the GI immune system are localized in the two ends of the GI tract: the oral cavity with its important salivary glands and its flora, and the large intestine with its complex flora. Measures to control APR and regulate immune functions mean not only early enteral nutrition, but also efforts to maintain GI secretions, including a rich salivation and normal gastric, pancreatic, and intestinal secretions. These secretions are all rich in factors controlling the immune reaction, infection, and growth.

Intestinal Starvation: A Key to Morbidity

It is important to realize that the body has two separate digestive systems: one based on normal GI enzymes provided through gastrointestinal secretions, the other based on enzymatic breakdown of fibers and complex proteins by the commensal flora, mainly in the colon. It is essential to provide the substrate for daily microbial degradation, and enteral nutrition should meet the special needs of the colon. For example, at least 10% of calories, roughly corresponding to 20% of the food volume, should consist of nutrients (plant fibers) destined for the large intestine—"colonic foods." For this reason, every ICU should make strong attempts to provide these "colonic foods."

Lack of enteral nutrition has several immediate negative consequences:

1. Inhibition of saliva and digestive tract secretions
2. Inhibition of GI motility and splanchnic circulation
3. Increased virulence of potentially pathogenic microorganisms in the subflora
4. Reduction and inhibition of the protective flora
5. Atrophy of the mucosa of the small intestine and colon
6. Increased microbial translocation
7. Reduced supply of important antioxidants, flavonoids, phytoestrogens, and other important components, known or still unknown, that influence the rate and severity of postoperative and posttrauma morbidity.

Immunostimulatory Nutrition Is Complex

Numerous attempts have been made in recent years to compare the efficacy of EN and to PN, sometimes with conflicting results. Many of the human studies presented in the literature seem to lack the necessary knowledge, understanding, and respect for the complex physiology and immunology of the GI tract, and have been undertaken without any clear criteria by which to evaluate the role of enteral nutrition.

There are at least five important cornerstones in immunostimulatory nutrition[15] that must be seriously considered if the goal is to use EN to control APR and immune functions:

1. *EN must be instituted early.* If possible, EN should be underway before the injury/operation, but always as early as possible after the onset of disease or infliction of injury. Significant alterations in APR are already occurring during the first minutes and hours. With early intervention, the common preoperative and postoperative enteral starvation period—often 12 to 20 hours—can be made significantly shorter.
2. *EN must always include fiber.* A significant part of the immune system resides in the large intestine, with its immunologically most active cells: flora,

mucosal cells, and gut associated lymphoid (GALT) cells. EN solutions should, if possible, always contain substrate (fiber) for commensal flora fermentation and local production of needed immunoregulatory nutrients (short chain fatty acids [SCFAs], polyamines, amino acids, antioxidants, vitamins, etc.). Most published clinical studies do not include fibers in the formulas for enteral nutrition. The choice of type of fiber is equally important, because flora can only produce the various necessary nutrients, antioxidants, coagulation, and growth factors if the substrate contains necessary precursors (see Chapter 34).

3. *Saturated fat must be avoided.* Saturated fat is known to be immuno-depressive. More generally, fat in the diet has been shown to significantly influence health. (For further information, see Chapter 34.)
4. *Preservation of the commensal flora is essential.* Fiber alone does not always affect diarrhea in sick patients, because the flora is often suppressed and fermentation does not take place. Flora is almost always depressed in the sick patient, and antibiotics only make matters worse. To the extent possible, flora-reducing antibiotics and other pharmaceuticals with immuno-depressive effects should be avoided. When necessary, re-supply of flora should be considered. (See Chapter 34.)
5. *Antioxidants must always be considered.* The unavoidable large production of free radicals in severely sick patients consumes large amounts of antioxidants. Serum levels of key antioxidants such as glutathione and vitamin C are known to be sensitive indicators of disease. Plasma vitamin C in healthy individuals, for example, averaged 62 μmol/L (range 55–72) in one study, but decreased in patients with gastritis to about 47 μmol/L, in diabetes to 45 μmol/L, and in ICU patients to as low as 11.0 μmol/L (range 8–22).[13] Patients who later developed MOF demonstrated extremely low levels of vitamin C (MOF:3.8 $\pm$ 1 vs. no MOF:11.2 $\pm$ 1.8).[16] Low serum levels of antioxidants are associated with extreme elevations in cytokines such as IL-6 and TNF-α, and in acute-phase proteins—and indicate an ongoing exaggerated inflammation. It is reasonable to anticipate that numerous other antioxidants, not yet systematically studied, such as glutathion or various carotenoids and flavonoids, are also sensitive markers of inflammation in injury and infection.

Supply of Antioxidants Essential

It is unfortunate that the sickest patients in the ICU receive nutrition that is artificial and incomplete in content of nutrients. Usually no attempts are made within the ICU to substitute for the absence of normal food, especially fresh fruits and vegetables. It is true that some formula producers claim that their feeding formulas are based on normal food, but even if industry-made formulas have been much improved, they cannot match the benefits of fresh fruits and vegetables.

Enteral nutrition formulas are essentially a mixture of chemicals. Hospital-made formulas are no longer used in the developed world, but are still frequently used in developing countries. It is clear that industry-made formulas have many advantages, especially from a hygienic point of view; however, they lack quite a few important nutritional ingredients. **It is not unreasonable to assume that hospital-made formulas have better antioxidant capacity and immuno-stimulatory effects than industry-made EN solutions.** If five to eight servings of fruit and vegetables are important for health in normal individuals, they might be even more important in the very sick. One encouraging trend is the effort in ICU units around the world to complement "synthetic" formula nutrition with fresh fruits and vegetable juices, prepared by juicing machines by the ICU staff.

Food is complex, with hundreds of thousands of important nutrients and micronutrients. Ingredients such as glutamine, arginine, nucleotides, n-3 fatty acids, vitamin E, and glutathione have in the past been lacking in feeding formulas. Many important vitamins, antioxidants, and other nutritional ingredients do not tolerate processing; drying, heating and freezing destroy an average 80% of the content of vitamins and antioxidants as well as some amino acids and other nutrients.[17] For example, glutamine, the dominating amino acid in muscles, and glutathione, sometimes referred to as the master antioxidant, often disappear totally when food is processed.

Although the human body has a limited ability to synthesize glutathione, it is usually not enough for the needs of the sick, and glutathione deficiencies are often reported in sick and malnourished patients. Glutathione deficiency has been regarded as an early indicator of disease and poor outcome. A recent study reported glutathione deficiency in skeletal muscle just 24 hours after trauma in otherwise healthy, well-nourished individuals.[18] Fresh meat and fresh vegetable products are usually rich in glutathione.[19] It is especially abundant (>300 nmol/g food) in fresh pork and beef, but also in broccoli, spinach, parsley, and yellow squash (Table 33.1). Fruits like oranges and tangerines contain >100 nmol/g. But fruits and vegetables also contain, as mentioned above, large amounts of other strong antioxidants, including more than 4,000 flavonoids and more than 500 carotenoids, some of which have an antioxidant effect 5 to 10 times stronger than vitamin C or E.

Modulation of the Acute Phase Response

To a large extent, the alarm reaction, triggered by psychological and physical challenges such as microbial invasion, allergic reaction, surgical operation, trauma, burn, tissue ischemia, tissue infarction, strenuous exercise, and childbirth, is modulated by the hypothalamo-pituitary-adrenal (HPA) axis. The gut and the liver also play important roles.

During the early phase of APR, gut-derived bacteria, toxins, and various signal substances (bacteriokines, cytokines) are responsible for a number of critical functions. For example, they activate important neuroendocrine mechanisms. They also influence tissues such as the gut mucosa, the gut—associated lymphoid tissues (GALT), T-cells, B-cells, NK-cells, the free macrophages and fixed macrophages of the liver (Kupffer cells), spleen, and the hepatocytes. Local production and release of cytokines is important to the initiation and resolution of inflammation. Release of nitric oxide is critical for regulation of gastrointestinal motility, mucosal and splanchnic blood flow, bile production, and for various anti-infection mechanisms.

TABLE 33.1

Glutathione in Foods[19]

	Nmol/g
Pork	630
Broccoli (flower)	440
Parsley (leaf)	400
Spinach	400
Yellow squash (fresh)	320
Yellow squash (frozen)	70
Potato (raw)	230
Beef (ground)	230
Potato (boiled 15 min)	110
Tomato	170
Green pepper	170
Chicken	160
Tangerine	140
Broccoli (stem)	140
Cauliflower	130
Orange	130
Corn meal	130
Peas	90
Carrot	70
Pear	40
Banana	20
Apple	20
Rye bread	20
Fish	20
Green beans	15
Milk	<1
Butter	<1
Egg	<1
Oatmeal	<1
Corn flakes	<1

The Acute Phase Response Is Instantaneous

The largest proportion of the human immune system is localized in the gut, and the gut produces most of the body's IgA, which is transferred each day to the lumen of the gut. The synthesis of IgA is highly dependent on T-cells as well as on several cytokines, particularly TGF-β, which influences the IgA differentiation.[20] Deficiencies in IgA are strongly associated with pronounced increase in morbidity and mortality after major surgery, and with increased rejection after liver transplantation.[21]

The APR is instantaneous! Therefore, attempts to modulate APR should be instituted, if not before, at least immediately on arrival in the emergency department, ICU, or postanesthesia unit (PACU). Figure 33.2, reproduced from a classic study published in 1972, demonstrates the changes in some acute phase proteins (APPs) after a standard elective cholecystectomy.[22] Some key APPs are significantly elevated just 4 to 8 hours following the operation. With more sensitive diagnostic tools today, however, it has become evident that the APR reaction is rapid, and immediate elevations in serum levels of some cytokines (especially TNF and IL-6), coagulation, and growth factors are seen.[23] This immediate immune response also occurs at the cellular level: platelets and leucocytes increase almost immediately after trauma or surgery.[23] The increase can be dramatic, with some APPs increasing up to 1,000 times.

A Narrow Therapeutic Window

Serum levels of norepinephrine, cortisol, and excretion of lactulose (indication of increased intestinal mucosa permeability) increase almost immediately when endotoxin is injected in human volunteers.[24] Increases in cytokines such as TNF and IL-6 have also been ob-

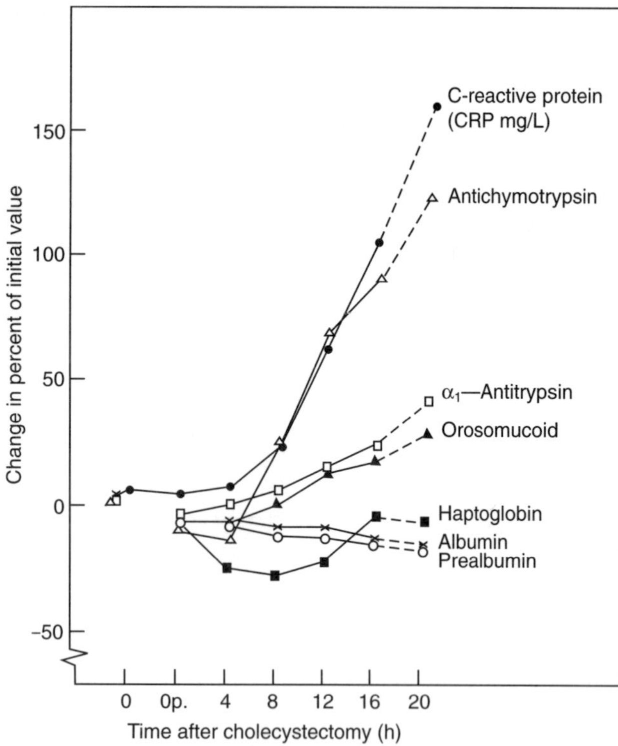

Figure 33.2

Fast Quantitative Changes in Acute Phase Reactants During the First 20 Hours After Cholecystectomy

Reprinted with permission Aronsen KF, Ekelund G, Kindmark CO, et al. Sequential changes of plasma proteins after surgical trauma. *Scandinavian Journal of Clinical & Laboratory Investigation*. 1972;29,(Suppl)124:127–136l.

served during the late phase of liver transplantation.[25] A six-fold or greater increase of these cytokines appears to be a strong predictor for development of postoperative septic complications. IL-6 samples taken in 61 patients one hour after ERCP showed a significant elevation in 9 patients who subsequently developed clinical post-ERP pancreatitis.[26] The state of gastrointestinal mucosal metabolism during the first 12 hours after surgery seems to relate to outcome as well; death is likely to occur if the mucosa continues to remain acidotic after 12 hours.[27,28]

In experimental pancreatitis, significant elevations in serum IL-6, IL-8, and serum amylase can be observed at the earliest time-point measured, 30 minutes.[29] Reduced bowel motility and leakage of plasma proteins into the peritoneum can occur within 3 hours.[30] As early as 6 hours from induction of pancreatitis, a significant decrease in the number of anaerobic bacteria, especially lactobacilli, can be demonstrated both in the ileum and colon.[31] Signs of translocation of bacteria to mesenteric lymph nodes (MLN) and to the inflamed pancreatic tissue occur as well,[32] followed by an immediate and significant overgrowth of potentially pathogenic microorganisms such as E. coli in the distal ileum and the colon.[31]

Norman[33] suggests that, in acute pancreatitis, there exists a therapeutic window of not much more than 24 to 36 hours from the onset of disease. A similar, equally narrow window probably exists in other conditions following surgery and trauma—reinforcing the need for early and aggressive efforts to modulate the acute phase response. Wherever possible, therefore, patients should receive aggressive nutritional control of APR immediately after arriving in the emergency or recovery room. In the case of a scheduled operation, nutritional support should be provided before the surgical procedure.

Exaggerated Cytokine Response a Prognosticator

Nuclear factor-κB (NK-κB) is receiving increasing attention for its important role in the inflammatory process. This factor is known to activate several genes of importance in the inflammatory response, including the IL-6 gene, especially in B cells, T cells, and monocytes.[34,35] Increasing evidence suggests that IL-6 plays a specific role in both acute and chronic inflammation. IL-6, as well as PAI-1, is regarded as a prognosticator of outcome in such chronic inflammatory conditions as myocardial infarction, acute pancreatitis, and Alzheimer's, and in acute conditions following operation or trauma.

Many of the manifestations of the inflammatory response are reproducible by administration of cytokines, particularly IL-6.[36] High levels of IL-6 are observed in conditions associated with sepsis such as fatigue, somnolence, mental depression, anorexia, and daytime sleepiness. By administering cytokines in experimental studies, it is possible to mimic the inflammatory response and observe its effects in hypermetabolism; changes in carbohydrate, lipid, and protein metabolism; and hormonal changes such as insulin resistance. These cytokines include not only IL-6, but also TNF, IL-1, IFN-γ and LIF (leukemia inhibitory factor).[37] IL-6 is usually secreted after IL-1 and TNFα, but unlike these cytokines, it circulates freely in the plasma.[38]

Several types of cells, including enterocytes and visceral fat cells, produce IL-6. IL-6 is produced by the murine enterocyte in response to endotoxin[36] and by the human enterocyte in response to interleukin-1β (IL-1B).[39,40] Observations confirm that IL-6 and PAI-1 are secreted more from visceral than subcutaneous fat cells, which may explain why people with visceral obesity suffer a much higher risk of disease,[41] especially as the amount of fat in the abdomen can vary from a few milliliters to about six liters in persons with gross obesity.[42] This fact explains the individual variations in the amounts of both IL-6 and PAI-1 released in response to identical stimuli or injury. Chronically elevated IL-6 and PAI-1 are strongly associated with metabolic syndrome, particularly insulin resistance,[43] and increased risk of morbidity and mortality following surgery and trauma.

Patients who display a sustained rise in acute phase proteins often later develop signs of postoperative infections. This pattern contrasts sharply to the quick rise and fall observed in patients with uncomplicated surgery.[44] CRP and α_1-antichymotrypsin are shown to be considerably higher in patients who later develop post-operative complications as well.[45] It is the changes in serum IL-6 that have attracted the greatest interest, since exaggerated IL-6 response (both significantly prolonged and with extreme elevations) is associated with adverse clinical events such as acute respiratory distress (ARDS) and multiple organ failure in patients suffering from such conditions as infection, burns, or trauma.[46] Other changes associated with an exaggerated IL-6 response are augmented endothelial adhesion of polymorph nuclear (PMN) cells, increased production of intracellular adhesion molecule-1 (ICAM-1), priming of the PMNs for an oxidative burst, release of pro-inflammatory platelet activating factor (PAF), and delay in PMN apoptosis.[46]

Need of Calories and Nitrogen Balance Overrated

Parenteral supply of large amounts of calories to critically ill patients is no longer the praxis. Instead, we are increasingly aware that overfeeding macronutrients to the critically ill, as to healthy individuals, is often dangerous. Excessive nutrition, whether parenteral or enteral, often seems to lead to serious, sometimes fatal metabolic consequences.[47] TPN is rarely indicated in peri-operative nutrition today, at least not during the first 2 weeks after surgery. A recent well-designed randomized study with 300 patients undergoing major general surgery compared TPN with IV supply of only 1000–1500 kcal/d as glucose, supplied when necessary for up to 15 postoperative days.[48] No differences could be demonstrated between the two groups, either in morbidity or mortality. The nitrogen loss during the first week was reduced to about half in the glucose group compared to the TPN group. Most patients, who were back to eating normally within one week, seemed to do well. However, TPN could be lifesaving for about 20% of the patients who could not go back to normal eating after 2 weeks. The authors conclude that "overfeeding seemed to be a larger problem than underfeeding."

Another recent, similarly designed study performed at Memorial-Sloan-Kettering Cancer Center in New York seems to reach similar conclusions. One hundred ninety-five patients undergoing resection for upper gastrointestinal malignancies were randomized to receive either enteral supplementation with immuno-enhancing diet (Impact®, Novartis, Minneapolis, MN) or only IV crystalloid infusions (CON).[49] The EN feeding, with no supplemental fiber, started within 24 hours of the operation. There was no information on antibiotic policy. The caloric intake was low in the two groups, 61% and 22% of the defined goals (25 kcal/kg/d; e.g., in an 70 kg person about 1000 kcal in the EN group and in the CON group about 400 kcal). No differences were observed between the groups in terms of minor (Impact® 26/97, CON 16/98), major (Impact® 27/97, CON 25/98), or infectious wound (Impact® 20/97, CON 23/97) complications. Nor were there any differences in mortality (Impact® 2/97, CON 3/98) or in length of stay (median 11 days for each group). A study of the same patient population for protein kinetics found a significant decrease in fat oxidation and protein catabolism, and an improved net nitrogen balance in the enterally fed "immuno-enhanced" group.[50] By the fifth postoperative day, the insulin/glucagon quotient and the level of growth hormone were significantly increased in the enterally fed/immuno-enhanced group, when both the insulin/glucagon quotient and the level growth hormone were increased. None of these changes seemed to have any significant influence on outcome.

Immune Control More Important

Judging from recent literature, maintaining calorie and nitrogen balance in typical surgical patients seems to have lost some importance. Instead, nutrition, or at least enteral nutrition, appears more important as a tool for modulation of the immune system. Two recent studies support this assumption. When parenteral hyperalimentation (PN) was compared with enteral nutrition (EN) in liver resection patients, no differences could be observed among such nutritional parameters as RBP, transferrin, prealbumin, or 3-methylhistidine. However, the study found significant differences in such immunological parameters as lymphocyte numbers (114 vs. 66 $p<0.05$), response to phytohemagglutinin (PHA) (103 vs. 78 $p<0.05$), and natural killer cell activity (106 vs. 49 $p<0.05$).[51] Most important, the incidence of infectious complications was 8% in the EN group compared to 31% in the PN group. A study in acute pancreatitis reached similar results.[52] Here, disease severity scores (APACHE II) (6 vs. 8 $p<0.0001$), C-reactive protein (CRP) (84 vs. 156 $p<0.005$), IgM anticore endotoxin antibodies (EndoCAB, –1.1 vs. +29 $p<0.05$), and total antioxidant index (TAC, +33 vs. –28% $p<0.05$) were significantly better in the EN group compared to PN. In addition, the systemic inflammatory response (SIRS), sepsis rate, incidence of organ failure, and length of stay in the intensive care unit were significantly better in the EN group.

Preoperative Enteral Starvation to Be Reduced

The routine of preoperative enteral starvation has been practiced since the early days of surgery and inhalation anesthesia—primarily to avoid vomiting and the risk of aspiration with the introduction of anesthesia. This relic from the past persists, even though denial of food before surgery has largely lost its importance in preventing vomiting and aspiration. Instead, several investigations show negative metabolic and psychological consequences of preoperative starvation.

The time needed to obtain an empty stomach is clearly overrated. Studies show that at least 50% of a liquid meal has left the stomach already after 22 ± 3 minutes.[53] Numerous foods can be supplied as a liquid, some of which are even water-soluble; moreover, all fibers can be mixed with liquids. It has been claimed that some patients, especially the obese, often have residuals in their stomach; but a recent study could not find any differences in residual gastric content between lean and obese patients.[54]

Attempts were made as early as 15 years ago to introduce a preoperative breakfast. The volume of gastric content, the median pH of gastric content, and the number of patients with pH of >3 did not differ when a light breakfast (buttered toast, tea/coffee and milk) was offered to the patients three hours before induction of anesthesia. No other negative effects were observed when compared to patients who fasted from midnight.[55] A recent survey of the policy at four British hospitals shows that elective patients regularly fast at least from midnight, and preoperative starvation periods of up to 12 hours are not uncommon.[56] There are no indications that the policies are better at other hospitals or in other countries. Long preoperative starvation periods, with a mean of 10 hours, remain the dominating praxis in pediatric practice as well.[57]

It is clear that this praxis handicaps both the barrier and immune functions prior to surgery. The reason for this seemingly negligent attitude is the continued belief that PN and IV glucose infusion can safely replace EN, at least in the immediate peri-operative period. Children, elderly, outpatients, and surgical patients—especially those with reduced immune systems—suffer the most. Many attempts have been made to overcome the metabolic and psychological harm of preoperative enteral starvation, especially in children, and "new" regimens for preoperative enteral feeding have been tried, such as enteral supply of glucose, eating porridge,[58] and "ultra short" (no more than 2 hours) preoperative starvation.[59] It is reported that children became less irritable, and easier to deal with, with no other negative consequences, when the preoperative starvation period is reduced to 2 hours.[59] Unfortunately, these attempts have not received enough attention to change the general routine.

National professional organizations regard present routines as unsatisfactory and recommend at least modest changes in praxis. It is my opinion that the time is ripe for strong efforts to discontinue avoidable physical and psychological harm by withholding food from patients needing surgery under general anesthesia.[60]

Uninterrupted Jejunal Feeding

Timing and content of the nutritional supply seem to be equally important for successful immune-nutrition. There are some good reasons to suggest that optimal control of APR and immune functions result from never fully discontinuing the enteral supply of nutrients. The concept of uninterrupted enteral nutrition (UEN) was developed for management of patients with thermal injuries, patients who require repeat operations, and a group of patients who suffer significantly from the frequent interruptions in supply of enteral nutrients.

Uninterrupted jejunal tube-feeding was introduced in the early 1990s and tried in 47 patients with thermal injuries.[61] The patients tolerated continuous enteral tube feeding well during the operation, and no unwanted effects could be observed. Furthermore, no increase in gastric residuals could be observed at the end of the operation.[61] The authors of the study concluded that "cessation of enteral feeding of even extensively burned patients during operation is not required." A subsequent controlled study compared 40 patients, who were tube-fed without interruption during 161 surgical procedures, with 40 patients managed traditionally with a return to parenteral feeding during 129 operations.[62] Despite slightly more extensive burns (27.0 ± 2.4 vs. 22.0 ± 2.9%, $p<0.03$), the patients fed enterally without interruption demonstrated significant improvements: lower caloric deficit (cumulative caloric balance: +2673 ± 2147 vs. −7899 ± 3123, $p<0.006$), less albumin supplementation to maintain a minimum serum level of 2.5 g/dL (732 ± 124 mL vs. 1528 ± 376, $p<0.04$), and a lower incidence of wound infections (2/40 vs. 9/40 patients, $p<0.02$).

It seems reasonable to assume that uninterrupted EN is of value for other types of patients as well, especially those undergoing extensive cancer surgery or organ transplantation. Some medical centers are trying UEN, and reports from extensive oropharyngeal, pancreatic, and hepatic operations are encouraging.[63] If UEN is to be widely practiced, efficient and easy-to-manage jejunal feeding must be available. Such tubes should have a high rate of "spontaneous" post-pyloric placement (without assistance by endoscopy or X-ray), with their tip reaching the region of the ligament of Treitz within a few minutes or hours. It is also necessary to reduce considerably the rate of unintentional dislodgement (regurgitation or accidental removal). The tubes used in the past have a bad record: spontaneous postpolyric placement with conventional tubes was obtained in only about 33% of the patients after 24 hours and about 66% after 72 hours.[64] Furthermore, at least half the conventional tubes are dislodged within one week.[64]

GI Secretions Important in Immune Defense

It has often been forgotten that gastrointestinal secretions, especially saliva, are full of immunostimulatory and infection-preventive factors, as well as important growth and coagulation factors. The nitrate content of the saliva in a healthy person is comparatively high, which is of special interest, since this molecule acts as a donor molecule for gastric production of nitric oxide. Nitric oxide, in turn, is essential for stimulation of GI motility and mucosal and splanchnic blood flow, and for bacteriostasis in the stomach.[65,66]

The daily production of saliva and gastrointestinal juices is large and most likely more than 10 liters; saliva 2.5 liters, gastric secretion 2.5 liters, bile 0.5 liter, bile 0.5 liter, pancreatic secretion 1.5 liters small intestinal secretion and colonic secretion between 1.0 and 5.0 liters. This is important to remember, especially when the oral cavity and stomach are bypassed by jejunal feeding. It is said about saliva that it possesses "a multiplicity of defense systems for antibacterial warfare that the Pentagon can envy."[67] This is also true for the other secretions. To a large extent, the composition of saliva, like some other secretions, resembles breast milk. Both saliva and breast milk are rich in immunologically important factors such as IgA, lactoferrin, lactic dehydrogenase, lysozyme, mucins, and surfactants, and other important compounds (Table 33.2).[68–71] Saliva appears to provide the same mucosa-protective function as breast milk—albeit from early infancy to old age. Sialoadenectomy, for example, leads to in-

TABLE 33.2

Salivary Constituents

1. Proteins	2. Small Organic Molecules	3. Electrolytes
Albumin	Creatinine	Ammonia
Amylase	Glucose	Bicarbonate
B-glucuronidase	Lipids	Calcium
Carbohydrases	Nitrogen	Chloride
Cystatins	Sialic acid	Fluoride
EGF	Urea	Iodide
Esterases	Uric acid	Magnesium
Fibronectin	Nitrate	Non-specific buffers
Gustin		Phosphates
Histamins		Potassium
Immunoglobulin A		Sodium
Immunoglobulin G		Sulphates
Immunoglobulin M		Thiocyanate
Kallikrein		
Lactoferrin		
Lipase		
Lactic dehydrogenase		
Lysozyme		
Mucins		
Nerve growth factor		
Parotid aggregins		
Peptidases		
Phosphatases		
Proline-rich proteins		
Ribonucleases		
Salivary peroxidases		
Secretory component		
Secretory IgA		
Serum proteins (trace)		
Tyrosine-rich proteins		
Vitamin-binding proteins		

Adapted from Sreebny LM, Banoczy J, Baum BJ, et al. Saliva: its role in health and disease. *International Dentistry Journal.* 1992;42:291–304. Reprinted with permission from World Dental Press, Ltd.

testinal ulcerations and delayed healing of wounds both at the skin, in the mouth, and in the stomach. Absence of salivation is also associated with decreases in rate of liver regeneration. In addition, the large secretion of protein through the pancreas—about the size of the daily protein intake—is of great importance for the metabolism of colonic flora and should not be inhibited.

A child of only 5 years of age produces 0.5 L of saliva/d.[72] Salivation is minimal during rest (adults appr 25 mL/h) but increases about 20 times on stimulation by chewing. It is reasonable to assume that it is favorable to stimulate the patient's salivation when on jejunal tube feeding through chewing gums, or eating fruits and vegetables. Salivation is known to particularly increase when nitrate-rich vegetables (see p. 376) are chewed. Alternatively salivation can be pharmacologically stimulated by repeat pilocarpin injections (5 mg × 3).[73]

Secretion Inhibited by Drugs

Both mucosal and glandular cells in the digestive tract are extremely sensitive to modern drugs, and drug side effects seem to be more common in the GI tract than in other organs. Standard ICU practice seems to promote inhibition of GI secretion, and many of the drugs used in the ICU produce dry mouth as a side effect (Table 33.3),[68] along with nausea, vomiting, diarrhea, or constipation. Although not thoroughly studied, one can assume that inhibition of secretions is not specific to the salivary glands, but occurs throughout the entire GI tract. These reduced secretions not only weaken the immune defense significantly, but also actively contribute to increased microbial translocation. For these reasons, drugs that reduce gastrointestinal secretions should kept to an absolute minimum.

Mucin possesses properties that enable it to become concentrated on mucosal surfaces[69] and form an effective barrier against environmental insults. Mucus covers ingested foods and builds a mucosa-protective shield on the mucosal face from the oral cavity to the anus. The density of mucus-producing Goblet cells is rather low in the upper GI tract but increases considerably with distance from the oral cavity. For this reason, the upper GI tract is greatly dependent on salivary-gland mucus for maintaining integrity of the mucosa.[70] The content of mucus is reduced in experimental animals by about 80% also in the lower oesophagus after extirpation of the salivary glands,[71] and is most likely the same in humans.

TABLE 33.3

Xerogenic Pharmaceuticals[72]
Analgesics
Meperedine HCl (Demerol)
Alprazolam (Xanax)
Diazepam (Valium)
Triazolam (Halcion)
Anorexic (Amphetamine)
Methamphetamine HCl (Dexosyn)
Anorexic (Non-amphetamine)
Phendimetrazine tartrate (Adipex, Obezine, Trimtabs)
Anti-acne preparation
Isotretion (Accutane)
Antiarthritic
Piroxicam (Feldene)
Anticholinergic; Antispasmodic (G.I.)
Artropine sulphate
Clidinium bromide (Quarzan)
Dicyclomine (Bentyl)
Glycopyrrolate (Robinul)
Hyoscyamine sulphate (Anaspaz)
Propanteline bromide (pro-Banthene)
Combination drugs (Donnatal)
Anticholinergic: Antispasmidic (Urinary)
Oxybutynin chloride (Ditropan)
Combination drugs (Cytospaz, Urised)
Antidepressant
Tricyclics (Elavil, Pamelor, Tofranil)
Antidiarrheal
Diphenoxylate HCl and atropine (Lomotil)
Antihistamine
Diphenhydramine HCl (Benadryl)
Brompheniramine maleate (Dimetane, Veltane)
Combination drugs (Triaminic, Historal, Dimetapp)
Antihypertensive
Clonidine HCl (Catapres)
Prozosin HCl (Minipress)
Antihypertensive & Diuretic
Chlonidine HCl & Chlorthalidone (Combipres)
Naldolol & bendroflumethazid (Corzide)
Propanolol HCl & hydrochlorothiazide (Inderdide)
Antiparkinson
Biperden HCl & Biperden lactate (Akineton)
Benztropine mesyltate MSD (Cogentin)
Antipsychotic
Lithium carbonate (Lithobid)
Thioridazine (Mellaril)
Trifluoperazine (Stelazine)
Diuretics
Chlorthiazide (Diuril)
Hydrochlorthiazide (Esidrex, HydroDIURIL)
Triamterene & hydrochlorothiazide (Dyazide)
Psychotherapeutic agent
Alprazolam (Xanax)
Diazepam (Valium)
Triazolam (Halcion)

Adapted with permission from Sreebny LM, Banoczy J, Baum BJ, et al. Saliva: its role in health and disease. *Int Dent J.* 1992;297:Table 6.

Gastric Secretion Important in Infection Control

Low gastric pH constitutes an important barrier to invading microorganisms. With the exception of some lactic-acid bacteria, few microorganisms seem to survive at a pH below 3.5. Unacidic conditions in the stomach are known to promote an early colonization of the stomach with microorganisms that constitute a potential threat for infections not only in the GI tract but also in the nasopharynx and chest.[74] The stomach is also a reservoir for bacteria that cause pneumonia,[73–77] and reduction or elimination of stomach acidity promotes colonization and development of pneumonia.[76] The risk of colonization is significantly increased in the presence of foreign material such as feeding or drainage tubes in the stomach. Nosocomial pneumonia, the second most common hospital-acquired infection,[75] is a significant burden to the ICU.

Studies of ICU patients show that Gram-negative bacilli can be recovered in more than half of the patients with inhibited gastric acidity; in 59% when the pH is >4 compared to only 14% when it is <4.[78] The scientific support for routine use of stress-ulcer prophylaxis both postoperative and in the ICU, not long ago a standard practice, seems no longer to exist. No difference in incidence or severity of bleeding related to stress ulcer could be found in a controlled study performed in 300 ICU patients when treated with Sucralfate, Cimetidine, or no treatment at all. The incidences of nosocomial pneumonia in these patients were 12%, 13%, and 6% respectively, suggesting that routine prophylaxis possibly is not warranted.[79] A second study reported the same experience.[80] In a series of 106 burn patients,[81] the use of early enteral feeding reduced the incidence of nosocomial infections and eliminated the need for stress-ulcer prophylaxis.

It is important to consider that uninterrupted tube feeding, especially into the stomach, has the potential to contribute to stomach colonization and prevent disruption of the important gastric mucosal barrier.[82] Using a gastric feeding tube, the feeding should be intermittent to allow reduction of the pH level between the feeding episodes.[82] However, tube feeding into jejunum appears a more attractive alternative. Should additional mucosa protection be desired, special food ingredients, especially those rich in phospholipids and pectin (e.g., normal ingredients in a green unripe banana) will act as a pseudomucus and offer effective gastric mucosa protection.[83] (See Chapter 34.)

Nitric Oxide—The Key to GI Motility and Blood Flow

As noted earlier, the normally high nitrate content in saliva is noteworthy, as this molecule acts as a donor for gastric production of nitric oxide (NO), which is essential for stimulation of GI motility, mucosal and splanchnic circulation, and gastric bacteriostasis. Recently, an important entero-salivary circulation of nitrate has been discovered.[84,85] Nitrate secreted by the salivary glands, and/or ingested nitrate (mainly from nitrate-rich vegetables or meat), is reduced to nitrite through action of a facultative anaerobic bacteria at the posterior third of the tongue. However, the reduction does not occur in germ-free animals and is significantly reduced in antibiotic-treated patients. Nitrite swallowed into an acified stomach will immediately produce a large cascade of NO into the lumen of the stomach—if the gastric pH is not elevated by treatment with H_2-blockers or proton inhibitors. This release of NO has been calculated to be significantly larger than could be generated through intrinsic NO synthase.[84] At a pH of around 2, about 600 nM of NO will be produced, which is regarded as "several orders of magnitude greater than required for stimulation of mucosal blood flow, mucus formation, to influence motility, and for bacteriostasis." It has been suggested that such an NO release is important to prevent colonization of the stomach with pathogenic flora, since acidified nitrite is known to effectively eliminate Candida albicans, Escherichia coli, Shigella, Salmonella, and Helicobacter pylori—as well as conditions such as amoebic dysentery and chronic intestinal parasitism.[65,66] A recent study in vitro showed that adding 1 mM of nitrite to an acidic solution (pH 2) produces a complete kill of Helicobacter pylori (p<0.001) within 30 minutes.[85]

In dogs with induced endotoxemia, jejunal tube feeding of a standard nutrition formula produces an immediate and significant increase in hepatic artery, portal vein, and superior mesenteric artery blood flow. It also causes significant improvements in mucosal and hepatic microcirculation, intestinal mucosal pH, and hepatic tissue oxygen pressure and energy charge.[86] A supply of an enteral formula especially made to contain donor molecules for production of NO in the upper and lower GI tract is likely to result in even more pronounced and long-lasting effects. Nitrate/nitrite seems to be important as a donor molecule mainly in the upper GI tract, especially the stomach, but might also be a complement to arginine—the main donor molecule in the lower gastrointestinal tract. Flora is likely to play a key role in the release of arginine from arginine-rich foods, and in the production of NO from arginine. To reach the colon in large enough quantities, the donor molecules should be supplied in a "wrapped" form, e.g., as arginine-rich colonic foods (Table 33.4).

NO produced by acidified nitrite is used to control microbial overgrowth, maintain and improve mucosal and splanchnic blood flow, and stimulate gastrointestinal motility. It can also be used to promote a fast introduction of feeding tubes. Similar effects can be obtained if patients are encouraged to chew fruits and vegetables rich in nitrate, or to let them slowly "wash the mouth" with fresh juices made from nitrate-rich vegetables and fruits (see Table 33.5 for suggestions). Animals with induced pancreatitis, treated with a 10% rhubarb decoction (rhubarb is rather rich in nitrate) displayed significant reductions in the rate of translocation to mesenteric lymph nodes and pancreatic tissue (treated 25% vs. controls 100%), mortality (1/8 vs. 5/8 animals), and serum endotoxin levels (rhubarb treated: 5.41 ± 3.6 pg/L vs. controls: 61.36 ± 28.3 pg/L, $p<0.001$).[87] The authors also saw a "remarkable inhibition of gut motility observed in the control group, while gut motility was significantly improved by administration of rhubarb." Attempts to use rhubarb decoction in the ICU to promote motility when introducing feeding tubes have been successful.[88] An alternative is canned vegetable juice, such as V8 (Campbell Soup Company, Camden, NJ), which is also rich in nitrate.

TABLE 33.4

Arginine-Rich Foods	mg/100 gram
Gelatine	6000
Pumpkin seeds	4030
Soy protein	3760
Peanuts	3600
Sesame seeds	3330
Soy beans	2730
Almonds	2500
Sunflower seeds	2400
Brazil nuts	2390
Peas, lentils	2050
Shrimp	2000
Baker's yeast	2000
Parmesan cheese	1560
Meat, fish	1500

TABLE 33.5

Nitrate-Rich Foods	mg/kg
Fennel	3200
Lettuce	2900
Celery	2700
Mangold	2600
Dill	2400
Spinach	1900
Beetroot	1700
Nettle	1600
Radish	1300
Chinese cabbage	1300
Leek	720
Rhubarb	700
Chives	670
White cabbage	620
Squash	580
Broccoli	490
Horseradish	390

EN and LAB Might Modulate Rejection

The gastrointestinal tract is not only a major target organ for acute graft-versus-host disease, but also a critical amplifier of the "cytokine storm" characteristic to this condition.[89] Observations in human liver transplantation indicate that early and aggressive enteral nutrition reduces the rate of early rejection from 44% in patients fed parenterally to 7% in patients fed enterally.[90] Furthermore, animal studies performed in the 1970s demonstrated that death after bone marrow transplantation can be prevented by normalization of the gut flora.[91]

A key to success is to inhibit the process of GI tract damage. Endotoxin seems to be a key factor behind the breakdown of the gastrointestinal mucosa and gut-associated lymphoid tissue. Endotoxin is also responsible for the increased translocation and frequency and severity of graft-versus-host disease. Supplying probiotics reduces and sometimes even eliminates serum endotoxin. One could therefore speculate that supplying of probiotics to transplant patients will not only reduce the rate of infection, but also the frequency and severity of rejection.

It has become increasingly evident that NF-κB is a major player in the inflammatory response.[92] This transcription factor is normally bound to its inhibitor IκB. Recent studies suggest that pathogenic bacteria activate NF-κB and switch on genes for TNF and IL-8, which leads to an amplification of the inflammatory immune response. But exposure to nonpathogenic bacteria (probiotic bacteria) prevents ubiquitination and hence degradation of the inhibitor IκB, and blocks an exaggerated immune response.[93,94]

Use of Special Immunomodulatory Nutrients

Clearly, some important mediators are deeply involved in the inflammatory reaction and are responsible for the development of a super-inflammation, which induces the general systemic inflammatory response (SIRS). Further down the road, SIRS leads to MOF and MODS, which has stimulated numerous attempts to produce molecules with inhibitory effects for specific key mediators. Such attempts, unfortunately, have been largely unsuccessful.[95–97] One reason could be that most mediators do normally function in large consortia, "as instruments in a large immuno-modulatory orchestra." If so, mono-therapy, consisting of inhibition of only one or two modulators, no matter how important, cannot be expected to lead to any radical improvement. Furthermore, treatment with various inhibitors is often instituted late in the disease process, when the super-inflammation is already established. It is clear that the opportunity to influence the acute phase response and prevent it from overreacting is limited to the very early phase of disease—in the case of surgery to the intra-operative and immediate early postoperative period.

Conclusions

The positive immuno-modulatory effects of enteral nutrition is well documented, but must be done properly to be effective. Both timing and content of the formula are equally important. Patients who have been starving overnight are already immunologically handicapped at the beginning of the operation. As long ago as 40 years, it was shown that the depletion of glycogen stores, which occurs during preoperative starvation, reduces resistance to complications and increases the risk of morbidity.[98] Furthermore, due to the high adrenergic activity during anesthesia, no glycogen synthesis is likely to occur during the immediate hours after surgery, either in the liver or in the muscles.[98] However, the GI mucosa is able to absorb nutrition directly from the lumen. The uninterrupted and continuous supply of nutrients and antioxidants is important for maximal function of the enterocytes and their associated GALT-system. Supply of fiber is essential for maintenance of the mucosal function in the lower gastrointestinal tract, although it is the probiotic flora that processes the fibers and provides the necessary nutrients and antioxidants to the mucosal cells. This will be further discussed in Chapter 34.

References

1. Hippocrates. *Aphorisms.* English translation. Jones WHS, ed. London: Heineman; 1931.
2. Andresen AFR. Immediate jejunal feeding after gastroenterostomy. *Ann Surg.* 1918;67:565–566.
3. Mulholland JH, Tui C, Wright AM, et al. Nitrogen metabolism, caloric intake and weight loss in postoperative convalescence. *Ann Surg.* 1943;117:512–534.
4. Riegel C, Koop CE, Drew J, et al. The nutritional requirements for nitrogen balance in surgical patients during early postoperative periods. *J Clin Invest.* 1947;26:18–23.
5. Shepherd AP. Intestinal blood flow autoregulation during foodstuff absorption. *Am J Physiol.* 1980;239:561–562.
6. Roediger WEW. Role of anaerobic bacteria in the metabolic welfare of the colonic mucosa in man. *Gut.* 1980;21: 793–798.
7. Hoover HC, Ryan Jr JA, Anderson EJ, Fischer JE. Nutritional benefits of immediate postoperative jejunal feeding of an elemental diet. *Am J Surg.* 1980;139:153–159.
8. Alexander JW, MacMillan BG, Stinnett JD, et al. Beneficial effects of aggressive protein feeding in severely burned children. *Ann Surg.* 1980;192:505–517.
9. Ryan Jr JA, Page CP, Babcock L. Early postoperative jejunal feeding of elemental diet in gastrointestinal surgery. *Amer Surg.* 1981;47:393–403.
10. Moore FA, Feliciano DF, Andrassy JR, et al. Early enteral feeding compared with parenteral, reduces postoperative septic complications: the result of a meta-analysis. *Ann Surg.* 1991;216:172–183.
11. Kudsk KA, Groce MA, Fabian TC, et al. Enteral versus parenteral feeding: effects on septic morbidity after blunt and penetrating abdominal trauma. *Ann Surg.* 1992;215: 503–513.
12. Bengmark S. Progress in perioperative enteral tube feeding. *Clin Nutr.* 1998;17:145–153.
13. Bengmark S, Andersson R, Mangiante G. Uninterrupted perioperative enteral nutrition. *Clin Nutr.* 2001;20:11–19.
14. Brandtzaeg P, Halstensen TS, Krajci P, et al. Immunobiology and immunopathology of human gut mucosa: humoral immunity and intraepithelial lymphocytes. *Gastroenterology.* 1989;97:1562–1584.
15. Bengmark S. Gut microenvironment and immune function. *Current Opinion in Clinical Nutrition and Metabolic Care.* 1999;2;83–85.
16. Schorah CJ, Downing C, Piripitsi A. Total vitamin C, ascorbic acid, and dehydroascorbic acid concentrations in plasma in critically ill patients. *Am J Clin Nutr.* 1996;63: 760–765.
17. Schroeder HA. Losses of vitamins and trace minerals etc. *Am J Clin Nutr.* 1971;24:562–573.

18. Luo J-L, Hammarquist F, Andersson K, et al. Skeletal muscle glutathione after surgical trauma. *Ann Surg.* 1996; 223:420–427.
19. Wierzbicka GT, Hagen TM, Jones DP. Glutathione in food. *J Food Comp Analys.* 1989;2:327–337.
20. Brandtzaeg P. Molecular and cellular aspects of the secretory immunoglobulin system. *APMIS.* 1995;103:1–19.
21. Van Thiel DH, Finkel R, Friedlander L. The association of IgA deficiency but not IgG or IgM deficiency with a reduced patient and graft survival following liver transplantation. *Transplantation.* 1992;54:269–273.
22. Aronsen KF, Ekelund G, Kindmark CO, et al. Sequential changes of plasma proteins after surgical trauma. *Scand J Lab Invest.* 1972;29; (Suppl) 124:127–136.
23. van Deventer SJH, Büller HR, ten Cate JW, et al. Experimental endotoxemia in humans: Analysis of cytokine release and coagulation, fibrinolytic and complement pathways. *Blood.* 1990;76:2520–2526.
24. O'Dwyer ST, Michie HR, Ziegler TR. et al. A single dose of endotoxin increases intestinal permeability in healthy humans. *Arch Surg.* 1994;123:1459–1464.
25. Sautner T, Függer R, Götzinger P et al. Tumour necrosis factor-α and interleukin-6: early indicators of bacterial infection after human orthotopic liver transplantation. *Eur J Surg.* 1995;161:97–101.
26. Messmann H, Vogt W, Holstege A, et al. Post-ERP pancreatitis as a model for cytokine induced acute phase response in acute pancreatitis. *Gut.* 1997;40:80–85.
27. Fiddian-Green RG, Baker S. Predictive value of the stomach wall pH for complications after cardiac operations: comparison with other monitoring. *Crit Care Med.* 1987; 15:153–156.
28. Doglio GR, Pusajo JF, Egurrola MA, et al. Gastric mucosal pH as a prognostic index of mortality in critically ill patients. *Crit Care Med.* 1990;19:1037–1040.
29. Takács T, Farkas G, Czako L, et al. Time-course changes in serum cytokine levels in two experimental acute pancreatitis models in rats. *Res Exp Med.* 1996;196:153–161.
30. Leveau P, Wang X, Soltesz V, et al. Alterations in intestinal permeability and microflora in experimental acute pancreatitis. *Int J Pancreatology.* 1996;20:119–125.
31. Andersson R, Wang X, Ihse I. The influence of abdominal sepsis on acute pancreatitis in rats: a study on mortality, permeability, arterial blood pressure and intestinal blood flow. *Pancreas.* 1995;11:365–373.
32. De Souza LJ, Sampietre SN, Figueiredo S, et al. Bacterial translocation during acute pancreatitis in rats. (In Portuguese, with English summary) *Rev Hosp Clin Fac Med S. Paolo.* 1996;51:116–120.
33. Norman J. The role of cytokines in the pathogenesis of acute pancreatitis. *Am J Surg.* 1998;175:76–83.
34. Parikh AA, Salzman AL, Fischer JE, et al. Interleukin-1β and interferon-γ regulate interleukin-6 production in human intestinal cells. *Shock.* 1997;8:249–255.
35. Liebermann TA, Baltimore D. Activation of interleukin-6 gene expression through the NF-κB transcription factor. *Mol Cell Biol.* 1990;10:2327–2334.
36. Akira S, Hirano T, Taga T, et al. Parenteral nutrition in patients receiving cancer chemotherapy. *FASEB J.* 1990;4: 734–736.
37. Argilés JM, López-Soriano FJ. The role of cytokines in cancer cachexia. *Med Res Rev.* 1999;3:223–248.
38. Keller U. Pathophysiology of cancer cachexia. *Support Care Cancer.* 1993;1:290–294.
39. Meyer TA, Noguchi Y, Ogle CK, et al. Endotoxin stimulates interleukin-6 production in intestinal epithelial cells. *Arch Surg.* 1994;129:1290–1295.
40. Meyer TA, Tiao GM, James JH. Nitric oxide inhibits LPS-induced IL-6 production in enterocytes. *J Surg Res.* 1995;58:570–575.
41. Fried SK, Bunkin DA, Greenberg AS. Omental and subcutaneous adipose tissues of obese subjects release interleukin-6: depot difference and regulation by glucocorticoid. *J Clin Endocrinol Metabol.* 1998;83:847–840.
42. Thomas EL, Saeed N, Hajnal JV, et al. Magnetic resonance imaging of total body fat. *J Appl Physiol.* 1998;85: 1778–1785.
43. Landin K, Stigendal L, Eriksson E, et al. Abdominal obesity is associated with impaired fibrinolytic activity and elevated plasminogen activator inhibitor-1. *Metabolism.* 1990;39:1044–1048.
44. Crockson RA, Payne CJ, Ratcliff AP, et al. Time sequence of acute phase proteins following surgical trauma. *Clin Chim Acta.* 1966;14:435–441.
45. Shakespeare PG, Ball AJ, Spurr ED. Serum protein changes after abdominal surgery. *Ann Clin Biochem.* 1989;26:49–57.
46. Biffl WL, Moore EE, Moore FA, et al. Interleukin-6 delays neutrophil apoptosis via a mechanism involving platelet-activating factor. *J Trauma, Injury, Infect & Crit Care.* 1996;40:575–579.
47. Klein CUJ, Stanek GS, Wiles CE. Overfeeding macronutrients to critically ill adults: metabolic complications. *J Am Diet Assoc.* 1998;98:795–806.
48. Sandström R, Drott C, Hyltander A, et al. The effect of postoperative intravenous feeding (TPN) on outcome following major surgery evaluated in a randomized study. *Ann Surg.* 1993;217:185–195.
49. Heslin MJ, Latkany L, Leung D, et al. A prospective randomized trial of early enteral feeding after resection of upper gastrointestinal malignancy. *Ann Surg.* 1997;226: 567–580.
50. Hochwald SN, Harrison LE, Heslin MJ, et al. Early postoperative enteral feeding improves whole body protein kinetics in upper gastrointestinal cancer patients. *Am J Surg.* 1997;174:325–330.
51. Shirabe K, Matsumata T, Shimada M, et al. A comparison of parenteral hyperalimentation and early enteral feeding regarding systemic immunity after major hepatic resection —the result of a randomized prospective study. *Hepato-Gastroenterology.* 1997;44:205–209.
52. Windsor ACJ, Kanwar S, Li AGK, et al. Compared with parenteral nutrition, enteral feeding attenuates the acute phase response, and improves disease severity in acute pancreatitis. *Gut.* 1998;42:431–435.

53. Bateman DN, Whittingham TA. Measurement of gastric emptying by real-time ultrasound. *Gut.* 1982;23:524–527.

54. Harter RL, Kelly WB, Kramer MG, et al. A comparison of the volume and pH of gastric contents of obese and lean surgical patients. *Anesth Analg.* 1998;86:147–152.

55. Miller M, Wishart HY, Nimmo WS. Gastric contents at induction of anesthesia. Is a 4-hour fast necessary? *Br J Anesth.* 1983;55:1185–1188.

56. Groves H. Preoperative patient fasting regimes. *Br J Theatre Nurs.* 1994;4:14–16.

57. Maclean AR, Renwick C. Audit of pre-operative starvation. *Anesthesia.* 1993;48:164–166.

58. Kushikata T, Matsuki A, Murakawa T, et al. Possibility of rice porridge for preoperative feeding in children. *MATSUI.* 1996;45:943–947.

59. Schreiber MS, Triebwasser A, Keon TP. Ingestion of liquids compared with preoperative fasting in pediatric outpatients. *Anesthesiology.* 1990;72:593–597.

60. Hung P. Pre-operative fasting. *Nursing Times.* 1992;25: 57–60.

61. Buescher TM, Cioffi WG, Becker WK, et al. Perioperative enteral feedings. *Proc Am Burn Assoc.* 1992;22:abstract 162.

62. Jenkins ME, Gottschlich MM, Warden GD. Enteral feeding during operative procedures in thermal injuries. *J Burn Care Rehabil.* 1994;15:199–205.

63. Mangiante G, et al. Personal communication.

64. Levenson R, Turner Jr WW, Dyson A, et al. Do weighted nasoenteric feeding tubes facilitate duodenal intubations? *J Parenter Enteral Nutr.* 1988;12:135–137.

65. Duncan C, Dougall H, Johnston P, et al. Chemical generation of nitric oxide in the mouth from the enterosalivary circulation of dietary nitrates. *Nat Med.* 1995;1: 546–551.

66. Lundberg JON, Weitzberg E, Lundberg JM, et al. Intragastric nitric oxide production in humans: measurement in expelled air. *Gut.* 1994;35:1543–1546.

67. Mandel ID. The function of saliva. *J Dent Res.* (Spec Iss) 1987;66:623–627.

68. Sreebny LM, Banoczy J, Baum BJ, et al. Saliva: Its role in health and disease. *Int Dent J.* 1992;42:291–304.

69. Pollack JJ, Lotardo S, Gwinnett AJ, et al. Antimicrobial interactions of salivary cationic proteins. In Mergenhagen SE, Rosan B, eds. Molecular basis of oral microbial adhesion. *Am Soc Microbiol.* 1985:136–143.

70. Tabak LA, Levine MJ, Mandel ID, et al. Role of salivary mucins in the protection of the oral cavity. *J Oral Pathol.* 1982;11:1–17.

71. Sarosiek J, Feng TT, McCallum RW. The interrelationship between salivary epidermal growth factor and the functional integrity of the mucosal barrier in the rat. *Am J Med Sci.* 1991; 302: 359–363.

72. Watanabe S, Ohnishi M, Imai K, et al. Estimation of the total saliva volume produced per day in five-year-old children. *Archs Oral Biol.* 1995;40:781–782.

73. Fox PC, van der Ven PF, Baum BJ, et al. Pilocarpine for the treatment of xerostomia associated with salivary gland dysfunction. *Oral Surg.* 1986;61:243–248.

74. Wilder-Smith CH, Spirig C, Krech T, et al. Bactericidal factors in gastric juice. *Eur J Gastro Hepatol.* 1992;4:885–891.

75. Horan TC, White JW, Jarvis WR. Nosocomial infection surveillance. *MMWR.* 1986;35:17–29.

76. Atherton ST, White DJ. Stomach as source of bacteria colonizing the respiratory tract during artificial respiration. *Lancet.* 1978;1:2968–2969.

77. Heyland D, Mandell LA. Gastric colonization by Gram-negative bacilli and nosocomial pneumonia in the intensive care unit patients. *Chest.* 1992;101:187–193.

78. Donowitz GL, Page ML, Mileur BL. Alteration of normal gastric flora in critical care patients receiving antacid and cimethidine therapy. *Infect Control.* 1986;7:23–26.

79. Ben-Menachen T, Fogel R, Patel RV, et al. Prophylaxis for stress-related gastric hemorrhage in the medical intensive care unit. A randomized controlled, single-blind study. *Ann Int Med.* 1994; 121: 568–575.

80. Cook DJ, Fuller HD, Guyatt GH, et al. Gastrointestinal bleeding in the critically ill: stress ulcer prophylaxis is not for everyone. *N Engl J Med.* 1994;330:377–381.

81. McDonald WS, Sharp CW, Deitsch EA. Immediate enteral feeding in burn patients is safe and effective. *Ann Surg.* 1991;214:177–183.

82. Bonten MJM, Gaillard CA, van Thiel FH, et al. Continuous enteral feeding counteracts preventive measures for gastric colonization in intensive care patients. *Crit Care Med.* 1994;22:939–944.

83. Bengmark S, Larsson K, Molin G. Gut mucosa reconditioning with species-specific lactobacilli, surfactants, pseudomucus, and fibers—an invited review. *Biotechnol Therapeut.* 1995;5: 171–194.

84. McKnight GM, Smith LM, Drummond RS. Chemical synthesis of nitric oxide in the stomach from dietary nitrate in humans. *Gut.* 1997;40:211–214.

85. Dykhuizen RS, Fraser A, McKenzie H, et al. Helicobacter pylori is killed by nitrite under acidic conditions. *Gut.* 1998;42:334–337.

86. Kazamias P, Kotzampassi K, Koufogiannis D, et al. Influence of enteral nutrition-induced splanchnic hyperemia on the septic origin of splanchnic ischemia. *World J Surg.* 1998;22:6–11.

87. Lin BF, Huang CC, Chiang BL, et al. Dietary fat influences Ia antigen expression, cytokines and prostaglandin E_2 production in immune cells in autoimmune-prone NZBxNZW F1 mice. *Brit J Nutr.* 1996;75:711–722.

88. Mangiante G, Nicoli N, Marchiori L, et al. Uninterrupted perioperative enteral nutrition: a safe procedure in surgical practice. *Eur Surg Res.* 2000:32:11.

89. Hill GR, Ferrara LM. The primacy of the gastrointestinal tract as a target organ of acute graft-versus-host disease: rationale for the use of cytokine shields in allogenic bone marrow transplantation. *Blood.* 2000;95:2754–2759.

90. Sharpe MD, Pikul J, Lowndes R, et al. Early enteral feeding (EEF) reduces incidence of early rejection following liver transplantation (abstract). *Joint Congress of Liver Transplantation.* London;1995.

91. van Bekkum DW, Rodenburg J, Heldt PJ, et al. Mitigation of secondary disease of allogeneic mouse radiation chimeras by modification of the intestinal flora. *J Natl Cancer Inst.* 1974;52:401–404.

92. Karin M, Ben-Neriah Y. Phosphorylation meets ubiquitination: the control of NF-[kappa]B activity. *Annu Rev Immunol.* 2000;18:621–63.

93. Neish AS, Gewirtz AT, Zeng H, et al. Prokaryotic regulation of epithelial responses by inhibition of IκB-α ubiquitination. *Science.* 2000;289:1560–1563.

94. Xavier RJ, Podolsky DK. How to get along—friendly microbes in a hostile world. *Science.* 2000 Sep 1;289:1483–1484.

95. Abraham E, Anzueto A, Gutierrez G, et al. Double-blind randomized controlled trial of monoclonal antibody to human tumour necrosis factor in the treatment of septic shock. *Lancet.* 1998;351:929–933.

96. Van Dissel JT, van Langevelde P, Westendorp RG, et al. Antiinflammatory cytokine profile and mortality in febrile patients. *Lancet.* 1998;351:950–953.

97. Vincent JL. Search for effective immunomodulating strategies against sepsis. *Lancet.* 1998;28:922–923.

98. Sunzel H. The importance of liver glycogen in preventing the development of liver lesions at operation. *Acta Chir Scand.* 1963;(Suppl)304:1–128.

CHAPTER

34

Probiotics, Prebiotics, and Synbiotics in the Intensive Care Unit

Stig Bengmark, M.D., Ph.D.

THE MICROBIAL ORGAN 381
FIBERS ARE PREBIOTICS 382
Pectin 382
Betaglucans 382
Resistant Starch 383
Fructooligosaccharides 383
Algal Fibers 383
Glucomannans 383
A COMPLEX FLORA 383
COMMENSAL FLORA REDUCED EARLY IN DISEASE 384
POSTOPERATIVE MORBIDITY STILL HIGH—AND UNCHANGED? 384
A LIFESTYLE-ASSOCIATED PREDISPOSITION? 384
DIET-INDUCED SUPERINFLAMMATION 385
THE MAJORITY OF IMMUNE SYSTEM IS IN THE GUT 385
NEUROENDOCRINE REGULATION OF THE ACUTE PHASE RESPONSE 386
IMMUNO-ENHANCING NUTRITION SOLUTIONS CONTROVERSIAL 386
LACTIC ACID BACTERIA 387
Initiates Immunoglobulin Production 387
Restore Macrophage Function 387
Stimulate Apoptosis 387
Modulate Lymphocyte Functions 388
Modulate Cytokine Release 388
Increase Mucin Production 389
Eliminate Toxins and Mutagens 389
Stimulate Mucosal Growth 390
Prevents/Reduces Diarrhea 390
Prevents/Reduces Severity of Colitis 391
In Intensive Care Patients 391
To Patients with Fulminant MOF 392
CONCLUSIONS 394
REFERENCES 395

The Microbial Organ

Not long ago, the large intestine was regarded as an organ with only one primary function—to reabsorb water and electrolytes. Only recently have clinicians recognized that the colon is a highly active organ in which numerous metabolic processes take place and myriad nutrients are released and absorbed. It is here, for example, that enzymes produced by *probiotic* bacteria metabolize *prebiotics* (various fruit and vegetable fibers, gastrointestinal secretions, and apoptotic cells).

The countless numbers of products being released and absorbed in the GI tract are increasingly referred to as *synbiotics*.

Today, the colon is known as a metabolic organ with functions that are both larger in number and more complex than the rest of the gastrointestinal tract. Here chemical processes are promoted by enzymes produced by bacteria—instead of by eukaryotic cells. An indication of the complexity of the metabolic activities in the large intestine is the fact that the colonic "microbial organ" contains about 300,000 genes —compared to about 65,000 genes in the rest of the human body. Numerous substances—several hundred thousand if not millions—are produced, released, and absorbed at the level of the lower small intestine and the large intestine. Among these are various fatty acids, especially short-chain fatty acids (SCFAs), carbohydrates, amino acids, polyamines, vitamins, antioxidants, phytoestrogens, and coagulation and growth factors. Among these are for example polyphenols such as flavonoid which make up more than 4,000 compounds and carotenoids which comprise another approximately 600 compounds.

Although the word synbiotics was coined to describe the combined action of pre- and probiotics, e.g. like the ability of antibiotics to control infection, the term today is increasingly used in a wider sense: as a name for all the substances released by microbial fermentation in the lower gut. One obvious reason is that most of the substances released seem to influence the immune defense, increase resistance to disease, and most important, prevent complications to surgery such as infections and thrombosis.

The food ingredients (fibers, complex proteins, etc.) that reach the colon largely unchanged are usually referred to as "colonic foods." It is recommended that at least 10% of the total calorie intake should be of this type, a goal difficult to meet in the critically ill patient. Since prebiotic fibers are low-calorie, at least one-fourth of the food eaten under healthy conditions should be "food destined for the colon," e.g., food ingredients that not are broken down by gastrointestinal enzymes and absorbed in the upper small intestine. In the past, it was usually regarded as more or less impossible to provide colonic foods to patients in the ICU. In recent years, however, this view has been revised.

Fibers Are Prebiotics

Research regarding various probiotics has exploded in recent years, and information about the various probiotic bacteria is rapidly expanding. Since the availability and content of prebiotic fibers influence the production of these bacterium compounds, prebiotics are now regarded as important as probiotics.

Fibers are carbohydrates derived from plant-cell walls. Dietary fibers are usually classified into three groups: *soluble fibers* such as pectins and various gums, *insoluble fibers* such as cellulose, and *mixed-type fibers* such as brans. The most important characteristic for them all is that they are resistant to hydrolysis by human alimentary-tract enzymes, which make some of them ideal as substrate for microbial fermentation in the lower GI tract. Soluble fibers (prebiotics) constitute an important source for bacterial fermentation and microbial production of nutrients, antioxidants, vitamins, and growth and other important factors. Thus far, the main interest has focused on the production of various short-chain fatty acids (SCFAs), and fermentation byproducts such as hydrogen, methane, and carbon dioxide. But the content of other nutrients—various bioactive amino acids, polyamins, antioxidants, and various growth factors—are equally important.[1–5]

Prebiotic fibers are slow carbohydrates, which have a strong influence on glucose and fat metabolism and cause reductions in postprandial glycemia, concentration of free fatty acids, and serum cholesterol levels.[6,7] An increase in proliferation of mucosa epithelial cells will occur in the caecum and in the colon as a result of increased fiber consumption. This proliferation is associated with a significant decrease in intraluminal pH.[6] Fibers also have their own direct physiological effects. Soluble and viscous fiber delay gastric emptying, increase intestinal transit time, and improve glucose tolerance. Soluble dietary fibers also sequestrate bile salts and significantly affect lipid absorption.

The following is a short introduction to some interesting bioactive fibers.

Pectin

Our group has observed, when studying a pectin solution in water, that when pH is reduced to a level of 1.0, e.g., the pH seen in the stomach, a so-called two-phase separation will occur,[8] leading to formation of a gel phase and a watery phase. It is likely that, when this separation occurs in the stomach, the gel phase will adhere to the mucosa layer and increase the protective capacity of the mucus. Banana, especially when green and immature, is rich in both pectin and phospholipids—both known to have strong protective effects against peptic ulcer.[9–10] The effects of using concentrations greater that those normally seen in fruit did not differ much from the effects obtained by established drugs such as H_2-blockers, proton inhibitors, and surface-protecting agents.[11,12]

Another interesting feature of pectin is that it is a strong antioxidant, which offers mucosal protection against all three main types of oxidation damage: peroxy, superoxide, and hydroxyl radical.[13] This could be the mechanism by which pectin stimulates the GALT system and prevents disruption of the intestinal microflora.[14] A disadvantage with pectin is that it is difficult to use in tube-feeding, as it has a tendency to clog the tube.

Betaglucans

Another most interesting group of fibers is the betaglucans, unique water-soluble fibers often extracted from oat, which contain up to as much as 17% of betaglucans.[15] This gum fiber compares favorably with other high viscosity polysaccharides such as substituted celluloses, guar gums, and locust-bean gums. The clinical effects of oat gums have not yet been explored to the same extent as those of pectin, but are likely to be similar. Most clinical studies have concentrated on oat's unique cholesterol-lowering effects[60] and its unique and strong antioxidant effects, extensively used in the past for food-stabilizing purpose.

Resistant Starch

Resistant starch, unlike most starches, resists digestion in the small intestine and reaches the colon. Resistant starch, which is one of the main sources of carbohydrate substrates for colonic microflora, is a good determinant of human large bowel function. It is known to release large quantities of butyrate when fermented—butyrate being the primary fuel for the colonocyte.

Fructooligosaccharides

Fructooligosaccharides (FOS), composed of one molecule of glucose and one to three molecules of fructose, have been shown to have unique abilities to stimulate the intestinal flora effectively.[17] Fructooligosaccharides exist naturally in many kinds of plants such as onions, asparagus roots, tubers of Jerusalem artichoke and wheat, as well as in banana, beer, burdock, Chinese chives, garlic, graminae (fodder grass), honey, oat, pine, rye, chicory, stone leak—and even in bacteria and yeasts. In a recent survey, the daily intake of inulin and oligofructose by the North American population has been estimated to be 2 g to 8 g.[18] It is important to recognize that only few lactic-acid bacteria strains have the ability to ferment fructans such as phlein and inulin. When 712 LAB strains were tested, only 16 could utilize phleins and only 8 inulins.[71] Of these, *L plantarum*, followed by *L paracasei* was the most effective both to ferment the fibers and to reduce pH.[19] Beneficial effects of fructooligosaccharides on serum cholesterol, triglyceride levels, and blood pressure in elderly patients with hyperlipemia have been reported.[20]

Algal Fibers

Algal polysaccharides are receiving renewed and increasing interest. Most of these fibers are resistant to hydrolysis by human digestive enzymes[21–23] and should be suitable as dietary fibers. Their physiological effects have only recently begun to be investigated.[24] Most recent studies deal with their fermentative degradation by the colonic flora.[25] The soluble fibers in seaweed, for example, consist of *laminarans* (a sort of β-glucans associated with mannitol residues), *fucans* (sulphated polymers associated with xylose, galactose, and glucoronic acid), and *alginates* (mannuronic and guluronic acid polymers). By contrast, the *insolubles algal fibers* are essentially cellulose. Fermentation of alginates result in a high acetate production (80%), and laminarans have a very high yield of butyrate. Seaweed, with its high content of fermentable fibers, its documented ability to produce large quantities of SCFAs, and its high content of omega-3 fatty acids, should be an interesting source of medical fibers—and most likely will soon be explored more fully by researchers.

Glucomannans

Glucomannan, a nonabsorbable polysaccharide (glucose/mannose polymer) derived from *Amorphophallus konjak* (English names: devil tongue, elephant yam, umbrella arum) is also receiving increasing attention for its potential health effects, most likely associated with its unique hydroscopic ability. On contact with water, it swells and becomes a viscous gel.[26] Like other soluble fibers, it delays both the gastric emptying and intestinal transit time. It is also effective in decreasing the intake of digestible energy.[27] Glycomannans are frequently used in Japan for conditions such as hypercholesterolemia, hypertension, and diabetes.[98,99]

A Complex Flora

It has been calculated that the human body contains more than 10 times as many bacterial cells (10^{14}) as eukaryotic cells (10^{13}). The large intestine is supposed to contain, when on Western-type diet, about one kilogram of bacteria. However, individuals living in rural areas and consuming larger amounts of fruits and vegetable fibers—as well as more live lactobacilli—often harbor about two kilograms of live bacterial flora in their large intestine. But it is not only the gut that has a "protection layer" of probiotic bacteria. There are approximately 200 grams on our skin; about 20 grams each in the mouth, the lung, and the vagina; 10 grams in the nose; and about 1 gram in the eyes. This protection layer is most often lost in the environment of ICU—especially when treated with antibiotics and cytostatics.

About 400 bacterial species are normally found in the fecal/colonic microflora of a healthy individual, but 30 to 40 species seem to constitute 99% of the collection in any one human subject.[28] The bacterial genera, which are common components of the human intestinal microflora, are *Bacteroides, Bifidobacterium, Clostridium, Enterococcus, Eubacterium, Fusobacterium, Peptostreptococcus, Ruminococcus, Lactobacillus* and *Escherichia.* It is suggested that each human being has his or her own unique microbial collection, especially of strains such as *Bifidobacterium* and *Lactobacillus*, and that it should be possible to identify an individual on the basis of his or her personal intestinal microflora.[28]

The most common LAB strains found on the rectal mucosa of healthy humans living a Western lifestyle are *Lactobacillus plantarum*, *Lactobacillus rhamnosus* and *Lactobacillus paracasei* ssp *paracasei*, isolated in 52%, 26%, and 17% of tested individuals respectively.[29] In the same study, the colonization rate of commonly used milk-born probiotic bacteria such *Lactobacillus casei*, *Lactobacillus reuteri*, and *Lactobacillus acidophilus* was only 2%, 2%, and 0% respectively. *Lactobacillus plantarum* is likely to more often colonize vegetarians (approximately 66% of that population) than omnivores (approximately 25% of that population).[30] Lactic-acid bacteria (LAB) seem not to tolerate well in a modern, so-called Western lifestyle well. Swedish children, for example, have a different and less rich flora than Parkistani[31] or Estonian children.[32]

Commensal Flora Reduced Early in Disease

On return from space flights, cosmonauts are reported to have lost most of their commensal flora, including *Lactobacillus* species such as *Lactobacillus plantarum* and *Lacobacillus casei* (down almost 100%), *Lactobacillus fermentum* (reduced 43%), *Lactobacillus acidophilus* (reduced 27%), *Lactobacillus salivarius* (reduced 22%) and *Lactobacillus brevis* (reduced 12%).[33] These changes are attributed to poor eating (dried food, no fresh fruits and vegetables) and reduced supply of fiber and antioxidants, but also lack of exercise and mental and physical stress. In many ways this is analogous to the ICU patient. The flora always seems to be significantly reduced in the sick, especially in connection with severe disease, but also as a result of care in ICU, and in patients with little food intake or on parenteral nutrition.

The reduction of the commensal flora occurs early in disease. In experimental pancreatitis, for example, anaerobic bacteria and lactobacilli are significantly reduced both in the distal small bowel and in the colon within 6 to 12 hours after induction of disease. The changes in patterns of probiotic flora are almost instantly followed by significant increase in numbers of potentially pathogenic microorganisms (PPMs) such as *Escherichia coli*. Dramatic increases in mucosal barrier permeability (lumen to blood) and in endothelial permeability (blood to tissue) also occur.[34,35] Both are associated with increased microbial translocation and microbial growth of mesenteric lymph nodes and, in the case of pancreatitis, the pancreatic tissue.[36]

Postoperative Morbidity Still High—And Unchanged?

The incidence of major complications following trauma and surgical treatment does not appear to have been reduced at all in recent years—or at least not as much as expected. These complications include infections, venous thrombosis, and major sequelae such as formation of serosal adhesions. As a result, almost every second patient subjected to transplantation suffers episodes to infection, especially bone marrow, liver, pancreas, and intestinal transplantation. Infections strike every third patient subjected to major liver and pancreas resection, and every fifth patient having extensive gastric and large intestinal surgery.[37,38] Moreover, laryngopharyngeal, orthopedic, and cardiac surgery often report a double digit incidence of infections. Accumulating evidence suggests that the occurrence of septic complications is intimately associated with a reduced immunological protection of the patient, and a large proportion of the complications are seen in patients over the age of 65 and in immuno-compromised patients.

Venous thrombosis is a frequent complication even today. It is true that clinical manifestations of thrombosis can successfully be eliminated by prophylactic use of various anti-thrombotic agents, but 50% to 70% of the patients will, if phlebography is performed, show signs of venous thrombosis. High incidence of thrombosis seems particularly to be associated with parenteral nutrition (PN), and especially total parenteral nutrition (TPN). Thrombosis and infection seem to be interrelated, and it has recently been suggested that "one common complication may facilitate the occurrence of another common complication by synergistic stimulation of the coagulation system."[39] Also, the incidence of serosal adhesions in cavities such as the peritoneum, pleura, pericardium, and around tendons remains high following surgery. These adhesions make re-operations more difficult and sometimes impossible, and can also lead to other severe health problems such as intestinal obstruction and infertility.

A Lifestyle-Associated Predisposition?

There is accumulating evidence that a Western lifestyle, especially Western food habits, predisposes patients to super-inflammation and to subsequent clinical complications. It is a rather old observation, for example, that men eating large amounts of fiber are protected from postoperative venous thrombosis.[40,41] It has also been reported that men living in rural areas and consuming large quantities of cellulose and vegetable fibers, plus live lactobacilli (fermented milk), have a significantly longer mean clotting time and soft jelly-like clots compared to those living in urban areas.[42] Reduced plasma levels of fibrinogen and factor X have been observed in baboons on a "Western diet" when supplemented with a fiber such as konjak-glucomannan.[43] Decreased levels of plasma viscosity and fibrinogen are found in diabetic children supplemented with another fiber, guar-gum.[44]

Serosal adhesions are associated with an increased endotoxin production and with over-expression of TGFβ[45]; germ-free animals do not develop serosal adhesions.[46] Both observations support an assumption that peritoneal adhesions resulting from trauma are associated with alterations in the intestinal environment and in the immune defense.

Increased coagulation is associated with dyslipidemia, glucose intolerance, and intravascular coagulation and thrombosis. Diabetic and obese rats with insulin deficiency show raised levels of circulating free fatty acids (FFA).[47] Raised levels of circulating saturated FFAs stimulate fibrinogen synthesis.[48] Insulin resistance, research suggests, can promote increased levels of FFA and increased fibrinogen synthesis.[49] Fibrinogen synthesis can be prevented by increased intake of prebiotics. These dietary fibers, such as cellulose, pectin, hemicellulose, and some starches, are all substrates for production in the large intestine of short-chain fatty acids (SCFA), which improve insulin sensitivity.[50]

Diet-Induced Superinflammation

Consumption of saturated fatty acids, as well as trans-fatty acids, induces significant alterations in the immune response,[51] inhibits the macrophage functions,[52] and stimulates Th2 response relative to the Th1 response. A recent study in mice observed higher IgM and IgG antibody levels, worsened proteinuria, and shortened life span in mice fed a high-fat diet (200 g fat/kg food) compared to those fed a low-fat diet (50 g fat/kg food). In vitro LPS stimulation of peritoneal macrophages from the two groups showed significantly higher release of IL-6 (134 vs. 59 ng/10^6 cells, p=0.02), TNF-α (311 vs. 95 pg/10^6 cells, p =0.001) and PGE_2 (906 vs. 449 pg/10^6 cells, p=0.01) in the group fed a high-fat diet.[53]

In the absence of adequate oral/enteral nutrition supply—as a result of bowel rest or TPN, for example—the response of splanchnic cytokines to a challenge with endotoxin is significantly enhanced. It has been postulated that lack of luminal nutrition amplifies injury-induced metabolic and immunological responses. Accumulating evidence suggests that IL-6, in particular, is a key mediator to a superinflammation during the acute phase response (APR). It is well known that an exaggerated IL-6 response (e.g., prolonged and/or extreme elevations of circulating IL-6) is associated with adverse clinical events such as acute respiratory distress (ARDS) and multiple organ failure (MOF) in patients suffering from conditions such as infection, burns, or trauma.[54] Among the effects associated with an exaggerated IL-6 response are augmented endothelial adhesion of polymorphonuclear (PMN) cells, increased production of the intracellular adhesion molecule-1 (ICAM-1), priming of the PMNs for an oxidative burst, release of pro-inflammatory platelet activating factor (PAF), and associated with this, a delay in PMN apoptosis.[54] Observations made in liver transplant patients are of special interest. It was observed that patients who show a six-fold or more increase in cytokines such as TNFα and IL-6 as early as the final phase of the operation will almost certainty develop sepsis in the subsequent postoperative days.[55]

The Majority of Immune System Is in the Gut

About 80% of the total immunoglobulin-producing cells of the body are localized in lamina propria of the gut,[56] and large quantities, especially of IgA, are released each day to the gut lumen. The synthesis of IgA is highly dependent on T-cells and several cytokines produced by activated lymphocytes influence different steps in the IgA differentiation pathway.[57] Transforming growth factor-β (TGF-β) has been, at least in the mice, found to be a crucial "switch" factor. However, cytokines such as IL-2, IL-5, and IL-10 are also known to be involved.[58] Changes in nutrition, physical activity, sleep, mood, age, gender, circadian rhythm, body temperature, consumption of drugs, and illness are known to influence lymphocyte function and the production of immunoglobulins, thereby affecting resistance to disease.

Care in the ICU setting is not only associated with dramatic changes in nutrition, but also in physical activity, body temperature, sleep, mood, circadian rhythm, and other innate functions—as well as with increased consumption of drugs. All these factors have a profound influence on the immune response of the patient. It is suggested in the literature that supply of both pre- and probiotics can modify functions such as appetite, sleep, mood, and circadian rhythm—most likely through metabolites produced by microbial fermentation in the gut.[59–62] Supply of LAB can also significantly reduce serum levels of a variety of toxins such as endotoxin—(see below).

Neuroendocrine Regulation of the Acute Phase Response

Functions such as resistance to disease and size and extent of the acute phase response are unquestionably regulated from the gut, but also by the liver and, to a large extent, by neuro-endocrine mechanisms. During the last decade, knowledge has rapidly increased about the complex adaptive mechanisms that regulate psychobiological states (mood, sleep, appetite, libido, etc.) in response to both psychological and physical stressors such as noxious antigenic toxins and invasive microbiological organisms. Evidence is mounting that nervous, endocrine, immune, and inflammatory systems are both anatomically and functionally interconnected. Stressors influence the immune functions and the inflammatory response to a large extent via the sympathetic nervous system and the hypothalamic-pituitary-adrenal (HPA) axis.[64] Excessive cytokine production (IL-1, TNFα, but also IL-6) is normally down-regulated by corticosteroids. Various defects in the interaction of these systems will undoubtedly lead to increased morbidity in acute conditions such as Systemic Inflammatory Response Syndrome (SIRS), Multiple Organ Dysfunction Syndrome (MODS), and Multiple Organ Failure (MOF), and in chronic conditions such as autoimmune diseases. Elimination of neuroendocrine by adrenalectomy and subsequent "unrestricted" production of inflammatory cytokines increases lethality on challenge with LPS 500-fold.[65] Whereas acute stressors in general seem to stimulate immunity, chronic stress (environmental, social, physiological, or nutritional) is generally considered to down-regulate the immune system.[66]

Today, enteral nutrition is regarded as a more important a tool to control APR and immune response than as a means of providing calories and nutrients to the very sick patient. Recent studies in surgical patients support such an assumption. In a recent study comparing parenteral hyperalimentation (PN) and early enteral feeding (EN) after major liver resection, no differences were found between the groups when studying nutritional parameters. However, significant differences were observed when studying immunological parameters such as natural killer cell activity, lymphocyte numbers, response to phytohemagglutinin (PHA), and natural killer cell activity. Most important, the incidence of infectious complications was 8% in the EN group compared to 31% in the PN group.[67] Similar results have been reported in patients with severe acute pancreatitis. The changes in C-reactive protein (CRP) and disease-severity scores (Apache II) were significantly improved with EN compared to PN.[68] The IgM anticore endotoxin antibodies (EndoCAb) and total antioxidant potential (TAC) were both significantly better in the EN group than PN. But most important, SIRS, sepsis, organ failure, and stay in intensive care were globally improved in the EN-fed patients.[68]

Immuno-Enhancing Nutrition Solutions Controversial

The knowledge that some nutritional components such as some amino acids, polyunsaturated fatty acids, vitamins, and antioxidants have all strong immuno-modulatory effects led to commercial production of special immune-enhancing nutrition solutions with various nutritional components. The experience so far has not been what was originally expected—for review see Barton,[69] Dickerson,[70] and Bengmark.[71] Despite the fact that some compelling data have been presented in the literature, there is much to support the view of these reviewers and others that at present, "*routine* use of these formulas cannot be recommended."

There seem to be several reasons why the success has not been as expected. The most important is probably that the need for supply of various immuno-stimulatory components to the colon has been neglected, since these formulas do not contain substrate (fibers) for microbial fermentation, and for supply of immuno-stimulatory nutrients from microbial fermentation at the level of the colonic mucosa. It is reasonable to assume that adding fibers (prebiotics) and lactic-acid bacteria (probiotics) can significantly improve the efficacy of these nutrition solutions.

In addition, EN is also often instituted too late to significantly affect APR. It is also often combined with nutrition solutions rich in fat, which at least in theory should inhibit immune functions and counteract the purpose of EN. Furthermore, EN is often combined with treatment with antibiotics, which reduces or even eliminates the important commensal flora.

Lactic Acid Bacteria

Initiates Immunoglobulin Production

It has been suggested that LAB during fermentation may release components that possess immuno-modulatory activities. The ability of bifidobacteria to induce production of more significant quantities of IgA by Peyer's patches has been studied in vitro. It is interesting to note that only 3 of 120 strains tested, all isolated from human feces, had such an ability.[72] Two of them were identified as *Bifidobacterium breve* and one as *B. longum*. As far as I am aware, no similar study has compared the ability of various *Lactobacillus* to initiate production of IgA. There are, however, studies showing that at least some LAB do possess the ability to induce production of IgA. *Lactobacillus* GG is reported to significantly increase the IgA immune response in Crohn's disease[73] and to enhance the IgA response to rotavirus.[74] Human intake of *Lactobacillus acidophilus* is also known to result in a greater than fourfold increase in IgA response when challenged by *S typhi*.[75] Supplementation of both *Lact. reuteri* (R2LC) and *Lact. plantarum* (299 V, DSM 9843) in animals with methotrexate-induced colitis does, in addition to elevating the numbers of both CD4 and CD8 T-cells, significantly increase small- as well as large-bowel IgA secretion, both the soluble and insoluble fractions.[76]

Restore Macrophage Function

The ability of special cells to engulf, kill, and eliminate invading microorganisms and/or defective cells, and to eliminate toxins, mutagens, and other poisonous substances is important to health and to outcome in ICU patients. That enteral and/or parenteral supply of fat, as mentioned above, has a profound effect on APR and inhibits immune functions is supported by several clinical observations. It is also observed that intravenous infusion of 20% of fat emulsions (Intralipid) significantly activates endotoxin-induced coagulation.[77] But a diet too rich in polyunsaturated fatty acids can also be negative. Studies in mice with standardized thermal injuries showed a significantly increased mortality on challenge with *Pseudomonas aeruginosa* when as much as 40% of total calories were supplied as fish oil.[78]

Modern man is commonly exposed to chemicals, especially pharmaceuticals. Many of these inhibit macrophage functions, the bactericidal function, and the production and secretion of cytokines—effects that have not been studied to the extent they should be. Antibiotics are no exception. Supply of antibiotics (150 mg/kg body weight of Mezlocillin, Bayer) did result in suppression of the various macrophage functions as demonstrated by studies of chemiluminescence response, chemotactic motility, bactericidal and cytostatic ability, and lymphocyte proliferation.[79] Subsequent work has demonstrated that the reduction in peritoneal macrophage function and in lymphocyte proliferation after microbial decontamination of the digestive tract is significantly restituted by supply of low molecular weight peptides obtained from indigenous gastrointestinal tract microflora species such as *Bacteroides sp.*, *Clostridium sp.*, *Propionebacterium sp.*, and from *Lactobacillus sp.*[80]

Other studies demonstrate that supply of live or nonviable bacteria or bacterial-wall components such as peptidoglucan stimulates macrophage recruitment and function,[81] and cell-free extracts of both *Bifidobacterium longum* and *Lactobacillus acidophilus* have been shown to significantly enhance phagocytosis of both inert particles and viable *Salmonella*.[82] However, not all LAB are capable of activating macrophages. As an example, an increased macrophage activation (increased expression of Ia antigen on the surface) was observed in mice after intraperitoneal administration of *Lactobacillus casei* or *Corynobacterium parvum*, but not after administration of *Lactobacillus fermentum*.[83]

Stimulate Apoptosis

Programmed cell death is one of the important mechanisms by which the body controls infections, especially those of viral origin, but also those resulting from neoplastic transformation. Dairy products, rich in saturated fat and various growth factors[84,85] including insulin growth factor 1 and various cow oestrogens and sometimes xenoestrogens (from pesticides), have been suggested to inhibit or delay apoptosis and to promote malignant cell proliferation. These changes are associated with increased luminal concentrations of bile acids[86] and with modifications in composition of bowel microflora.

Several reports demonstrate that increased consumption of prebiotics—plant fibers such as pectin, oat, wheat, rye, or chicory fibers (inulin)[87]—significantly increases the rate of apoptosis. Also, cells infected with a virus are supposed to undergo apoptosis in order to prevent spreading of the viral infection.[88] These various processes seem to be enhanced by supply of both fiber and LAB (synbiotics), most likely through production of SCFAs, known to enhance the process of apoptosis.[89,90] For example, it has been observed that feeding beans to experimental animals increases the SCFA production sevenfold.[91]

MODULATE LYMPHOCYTE FUNCTIONS

Lymphocyte-proliferation studies are commonly used to evaluate the efficacy of immuno-suppressive or immuno-enhancing therapies, to test chemicals for their potential immuno-toxicity, and to monitor congenital immunological effects. Four probiotic lactic acid bacteria were recently tested in an animal model. Interestingly, *Lactobacillus acidophilus* ATCC 4356 did enhance basal proliferation by 43%. However, *Lactobacillus casei* (Yakult), *Lactobacillus gasseri* ATCC 33323 and *Lactobacillus rhamnosus* DSM 7061 inhibited both basal (by 14%–51%) and mitogen-stimulated proliferation by the mitogen concanavalin A (by 43%–68%) and by LPS (by 23%–63%), and particularly at supra-optimal concentrations.[92] As it appears from this study, various LAB have different immune effects and experience cannot be extrapolated from one *Lactobacillus* to another *Lactobacillus* strain or species, even if they are closely related.

It is suggested that a balance between Th1 lymphocytes, primarily associated with cellular immunity, and Th2 lymphocytes, mainly associated with humoral immunity, is essential for maintenance of health. Most of the studies on this balance have been done in atopic persons—individuals who also suffer an aberrant inflammation. Implications for studies of this balance in the ICU patient should be obvious and future studies warranted.

Reduced microbial stimulation during early infancy and childhood, especially in developed countries, has been associated with the considerably increased prevalence of atopic diseases in children and young adults.[93] Reduced microbial stimulation is associated with slower postnatal maturation of the immune system, a delayed development, and lack of balance between Th1 and Th2 immunity.[94] Swedish infants, as already mentioned, have a significantly different gut flora than both Parkistani[31] and Estonian children.[32] Children prone to develop allergies are also more sensitive to infections when in the ICU.

The super-inflammation seen in atopic diseases is thought to be caused by inappropriate generation and activation of Th2 cells, a process inhibited by IFN-γ, but also by IL-12. It is of special interest to know that some *Lactobacillus* species—evidently only a few—have the ability to stimulate both IFN-γ and IL-12 production, as well as to promote Th1-type response, inhibit Th2-type immune response, and restore the Th-1/Th-2 balance.[96] It was observed that stimulation of human peripheral blood mononuclear cells (PBMC) using *Lactobacillus rhamnosus* or *Lactobacillus bulgaricus* strains led to induction of Th1 type cytokines IL-12, IL-18, and IFN-γ.[97] It was also observed that supply of *Lactobacillus casei*[98] and *Lactobacillus plantarum*[96] totally inhibited antigen-induced IgE secretion in ovalalbumin- and casein-primed mice, an effect not obtained with *Lactobacillus johnsonii.* Furthermore, IL-12 production by peritoneal macrophages was enhanced and IL-4 production of concanavalin A-stimulated spleen cells suppressed in animals treated with *Lactobacillus plantarum.*[96]

MODULATE CYTOKINE RELEASE

Oral administration of LAB seems to determine the direction and efficacy of the humoral response, a response that is differently modulated by different LAB. Most of the attention has so far been given to the cytokine production by monocytic cells such as macrophages, but mononuclear eukaryotic cells are also important sources of cytokines. It has thus become increasingly clear that tissues such as intestinal epithelial cells[99,100] and prokaryotic cells such as commensal flora and/or supplemented probiotic bacteria,[101,102] when challenged, will secrete a spectrum of chemo-attractants and cytokines or cytokine-like molecules (sometimes called bacteriokines). As an example, it has been demonstrated in cell cultures that intestinal epithelial cells on challenge with LPS and PGE_2 produce significant amounts of IL-6, a process that can be blunted by supply of indomethacin[103] and inhibited by nitric oxide.[104]

Supplementation with some LAB seems to significantly influence the expression of cytokines, but the response varies with strain of LAB supplied. The activity in blood mononuclear cells in healthy subjects of 2'–5' synthetase, an expression of interferon-gamma (IFN-γ), is significantly increased (approximately 250%) 24 hours after a LAB-containing meal.[75] Significant increases in cytokine activity compared to controls are also observed when human mononuclear cells are incubated in the presence of the yogurt bacteria; *Lb bulgaricus (BUL)*, and *S. thermophilus (Ther)*, alone or in combination (Yog); *INF-γ: Bul* 775%, *Ther* 2100%, Yog 570%, *TNF-α: Bul* 1020%, *Ther* 3180% Yog 970%, and in IL-1β: *Bul* 2120%, *Ther* 1540%, and Yog 1920%—all indicating a significant immuno-activation after supply of these LAB.

Another recent study, using both a macrophage model and a T-helper-cell model, examined the in-vitro ability to induce cytokine production by some LAB used by the dairy industry for yogurt production.[105] Although there was a considerable variation in response between various *S. thermophilus* strains, this LAB seemed to stimulate macrophage and T-cell cytokine production to a somewhat greater extent than did *Lactobacillus bulgaricus*, *Bifidobacterium adolescentis*, and *Bifidobacterium bifidum*.[105] In addition, heat-killed *Lactobacillus acidophilus* (LA 1) has been shown in vitro to increase the mouse macrophage production of IL1-α (approximately 300%) and TNF-α (approximately 1000%) to a considerably greater extent than other *Lactobacillus* and *Bifidobacteria* tried.[106]

It is mainly effects of milk-born LAB that have been studied in recent years—understandably, since it is primarily the dairy industry that has had a longstanding interest in producing food products containing live LAB. One can expect, as interest in LAB with specific ability to ferment plant fibers gains popularity, that studies will be undertaken with LAB such as *Lactobacillus plantarum*, *Lactobacillus paracasei*, various *Lactococcus*, *Pentococcus* strains, and other related LAB, known for their special ability to metabolize fibers.

Increase Mucin Production

Numerous studies have demonstrated that nonpathogenic bacteria of various kinds, including LAB, have the ability to prevent infections and/or improve recovery times. Several mechanisms have been suggested, such as release of various bacteriokines (cytokine-like molecules), nitric oxide, free radicals, and lowering pH. Two other mechanisms have recently been suggested: blocking of receptors and inhibition of attachment to epithelial cells by intestinal mucins. While the adherence of most LAB are via protease-sensitive mechanisms or via lipid (lactosylceramide) receptors, *Lactobacillus plantarum* seem to adhere via carbohydrate (mannose) adhesion mechanisms, e.g. the same receptors as Gram-negative bacteria like *E. coli*, *Enterobacter*, *Klebsiella*, *Salmonella*, *Shigella*, *Pseudomonas*, and *Vibrio cholerae*.[107] This fact offers unique possibilities for preventing infections and reducing endotoxemia.

Binding of pathogens to mucosal epithelial cell mucins is an important defense mechanism for the host.[108] The density of Goblet cells and the intestinal mucus production seem to increase with distance from the mouth. Several human genes are involved in mucin production, but MUC2 and MUC3 are the predominant ileo-colonic mucins. Both mucins show expression in Goblet cells in the large and small intestine, but MUC2 is suggested to be the major secreted mucin component of the colon.[109] Increased MUC2 and MUC3 mRNA expression—and inhibition of adherence of pathogenic *Escherichia coli* to HT29 intestinal cells, but not to non-intestinal cells—has recently been demonstrated in vitro, when the cells were incubated with *Lactobacillus plantarum* 299v.[110] This suggests that the ability of probiotic agents such as *L. plantarum* to inhibit adherence of attaching and effacing organisms to intestinal epithelial cells is also mediated through their ability to increase expression of MUC2 and MUC3 intestinal mucins.

Eliminate Toxins and Mutagens

Several studies show strong effects of various lactobacilli to reduce significantly and sometimes eliminate various toxins and mutagens. Several *lactobacillus*[111] and *bifidobacteria*[112] strains have proven to non-covalently bind and sequestrate very potent endotoxins such as aflatoxin B, both in vitro and in vivo. Other bacterial toxins such as *E. coli* endotoxin are also effectively reduced by probiotic bacteria. This is important as translocation of endotoxin and pathogenic bacteria occurs frequently in critical conditions such as burns, hemorrhagic shock, severe pancreatitis, and after larger operations such as transplantation.

Infections and endotoxemia are regarded as critical factors for hemodynamic alterations that lead to increased risk of bleeding in subjects with liver cirrhosis, esophageal varices, and portal hypertension.[113] This is the reason why it is suggested that antibiotic treatment might prevent bleeding. Supplementing *Lactobacillus* has been shown to reduce endotoxemia and severity of experimental alcoholic liver disease.[114] Strong effects of supplied *Lactobacillus*, for example, can be observed in galactosamine-induced chemical hepatitis. Supplemented *Lactobacillus rhamnosus* DSM 6594 (= strain 271), *Lactobacillus plantarum* DSM 9843 (= strain 299v), *Lactobacillus fermentum* DSM 8704:3 (= strain 245), and *Lactobacillus reuteri* (= strain 108) did significantly reduce the extent of liver injury as well as reduce bacterial translocation. Again, the most pronounced effect was seen when supplementing *Lactobacillus plantarum*, especially if combined with arginine. Significant reduction in release of liver enzymes, extent of hepatocellular necrosis, inflammatory cell infiltration, and bacterial translocation were observed parallel with a significant reduction in number of *Enterobacteriaceae*, both in caecum and colon.[115]

A subsequent study could demonstrate that the extent of liver injury and bacterial translocation is increased after supply of *Bact. fragilis* and *E. coli*, but again significantly inhibited by *Lact. plantarum*.[116] A recent study, undertaken in one patient, is of particular interest. Supply of a cocktail of seven probiotic bacteria—LAB most likely chosen at random, and without any deeper knowledge about the immunological and other cellular effects of each of the bacteria—seemed to result in a greatly increased blood velocity and flow when studied one month after the initiation of treatment.[117] If this proves to be reproducible, an umbrella of supplemented probiotics could provide patients with liver cirrhosis a tool to reduce septic manifestations as well as the incidence of bleeding.

Stimulate Mucosal Growth

Reduced epithelial cell proliferation and mucosal atrophy are associated with increased invasion of various pathogens to peritoneal lymph nodes and to interior organs, which produces a risky situation in critically ill patients, especially those on parenteral nutrition or elemental diet.[118,119] Local degrading in the gut by microbial fermentation of fibers and proteinous material constitute the mechanisms by which SCFAs as well as lactic acid, succinic acid, and ammonia are made available throughout the lower gastrointestinal tract. In addition to providing fuel for the enterocytes, SCFAs promote sodium and water absorption and suppress colonic propulsive motility, thereby reducing diarrhea (mainly propionic and η-buturic acid). SCFAs derive mainly from carbohydrate degradation, ammonia, and iso-valeric acid from degradation of proteinous material. It seems reasonable to assume that, in the absence of a supply of fibers for SCFA production, the remaining bacteria will ferment proteinous material, which is always available (gastrointestinal secretions, apoptotic cells), producing more ammonia, which is highly unwanted in the cirrhotic patient, especially when treated in the ICU for liver failure.

A recently published study[120] suggest that probiotic bacteria, even in the absence of prebiotics, are capable of stimulating growth of the mucosa in the lower gastrointestinal tract. Three groups of animals, all kept on elemental diet without any supply of fibers, were studied. One group served as the control; the other two were treated with two different LAB. The cell-crypt production rate was about 25%–40% higher in the jejunum and ileum, 70% higher in the caecum, and more than 200% higher in the distal colon in LAB-supplied than in control rats. The effect was more pronounced in jejunum when treated with *Lactobacillus casei* and in the colon when supplied *Clostridium butyricum*,[120] again suggesting that a combination of a few LAB could be advantageous (see Table 34.2).

TABLE 34.1

A Summary of Some Documented Molecular Effects of Probiotics

Probiotics—Molecular Effects

- Stimulates sIgA production
- Inhibits IgE production
- Modulates Th1/Th2 response
- Modulates cytokine response
- Stimulates nitric oxide production
- Stimulates macrophage function
- Stimulates NK cell activity
- Activates the MALT system
- Stimulates apoptosis
- Promotes growth and regeneration
- Controls PPMs
- Reduces endotoxin production
- Reduces mutagenicity
- Produces antioxidants, nutrients (synbiotics) and various growth and clotting factors

TABLE 34.2

A Summary of Some Potential Clinical Effects of Probiotics

Probiotics—Clinical Effects

- Prevents or reduces duration of diarrhea (rotavirus)
- Reduces atopic dermatitis
- Induces remission of IBD
- Reduces symptoms in irritable colon
- Delays onset of diabetes (animals)
- Reduces the rate of colonic cancer (animals)
- Prevents or reduces Helicobacter infections (animals)
- Reduces the incidence and severity of pancreatic sepsis in pancreatitis (animals)
- Reduces the incidence and severity of ICU sepsis
- Reduces the incidence and severity of sepsis after major surgery
- Reduces biofilm

Prevents/Reduces Diarrhea

There seems to be no condition in which LAB (and fibers) have been as extensively tried as in diarrhea of various kinds, varying from rather simple tourist diarrhea to severe and life-threatening conditions such as antibiotic-associated and radiotherapy-induced diarrhea. It is clear from all these studies that LAB provides a simple, inexpensive, and effective tool, with no documented side effects, which can be used both in prevention and treatment of all forms of diarrhea. For more details, see a recent review by Heyman.[121] It is obvious that LAB are effective in controlling diarrhea of both bacterial and viral origin, but seem to be slightly more effective in virus-induced diarrhea. This is promising, as an increasing number of infections today are of viral origin, both in connection with extensive surgery such as transplantation and severe chronic disease such as HIV.

A larger European multi-center trial in children 1 month to 3 years of age was recently reported. One group consisting of 140 children was randomly allocated to oral rehydration + placebo, the other group of 147 children to oral rehydration + supply of 10^{10} cfu of Lactobacillus GG. The duration of diarrhea was 58.3 ± 27.6 hours in the LAB-treated group vs. 71.9 ± 35.8 hours (p=0.03). In rotavirus-positive children in the LAB-treated group, the diarrhea lasted 56.2 ± 16.9 hours vs. 76.6 ± 41.6 in the control group (p=0.008).[122]

Prevents/Reduces Severity of Colitis

Experimental studies, as well as clinical observations, suggest that the contents of the intestinal luminal environment are responsible for the initiation and/or perpetuation of inflammatory bowel disease. It has been convincingly demonstrated that the concentrations of endogenous *Lactobacillus* and *Bifidobacteria* are significantly reduced in patients with active Crohn's disease, ulcerative colitis, pouchitis, and experimental colitis.[123–126] These observations have stimulated interest in trying various probiotic bacteria in inflammatory bowel disease (IBD). A series of experimental studies[124] and several uncontrolled clinical studies support the idea of using probiotics in patients with IBD, but so far few controlled studies have been reported.

A cocktail called VSL#3 was recently tried in an uncontrolled study in patients with ulcerative colitis.[127] It consisted of four lactobacillus strains, three bifidobacteria strains, plus *Streptococcus salivarius* ssp *thermophilus* (5×10^{11} cells/g)—most probably chosen at random without any further documentation of the molecular/immonological effects of each of the LAB. The patients were given 3 grams a day during 1 year and 15/20 patients remained in remission; one was lost to follow up and 4/20 had signs of relapse. The same LAB cocktail was also tried in a small controlled study in patients with pouchitis.[128] Twenty patients served as controls, all showed remission within 9 months. In sharp contrast to this, only 3/20 patients developed remission during the same time period when supplied with VSL#3 probiotic cocktail.[128] It is reasonable to assume that with a cocktail of LAB where each bacteria would be chosen based on well-documented metabolic and immunological effects, even better results should be expected.

A recently published Colombian study[129] compared the outcome of 1,237 newborns (inpatients and transfer patients) who all received daily 250 million live *Lactobacillus acidophilus* and 250 million live *Bifidobacterium infantis* until they were discharged, usually after about 1 week. Similar children treated during the previous year served as controls. The incidence of necrotizing enterocolitis with probiotic prophylaxis was reduced to one third (18 vs. 47, p<0.0005) in the inpatient group, and by half (19 vs. 38, p<0.03) in the patients transferred from other hospitals (which most likely came under treatment late).[129] It is most important to observe that no complications could be attributed to the use of probiotic preparations even in these very sick newborn children weighing on average 2600 gr (range <1000 to >4000 g), where as much as one-third of the babies suffered from severe conditions such as sepsis, pneumonia, or meningitis. It was incidentally observed that the LAB-treated children suffered significantly less diaper dermatitis.

In Intensive Care Patients

Few studies have been performed in a mixed ICU patient population. A small study was performed by a nurse in Hong Kong as a thesis for B Sc Degree in Health Studies.[130] From within 12 hours of arrival at the ICU, 19 patients received daily 10^{10} of *Lactobacillus plantarum* 299, another 19 patients heat-killed *Lactobacillus plantarum* 299 (controls); 5/19 (26%) died in the treated group vs. 8/19 (42%) in the control group; the difference did not reach statistical significance. However, the study encouraged the physicians at the unit to undertake a larger study, which is underway.

A somewhat larger prospective, randomized placebo controlled study was undertaken in a mixed abdominal-surgery patient population at the University of Berlin.[131] Thirty patients were treated with *Lactobacillus plantarum* 299 in a daily dosis of 10^{10}, compared to 30 patients receiving inactivated heat-killed *Lactobacillus plantarum* 299. Another 30 received parenteral nutrition (PN). The rate of complications for the various groups was: PN 30%, heat-inactivated lactobacilli 17% and active lactobacilli 13%. Infections developed in 3/30 (10%) patients in each of the two treated groups vs. 9/30 (30%) in the PN group (p=0.001). Furthermore, significantly more antibiotics were administered to the PN group. The difference was even larger when the subgroup of patients having more extensive surgery (gastric and pancreatic surgery, mainly resections) was separately analyzed. One of 15 patients (7%) developed infections in the group receiving *Lactobacillus plantarum* vs. 3/17 (17%) in the group receiving heat-inactivated *Lactobacillus plantarum*, and 8/16 (50%) in the group on parenteral nutrition.

A separate study was undertaken by the same group at Virchow Clinic, Charité University Hospital in patients undergoing liver transplantation.[132] Treatment with active as well as heat-killed *Lactobacillus plantarum* 299 with inulin fiber added was compared to selective bowel decontamination (SBD), which during several years was the gold standard of the clinic. Infections developed within 30 days (p=0.017) at the following rates: 4 of 31 patients (13%) in the group receiving active *Lactobacillus plantarum*, 11/32 (34%) in the group receiving inactivated *Lactobacillus plantarum*, and 15/32 (48%) in the group treated by SBD.

A randomized study was just concluded in Györ, Hungary, of patients with severe pancreatitis.[133] The rate of septic complications was significantly reduced in the group supplied live *Lactobacillus plantarum* 299 compared to the group supplied heat-inactivated *Lactobacillus plantarum* 299; 4.5% (1/22) vs. 30.4% (7/23), p<0.05. Similarly, the rate of re-operation was significantly reduced; 4.5% (1/22) vs. 26.1% (6/23), p<0.05.

General Comments

Table 34.3 summarizes the present limited experience in ICU patients. All studies have been performed with a single, but well-documented bioactive LAB, *Lactobacillus plantarum* 299. Some of the studies discussed above were not large enough to allow statistical significance, but the trend is the same in all studies: the lowest mortality or the lowest infection rate was always obtained in the group receiving supply of LAB and fiber. But the differences observed are impressive: in extensive gastric and pancreatic surgery 7% infection with and 50% without supply of pro- and prebiotics (p<0.05); in liver transplant 13% with and 48% (p=0.017) without supply of pro- and prebiotics; and acute pancreatitis 4.5% vs. 30.4% (p<0.05).

It has been calculated, based on the present Berlin experience, that groups of approximately 30 patients are needed to reach statistical significance with mixed patient populations. Several such studies are on the way. In very sick patients, however, statistical significance seems to occur with smaller groups; for example, gastric and pancreatic surgery and severe pancreatitis—approximately 20 in each group. It is important to stress at this stage that the limited documentation of clinical efficacy of treatment with *Lactobacillus* in very sick patients is further supported by extensive studies in experimental animals, using a variety of models.[1–5]

It has thus far been necessary to accept that treatment of patients with *Lactobacillus* is done in parallel to treatment with strong antibiotics, which most likely reduces the efficacy of LAB treatment. Although the doses of *Lactobacillus* supplied in the above studies were large compared to what has been given in other probiotic treatments, an even larger dose could eventually further improve the outcome. The treatment was also often instituted late and the supply of substrate (fibers) was never optimal. The supply of fibers could be both larger and more diverse, e.g., contain several different bioactive fibers.

To Patients with Fulminant MOF

Lactobacillus was supplied as a desperate action to five patients suffering from severe MOF after gastrointestinal surgery (Figure 34.1). The mean Apache II score fell from a mean 18 before institution of treatment to 12 and 9, after 5 and 10 days of treatment respectively.

TABLE 34.3

Summary of Present Experience with Pro- and Prebiotics in the ICU

Lactic Acid Bacteria in the Settings of ICU—Collected Experience

Site of study	Type of patients	TPN	SBD	LAB + FIBER	Inactivated LAB + FIBER
Mortality:					
Hong Kong[130]	mixed ICU			26% (5/19)[¤]	42% (8/19)
Rate of infections:					
Berlin[131]	Abdom. surg	30% (9/30)		10% (3/30)[¤¤]	10% (3/30)
Berlin[132]	Gastr+pancr	50% (8/16)		7% (1/15)[¤¤]	17% (3/17)
Berlin[132]	Liver transpl		48% (15/32)	13% (4/31)[¤¤¤]	34% (11/32)
Györ[133]	Acut pancreat			4.5%(1/22)[¤¤¤¤]	30% (7/23)

Abdom. TPN=total parenteral nutrition, SBD=selective bowel decontamination, Abdom Surg=abdominal surgery patients, Acut pancreat=acute pancreatitis, Gastr=gastric surgery patients, Liver transpl=liver transplant patients, Pancr=pancreatic surgery patients, Mixed ICU=mixed group of various ICU patients.
[¤]=not statistically significant, [¤¤] p<0.0001, [¤¤¤] p=0.017, [¤¤¤¤] p=<0.05.

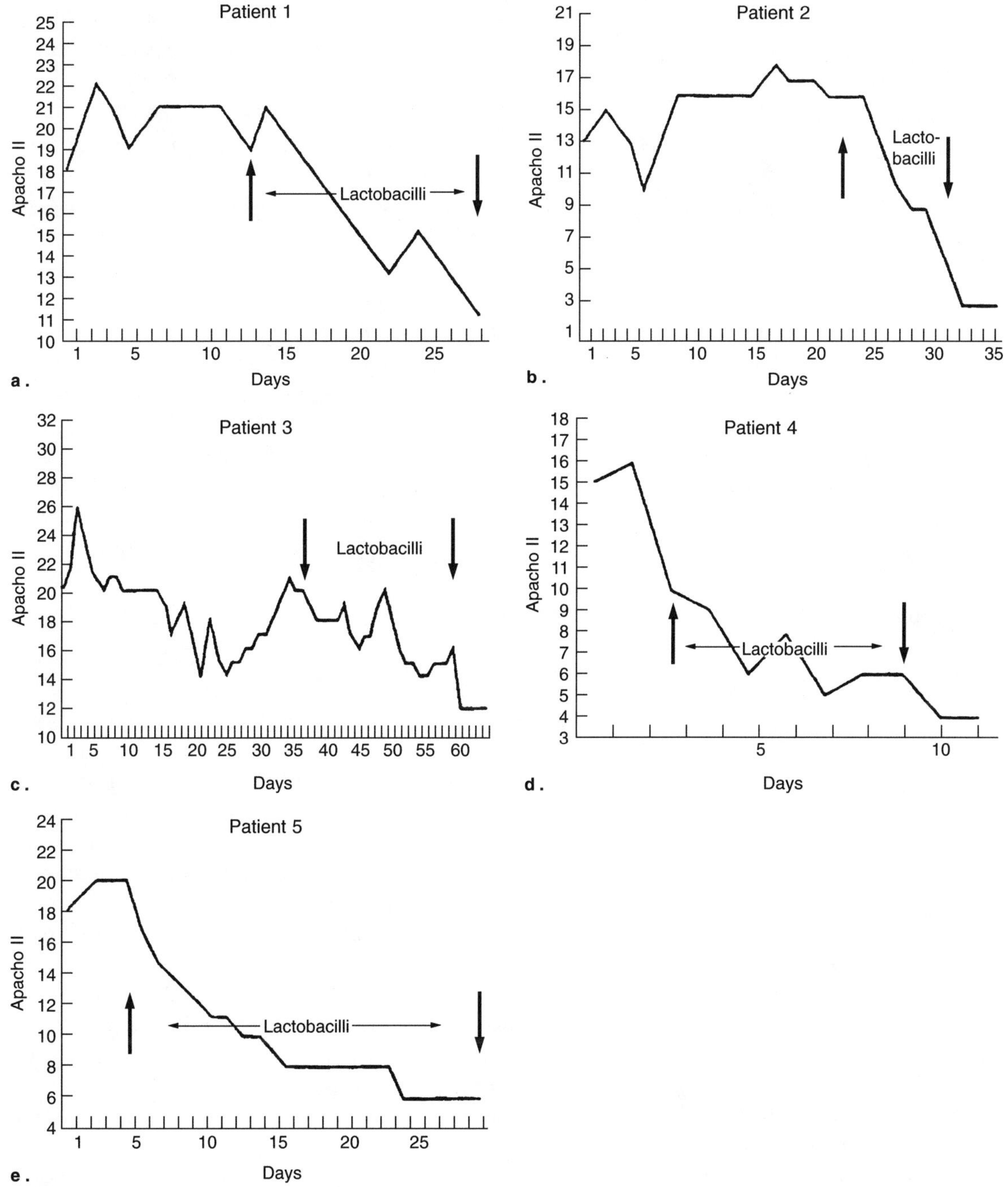

Figure 34.1

Changes in Apache-II Scores in Five Patients with Multiorgan Dysfunction and Treated with Pre- and Probiotics

All patients left the ICU unit in improved condition. A short description of each of the patients follows:

Patient 1

(Figure 34.1a) 74-year-old man with Parkinson's disease suffering severe upper GI bleedings. No source of bleeding could be found at emergency laparotomy. After the laparotomy, severe gastric-wall necrosis, wound dehiscence, and peritonitis developed. An emergency gastric resection was performed and a feeding jejunostomy applied. The patient was referred to the university hospital with severe sepsis and signs of pulmonary and renal insufficiencies. *Lactobacillus* and oat fiber were administered via a jejunal feeding tube. Dramatic recovery was observed and the patient could be weaned off the ventilator after 10 days and leave the ICU.

Patient 2

(Figure 34.1b) 65-year-old man initially operated on for perforated duodenal ulcer and diffuse peritonitis. He postoperatively developed severe sepsis with pulmonary insufficiency. Repeated scans showed no signs of abscesses, and exploratory laparotomy was performed on two occasions. His general condition deteriorated with increasing leukocytosis and plasma-creatinine levels. Daily enteral supply of *Lactobacillus* and oat fiber was instituted from the 22nd day and a slow recovery began. He left the ICU after about 2 weeks of treatment.

Patient 3

(Figure 34.1c) 52-year-old man was operated on at a local hospital with an emergency partial gastrectomy and later referred to the university hospital with a leaking duodenal stump. He was re-operated on, gastrostomy performed, and drainage of the retroduodenal stump and PTC applied. Despite these measures, the condition quickly deteriorated and the patient developed high fever, leucocytosis, and signs of pulmonary, renal, and hepatic insufficiencies. Treatment with *Lactobacillus* and oat fiber was instituted from the 45th day. An immediate but slow recovery began and continued over the following 3 weeks. The function of the organs steadily improved, and he could be weaned off the ventilator and leave the ICU.

Patient 4

(Figure 34.1d) 43-year-old man who had an emergency sigmoid resection for a perforated diverticulitis. He postoperatively developed anastomotic dehiscence with fecal peritonitis, and was re-operated on with a Hartmann procedure. He continued to deteriorate, developing high fever and signs of ventilatory insufficiency, and was referred to the university hospital for care in the ICU. Probiotic treatment was instituted and he could leave the ICU after about one week on *Lactobacillus* and oat.

Patient 5

(Figure 34.1e) 63-year-old woman suffering from diabetes who received on with an emergency colectomy and ileostomy due to a colonic ischemia with colonic-wall necrosis. She postoperatively developed abdominal abscesses, wound dehiscence, and small-bowel fistulas, along with increasing signs of circulatory, ventilatory, and renal insufficiencies. Treatment with *Lactobacillus* and oat was instituted. The patient recovered slowly during the following weeks and was able to leave the ICU after 24 days on pro- and prebiotics.

General Comments

None of the patients had positive blood cultures before or during the treatment. They all developed clinical signs of sepsis and organ dysfunction despite treatment with broad-spectrum antibiotics, which continued in parallel with the *Lactobacillus* and fiber treatment. All patients had received TPN before the institution of enteral nutrition with *Lactobacillus* and oat. TPN was often continued in parallel with the enteral nutrition. A dramatic improvement in general condition and Apache II scores occurred from the day *Lactobacillus* and oat treatment was instituted in all cases. Especially encouraging is that recovery was obtained even when the treatment was instituted late in the disease process (22 days in case 2; 45 days in case 3).

Conclusions

The molecular effects of pre-, pro- and synbiotics are well documented in the literature. The documentation of clinical effects is presently thin for all indications except diarrheal diseases. It is encouraging that the treatment seems to be even more effective in preventing viral diseases. This is important, especially in transplantation, where viral complications are increasingly common. It offers hope that the treatment can be of benefit in viral diseases such as HIV—positive experience has also been reported in this disease[134] (see Table 34.4).

As mentioned above, the protection layer of lactobacillus does not exist only on the GI tract mucosa; it is important at all exterior body surfaces including those of the eye, nose, mouth, respiratory tract, vagina, and skin. It is clearly reduced at all sites when the patient is in the ICU with its special hygienic conditions and supply of antibiotics and other drugs. Some observations support the view that an overflow of probiotic bacteria continuously occurs under normal hygienic conditions from the GI tract to all the other sites mentioned, but this is more unlikely to occur in the ICU with its vigorous hygienic conditions. For that reason, in the future it may be indicated that the gastrointestinal supply be complemented by use of LAB-containing gels on sensitive body surfaces, and of LAB-containing aerosols for the respiratory tract, where this protection layer is much needed. (The incidental observation that LAB supplementation reduces the incidence of diaper dermatitis is of interest in this

TABLE 34.4

Potential Candidates of Pre- and Probiotic Treatment
Prematures
Infants
As alternative to antibiotics
"Astronauts," e.g., those with insufficient intake of fresh fruits and vegetables
When treated with antibiotics or chemotherapeutics
When irradiated or treated with cytostatics
When treated with renal or peritoneal dialysis
Biliary obstruction
Liver cirrhosis, portal hypertension
Cancer
When allergy
When immunodepressed
Hematological malignancies
HIV/Aids
Inflammatory bowel disease
Irritable bowel disease
Rheumatoid arthritis
Hepatitis
Pancreatitis
Stomatitis
Diarrhea
When infected
After trauma
In major surgery, especially transplantation
In intensive care

connection.) It is also interesting that two recent reports suggest that consumption of LAB-containing drinks prevents formation of biofilm and removes both yeast and bacteria from prostheses—in this case silicon rubber voice prostheses,[135,136] suggesting that LAB could be effective also in the prevention of catheter infections.

As the problems with antibiotic-associated microbial resistance increase, the medical world is increasingly looking for a tool to replace antibiotics, especially in the sensitive and very artificial microbial world of the ICU. Such a tool exists in combined use of pre- and probiotics. It is also necessary to remember that all fibers are not identical—that they are each precursors for their special nutrients. It seems therefore important to provide several types of fibers and, if in any way possible, fresh fruits and vegetables. Nor do all lactic-acid bacteria have similar effects. It is said the genetic differences between two LAB can be greater than those between a fish and a human being. In addition, many ingested LAB do not survive the acidity of the stomach or the bile acids of the small intestine, nor do they adhere to the intestinal mucosa. Each LAB has its own narrow metabolic spectrum, which is why the LAB are more effective in consortia. This supports the idea that a composition of several LAB could have stronger effects than from administration of a single strain.

LAB cocktails for medical purpose must not only be composed of bacteria with scientifically well-documented bioactivities, but also demonstrate qualities such as strong mucus adhesivity, great ability to ferment semi-resistant fibers such as inulin, strong antioxidant capacity, and strong ability to modulate the immune response. Such LAB are normally not found in milk products, where LAB in general tend to have comparatively weak bioactivities. Instead, they are found in fiber ferments such as sauerkraut, sourdoughs, and exotic dishes of fermented fruits and fermented vegetables.

An attempt to construct such a scientifically based composition of fibers and LAB, chosen on the basis of documented bioactivities, is Synbiotic 2000. It consists in four bioactive LAB (containing 10^{10} of each of four LAB *Lactobacillus plantarum*, *Lactobacillus paracasei* subsp *paracasei*, *Pediacoccus pentoceus*, and *Lactococcus raffinolactis*) and is combined with 10 grams of bioactive fibers (2.5 grams each of betaglucan, inulin, pectin and resistant starch). It is presently the object of extensive studies around the world.

It is likely that the settings and premises of ICU, as we move further into the new millennium, will be designed to look less artificial than at present. The physical and psychological environment will most likely be dramatically improved. Strong attempts will also be made to reduce the amount of pharmaceuticals and increase the amounts of natural foods. The goal will be to reduce the stay in ICU and to use the home of the patient as much as possible. Patients who not long ago were treated for long periods of time in the ICU, such as bone-marrow transplant patients, are increasingly treated in a much more ecologically friendly place—their own home. Ecoimmunonutrition with pre-, pro-, and synbiotics offers substantial promise as tools in this continuously changing process.

References

1. Bengmark S. Ecological control of the gastrointestinal tract. The role of probiotic bacteria. *Gut.* 1998;42:2–7.
2. Bengmark S. Immunonutrition: role of biosurfactants, fiber and probiotic bacteria. *Nutrition.* 1998;14:585–594.
3. Bengmark S. Gut and the immune system: enteral nutrition and immunonutrients. In: Baue AE, Faist E, Fry D, eds. *SIRS, MODS and MOF—Systemic Inflammatory Response Syndrome, Multiple Organ Dysfunction Syndrome, Multiple Organ Failure—Pathophysiology, Prevention and Therapy*. New York: Springer; 2000:408–424.

4. Bengmark S. Refunctionalization of the gut. In: Baue AE, Faist E, Fry D, eds. *SIRS, MODS and MOF—Systemic Inflammatory Response Syndrome, Multiple Organ Dysfunction Syndrome, Multiple Organ Failure—Pathophysiology, Prevention and Therapy*. New York: Springer; 2000:435–446.
5. Bengmark S. Prospect for a new and rediscovered form of therapy: probiotic and phage. In: Andrew PW, Oystron P, Smith GL, Stewart-Tull DE, eds. *Fighting Infection in the 21st Century*. Blackwells; 2000:97–132.
6. Macfarlane GT, Cummings JH. The colonic flora, fermentation and large bowel digestive function. In: Phillips SF, Pemberton JH, Shorter RG, eds. *The Large Intestine: Physiology, Pathophysiology and Disease*. New York: Raven Press; 1991:51–92.
7. Roberfroid M. Dietary fiber, inulin and oligofructose: a review comparing their physiological effects. *Crit Rev Food Sci Nutr.* 1993;33:103–148.
8. Bengmark S, Larsson K. to be published
9. Best R, Lewis DA, Nasser N. The anti-ulcerogenic activity of the unripe banana (Musa species). *Br J Pharmacol.* 1984;82:107–116.
10. Hills BA, Kirwood CA. Surfactant approach to the gastric mucosal barrier: protection of rats by banana even when acidified. *Gastroenterology.* 1989;97:294–303.
11. Dunjic BS, Svensson I, Axelsson J, et al. Is resistance to phospholipase important to gastric mucosal protective capacity of exogenous phosphatidylcholine? *Eur J Gastroenterol Hepatol.* 1994;6:593–598.
12. Dunjic BS, Svensson I, Axelsson J et al. Green banana protection of gastric mucosa against experimentally induced injuries in rats—a multicomponent mechanism? *Scand J Gastroenterol.* 1993;28:894–898.
13. Kohn CL, Keithly JK. Enteral nutrition: potential complications and patient montoring. *Nurs Clin North Am.* 1989; 24:339–353.
14. Zaporozhets TS, Besednova NN, Liamkin GP, et al. I Antibacterial and therapeutic effectiveness of a pectin from sea grass zostera. II Immunomodulating properties of pectin from seawater grass zostera. *Antibiot Khimother.* 1991;36:24–26 and 31–34.
15. Hohner GA, Hyldon DJ. Oat groat fractionation process. US Patent 4,028,468.
16. Beer MU, Arrigino E, Amado R. Effects of oat gum on blood cholesterol levels in healthy young men. *Eur J Clin Nutr.* 1995;49:517–522.
17. Wang X, Gibson GR. Effects of the in vitro fermentation of oligofructose and inulin by growing bacteria in the human large intestine. *J Appl Bacteriol.* 1993;75:373–380.
18. Egan SK, Petersen BJ. Estimated consumption of inulin and oligofructose by the US population. Technical Assessment Systems Inc. Washington, DC; 1992.
19. Müller M, Lier D. Fermentation of fructans by epiphytic lactic acid bacteria. *J Appl Bacteriol.* 1994;76:406–411.
20. Fiordaliso M, Kok N, Desager J-P, et al. Dietary oligofructose lowers triglycerides, phospholipids and cholesterol in serum and very low density lipoproteins of rats. *Lipids.* 1995;30:163–167.
21. Southgate DAT. The definition and analysis of dietary fibre. *Nutr Rev.* 1977;35:31–37.
22. Salyers AA, Palmer JK, Wilkins TD. Degradation of polysaccharides by intestinal bacterial enzymes. *Am J Clin Nutr.* 1978;31(suppl):S128–S130.
23. Anderson DMW, Brydon WG, Eastwood MA, Sedgwick DM. Dietary effects of sodium alginate in humans. *Food Add Contam.* 1991;8:225–236.
24. Torsdottir I, Alpsten M, Holm G, et al. A small dose of soluble alginate-fiber affects postprandial glycemia and gastric emptying in humans with diabetes. *J Nutr.* 1991; 121:795–799.
25. Gibson GR, Macfarlane S, Cummings JH. The fermentability of polysaccharides by mixed human faecal bacteria in relation to their suitablity as bulk-forming laxatives. *Lett Appl Microbiol.* 1990;11:251–254.
26. Garcia MJ, Charlez M, Fauli C, et al. Physicochemical comparison of the dietary fibres glucomannan, galactomannan, carboxymethyl cellulose, pectin and wheat bran. *Curr Ther Res.* 1988;43:1010–1013.
27. Biancardi G, Palmiero L, Ghirardi PE. Glucomannan in the treatment of overweight patients with osteoarthrithosis. *Curr Ther Res.* 1989;46:908–912.
28. Tannock GW. Probiotic properties of lactic-acid bacteria: plenty of scope for fundamental R&D. *Trends in Biotechnology* (TIBTECH). 1997;15:270–274.
29. Ahrné S, Nobaek S, Jeppsson B, et al. The normal *Lactobacillus* flora in healthy human rectal and oral mucosa. *J Appl Microbiol.* 1998;85:88–94.
30. Finegold SM, Sutter VL, Mathisen GE. Normal indigenous intestinal flora. In: Hentges DJ, ed. *Human Intestinal Microflora In Health And Disease.* London: Academic Press; 1983:3–31.
31. Adlerberth I, Carlsson B, deMan P, et al. Intestinal colonization with *Enterobacteriaceae* in Parkistani and Swedish hospital-delivered infants. *Acta Pediatrica Scandinavica.* 1991;80:602–610.
32. Sepp E, Julge K, Vasur M, et al. Intestinal microflora of Estonian and Swedish infants. *Acta Pediatrica.* 1997;86: 956–961.
33. Lencner AA, Lencner CP, Mikelsaar ME, et al. Die quantitative zusammensetzung der lactoflora des verdauungstrakts vor und nach kosmischen flügen unterschiedlicher dauer. *Die Nahrung.* 1984;28:607–613.
34. Andersson R, Wang X, Ihse I.The influence of abdominal sepsis on acute pancreatitis in rats: a study on mortality, permeability, arterial blood pressure and intestinal blood flow. *Pancreas.* 1995;11:365–373.
35. Leveau P, Wang X, Soltesz V et al. Alterations in intestinal permeability and microflora in experimental acute pancreatitis. *Int J Pancreatology.* 1996;20:119–125.
36. De Souza LJ, Sampietre SN, Figueiredo S, et al. Bacterial translocation during acute pancreatitis in rats. (In Portuguese, with English summary.) *Rev Hosp Clin Fac Med.* S. Paolo: 1996;51:116–120.
37. Schwartz MN. Hospital-acquired infections; diseases with increasingly limited therapies. *Prox Natl Acad Sci USA.* 1994;91:2420–2427.

38. Hasse JM, Blue LS, Crippin JS, et al. The effect of nutritional status on length of stay and clinical outcomes following liver transplantation. Abstract: *J Am Diet Assoc.* 1994;88:143–145.

39. van der Poll T, Levi M, Braxton CC, et al. Parenteral nutrition facilitates activation of coagulation but not fibrinolysis during human endotoxemia. *The Journal of Infectious Diseases.* 1998;177:793–795.

40. Frohn MJN. Letter to the editor. *Lancet.* 1976;11:1019–1020.

41. Latto C. Postoperative Deep-vein thrombosis, pulmonary embolism, and high-fibre diet. *The Lancet.* 1976;11:1197.

42. Malhotra SL. Studies in blood coagulation, diet and ischemic heart disease in two population groups in India. *British Heart Journal.* 1968;30:303–308.

43. Vorster HH, Kruger HS, Fryllinck S, et al. Physiological effects of the dietary fiber component konjac glucomannan in rats and baboons. *J Plant Food.* 1985;6:263–274.

44. Koepp O, Hegewisch S. Effects of guar on plasma viscosity and related parameters. *Europ J Pediatr.* 1981;137:31–33.

45. Chegini N. The role of growth factors in peritoneal healing: transforming growth factor beta (TGF-betaq). *Eut J Surg* (suppl). 1997:17–23.

46. Bothin C, Okada M, Midtvedt T, Perbeck L. The intestinal flora influences adhesion formation aqround surgical anastomoses. *Br J Surg.* 2001;1:143–145.

47. Antoniades HN, Westmoreland N. Metabolic influences in experimental thrombosis. *Ann N Y Acad Sci.* 1976;275: 28–46.

48. Pilgeram LO, Pickart RL Control of fibrinogen biosynthesis: the role of free fat acid. *J Atheroscler Res.* 1968;8: 155–66.

49. Venter CS, Vorster HH. Possible metabolic consequences of fermentation in the colon for humans. *Medical Hypothesis.* 1898;29:161–166.

50. Randle PJ, Hales CN, Garland BP, Newsholme EA. The glucose fatty-acid cycle. Its role in insulin sensitivity and the metabolic disturbances of diabetes mellitus. *The Lancet.* 1963;1:785–89.

51. Wang H, Storlien LH, Huang XF. Influence of dietary fats on c-fos-like immunoreactivity in mouse hypothalamus. *Brain Research.* 1999;843:184–192.

52. Watanabe S, Onozaki K, Yamamoto S, Okuyama H. Regulation by dietary essential fatty acid balance of tumor necrosis factor production in mouse macrophages. *J Leukoc Biol.* 1993;53:151–156.

53. Lin BF, Huang CC, Chiang BL, Jeng SJ. Dietary fat influences Ia antigen expression, cytokines and prostaglandin E_2 production in immune cells in autoimmune-prone NZBxNZW F1 mice. *British Journal of Nutrition.* 1996; 75:711–722.

54. Biffl WL, Moore EE, Moore, FA, Barnett CC. Interleukin-6 delays neutrophil apoptosis via a mechanism involving platelet-activating factor. *The Journal of Trauma, Injury, Infection and Critical Care.* 1996;40:575–579.

55. Sautner T, Függer R, Götzinger P et al. Tumour necrosis factor-α and interleukin-6: Early indicators of bacterial infection after human orthotopic liver transplantation. *Eur J Surg.* 1995;161:97–101.

56. Brandtzaeg P, Halstensen TS, Kett K, et al. Immunobiology and immunopathology of human gut mucosa: humoral immunity and intraepithelial lymphocytes. *Gastroenterology.* 1989;97:1562–1584.

57. Kiyono H, McGhee JR. T helper cells for mucosal immune responses. In: Ogra PL, Mestecky J, Lamm ME, et al., eds. *Handbook of Mucosal Immunology.* Orlando, Florida: Academic Press; 1994:263–274.

58. Brandzaeg P. Molecular and cellular aspects of the secretory immunoglobulin system. *APMIS.* 1995;103:1–19.

59. Bermann JF, Chassany O, Perit A, et al. Correlation between echographic gastric emptying and appetite: influence of psyllium. *Gut.* 1992;33:1041–1043.

60. Rhee YH, Kim HI. The correlation between sleeping-time and numerical change of intestinal normal flora in psychiatric insomnia patients. *Bull Nat Sci.* Chungbuk Natl Univ: 1987;1:159–172.

61. Brown R, Price RJ, King MG, et al. Are antibiotic effects on sleep behavior in the rat due to modulation of gut bacteria? *Physiol Behav.* 1990;48:561–565.

62. Meiselman HL, Lieberman HR. In: Goldberg I, ed. Mood and performance foods, chapter 7. *Functional Foods, Designer Foods, Pharmafoods, Nutraceuticals.* Chapman and Hall: 1994;126–150.

63. Del Aguila LF, Claffey KP, Kirwan JP. TNF-alpha impairs insulin signaling and insulin stimulation of glucose uptake in C2C12 muscle cells. *Am J Physiol.* 1999;39:E849–855.

64. Bertini R, Bianci M, Ghezzi P. Adrenalectomy sensitizes mice to the lethal effects of interleukin-1 and tumor-necrosis factor. *J Exp Med.* 1988;167:1702–1712.

65. Ramachandra RN, Sehon AH, Berczi I. Neuro-hormonal host defence in endotoxin shock. *Brain Behav Immun.* 1992;6:157–169.

66. Olff M. Stress. Depression and immunity: the role of defense and copying styles. *Psychiatry Res.* 1999;85:7–15.

67. Shirabe K, Matsumata T, Shimada M, et al. A comparison of parenteral hyperalimentation and early enteral feeding regarding systemic immunity after major hepatic resection—the results of a randomized prospective study. *Hepato-Gastroenterology.* 1997;44:205–209.

68. Windsor ACJ, Kanwar S, Li AGK, et al. Compared with parenteral nutrition, enteral feeding attenuates the acute phase response, and improves disease severity in acute pancreatitis. *Gut.* 1998;42:431–435.

69. Barton RG. Immune-enhancing enteral formulas: are they beneficial in critically ill patients? *Nutrition in Clinical Practice.* 1997;12:51–62.

70. Dickerson RN. Immune-enhancing enteral formulas in critically ill patients. *Nutrition in Clinical Practice.* 1997;12:49–50.

71. Bengmark S. Gut microenvironment and immune function. *Current Opinion in Clinical Nutrition and Metabolic Care.* 1999;2:83–85.

72. Yasui H, Nagaoka N, Mike A, et al. Detection of *Bifidobacterium* strains that induce large quantities of IgA. *Microb Ecol Health Dis.* 1992;5:155–162.

73. Malin M, Suomalainen H, Saxelin M, Isolauri E. Promotion of IgA immune response in patients with Crohn's disease by oral bacteriotherapy with *Lactobacillus* GG. *Annals of Nutrition and Metabolism.* 1996;40:137–145.

74. Kaila M, Isolauri E, Soppi E, et al. Enhancement of the circulating antibody secreting cell response in human diarrhea by a human *lactobacillus* strain. *Pediatric Research.* 1992;32:141–144.

75. Solis-Pereyra B, Aattouri, N, Lemonnier, D. Role of food in the stimulation of cytokine production. *Am J Clin Nutr.* 1997;66:521S–525S.

76. Mao Y, Nobaek S, Kasravi B, et al. The effects of *Lactobacillus* strains and oat fiber on methotrexate-induced enterocolitis in rats. *Gastroenterology.* 1996;111:334–344.

77. van der Poll T, Coyle SM, Levi M, et al. Fat emulsion infusion potentiates coagulation activation during human endotoxemia. *Thrombosis and Heamostasis.* 1996;75:83–86.

78. Peck MD, Alexander JW, Ogla CK, Babcock GF. The effect of dietary fatty acids in response to *Pseudomonas* infection in burned mice. *J Trauma.* 1990;30:445–452.

79. Roszkowski K, Ko KL, Beuth J, et al. Intestinal microflora of BALB/c-mice and function of local immune cells. *Zeitschr Bakteriol Hygien.* 1988;270:270–279.

80. Pulverer G, Ko HL, Roszkowski W et al. Digestive tract microflora liberates low molecular weight peptides with immunotriggering activity. *Zentralbl Bakteriol.* 1990;272: 318–327.

81. Kilkullen, JK, Ly OP, Chang, TH, et al. Nonviable *Staphylococcus aureus* and its peptidoglucan stimulate macrophage recruitment, angiogenesis, fibroplasia and collagen accumulation in wounded rats. *Wound, Repair and Regeneration.* 1998;6:149–156.

82. Hatcher GE, Lamprecht RS. Augmentation of macrophage phagocytic activity by cell-free extracts of selected lactic acid-producing bacteria. *J Dairy Scien.* 1993;76: 2485–2492.

83. Kato I, Yokokura T, Mutai M. Correlation between increase in Ia-bearing macrophages and induction of T-cell-dependent antitumor activity by *Lactobacillus casei* in mice. *Cancer, Immunology and Immunotherapy.* 1988;26:215–221.

84. Outwater JL, Nicholson A, Barnard N. Dairy products and breast cancer: The IGF-1, estrogen and bGH hypothesis. *Medical Hypotheses.* 1997;48:453–461.

85. Westin JB, Richter E. The Israeli breast-cancer anomaly. *Ann NY Acad Scien.* 1990;609:269–279.

86. Hague A, Manning AM, Hanlon KA, et al. Sodium butyrate induces apoptosis in human colonic tumour cell lines in a p53-independent pathway: implications for the possible role of dietary fiber in the prevention of large-bowel cancer. *Int J Cancer.* 1993;55:498–505.

87. Hong MY, Chang WC, Chapkin RS, Lupton JR. Relationship among colonocyte proliferation, differentiation, and apoptosis as a function of diet and carcinogen. *Nutrition and Cancer.* 1997; 28;20–29.

88. Solary E, Dubrez L, Eymin B. The role of apoptosis in the pathogenesis and treatment of diseases. *Eur Resp J.* 1996;9:1293–1305.

89. Heerdt BG, Houston MA, Augenlicht LH. Potentiation by specific short-chain fatty acids of differentiation and apoptosis in human colonic carcinoma cell lines. *Cancer Research.* 1994;54:3288–3294.

90. Marchetti MC, Graziella M, Rosalba M, et al. Possible mechanisms involved in apoptosis of colon tumor cell lines induced by deoxycholic acid, short-chain fatty acids, and their mixtures. *Nutrition and Cancer.* 1997;28(1):74–80.

91. Key FB, Mathers JC. Digestive adaptations of rats given white bread and cooked haricot beans (phaseolus vulgaris): large bowel fermentation and digestion of complex carbohydrates. *Brit J Nutr.* 1995;74:93–406.

92. Kirjavainen PV, El-Nezami HS, Salminen SJ, et al. The effect of orally administered viable probiotic and dairy lactobacilli on mouse lymphocyte proliferation. *FEMS Immun and Med Microbiol.* 1999;26:131–135.

93. Björksten, B. Risk factors in early childhood for the development of atopic diseases. *Allergy.* 1994;49:400–407.

94. Lucey DR, Clerici M, Shearer GM. Type 1 and type 2 cytokine dysregulation in human infections, neoplastic and inflammatory diseases. *Clin Microbiol Rev.* 1996;9:532–562.

95. Björksten B. Allergy priming early in life. *Lancet.* 1999; 353:167–168.

96. Murosaki S, Yamamoto Y, Ito K, et al. Heat-killed *Lactobacillus plantarum* L-137 suppresses naturally fed antigen-specific IgE production by stimulation of IL-12 production in mice. *J Allerg Clin Immunol.* 1998;102:57–64.

97. Miettinen M, Matikainen S, Vuopio-Varkila J, Pirhonen J, et al. Lactobacilli and Streptococci induce Interleukin-12 (IL-12), IL-18, and gamma interferon production in human peripheral blood mononuclear cells. *Infect Immun.* 1998;66:6058–6060.

98. Shida K, Makino K, Takamizawa K, et al. *Lactobacillus casei* inhibits antigen-induced IgE secretion through regulation of cytokine production in murine splenocyte cultures. *Internat Arch Allerg Immunol.* 1998;115:278–287.

99. Eckmann L, Kagnoff MF, Fierer J. Intestinal epithelial cells as watchdogs for the natural immune system. *Trends Microbiol.* 1995;3:118–120.

100. Ogle CK, Guo X, Hasselgren PO, et al. The gut as a source of inflammatory cytokines after stimulation with endotoxin. *Europ J Surg.* 1997;163:45–51.

101. Henderson B, Poole S, Wilson M. Microbial/host interactions in health and disease: who controls the cytokine network? *Immunopharmacol.* 1996,35:1–21.

102. Henderson, B., Wilson, M., Wren, B. Are bacterial exotoxins cytokine network regulators? *Trends in Microbiology.* 1998;5:454–458.

103. Meyer TA, Noguchi Y, Ogle CK, et al. Endotoxin stimulates interleukin-6 production in intestinal epithelial cells. A synergistic effect with prostaglandin E_2. *Arch Surg.* 1994;129:1294–95.

104. Meyer TA, Tiao GM, James JH, et al. Nitric oxide inhibits LPS-induced IL-6 production in enterocytes. *J Surg Res.* 1995;58:570–575.

105. Marin ML, Tejada-Simon MV, Lee JH, et al. Stimulation of cytokine production in clonal macrophage and T-cell models by *Streptococcus thermophilus*: comparison with *Bifidobacterium* sp. and *Lactobacillus bulgaricus*. *J Food Protect.* 1998;61:859–864.
106. Rangavajhyala N, Shahani KM, Sridevi G, Srikumaran S. Nonlipopolysaccharide component(s) of *Lactobacillus acidophilus* stimulate(s) the production of interleukin 1α and tumor necrosis factor-α by murine macrophages. *Nutr Cancer.* 1997;28:130–134.
107. Adlerberth I, Ahrné S, Johansson ML, et al. A mannose-specific adhesion mechanism in *Lactobacillus plantarum* conferring binding to the human colonic cell line HT-29. *Appl Environ Microbiol.* 1996;62:2244–2251.
108. Forstner JF, Forstner GG. Gastrointestinal mucus. In: Johnson LG, ed. *Physiology of the Gastrointestinal Tract, 3rd ed.* New York: Raven Press; 1994:1255–1283.
109. van Klinken BJ, Tytgat KMAJ, Buller HA, et al. Biosynthesis of intestinal mucins: MUC1, MUC2, MUC3 and more. *Biochem Soc Trans.* 1995;23:814–818.
110. Mack DR, Michail S, Wei S, et al. Probiotics inhibit enteropathogenic *e. coli* adherence in vitro by inducing intestinal mucin gene expression. *Am J Physiol.* 1999;276 (*Gastrointest. Liver Physiol* 39):G941–G950.
111. Haskard C, Binnion C, Ahokas J. Factors affecting the squestration of aflatoxin by *lactobacillus rhamnosus* strain GG. *Chemico-Biological Interactions.* 2000:128:39–49.
112. Oatley JT, Rarick MD, Ji GE, Linz JE Binding of aflatoxin to bifidobacteria in vitro. *J Food Protect.* 2000;63: 1133–1136.
113. Goulis J, Patch D, Burroughs AK. Bacterial infection in the pathogenesis of variceal bleeding. *Lancet.* 1999;353: 139–142.
114. Nanji AA, Khetty U, Sadrzadeh SMH. *Lactobacillus* feeding reduces endotoxemia and severity of experimental alcoholic liver disease. *Proc Soc Exp Med Biol.* 1994;205:243–247.
115. Adawi D, Kasravi FB, Molin G, Jeppsson B. Effect of *Lactobacillus* supplementation with and without arginine on liver damage and bacterial translocation in an acute liver injury model in the rat. *Hepatol.* 1997;25:642–647.
116. Adawi D, Molin G, Ahrné S et al. Modulation of the colonic bacterial flora affects differently bacterial translocation and liver injury in acute liver injury model. *Microb Ecol Health Dis.* 1999;11:47–54.
117. De Santis A, Famularo G, De Simone C. Probiotics for the hemodynamic alterations in patients with liver cirrhosis. Letter to the editor. *AJG.* 2000;95:323–324.
118. Alverdy J, Aoys E, Moss G. Effects of commercially available defined liquid diets on the intestinal microflora and bacterial translocation from the gut. *J Parenter Enteral Nutr.* 1990;14:1–6.
119. Deitch E, Xu D, Naruhn M, et al. Elemental diet and IV-TPN-induced bacterial translocation is associated with loss of intestinal barrier function against bacteria. *Ann Surg.* 1995;22:299–307.
120. Ichikawa H, Kuroiwa T, Inagaki A et al. Probiotic bacteria stimulate epithelial cell proliferation in rat. *Dig Dis & Scien.* 1999;44:2119–2123.
121. Heyman M. Effect of lactic acid bacteria on diarrheal diseases. *J Am Coll Nutr.* 2000;19:S137–S146.
122. Guandalini, S, Pensabene L, Zikri MA et al. *Lactobacillus* GG administered in oral rehydration solution to children with acute diarrhea: a multicenter European study. *J Pediatr Gastr Nutr.* 2000;30:54–60.
123. Fabia R, Ar'Rajab A, Johansson ML et al. Impairment of bacterial flora in human ulcerative colitis and in experimental colitis in the rat. *Digestion.* 1993;54:248–255.
124. Fabia R, Ar'Rajab A, Johansson ML, et al. The effect of exogenous administration of *Lactobacillus reuteri* R2LC and oat fibre on acetic acid-induced colitis in the rat. *Scand J Gastroenterol.* 1993;28:155–162.
125. Favier C, Neut C, Mizon C, et al. Fecal β-D-galactosidase and bifidobacteria are decreased in Crohn's disease. *Dig Dis Sci.* 1997;42:817–822.
126. Sartor RB. Microbial factors in the pathogenesis of Crohn's disease, ulcerative colitis and experimental intestinal inflammation. In: Kirsner JG, ed. *Inflammatory Bowel Diseases, Fifth Edition.* Philadelphia: Saunders; 1999:153–178.
127. Venturi A, Gionchetti P, Rizzello F, et al. Impact on the composition of the faecal flora by a new probiotic preparation: preliminary data on maintenance treatment of patients with ulcerative colitis. *Aliment Pharmacol Ther.* 1999;13:1103–1108.
128. Gionchetti P, Rizello F, Venturi A, et al. Oral bacteriotherapy as maintenance treatment in patients with chronic pouchitis: a double-blind, placebo-controlled trial. *Gastroenterology.* 2000;119:305–309.
129. Hoyos AB. Reduced incidence of necrotizing enterocolitis associated with enteral administration of *Lactobacillus acidophilus* and *Bifidobacterium Infantis* to neonates in an intensive care unit. *Int J Infect Dis.* 1999;3:197–202.
130. Gomersall CM. Does the administration of lactobacillus to critically ill patients decrease the severity of multi-organ dysfunction or failure? *Thesis for B Sc degree in Health Studies.* London: University of Surrey, Roehampton Institute, School of Life Sciences; 1998.
131. Rayes N, Hansen S, Boucsein K, et al. Comparison of parenteral and early enteral nutrition with fibre and lactobacilli after major abdominal surgery—a prospective randomized trial. In manuscript.
132. Rayes, N, Hansen, S., Boucsein K, et al. Early enteral supply of *Lactobacillus* and fibre vs. selective bowel decontamination (SBD)—a controlled trial in liver transplant recipients. In manuscript (2001).
133. Oláh, Attila, et al. To be published.
134. Cunningham-Rundles S, Ahrne S, Bengmark S, et al. Probiotics and immune response. *Am J Gastroenterol.* 2000; 95(1 Suppl):S22–25.
135. Buscher HJ, Free RH, Van Weissenbruch R, et al. Preliminary observations on influence of dairy products on biofilm removal from silicon rubber voice prostheses in vitro. *J Dairy Science.* 1999;83:641–647.
136. van der Mei HC, Free RH, Elving GJ, et al. Effect of probiotic bacteria on prevalence of yeasts in oropharyngeal biofilms on silicone rubber voice prostheses in vitro. *J Med Microbiol.* 2000:49:713–718.

CHAPTER

35 Is It Cost Effective to Feed Patients in the Intensive Care Unit

Stanley A. Nasraway, Jr., M.D., F.C.C.M., Kris M. Mogensen, M.S., R.D.

Introduction	401	Conclusions	404
Cost of Artificial Nutrition	402	References	405
Cost Savings from Artificial Nutrition	402		

Introduction

Malnutrition is widely prevalent among hospitalized surgical and medical patients stricken with acute illness[1–5] and is associated with increased complications, poorer outcomes, and longer hospital stays, generating significantly higher costs to the health care system.[3–8] The preponderance of evidence indicates that artificial nutrition in severely malnourished and seriously ill patients can improve outcome,[9–12] although some investigators are not in agreement with this view.[13–14] Furthermore, some studies[15–19] would seem to suggest an advantage with the use of enteral nutrition (EN) over total parenteral nutrition (TPN), whereas other investigations have failed to confirm this.[20–25] Among available tube feeding options, immune enhancing formulations have generated the greatest interest in the past decade, holding the possibility of reducing infectious complications and perhaps hastening wound healing.

While academic debate continues over the central issues described above, there has been, at best, a modest published effort to determine the costs of delivering artificial nutrition, and whether particular routes of delivery or specific formulations are cost-effective, especially in the critically ill and injured patient.[26] Explicit documentation of cost savings is lacking in this literature, in part because few studies have included finance as a measured endpoint. The remainder of this chapter will focus on the economic impact of artificial nutrition in the intensive care unit (ICU). Because of the paucity of economic data, length of stay and, to a lesser degree, complication rate will be important surrogates by which to estimate costs. Where possible, literature directly related to study of the critically ill will be used; however, it will also be necessary to extrapolate from studies of acutely ill patients who were not necessarily in the ICU.

Before considering the costs of artificial nutrition, one might first stop to consider the costs of not feeding the malnourished patient. Reilly et al. performed a retrospective study[6] of 771 acutely ill patients, in which the incidence of malnutrition was approximately 55%. These investigators compared outcomes and costs between two cohorts, those patients likely to be malnourished and those who were not. Malnourished patients sustained 3 times as many complications and were 3.8 times as likely to die. Consequently, malnourished patients had a prolonged hospital length of stay; parameters of malnutrition were significantly correlated with a longer stay in the ICU. The malnourished cohort sustained an increase in direct variable costs, suggesting that malnourished patients require a greater intensity of care. Interestingly, the authors noted that TPN was 5.7 times more costly to administer than was EN.[6]

Apart from the malnutrition with which patients are encumbered at the time of ICU admission, there are also the perpetuation and worsening of malnutrition that take place in many patients *after* hospitalization. Investigators at the University of Illinois studied 404 patients after hospitalization and, by means of the subjective global assessment, quantified a decline in nutritional status in 31% of these patients.[4] They found that a decline in nutritional status was a stronger determinant of subsequent complications and increased costs than was even the degree of malnutrition on hospital admission.[4] Critical care providers need to be conscious of nutritional compromise both at the time of ICU admission and during the hospital course.

Cost of Artificial Nutrition

The cost of artificial nutrition is influenced by a multiplicity of factors. These include the acquisition costs of elemental constituents and for additives that are used to supplement EN and TPN formulations. Moreover, the labor involved in preparing and giving these formulations involves pharmacists, dietitians, and nurses. There are also costs related to the intravascular or intra-enteric insertion of catheters, procedures that require skilled nurses and physicians, and which may require special interventional assistance involving the use of fluoroscopy, endoscopy, or even surgery. Additional costs are related to radiographic confirmation of placement of enteric or parenteral catheters. The procedures themselves carry an extra economic and morbid burden when they are complicated by mechanical misadventures, such as inadvertent insertion of a nasoduodenal feeding tube into the lung, or by the catheter-related sepsis to which dedicated TPN catheters are predisposed. Nevertheless, many of these costs are "fixed," in that they represent the use of necessary hospital assets and personnel.

There are no published data, anywhere, which prove that the specific use of artificial nutrition in the critically ill can decrease "full-time equivalents," i.e., the number of hired personnel needed to care for patients in an ICU. The daily cost of care in an ICU can be gargantuan and can represent a figure that is typically underestimated. For example, in the late 1990s at Tufts-New England Medical Center in Boston, the Finance Department, using very sophisticated software, determined that the cost (*not charges*) of caring for a single patient in the Surgical ICU was $4,104 per day of ICU stay (personal communication, Marilyn Gustafson). The overwhelming majority of this staggering cost was attributable to the cost of labor, principally measured in nursing hours per patient per day. Because hospital structural and personnel assets are constant no matter the provision of artificial nutrition, the most important variable in the cost of artificial nutrition is that of the cost and preparation of the constituents themselves. This was shown by Italian investigators, who prospectively randomized a population of patients undergoing surgery for upper gastrointestinal cancer to standardized isocaloric and isonitrogenous formulations of TPN or EN for the purpose of comparing outcomes and costs.[20] There was no difference in outcome for this patient population receiving either TPN or EN. However, TPN was fourfold more costly than EN, with the primary difference found in the prescription preparation itself. This is best seen in

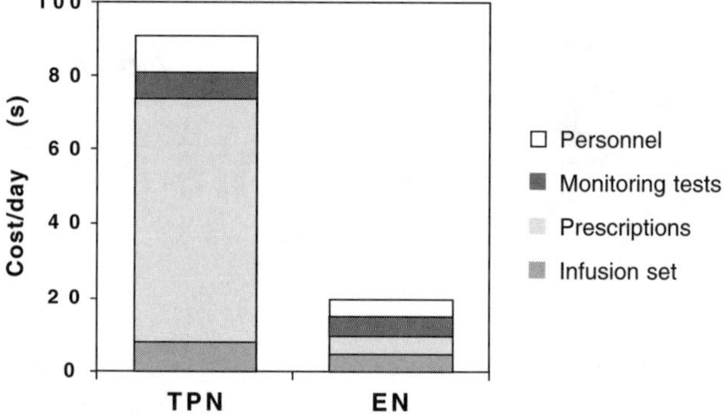

Figure 35.1

Cost Analysis of the Two Nutritional Regimens. TPN, total parenteral nutrition, EN, early enteral nutrition. Mean daily TPN cost, $90.60; mean daily EN cost $25.

Reprinted with permission from Braga M, Gianotti L, Gentilini O, et al. Early postoperative enteral nutrition improves gut oxygenation and reduces costs compared with total parenteral nutrition. *Crit Care Med.* 2001;29:242–248. ©Lippincott Williams & Wilkins.

Figure 35.1, adapted from the study by Braga et al.[20] By contrast, there was little difference in other costs, including the cost of infusion sets, monitoring tests, or personnel.[20] Other studies of critically ill patients, patients managed after liver transplantation, and patients managed on hospital wards have found a similar ratio in cost savings with respect to the use of EN.[6,24,27]

The acquisition costs of enteral and parenteral constituents at Tufts-New England Medical Center in Year 2000 are listed in Table 35.1. Consistent with the findings by others,[6,20,24,27] acquisition costs of constituents for TPN are about 4 times more expensive than for EN, when standardized by daily caloric intake.

Cost Savings from Artificial Nutrition

Since few studies in the nutritional support literature have incorporated a financial analysis into a prospective experimental design, one most often must use the decrease in "length of stay" as the surrogate measurement for cost savings. Fortunately, various studies have identified length of stay as an outcome measurement. The most ambitious attempt to answer the question of whether feeding malnourished patients was cost-effective has been the Malnutrition Cost Survey.[28] The Malnutrition Cost Survey was a retrospective study of 2,485 inpatients in 20 separate medical centers in the United States. A stepwise regression analysis of the factors influencing duration of hospitalization found that nutritional intervention was accompanied by a

TABLE 35.1

Acquisition Costs of TPN and EN*

TPN	Raw costs	Standardized**
Standard amino acid base solution***, 1 L	$23.82	$33.84
Intravenous lipid emulsions, 250 mL 20%	$ 7.28	$ 7.28
Trace elements, vitamins	$ 5.42	$ 5.42
Total cost per 1000 kcal	$36.52	$46.54
EN		
Standard polymeric:		
Osmolite HN® (Ross) cost per 1000 kcal	$ 6.48	$11.34
Standard Immune-enhanced:		
Impact® (Novartis) cost per 1000 kcal	$18.80	$32.90

TPN, total parenteral nutrition; EN, enteral nutrition

*Includes costs of solution, bag and pharmacy time for order entry, labor for preparation, April 2000, Tufts-New England Medical Center

**Standardized, to 25 kcal/kg, in a 70 kg patient, ideal body weight, i.e. caloric goal of 1750 kcal/day

***5% amino acids, 20% dextrose

20% decrease in mean length of stay.[28] Additionally, the earlier nutritional support was started, the greater was the decrease in length of stay.[28] Estimates from this study indicate that each 2 days of earlier nutritional intervention were accompanied by a decrease in 1 day of hospitalization.[28] Survey analysis found that for an average-sized medical center, early nutrition intervention resulted in savings of approximately 1500 patient days and more than 1 million dollars per year.[28]

The patients who have the most to gain from aggressive nutritional support are those who are the most malnourished. It is pivotal when interpreting the nutritional support literature to examine both the clinical outcome and the patient population that was studied. That is necessary because many studies of nutritional support are marred by the fact that patients who were not malnourished or who were only mildly malnourished are much less likely to sustain malnutrition-related complications, such as infection. The Veterans Affairs Cooperative Study[10] is an excellent example of a study in which the distinction of likelihood for benefit is made between patients with mild malnutrition and those who were severely malnourished. This is the largest prospective study to date of the value of aggressive nutritional restitution, examining how TPN might improve the hospital course of patients awaiting elective surgery.[10] Approximately 400 patients awaiting thoracic or abdominal surgery were randomly assigned to receive 7 to 10 days of TPN before surgery or allowed to rely solely on their oral diet.[10] Perhaps the most prominent finding from this study was that noninfectious postoperative complications, including wound or anastomotic dehiscence, were decreased by 88% ($p<0.03$) in the patients with severe malnutrition who received TPN; there was also a trend toward reduced infectious complications.[10] Unfortunately, the Veterans Affairs trial did not report length of stay, much less the financial implications of its results. A small trial of TPN for the first 7 postoperative days versus no artificial nutrition was conducted in 28 patients after liver transplantation; this trial, despite its small sample size, did demonstrate decreased ICU length of stay.[29]

A comprehensive meta-analysis comparing the value of "TPN in the critically ill patient" was conducted by Heyland et al.[13] This trial examined 26 prospective randomized trials spanning the period from 1976 to 1994; while comprehensive, conclusions are mitigated by the changing methods of care, the changing parenteral solutions involved, and the changing nutritional goals that evolved during this time period. Heyland's meta-analysis was mistitled, in that the vast majority of the included trials centered on patients undergoing major surgery. Many of these surgical patients were not critically ill; only 4 of the 26 studies included patients who might have been acutely ill or traumatized.[13] Moreover, many study patients were not seriously malnourished. While there was no mortality benefit overall, malnourished patients receiving TPN experienced a 48% reduction in complications (RR, 0.52: 95% CI, 0.30–0.91) according to subgroup analysis.[13] The major conclusion from this trial would be that short-term TPN probably does not improve outcome in patients having major surgery. What hasn't been answered is how long nutritional support with TPN can be delayed in critically ill patients who cannot be given enteral feeds.

Comparative trials between TPN and EN in the critically ill are relatively few, and are frequently experimentally flawed by unbalanced comparisons in nitrogen or caloric intake.[30] Nevertheless, the route of aggressive nutritional delivery seems to have a substantial impact on both the clinical outcome for the patient and for the costs involved in that patient's care. An increasingly compelling literature suggests EN is associated with fewer morbid events, largely infections, than TPN. This may be because of the immune-enhancing EN formulas that are increasingly used, or because TPN tends to be associated with greater degrees of hyperglycemia (see Chapter 11). The explanation for this undoubtedly resides in the finding that hyperglycemia, particularly in the chronically critically ill, is associated with higher mortality rates and greater degrees of septic complications and multiple organ failure.[31,32] In the Italian study[20] cited earlier, wherein a large sample of patients undergoing curative resection of upper gastrointestinal cancer was randomized to TPN or EN, there was no overall difference in survival between the two nutritional modalities. However, post hoc analysis of the severely malnourished cohort of patients receiving EN did demonstrate a significant decrease in length of stay, as well as a fourfold decrease in cost compared with patients receiving TPN.[20]

Two recent meta-analyses were conducted to examine the influence of immunonutrition therapy on mortality and infectious complications.[14,33] These meta-analyses reviewed randomized trials in which immune enhanced EN was compared with a standardized EN. The findings were similar, i.e., that immune enhanced EN significantly decreased hospital length of stay, lending credence to the idea that immune enhancing EN is more cost-effective than either standardized EN or TPN.[14,33] The Beale meta-analysis[33] centered on studies of the critically ill and found reductions in infectious complications and duration of mechanical ventilation. The Heyland meta-analysis[14] was larger, but included more heterogeneous patient populations including those after major surgery. This meta-analysis[14] also included unpublished data from the Ross Products Division of Abbott Laboratories, which in 1996 conducted a study that showed a curiously large mortality excess in the group of patients receiving the experimental immune-enriched formula (mortality: 23% vs. 9.6%, immune-enriched vs. standard EN). The inclusion of these unpublished and outlier data, according to subgroup analysis, may have tilted the results of the meta-analysis, which indicated an increased mortality in critically ill patients receiving immune-enriched EN. Since these data from the Ross study are still unpublished at the time of this writing, the validity of this conclusion from that single study, and from Heyland's meta-analysis,[14] cannot be verified and should otherwise be discounted until the data from the Ross study can be subjected to public scrutiny.

Unfortunately, most hospital administrators remain unconvinced of the potentially important benefits of organized and dedicated nutritional intervention. Reasons for this include: (1) A *dollar saved* is frequently not valued by hospital administrators as being as important as a *dollar generated* by increasing the revenue stream, in our experience. (2) Conventional hospital accounting systems do not track severity of illness or nutrition risk. (3) Any accumulated raw data on patients with malnutrition are rarely aggregated in a way that permits hospital-wide study of malnutrition-related costs. For these and other reasons, hospital administrators tend to be reluctant to invest in organized, dedicated nutritional support services. This is especially true in urban markets, suffering under the influence of managed care penetration in which cost pressures are very intense. In these circumstances, hospital administrators respond first to the fiduciary imperative of staying solvent. Investing in new programs that directly increase streams of revenues can still be attractive. Alternatively, investments in programs that may save dollars through indirect reductions in length of stay, based on somewhat cloudy evidence or rationale, require administrative "vision" and a leap of faith.[34] The evidence that aggressive nutritional support in the severely malnourished patient improves outcomes is not well appreciated and not well described. Nutritional support services are not glamorous, are not well reimbursed for time spent, and are generally underfunded, underappreciated and susceptible to budget cuts.

This lack of support for nutritional support, in hindsight, represents an "opportunity cost" to the medical center and its patients. When nutritional intervention in the ICU is unassisted by a dedicated support service, the application of nutrition is insufficient. A French study showed that nutritional intervention, prescribed by house officers under attending intensivist supervision in critically ill patients, was ineffectively prescribed and delivered.[35] These investigators concluded that it was advisable to develop a protocol for nutritional practice and apply it through the use of a multi-disciplinary team approach, including a pharmacist and dietitian, in order to obtain optimal nutritional care in the malnourished, catabolic critically ill patient.[35] The U.S. Agency for Health Care Policy and Research has provided a similar opinion, strongly encouraging the use of the dedicated dietitian, especially in transitioning the critically ill patient from the more costly TPN to EN.[36] The value of the nutrition support service was lent additional credence in a study of enteral feeding, by which it was determined that there was a benefit of $4.20 for every $1 invested in nutrition support team management.[37]

Conclusions

1. Malnutrition is associated with poor hospital outcomes and is costly as it relates to complications and prolonged length of stay. Nutritional depletion during hospitalization worsens outcomes, no matter the state of a patient's nutrition upon ICU admission.

2. Artificial nutritional repletion given to severely malnourished hosts is associated with improved outcomes and reduced length of stay, when compared to insufficient spontaneous oral caloric intake.
3. TPN by itself has not been shown specifically to improve survival outcomes in the critically ill, and therefore has not been demonstrated to be cost effective. There is, however, a trend towards a reduction in complications in selected circumstances.
4. Numerous individual studies of immune-enhancing EN in critically ill patients demonstrate reduced complications and decreased length of stay; the latter finding is also supported by meta-analysis.
5. TPN is approximately 4 times more expensive than EN, based primarily on the acquisition costs of the constituents.

References

1. Bistrian BR, Blackburn GL, Vitale J, et al. Prevalence of malnutrition in general medical patients. *JAMA.* 1976; 235:1567–1570.
2. Bistrian BR, Blackburn GL, Hallowell E, et al. Protein status of general surgical patients. *JAMA.* 1974;230:858–860.
3. Giner M, Laviano A, Meguid MM, et al. In 1995 a correlation between malnutrition and poor outcome in critically ill patients still exists. *Nutrition.* 1996;12:23–29.
4. Braunschweig C, Gomez S, Sheean PM. Impact of declines in nutritional status on outcomes in adult patients hospitalized for more than 7 days. *J Am Diet Assoc.* 2000; 100:1316–1322.
5. Naber T, Schermer T, de Bree A, et al. Prevalence of malnutrition in nonsurgical hospitalized patients and its association with disease. *Am J Clin Nutr.* 1997;66:1232–1239.
6. Reilly JJ, Hull SF, Albert N, et al. Economic impact of malnutrition: a model system for hospitalized patients. *J Parenter Enteral Nutr.* 1988;12:371–376.
7. Warnold I, Lundholm K. Clinical significance of preoperative nutritional status in 215 non-cancer patients. *Ann Surg.* 1984;199:299–305.
8. Windsor JA, Hill GL. Risk factors of postoperative pneumonia: the importance of protein depletion. *Ann Surg.* 1988;208:209–214.
9. Klein S, Kinney J, Jeejeebhoy K, et al. Nutrition support in clinical practice: review of published data and recommendations for future research directions. Summary of a conference sponsored by the National Institutes of Health, American Society for Parenteral and Enteral Nutrition, and American Society of Clinical Nutrition. *Am J Clin Nutr.* 1997;66:683–706.
10. The Veterans Affairs Total Parenteral Nutrition Cooperative Study Group: perioperative total parenteral nutrition in surgical patients. *N Engl J Med.* 1991;325:525–532.
11. Von Meyenfield M, Meijerink W, Rouflart M, et al. Perioperative nutritional support: a randomized clinical trial. *Clin Nutr.* 1992;11:180–186.
12. Cerra FB, Rios Benitez M, Blackburn GL, et al. Applied nutrition in ICU patients: a consensus statement of the American College of Chest Physicians. *Chest.* 1997;111: 769–778.
13. Heyland DK, MacDonald S, Keefe L, et al. Total parenteral nutrition in the critically ill patient: a meta-analysis. *JAMA.* 1998;280:2013–2019.
14. Heyland DK, Novak F, Drover JW, et al. Should immunonutrition become routine in critically ill patients? A systematic review of the evidence. *JAMA.* 2001;286: 944–953.
15. Kudsk DA, Croce MA, Fabian TC, et al. Enteral versus parenteral feeding. *Ann Surg.* 1992;215:503–513.
16. Moore FA, Feliciano DV, Andrassy RJ, et al. Total enteral feeding compared with parenteral reduces postoperative septic complications: the results of a meta-analysis. *Ann Surg.* 1992;216:172–183.
17. Hasse JM, Blue LS, Liepa G, et al. Early enteral nutrition support in patients undergoing liver transplant. *J Parenter Enteral Nutr.* 1995;19:437–443.
18. Chiarelli A, Enzi G, Casadei A, et al. Very early nutritional supplementation in burned patients. *Am J Clin Nutr.* 1990;51:1035–1039.
19. Hadfield RJ, Sinclair DG, Houldsworth PE, et al. Effects of enteral and parenteral nutrition on gut mucosal permeability in the critically ill. *Am J Resp Crit Care Med.* 1995; 152:1545–1548.
20. Braga M, Gianotti L, Gentilini O, et al. Early postoperative enteral nutrition improves gut oxygenation and reduces costs compared with total parenteral nutrition. *Crit Care Med.* 2001;29:242–248.
21. Adams S, Dellinger PE, Wertz MJ, et al. Enteral versus parenteral nutritional support following laparotomy for trauma: a randomized prospective trial. *J Trauma.* 1986; 26:882–891.
22. Dunham CM, Frankenfield D, Belzberg H, et al. Gut failure: predictor of or contributor to mortality in mechanically ventilated blunt trauma patients? *J Trauma.* 1994; 37:30–34.
23. Cerra FB, McPherson JP, Konstantinides FN, et al. Enteral nutrition does not prevent multiple organ failure (MOFS) after sepsis. *Surgery.* 1988;104:727–733.
24. Wicks C, Somasundaram S, Bjarnason I, et al. Comparison of enteral feeding and total parenteral nutrition after liver transplantation. *Lancet.* 1994;344:837–840.
25. Von Meyenfield M, Meijerink W, Rouflart M, et al. Perioperative nutritional support: a randomized clinical trial. *Clin Nutr.* 1992;11:180–186.
26. Twomey PL, Patching SC. Cost-effectiveness of nutritional support. *J Parenter Enteral Nutr.* 1985;9:3–10.

27. Sand J, Luostarinen M, Matikainen M. Enteral or parenteral feeding after total gastrectomy: prospective randomized pilot study. *Eur J Surg.* 1997;163:761–766.
28. Tucker HN, Miguel SG. Cost containment through nutrition intervention. *Nutr Rev.* 1996;54:111–121.
29. Reilly J, Mehta R, Teperman L, et al. Nutritional support after liver transplantation: A randomized prospective study. *J Parenter Enteral Nutr.* 1990;14:386–391.
30. Murray MJ. Confusion reigns: Enteral versus total parental nutrition. *Crit Care Med.* 2001;29:446.
31. Van den Berghe G, Wouters P, Weekers F, et al. Intensive insulin therapy in critically ill patients. *N Engl J Med.* 2001;345:1359–1367.
32. Pomposelli JJ, Baxter JK, Babineau TJ, et al. Early postoperative glucose control predicts nosocomial infection rate in diabetic patients. *J Parenter Enteral Nutr.* 1998;22:77–81.
33. Beale RJ, Bryg DJ, Bihari DJ. Immunonutrition in the critically ill: a systematic review of clinical outcome. *Crit Care Med.* 1999;27:2799–2805.
34. Hospital finds nutrition care pays off on all counts, cutting costs, complications, mortality. *Clin Resour Manag.* 2000;1(12):183–186.
35. De Jonghe B, Appere-De-Vechi C, Fournier M. A prospective survey of nutritional support practices in intensive care unit patients. *Crit Care Med.* 2001;29:8–12.
36. Critical literature review: Clinical effectiveness in allied health practices. Washington, D.C.: U.S. Dept of Health and Human Services; DHHS (PHS, AHCPR) publication 94:0029, 1993.
37. Hassel JT, Games AD, Shaffer B, et al. Nutrition support team management of enterally fed patients in a community hospital is cost beneficial. *J Am Diet Assoc.* 1994;94:993–998.

CHAPTER 36

The Team Approach to Nutrition Support in the Intensive Care Unit

Nicole M. Daignault, R.D., C.N.S.D., John R. Galloway, M.D., C.N.S.P., Glen F. Bergman, M.MSc., R.D., C.N.S.D., Elaina E. Szeszycki, Pharm.D., B.C.N.S.P., Therese McNally, R.N., B.S., B.S.N., Thomas R. Ziegler, M.D., C.N.S.P.

INTRODUCTION 407
PHYSICIAN 408
DIETITIAN 408
PHARMACIST 410
NURSE 411
PLACEMENT PROCEDURE FOR BEDSIDE POSTPYLORIC FEEDING TUBE PLACEMENT IN ICU PATIENTS 411
Patient Selection Criteria 412
Patient Preparation 412
Procedure 412
ADDITIONAL NST FUNCTIONS AND ACTIVITIES 412
RESEARCH 413
EFFICACY OF THE NST 413
REFERENCES 415

Introduction

The role of optimal nutrition in maintenance of good health is well documented in the literature. Malnutrition, a condition defined for purposes of this chapter as lack of an essential nutrient or nutrients, remains a common problem in many hospitalized patients.[1] In addition, many previously well-nourished patients are at risk for the development of malnutrition, particularly in intensive care unit (ICU) settings. The failure to diagnose and/or treat malnutrition can contribute to altered immune responses, compromise wound healing and tissue repair, increase the risk of infection, delay convalescence, and increase mortality.[1] Provision of enteral nutrition support as a means to supplement or satisfy nutritional requirements has been in practice for hundreds of years,[2] while parenteral nutrition support and current methods of tube feeding are relatively recent therapies in medical and surgical care. In 1968, Dudrick, Wilmore, Vars and Rhoads provided the initial demonstration of positive growth, development, and nitrogen balance with the long-term administration of total parenteral nutrition support in animal models and later in man.[3]

Historically, specialized nutritional support has been associated with several adverse events, particularly in ICU patients. For example, parenteral nutrition is commonly linked to various metabolic or central venous catheter-related mechanical or infectious complications.[1,2] In addition, enteral tube feeding may increase the incidence of aspiration or gastrointestinal intolerance and is associated with complications such as pneumothorax or bowel perforation with improper feeding tube placement.[4] Thus, over the past 3 decades of specialized nutrition support delivery, teams of health professionals that perform nutritional assessment, prescribe enteral and parenteral nutrient solutions, and monitor the response to therapy have been a standard of care in the hospital setting. The nutrition support team (NST) has classically been composed of dietitians, pharmacists, nurses, and physicians, representing the first use of a multidisciplinary team to help deliver complex medical care.[2,4]

In a landmark study, Nehme demonstrated that a significant reduction in catheter-related and metabolic complications was possible when parenteral nutrition support was managed by a multidisciplinary NST with defined guidelines of care.[5] Thus, the desire for the provision of safe and effective specialized nutrition support was an early impetus for the formation of interdisciplinary nutrition support teams.

The utilization of a multidisciplinary NST is likely to provide a particular benefit in the treatment of the complex ICU patient population. According to the Joint Commission 2000 Accreditation Manual for Hospitals, nutrition care monitoring is a collaborative process that requires the involvement of a formal NST or representatives from various disciplines.[6] NSTs in the ICU conform to this model of care, where decisions regarding the timing and the route of feeding critically ill patients can be made in a timely and cost effective manner. Ideally, members from each discipline on the NST offer unique skills, nutritional knowledge, and clinical experience to complete thorough nutritional assessments and formulate a comprehensive nutritional care plan. Cross training among team members is likely to improve the quality of patient care and may be cost effective for an institution. Moreover, order-writing privileges of team members within their individual scope of practice may enhance the efficiency and accuracy of the specialized nutrition support provided.[2,4] In our institution, the NST is involved in all patients requiring parenteral nutrition, most individuals requiring enteral tube feeding, and some complex patients receiving oral diet alone (e.g., post-abdominal surgery, inflammatory bowel disease). In our opinion, an NST functions optimally when it has responsibility for both parenteral and enteral nutrition support in an institution, particularly as most surviving ICU patients transition from specialized support to full oral feeding during the course of their hospitalization.

The role of each discipline on the NST in management of ICU patients varies according to the policies of the institution and the professional training and expertise of the practitioner. Certification in nutritional support by existing National Boards ensures that individuals possess a minimal level of competency in the area of specialized nutrition support. Although there is in practice often considerable overlap in day-to-day duties among team members, the responsibilities and expertise of NST members from multiple disciplines ensures that optimal care is provided. A summary of specific expertise and responsibilities for the classic disciplines involved in hospital-based nutrition support follows.

Physician

The physician on the nutrition support team often serves as a director of the NST and is an important liaison between the NST, house staff, attending physicians, and hospital administration. In addition, the physician provides the necessary expertise and clinical judgment required for physical examination, discussion of complex medical and surgical issues with the patient's primary medical/surgical team, and monitoring of emerging clinical problems. Although any member of a multidisciplinary NST may possess the pertinent leadership skills and clinical knowledge required to serve as team director, a strong physician advocate is best suited to successfully attend to political problems that may arise. In addition, this individual will have an understanding of complex clinical issues relevant to nutrition support.[7]

The physician nutrition specialist can also importantly increase awareness among hospital staff and other physicians as to the importance of nutritional status and nutritional support in medical/surgical recovery and can help to publicize the services offered by an NST. Likewise, the NST physician helps to broaden the nutrition support team's scope of practice by overseeing NST clinical, educational, and research activities.

As noted above, the NST physician can uniquely contribute to the initial assessment and monitoring of critically ill patients by performing nutritionally focused physical examinations. He or she also plays a key role in discussing pertinent clinical issues and reviewing nutrition assessments and therapeutic plans with the NST and primary or consulting physicians. In many institutions, the team physician is responsible for feeding tube or central venous catheter placement in the ICU setting. The NST physician participates in the ongoing clinical monitoring of the nutrition support patient and helps to identify the patient's response to nutrition therapies or clinical changes that may require alterations in the feeding regimen.

The physician may also contribute to NST activities by performing administrative responsibilities. As director of the team, the physician must ensure that the team is adequately represented by all key disciplines, in accordance with the needs of the institution.[7] In addition, it may be his or her responsibility to establish and assure compliance with nutrition support-related policies and procedures. Another key role of the NST physician in academic medical centers is to design and help carry out clinical research projects and nutrition education programs.[2,4,7]

Dietitian

The dietitian serves as a critical liaison between the NST and hospital or clinic staff dietitians and Food and Nutrition Services departments. Good communication between the NST and the staff dietitian promotes continuity of care and initiation of appropriate nutrition support in a timely fashion. Moreover, close interaction with Food and Nutrition Services departments clearly improves the accuracy of diet and nutritional supplement orders.

According to the 1997 American Dietetic Association position paper, "registered dietitians should make recommendations for nutrition support and implement them as needed in collaboration with other health care professionals."[8] The patient's primary service or the critical care medicine team in the ICU may consult the NST for the initiation of specialized nutrition support. The initial consult for NST is often generated by way of an ICU dietitian's nutrition screen or follow-up assessment, which identifies patients' nutritional status or risk.

Following consultation, the initial function of the NST dietitian is to perform a thorough nutritional assessment to determine nutritional status and risk. The NST dietitians should integrate dietary history, available body weight data (usual weight, current dry weight, temporal body weight pattern over the previous weeks and months), pertinent biochemical parameters, current medications (including vitamin, mineral, and herbal supplements), acute and chronic medical and surgical history, and discussion with primary and consultative physicians and other caregivers. Risk factors for malnutrition that may trigger initiation of specialized nutrition support include inadequate dietary intake relative to energy/protein needs for 7 days and/or involuntary body weight loss of 10% of usual weight over the previous several months. The use of parenteral versus enteral nutrition support and the nutrient prescription is determined based upon the nutritional assessment, ongoing discussion with the patient's primary and consulting physicians, and use of guidelines published by the American Society for Parenteral and Enteral Nutrition.[1,9]

In our institution, indications for parenteral nutritional support are the presence of the following:

1. The absence of a functional gastrointestinal tract (i.e., due to obstruction, peritonitis, intractable emesis, acute pancreatitis, ileus, short bowel, or other malabsorption syndromes)
3. The requirement for prolonged NPO status 7 days
3. Central venous or peripheral access

Many practitioners believe that hemodynamically unstable patients on vasopressor support may be poor candidates for enteral feeding due to the increased risk for gut ischemia. Thus, we typically provide parenteral feeding in hemodynamically unstable and hypotensive patients. Enteral feeding into the stomach is used in small amounts, in combination with parenteral feeding, and advanced as the hemodynamic status of the patient improves.

The indication for enteral nutritional support is based on one or more of the following:

1. Functional gastrointestinal tract
2. Hemodynamic stability
3. Inability to take adequate oral food due to dysphagia, mechanical obstruction, anorexia, altered mental status, or mechanical ventilation.[1]

Once the appropriateness of specialized nutrition support and the route of feeding have been determined, the NST dietitian may be responsible for developing and implementing a medical nutrition therapy care plan. The care plan will encompass nutrition recommendations pertaining to oral, enteral, or parenteral nutrition support. Based upon the findings obtained from the nutrition assessment, the care plan will specify goals and desired patient outcomes.[9]

The NST dietitian may be involved in many stages of the medical nutrition care plan implementation process, dependent upon his/her scope of practice, professional experience, licensure/credentials, and the rules and regulations of the institution. In addition to providing recommendations on oral diets and nutrient supplements, the NST dietitian may be involved in activities such as nasoenteric feeding tube insertion, feeding tube maintenance, and tube access site care. The dietitian may also be responsible for ensuring adherence to infection control guidelines with regard to enteral nutrition preparation, storage, and administration. Additionally, the NST dietitian may participate in the establishment and review of protocols to ensure that safe and effective nutrition support is provided.[9]

The NST dietitian, in close collaboration with other NST members, monitors the tolerance of and progress with the prescribed specialized nutritional support regimens (oral diet, supplements, tube feedings, and/or parenteral nutrition) by evaluating serial gastrointestinal function and symptoms, fluid status, biochemical parameters, and the patient's clinical course. The appropriateness of the route of specialized nutritional support will be frequently reassessed based upon changes in the patient's clinical or functional status. The NST dietitian has a primary role of assisting with the transition of parenteral or enteral nutrition to oral feedings by way of nutrient analysis, dietary modifications, and the provision of oral supplements or between-meal feedings.

The NST dietitian should also play a role in the termination of specialized nutrition support when medically indicated or dictated by advanced directives. This team member should be involved in establishing NST protocols for the deceleration or termination of nutrition support in the event of irreversible clinical conditions in which further medical treatment is futile, such as brain death, metastatic or unresectable cancer, or multiorgan failure. Protocols should be developed in accordance with city, state, and federal laws and should allow the practitioner flexibility in addressing issues of termination based upon clinical judgment and the patient's medical status.[9]

Pharmacist

In addition to participating in routine nutritional assessment, nutrient formulation recommendations and monitoring, the NST pharmacist acts as a liaison between the NST and the pharmacy department, especially the area responsible for compounding specialized parenteral nutrition (PN) solutions and other intravenous (IV) products. This helps to ensure accuracy and timeliness of parenteral nutrition orders. Order-writing privileges and direct communication with the IV room allow for earlier initiation of the compounding process and therefore a more timely delivery of the appropriate PN formula to the patient. This is particularly beneficial in the ICU population with its constantly changing clinical status.

The NST pharmacist's specific training is critical for the review of past and current medication orders and to identify nutrient-nutrient, drug-nutrient, drug-drug, and drug-disease/condition interactions that may be deleterious to the patient or incompatible in terms of PN compounding. Once specialized nutrition support has been initiated, the NST pharmacist can aid the physicians in ordering cost-effective medication dosage forms (i.e., crushable tablets that may be flushed via feeding tubes, etc.). The pharmacist should review medication administration records periodically for any drug-nutrient interactions, duplication, inappropriate dosages, and dosage forms. The pharmacist is in a unique position to provide drug information to the physicians and other health professionals caring for the patient, while helping to manage day-to-day nutrition support.

All disciplines on the NST play an integral part in developing a therapeutic plan for the patient, but the pharmacist's expertise in stability of parenteral nutrient solutions and compatibility of medications with parenteral and enteral formulas is required to ensure the provision of safe and effective specialized nutrition support. Recent reports[10] document the deleterious effect of precipitation within parenteral nutrition solutions (e.g., calcium-phosphorus precipitates). Therefore, it is paramount that strict institutional guidelines be developed and enforced when compounding these complex parenteral nutrition formulas. Pharmacists involved in specialized nutrition support should assume the responsibility of ensuring the compatibility of all PN solutions dispensed to the nursing unit.

Patients in the ICU receive multiple medications, so the need to co-infuse, co-administer, or even add medications with the specialized nutrition solutions commonly arises. It is the responsibility of the pharmacist to provide researched lists of compatible or incompatible medications to all hospital staff.[11] Knowing this information when writing specialized nutrition support orders in the ICU reduces time commitments and the potential for error. Early use of enteral feeding, cost reduction strategies with IV and oral medication conversion, inadequate intravenous access, and limited dosage forms of certain medications create challenges for the nurses and pharmacists involved in nutrition support. NST pharmacists should also be familiar with enteral tube feeding techniques, including de-clogging methods and techniques and strategies related to drug administration, taking into account specific pharmacokinetic properties of administered agents.

NST pharmacists practicing in the ICU should also be familiar with such medications as antidiarrheals, prokinetic agents, pancreatic enzymes, catheter-clearing agents, powdered specialty amino acid products that can be administered via feeding tubes (e.g., L-glutamine and L-arginine), and electrolyte/mineral products. Specialty intravenous amino acid products (e.g., branched-chain amino acid, glutamine-enriched, etc.) should be reviewed by the NST pharmacist to determine their appropriateness on the basis of cost and potential efficacy. Patients in the ICU have a multitude of electrolyte and mineral aberrations, so the pharmacist can assist with dosing patients appropriately via either the intravenous or enteral route. It is recommended that pharmacists involved with critically ill patients have particular expertise in fluid and electrolyte/mineral replacement, and in management of acid-base disorders.

Once the therapeutic plan is in place, the pharmacist assists in monitoring by ensuring that routine and as-indicated biochemical tests and specific nursing orders related to nutrient delivery are carried out. For example, it may be appropriate that acetaminophen be ordered as a "crush and flush" rather than as an elixir in tube-fed patients experiencing diarrhea due to the sorbitol content of elixir medications. These responsibilities, in addition to monitoring patient's clinical progress, clearly help to identify, prevent, and manage mechanical, metabolic, and infectious complications associated with specialized nutrition support.

Infections, hemodynamic instability, respiratory status, and wound healing are critical parameters to monitor in the ICU patient. The NST pharmacist thus needs to work closely with other NST members, nursing and respiratory staff, and all involved physicians to accurately assess the patient's progress. Discharge planning is not routinely required for critically ill patients, but extended hospitalization may require the pharmacist and other NST members to assist in determining the need for long-term intravenous or enteral access. Many factors are involved in this determination, but it is helpful to bring this to the attention of the primary physician as soon as the need is identified.

Nurse

The NST nurse acts as an important liaison between the patient's primary ICU nurse and the NST members. Both ICU and NST nurses are trained in physical examination, catheter care, mechanical complications associated with tube feeding, and biochemical and clinical assessment of complex medical/surgical problems, including identification of infection. The NST nurse thus plays a critical role to facilitate proper delivery of enteral and parenteral nutritional support regimens. Good communication between the NST and nursing helps to keep the team informed of changes in the clinical status in this dynamic patient population. In many institutions, the NST nurse assumes primary responsibility for catheter care in patients receiving PN. The NST nurse, like the NST physician, needs to be thoroughly familiar with the institutional policies for catheter care and is usually involved in continuing education activities and policy formulation regarding PN delivery and line care.

As with all nursing practice, the responsibilities of the nutrition support nurse involve 1) patient assessment, 2) development of a plan of care, 3) monitoring and evaluation of the patient's response to the treatment plan, and 4) updating and revising the plan of care as indicated by patients clinical condition and progress. Nutritional support nursing practice in the critical care setting is defined by the scope of practice, "patient focused, goal oriented, and outcome based."[12]

Because of their training in physical examination and assessment, nutrition support nurses play an important role in the initial evaluation of the critically ill patient. Professional training and experience with clinical assessment gives the nurse expertise in evaluating the patient's overall degree of critical illness, gastrointestinal function, fluid and electrolyte balance, and nutritional deficiency states. The NST nurse provides important expertise pertaining to access for and initiation of nutrition support.

Ideally, the nutrition support nurse should be competent in feeding tube placement, which in turn facilitates rapid initiation of enteral feedings in ICU patients. In our institution, the NST nurses are primarily responsible for bedside placement of all post-pyloric feeding tubes in ICU patients and in training other staff in this technique. This method is particularly useful in hemodynamically stable patients with delayed gastric emptying or unprotected airways at risk for pulmonary aspiration. This method has been found to be more cost-effective than fluoroscopic feeding tube placement and may be easier to perform in mechanically ventilated ICU patients.[13,14] Likewise, there is evidence to suggest that post-pyloric feeding tube placement decreases the risk of pulmonary aspiration of tube feeding associated with prolonged parenteral nutrition.[14]

Griffith et al. evaluated the efficacy of intravenous erythromycin as a means to facilitate small bowel feeding tube placement in the critically ill patient.[15] The study demonstrated a significant improvement of successful post-pyloric feeding tube placement and a significant reduction in nursing procedure time with the use of erythromycin.[15] The procedure developed by the Nutrition and Metabolic Support team at Emory University Hospital for small bowel feeding tube placement in the ICU is outlined below:

Placement Procedure for Bedside Postpyloric Feeding Tube Placement in ICU Patients

This procedure requires a physician's order and should not be attempted on patients with a large volume of nasogastric output, recent ear, nose, throat surgery, severe coagulopathies, or history of bleeding esophageal varices, or on patients who are combative.

Patient Selection Criteria

Indications

- Short-term (several weeks) tube feeding indicated
- History of tracheobrachial aspiration or patient at high risk for aspiration
- Gastric atony
- Inability to tolerate elevation of head (e.g., spinal surgery patients)
- Mechanical ventilator dependence
- Contraindications to transport to fluoroscopy

Contraindications

- Thrombocytopenia
- Active upper gastrointestinal bleeding, gastric or esophageal varices
- High output small bowel fistulas (>500cc/24 hour period)
- Hemodynamic instability
- Allergy to erythromycin

Patient Preparation

The rationale and basic steps of the procedure are explained to the patient (if awake and cognizant) or the family.

Procedure

1. If the patient has ordered nasojejunal feeding tube placement, obtain an order for 500 mg IV erythromycin mixed in 100 cc normal saline.
2. Infuse erythromycin via the central line over 20 minutes. (If the patient is allergic to erythromycin, 10 mg of IV metoclopramide may be substituted.)
3. Wash hands and don non-sterile gloves. (Follow standard infection control precautions.)
4. Position metal stylet securely into feeding tube.
5. Flush the feeding tube with water (10 French, 43 inch, non-weighted, hygromer-coated, feeding tubes made by Corpak Co., Wheeling, IL).
6. Measure the distance from the patient's nose to the earlobe to the xiphoid process. (This should be approximately 45–50 cm).
7. If the patient has a Salem sump for gastric decompression, it must be removed prior to the feeding tube placement.
8. Turn the patient onto his or her right side with the head of the bed elevated.
9. Place a generous amount of lubricant on the patient's nares.
10. Gently pass the feeding tube into the nasopharynx and proceed downward into the stomach. Coughing may indicate passage of the feeding tube into the trachea; if this occurs, pull the feeding tube back and re-advance slowly. If resistance is met, remove the feeding tube and notify the physician.
11. Verify gastric feeding tube placement by auscultation and/or aspiration of >20 cc of gastric secretions. Once gastric placement has been achieved, the head of the patient's bed should be lowered.
12. Advance the feeding tube slowly; if resistance is met, pull the feeding tube back and reattempt to advance (feeding tube may be coiled in the stomach).
13. Perform serial aspirations of gastric contents until translucent, yellow bile is obtained. Check pH with pH paper during serial aspirations; a step-up in gastrointestinal aspirate pH from acidic (5.0) to alkaline (6.0) indicates high probability of post-pyloric tube placement.[15]
14. Remove the stylet from the feeding tube.
15. Prep the patient's nose with skin prep, allow it to dry, and secure the feeding tube with nasogastric strip tape.
16. Obtain a KUB to verify feeding tube placement prior to initiation of enteral feedings.

In our institution, the NST nurse is responsible for writing and updating all nursing procedures related to nutrition support including maintenance and administration of central and peripheral parenteral nutrition central line dressing change, insertion of feeding tubes, and administration and maintenance of enteral nutrition. The nutrition support nurse also takes part in the education of nursing staff with regard to policy and procedure changes.[16]

Additional NST Functions and Activities

The NST ideally interacts daily with other teams and disciplines in the management of the critically ill patient. Ongoing communication with the patient's primary service, the critical care team, nursing, and other involved medical or surgical services promotes the coordination of patient care and helps to ensure that the patient's metabolic and nutritional needs are appropriately addressed. Collaboration with respiratory therapy may help to expedite the process of performing indirect calorimetry and facilitate better interpretation of the test results. Close contact with the wound, ostomy, and continence nurses provides valuable insight into the patient's fluid, electrolyte, and substrate requirements as well as progress with wound healing and management of gastrointestinal outputs. Lastly, a working relationship with rehabilitation therapies including speech pathology, physical therapy, and occupational therapy may enhance understanding of the patient's functional limitations and goals. Based on the patient's specific needs, nutritional therapies may be modified accordingly to improve patient tolerance, intake, and convenience.

The multidisciplinary structure of a nutrition support team is an ideal means of providing nutrition education. Specifically in the ICU setting, nutrition education can be focused on the unique nutritional and metabolic demands of the critically ill patient. Medical, pharmacy, and dietitian students, residents, and fellows may accompany the nutrition support team during ICU rounds in order to observe the expertise offered by each discipline of the team in patient assessment, monitoring, and formulation of specialized nutrition regimens. Observation of the team's interaction with other services and therapies helps to illustrate the importance of good communication among all pertinent healthcare providers to promote optimal patient management. Likewise, participation in nutrition support team rounds allows students the opportunity to gain valuable skills in clinical decision making. Formal lectures and in-services serve as additional methods to inform students, ancillary staff, and house staff on recent advances in clinical nutrition practice and research.

In our institution, a Nutrition Support Committee determines the specific functions and activities of the nutrition support team in the ICU and other units in the hospital. This committee is directed by the NST physicians and consists of representatives from Nursing, Food and Nutrition Services, Pharmacy, Critical Care, Infection Control, Medicine, and Surgery, in addition to the core members of the NST. The committee institutes the enteral formulary and evaluates the efficacy and cost of new enteral products. It also helps to establish parenteral formulary and ordering guidelines. Additionally, the committee is responsible for setting nutrition support policies and procedures, based upon the rules and regulations of the institution.[16]

Research

The ICU is an opportune setting to conduct clinical nutrition research. The complexity of the critically ill patient and the paucity of data on the nutritional and metabolic requirements during this period render this a desirable population to study. Patients in the ICU are frequently sedated, which promotes easier placement of post-pyloric feeding tubes when experimental enteral therapies are being investigated. They typically have central venous lines, which allow easy access for blood work and administration of PN or IV therapies required for the study protocol. The continuous monitoring that ICU patients receive may also provide pertinent data in following the patient's response to research treatments. A good working relationship of the NST with nursing, critical care medicine, and house staff aids in the identification of ideal study candidates and helps to facilitate proper administration of study protocol. Determination of research activities and protocol may be based upon input derived by each discipline of the NST. The team members may share in the responsibility of data collection and completion of patient consent forms. Involvement with clinical research also serves as an important means of education for the team on the recent advances and treatment modalities with respect to nutrition support.

Efficacy of the NST

The presence of a multidisciplinary NST has been shown to promote positive outcomes with regard to patient care and hospital costs. However, none of these studies, to our knowledge, have specifically addressed the efficacy of an NST in ICU patients. A study by Fisher and Opper revealed a dramatic reduction in PN-associated metabolic abnormalities and the provision of estimated nutritional requirements in a higher percentage of patients when a mandatory NST consult was obtained.[17] Trujillo et al. observed a significant decrease in the incidence of PN-related metabolic complications and the appropriateness of PN use when ordered by the NST versus the primary physician team.[18] PN was determined to be "indicated," "not indicated," or "preventable" based upon the ASPEN guidelines. Of the 209 parenteral nutrition starts evaluated, 33% were located in the intensive care unit. Patients who were being followed by the NST were found to have fewer metabolic complications (34% vs. 66% of PN days). Likewise, 62% of the PN starts were deemed to be indicated, as compared to 82% when an NST consult was obtained. The avoidable charges incurred due to the cost per day of PN that was "not indicated" or "preventable" were discovered to be significantly lower when the NST had been consulted. This translated into a substantial costs savings of one-half million dollars per year to the institution.[18] Hickey et al. investigated the effectiveness of an educational protocol and the services of a nutrition support consult service. Results revealed a decrease in the incidence of adverse events, a trend toward more appropriate use of PN, and reduced hospital length of stay.[19] To the contrary, ChrisAnderson et al., in a study of both ICU and non-ICU patients, found that an automatic consult with the nutrition support consultation service prior to the initiation of PN resulted in only a marginal effect on metabolic complications and costs of PN.[20] The researchers attributed these results to the nutrition support service's aggressive teaching efforts to the attending physicians and house staff on PN management and nutrition practice guidelines. The implementation of standard PN ordering forms was also thought to have played a role. It was further hypothesized that the results may have been more favorable had the NST been responsible for writing PN orders versus solely providing recommendations.[20]

Other studies have failed to show differences in metabolic complications with the services of an NST.[21,22] These negative results may be attributed to the use by prescribing physicians of standard PN ordering forms, which include routine monitoring guidelines (thus decreasing the potential for error) and/or to small study population size. Dalton et al. examined the effect of increased involvement of a consultative nutrition support service with respect to patient monitoring and verification of adherence to PN infection control guidelines on patient outcome.[23] The study revealed a significant reduction in metabolic complications, a decreased incidence of mechanical abnormalities, and no significant differences in the incidence of documented sepsis. The researchers noted however, that when compared to institutions in which the nutrition support team had complete control of PN management and order-writing privileges, there was still an excessive incidence of PN-related abnormalities.[23] Similarly, Gales and Riley demonstrated that patients who were managed by a multidisciplinary nutrition support team had a tendency to experience less metabolic abnormalities and were more likely to receive an adequate energy and protein intake.[24] These findings however, may have been more significant had the NST assumed a more active role, as only 52% of the team's recommendations were completely followed by the prescribing physician. It appears that the ability of a consultative-based NST to reduce the incidence of PN-associated metabolic and electrolyte abnormalities may be primarily related to the application of standardized PN solutions and ordering forms and increased clinical monitoring. It may be inferred that in order to optimize patient care and to minimize PN-related complications, it is important for institutions to develop a multidisciplinary NSS to assume the primary responsibility of managing PN patients rather than providing only a nutrition support consult service. These findings may be extrapolated to the critically ill, intensive care unit patient population, in which metabolic aberrations may be more prevalent. Nutrition support management by a trained interdisciplinary team is vital in this setting.

The impact of NST management of patients receiving enteral nutritional support as compared with the sole management by the primary physician is not well documented. Powers et al. demonstrated a decreased incidence of pulmonary, mechanical, metabolic, and gastrointestinal abnormalities in enterally fed NST patients versus their counterparts.[25] Likewise, Brown et al. found that patients who were followed by the NST were monitored more closely, suffered from fewer enteral nutrition (EN) related complications per day, had fewer untreated metabolic aberrations, and were more likely to receive minimal caloric goals of 1.2 × BEE in total calories.[26] In both studies, there were more frequent alterations in the EN solutions made in the NST group,[24,25] which suggests that the nutritional regimens were adjusted to accommodate the patient's specific needs or tolerance. Recent findings by Woodcock et al. revealed a higher overall mortality and increased incidence of inadequate nutritional intake in enterally fed vs. parenterally fed patients.[27] This appears to further support the need for an interdisciplinary nutrition team in the management of patients receiving enteral nutrition. Sufficient monitoring of tolerance and administration of EN regimens is vital to help reduce the incidence of complications and to ensure that nutritional requirements are met. Studies pertaining to the cost effectiveness of EN when the services of an NST are utilized remain indicated.

As a result of cuts in Medicare and health management organization (HMO) reimbursement, hospitals have made vigorous efforts to reduce costs. Labor expenditures account for the highest percentage of hospital costs. Nutrition support teams, which are labor intensive and typically non-revenue producing, have therefore suffered from these cost-cutting measures, as reflected by a reduction in team members or the elimination of entire teams. Goldstein et al. examined the effect on clinical and financial outcomes with the presence, the loss, and the subsequent reinstatement of a nutrition support nurse (NSN) position.[28] The study revealed an increased incidence in catheter-related sepsis, increased inappropriate TPN use and wastage, and a rise in hospital costs when the NSN position was vacant. The authors concluded that the cumulative financial losses and losses incurred due to diminished patient care far exceeded any cost savings derived from a reduction in labor expenditures.[28] Earlier studies have reported cost savings to the patient and the institution, which resulted from heightened NST involvement and the addition of a nutrition support pharmacist position.[29] Faubion et al. demonstrated a noticeable reduction in the incidence of central venous catheter (CVC) related sepsis due to an NST's use of protocols, staff training, and proper supervision.[30] This led to a substantial cost savings that likely exceeded the expenses required to staff and support the NST, dependent upon the cost allocated per episode of sepsis.[30] Cost savings produced from improvement with nutritional status or reductions in metabolic abnormalities are much more difficult to quantify. Documentation of cost savings should therefore be focused on measurable outcomes such as reduced hospital or ICU length of stay and hospital costs.

In order to survive in this era of healthcare reform, NSTs must be proactive and demonstrate their value added to the institution. It is vital that teams remain aware of evolving consumer trends and adapt to the needs of the institution. In addition to the traditional role of the NST, many teams have expanded their scope of services to include outpatient management, community nutrition education programs, and nutrition screening for inpatients. Ongoing data collection and documentation to demonstrate the effectiveness of the NST and its value to the institution is imperative. Outcome studies may be useful to illustrate cost savings, decreased length of stay, and improved quality of patient care. Teams that can document cost savings or revenue generated from team protocols or services in excess of the NST's administrative costs have a greater chance for longevity. It is also important that individual team members maintain good interdepartmental relations in order to avoid turf conflicts or resentment. Likewise, the NST may be faced with the challenge of differing philosophies with the primary physician in the approach to patient care. A tactful approach to potential conflicts and a thorough review of the rationale behind the suggested therapies is advised. Overall, remaining visible and maintaining healthy working relationships with colleagues, administrators, and physicians may help the team to achieve continued support.[7,31]

Given the importance of proper administration and close monitoring of specialized nutrition support regimens, many institutions have established multidisciplinary NSTs. However, relatively limited data on efficacy of NSTs specifically in ICU settings are available in the literature. Of interest, recent data demonstrate that very tight blood glucose control (103 ± 19 mg/dL) in ICU patients markedly decreases morbidity and mortality vs. patients with only modestly higher blood glucose values (153 ± 33 mg/dL).[32] Thus, proper administration of specialized nutrition support in ICU patients by an NST may dramatically decrease overfeeding, nutrition support related hyperglycemia, and related morbidity and mortality. Studies to test the hypothesis that the presence of an active NST reduces hyperglycemia in ICU patients receiving PN and/or tube feedings are indicated.

Review of the literature demonstrates that an NST may be cost effective, reduce complications associated with specialized nutrition support, and subsequently improve quality of patient care. It is important, however, to use caution when interpreting the data and comparing studies. There appears to be great variation in the diagnosis criteria and correction for metabolic and electrolyte disturbances among studies. Also, the basic nutritional goals of the older studies are much different than today's practice. Furthermore, many studies neglect to incorporate the costs necessary to fund an NST in their evaluation of cost savings. The research also indicates that an NST is most capable of facilitating positive outcomes when the team has direct control over the management of the specialized nutrition support provided. Additional studies are indicated to better ascertain the efficacy of a nutrition support team, specifically in the management of the critically ill patient.

References

1. A.S.P.E.N. Board of Directors. Guidelines for the use of parenteral and enteral nutrition in adult and pediatric patients. *J Parenter Enteral Nutr.* 2002;26:1SA–138SA.
2. Fish J, Chernoff R, Shronts EP, et al. Evolution of the nutrition support team. In: Gottschlich MM, Matarese LE, Shronts EP, eds. *Nutrition Support Dietetics Core Curriculum.* 2nd ed. Silver Spring, MD: The American Society for Parenteral and Enteral Nutrition; 1993:1–9.
3. Dudrick SJ, Wilmore DW, Vars HM, et al. Long-term total parenteral nutrition with growth, development and positive nitrogen balance. *Surgery.* 1968;64:134–142.

4. Buzby K, Colaizzo-Anas T. Nutrition support team. In: Matarese LE, Gottschlich MM, eds. *Contemporary Nutrition Support Practice: A Clinical Guide*. Philadelphia: WB Saunders; 1998:3–14.
5. Nehme AE. Nutritional support of the hospitalized patient: the team concept. *JAMA*. 1980;243:1906–1908.
6. Care of patients. Standards and intent statements for nutrition care. In: *The Joint Commission 2000 Hospital Accreditation Standards*. Oakbrook, IL: The Joint Commission on Accreditation of Healthcare Organizations; 2000:116–118.
7. Martin AL. The nutrition support team: survey and thriving in an era of reform. *Nutr Clin Prac*. 1994;9:226–232.
8. Mueller C, Shronts EP. The role of the registered dietitian in enteral and parenteral nutrition support—position of ADA. *J Am Diet Assoc*. 1997;97:302–304.
9. Fuhrman MP, Winkler M, Biesemeier C. The American Society for Parenteral and Enteral Nutrition (A.S.P.E.N.) standards of practice for nutrition support dietitians. *JADA*. 2001;101:825–830.
10. McGinnis TJ. Safety alert: hazards of precipitation associated with parenteral nutrition. *Am J Hosp Pharm*. 1994;51: 1427–1428.
11. Trissel LA. Everything in a compatibility study is important. *Am J Health Syst Pharm*. 1996;53:2990.
12. A.S.P.E.N. Standards of practice: nutrition support nurse. *Nutr Clin Prac*. 1996;11:127–134.
13. Griffith DP, McNally TA, Battey CH, et al. Efficacy of IV erythromycin for small intestinal feeding tube placement in the ICU: a double-blind, randomized, placebo controlled study. *J Parenter Enteral Nutr*. 1997;21:S3.
14. Taylor B, Schallon L. Bedside small bowel feeding tube placement in critically ill patients utilizing a dietitian/nurse team approach. *Nutr Clin Prac*. 2001;16:258–262.
15. Griffith DP, McNally T, Battey CH, et al. Intravenous erythromycin facilitates post-pyloric feeding tube placement in critically ill patients: A double-blind, randomized, placebo-controlled study. *Crit Care Med*. 2002 (in press).
16. Emory University Hospital Policy and Procedure Manual, revised May 2001.
17. Fisher GG, Opper FH. An interdisciplinary nutrition support team improves quality of care in a teaching hospital. *JADA*. 1996;96:176–178.
18. Trujillo EB, Young LS, Chertow GM, et al. Metabolic and monetary costs of avoidable parenteral nutrition use. *J Parenter Enteral Nutr*. 1999;23:109–113.
19. Hickey MM, Munyer TO, Salem RB, et al. Parenteral nutrition utilization: evaluation of an educational protocol and consult service. *J Parenter Enteral Nutr*. 1979;3:433–437.
20. ChrisAnderson D, Heimburger DC, Morgan SL, et al. Metabolic complications of total parenteral nutrition: effects of a nutrition support service. *J Parenter Enteral Nutr*. 1996;20:206–210.
21. Traeger SM, Williams GB, Milliren G, et al. Total parenteral nutrition by a nutrition support team: improved quality of care. *J Parent Enteral Nutr*. 1986;10:408–412.
22. Jacobs DO, Melnik G, Forlaw L, et al. Impact of a nutritional support service on VA surgical patients. *J Am Coll Nutr*. 1984;3:311–315.
23. Dalton MJ, Scheper G, Gee JP, et al. Consultative total parenteral nutrition teams: the effect on the incidence of total parenteral nutrition-related complications. *J Parenter Enteral Nutr*. 1984;8:146–152.
24. Gales BJ, Riley DG. Improved total parenteral nutrition therapy management by a nutritional support team. *Hosp Pharm*. 1994;29:469–475.
25. Powers DA, Brown RO, Cowan GS, et al. Nutritional support team vs. nonteam management of enteral nutritional support in a Veterans Administration medical center teaching hospital. *J Parenter Enteral Nutr*. 1986;10:635–638.
26. Brown RO, Carlson SD, Cowan GSM, et al. Enteral nutritional support management in a university teaching hospital: team vs. nonteam. *J Parenter Enteral Nutr*. 1987;11: 52–56.
27. Woodcock NP, Ziegler D, Palmer D, et al. Enteral versus parenteral nutrition: a pragmatic study. *Nutrition*. 2001;17: 1–11.
28. Goldstein M, Braitman LE, Levine GM. The medical and financial costs associated with termination of a nutrition support nurse. *J Parenter Enteral Nutr*. 2000;24:323–327.
29. Mutchie KD, Smith KA, Mackay MW, et al. Pharmacist monitoring of parenteral nutrition: clinical and cost effectiveness. *Am J Hosp Pharm*. 1979;36:785–787.
30. Faubion NC, Wesley JR, Khalidi N. TPN catheter sepsis: impact of the team approach. *J Parenter Enteral Nutr*. 1986;10:642–645.
31. Wesley JR. Nutrition support teams: past, present, and future. *Nutr Clin Prac*. 1995;10:219–227.
32. Van Den Berghe G, Wouters P, Weekers F, et al. Intensive insulin therapy in critically ill patients. *N Engl J Med*. 2001; 345:1359–1367.

Index

A

Abdominal trauma, 120–122, 140
Absorption interactions, 161–168
  feeding tube position and, 161
  presystemic binding/complexation, 166
  presystemic metabolism, 161–162
  presystemic transport, 162–166
  preventing incompatibilities, 166–168
Acetate, 108
Acetazolamide, 108
Acid-base abnormalities, 101–109, 206
Acidosis, 102, 103, 104–108
Acquired immunodeficiency syndrome (AIDS), 3, 6, 54, 339
Acute pancreatitis, 269–277
  acute phase response in, 370
  case study, 275–276
  identifying, 273–274
  jejunal feeding in, 270–271, 274, 275
  maintaining gut integrity, 271–273
  monitoring nutrition in, 274–275
  nutritional support, 123–124, 270, 273–275
  pancreatic rest for, 269–270
  probiotic flora reduced in, 384
Acute phase response
  described, 14, 51, 348–349
  modulation of, 369, 370, 377
  neuroendocrine regulation of, 386
  in parenteral vs. enteral nutrition, 126–127
  predisposition for, 192, 384–385
  protein malnutrition and, 192
Acute renal failure, 209–217
  causes of, 209–210
  dialytic therapy, 210–212
  enteral feeding formula for, 234
  low urine output from, 83
  malnutrition in, 6, 212
  nutritional support, 214–215
  nutrition assessment, 212–214
  overfeeding and, 113
  phosphate contraindicated for, 96
  renal replacement, 210–211
  sodium bicarbonate in, 106, 107
  in trauma patients, 239–240
Acute respiratory distress syndrome, 190–191
Adipose tissue, 14, 329–330
Advanced Cardiac Life Support guidelines, 107
AIDS (acquired immunodeficiency syndrome), 3, 6, 54, 339
Albumin
  immune enhancing diets and, 362
  in nutrition assessment, 26–27, 28, 176, 177, 212, 262
Aldosterone, 86
Algal fibers, 383
Alkalosis, 103, 104, 105, 107, 108–109
Aluminum, excess in children, 321
Alveolar hypoventilation, 104
American Academy of Pediatrics, 291
American Dietetic Association, 409
American Medical Association (AMA), 52, 56, 62
American Society for Parenteral and Enteral Nutrition (ASPEN), 47, 187, 233, 409
Amino acids. *See also* Arginine; Glutamine
  branched-chain formulas, 40, 202
  overfeeding, 113
  in parenteral nutrition, 40–41, 204
  in protein metabolism, 349–350
  in renal failure, 214
Anabolic agents, 347–356
  anabolic steroids, 351
  growth hormones, 241, 252, 351–354
  inflammatory responses, 348–349
  insulin, 351
  metabolic responses, 347–348
  nutritional modulation of, 349–351
  testosterone, 252–253, 351
Anabolic compounds, 241
Anthropometric measurements, 3, 25, 225, 312
Antibiotics
  feeding solutions and, 154
  food's effect on, 170
  infections and, 135, 366
  macrophage function reduced by, 387
  probiotic bacteria and, 281, 368, 383, 386, 395
  vitamin K deficiencies from, 55
Antioxidants
  in acute phase response, 51, 250
  in enteral nutrition, 368–369
  micronutrients as, 73
  pectin as, 382
Antiseptic skin preparation, 132
Apoptosis of cells, 349, 381, 387
Apovian, Caroline, 175–185
Arginine
  for burn trauma, 251–252
  foods rich in, 376
  in immune enhancing formulas, 231–232
  for intestinal diseases, 280
  in neutraceuticals, 358–359
  in protein metabolism, 350
Arnold, William, 139–151
Arterial blood gas, 102
Ascites, 22
ASPEN (American Society for Parenteral and Enteral Nutrition), 47, 187, 233
Azotemia, 83, 113

B

Barbiturates, 260
Basal metabolic rate, 31, 312–314
Beindorff, Mary Ellen, 341–346
Bell, David, 153–173
Bengmark, Stig, 265–380, 381–399
Bergman, Glen, 407–416
Beriberi heart disease, 224
Beta carotene, 54
Betaglucans, 382–383
Bhatia, Jatinder, 297–309
Bicarbonate buffers, 101
Binkley, Jeff, 111–118
Bioelectrical impedance analysis, 5, 25, 241
Biphosphonates, 95
Bistrian, Bruce, 39–49
Blood work, monitoring, 28, 29
Body fat, assessing, 22
Body mass index, 3, 25, 288–289, 326
Body water. *See also* Electrolytes; Fluids
  distribution, 80
  edema, 3, 17, 177
  monitoring hydration, 24
  as percentage of body weight, 79
  respiratory illness and, 5
Body weight. *See also* Lean body mass; Obese patients; Weight loss
  assessing, 24–25, 202, 212
  body mass index, 3, 25, 288–289, 326
  of children, 312
  in energy expenditure assessment, 34–35
  feeding weight, 45–46, 47
  fluid needs and, 82
  gain during pregnancy, 288–289
  ideal body weight, 25, 202
  in macronutrient assessment, 45–46
  in malnutrition assessment, 2, 3, 25, 177
  obesity assessed with, 325–326, 330
  refeeding syndrome and, 113, 114
Brain injuries, 260–262. *See also* Head injuries
Burns, David, 199–208

Burn trauma, 245–257
assessment and evaluation, 246–247
growth hormones for, 353–354
macronutrients for, 247–248
melatonin for, 253
metabolic and physiologic responses in, 245–246
micronutrients for, 249–252
molybdenum for, 253
nutritional support, 248–252, 372–373
pharmacokinetics in, 246
renal function in, 246
testosterone analogs for, 252–253
B vitamins, 64–65, 67, 73, 74

C

Calcium
abnormalities, 93–96, 99, 224, 299
needs during pregnancy, 291
Calories. *See* Energy requirements
Cancer, 359
Carbamazepine, 169
Carbohydrates. *See also* Fiber; Glucose
in burn trauma, 247
in hepatic failure, 202–203
high carbohydrate intake, 5
metabolism, 15–16, 350
monitoring, 28, 29
overfeeding, 111, 112
in parenteral nutrition, 41–42
in respiratory failure, 5, 192
Cardiac disease, 219–228
acute myocardial infarction, 219–221
cardiac arrest, 107
cardiac cachexia, 222–223
cardiopulmonary resuscitation, 106–107
congestive heart failure, 220, 221–222, 226
electrolyte/metabolic abnormalities in, 223–224
nutrient problems in, 343
nutritional support, 225, 226
nutrition needs in, 344
prevalence of, 219–220
refeeding complications in, 225–226
unstable angina, 219
Carlson, Chris, 335–340
Carnitine, 214
Catabolism
assessing, 26
described, 347
hypercatabolism in burn trauma, 245–246
loss of lean body mass during, 348, 349
nutritional modulation of, 349–351
nutrition support and, 27, 210
testosterone analogs for, 252–253
Catheterization
antibiotic-impregnated catheters, 135
catheter occlusion, 136
catheter related infections, 134–135, 240, 298
central venous catheterization, 131–132, 134, 135, 331–332
femoral venous catheterization, 134, 135–136
tunneled catheters, 132, 134
Centers for Disease Control, 135
Central venous catheterization, 131–132, 134, 135, 331–332
Cerebrospinal fluid, 260
Charney, David, 209–217
Charney, Pamela, 209–217
Chemotherapy, 359
Children. *See* Pediatric patients
Chloride, 100
Chromium, 73, 251
Chronic obstructive pulmonary disease, 4–5, 189–190, 191
Cisapride, 140
Cohen, Mylan, 219–228
Colitis, 391
Commensal flora, 368, 384
Continuous venous-venous hemodialysis, 239
Copper, 23, 54, 57–58, 68, 292
Corticosteroids, 168
Cortisol, 350
Cost. *See* Financial issues
Creatinine height index, 25
Cresci, Gail, 21–30, 259–267, 287–296
Cytokines
described, 13
in disease outcome, 370–371
interleukin-11, 253
in nutritional assessment, 176
probiotics and, 388–389
in the stress response, 13–14, 348, 369, 385
tumor necrosis factor as, 13, 14, 222

D

Daignault, Nicole, 407–416
Deal, Leonard, 187–197
DeLegge, Mark, 139–151
Deppe, Scott, 245–257
Dextrose, 45, 85, 177, 178, 298
Diabetes, 175–185. *See also* Hyperglycemia; Insulin
acute myocardial infarction and, 220
avoiding hypoglycemia, 179–180
case studies, 170–171, 183–184
comorbid disease assessment and, 237
glucose infusion rate for, 42
glycemic control in, 178–179
with hepatic failure, 204–206
insulin for, 179, 180, 181–183, 204–206, 238
with myocardial infarction, 181–182
nutritional assessment, 176–178
nutritional support, 178, 180, 181
physiology of, 175–176
sepsis in, 125
with stroke, 182
Diabetic ketoacidosis, 105–106
Dialysis, 75, 106, 210–212, 239
Diarrhea, 390–391
Dietary Reference Intake, 52, 56, 316, 317
Dobbhoff tubes, 140
Driscoll, David, 39–49, 219–228
Drug-nutrient interactions, 153–173. *See also* Absorption interactions; Drugs
case study, 170–171
elimination/clearance altered by, 169–170
ex vivo biopharmaceutical inactivations, 154
fed vs. fasted state and, 168
interaction pairs, 168
in nutrition support, 154–160, 166–169
populations at risk, 154
for valproic acid, 168–169
Drugs. *See also* Drug-nutrient interactions
enteral nutrition incompatibilities, 156–157, 160
gastrointestinal secretions reduced by, 374
immunosuppression drugs, 341–342
liquid medications, 163–165
renal clearance of, 169, 170
selection and administration, 160
slow-release capsules, 167
which should not be crushed, 158–159, 162, 167
xerogenic, 374
Dryden, Gerald, 269–277
Dyes, 162

E

Edema, 3, 17, 177
Einstein, Albert, 265
Electrolytes, 85–100. *See also* Potassium
abnormalities in intestinal disease, 281
assessing requirements for, 17, 24, 28
calcium abnormalities, 93–96, 99, 224, 299
chloride abnormalities, 100
distribution in the body, 80
diuretics effect on, 169–170
fluid loss and, 81–82
magnesium abnormalities, 98–99, 113, 223–224

measuring, 85–86
monitoring, 17, 28, 29
normal concentrations of, 86
for organ transplant patients, 345
phosphorus abnormalities, 96–98
in renal failure, 214
sodium, 86–89, 94, 106–108
Endoscopic tube placement
for guiding feeding tubes, 141
in obese patients, 332
percutaneous endoscopic gastrostomy, 143–144, 263–264, 280, 293, 337
Energy expenditure. *See also* Hypermetabolism
components, 31–32
energy equations for, 33–34
energy requirements vs., 35, 36
measuring, 32–34
in obesity, 34–35
resting energy expenditure, 2, 112, 191, 312–314
Energy requirements, 31–37. *See also* Energy expenditure
assessing, 27–28, 35, 112, 177–178, 349
basal energy requirements, 31, 312–314
energy expenditure vs., 35, 36
in hepatic failure, 202
hypocaloric feeding and, 35
nutrition support goals for, 35
for parenteral nutrition, 45–46
in pediatric patients, 312–314
in post-transplant patients, 343
in renal failure, 213
Enteral access, 139–151. *See also* Nasoenteric nutritional access
in brain injured patients, 263–264
in obese patients, 332–333
percutaneous access, 143–146, 263–264, 280, 293, 337
small bowel access, 144, 233, 411–412
surgically placed, 146–149
Enteral nutrition. *See also* Enteral access; Neutraceuticals; Parenteral vs. enteral nutrition; Perioperative enteral nutrition
in burn trauma, 248–249
in cancer patients, 338, 339
cost of, 402–404, 405
disadvantages, 6–7, 252
drug-nutrient interactions and, 154
feeding formulas, 71–72, 232–233, 234–235, 319, 358
feeding protocol, 233–238
formula categories, 215
indications for using, 409
intolerance for, 28–29, 233, 235–237, 252
malnutrition and, 7, 119–120
micronutrients in, 53, 71–72
for nontrauma patients, 122–124
nutrient formulas for, 357
for organ transplant patients, 345–346
parenteral nutrition vs., 139, 230–231, 263, 365–366
pros and cons, 178, 194
for respiratory failure, 194
sepsis reduced with, 124–128, 231, 338
supraphysiologic supplementation, 72–74
for trauma patients, 120–122, 230–231
Enterocutaneous fistula, 279, 280, 282
Erythromycin, 140, 411
Erythropoietin therapy, 74, 305
Essential fatty acid deficiency, 42–43, 203. *See also* Fatty acids
Estrogen, in pregnancy, 288
Eucaloric macronutrient intakes, 46, 47
Expenses. *See* Financial issues
Extracellular fluid, 79–80, 82
Ex vivo biopharmaceutical inactivations, 154–160

F

Fabling, Janet, 153–173
Fasting. *See* Hypocaloric feeding
Fat. *See also* Body fat; Fatty acids; Lipids
for burn trauma patients, 247–248
daily requirements, 16
infusion rates, 43, 44
overfeeding, 45, 112–113
oxidation, 328–329
in respiratory failure, 193
underfeeding and, 328–329
Fat-free mass, 2, 5, 25, 241
Fat-soluble vitamins, 55, 62, 63–64
Fatty acids. *See also* Lipids
deficiencies, 42–43, 203
immunity and, 191, 247–248
intravenous lipid emulsions, 42–43, 44, 387
metabolism, 350
omega-3 fatty acids, 191, 194, 247–248, 360–361
omega-6 fatty acids, 358, 360, 361
oxidation, 16
polyunsaturated, 360
principal fatty acid profiles, 42
saturated, 368, 385
Federal Drug Administration (FDA), 203
Feeding formulas. *See also* Neutraceuticals
for burn trauma, 248
criteria for selecting, 234–235
for enteral nutrition, 71–72, 232–233, 234–235, 319, 358
feeding protocol, 235
high protein formulas, 169, 234
hospital-made vs. industry-made, 368
immune enhancing, 232–233, 234, 248, 386, 404
micronutrients in, 71–72
for pancreatitis, 271
for parenteral nutrition, 47, 71, 72
for pregnant women, 293–294
for premature infants, 298
Feeding weight, 45–46, 47
Femoral venous catheters, 134, 135–136
Fiber
defined, 382
in enteral nutrition, 367–368
for intestinal disease, 280–281
pectin as, 382
as prebiotics, 382–383, 384–385
types of, 382–383
Financial issues, 401–406
of artificial nutrition, 402–404, 405
hospital cost-cutting measures, 414–415
of immunonutrition, 361–362
of malnutrition, 401, 402–403
nutritional support team and, 414
of obesity, 326
Fluids. *See also* Body water; Electrolytes; Urine
abnormalities in, 79–85, 100
assessing requirements for, 17, 24, 28
concentrated TPN solutions, 204
decreased need for, 85
effect on drug and nutrient absorption, 162
extracellur fluid depletion, 82, 83
fluid-overload, 46–47, 85
gains and losses, 81–82
in hepatic failure, 204
increased needs for, 82
maintaining acid balance, 101–102
monitoring, 17, 28, 29
refeeding syndrome and, 113, 114
for transplant patients, 345
volume and electrolyte concentrations, 81–82
Fluoroscopy, 132, 134, 135, 141, 411–412
Folate, 66, 74, 291
Food
effect on drug absorption, 162, 166, 168, 169
effect on urine pH, 170
fruits, 284, 368–369, 382, 383
grapefruit, 161, 166, 167
nitrate-rich, 376
seaweed, 383
vegetables, 368–369, 383, 384

Food and Nutrition Board, 61, 291, 350
Formulas. *See* Feeding formulas
Fosphenytoin, 169
Franga, Dion, 131–137
Friedman, Bruce, 245–257
Fructooligosaccharides, 383
Fruits, 284, 368–369, 382, 383
Fuhrman, M. Patricia, 51–60

G

Gadacz, Thomas, 279–285
Gallium nitrate, 95
Galloway, John, 407–416
Gastrointestinal tract. *See also* Gut; Intestinal diseases
  changes during pregnancy, 288
  colon as microbial organ, 381–382
  effect of starvation on, 367
  enteral access leakage, 148–149
  flora in, 383–384
  fluids in, 81–82
  immune defense secretions, 367, 373–375
  motility and emptying, 262–263
  as part of the immune system, 357, 366
  synbiotics and, 381, 382
Gastroparesis, 144
Glasgow Coma Scale, 122
Glucomannans, 383
Glucose. *See also* Carbohydrates; Diabetes; Hyperglycemia; Hypoglycemia
  in burn trauma, 247
  cardiac disease and, 225
  daily requirements, 15–16
  diabetes and, 175–176, 179
  excessive amounts, 45
  infusion rates, 42
  intolerance, 42, 45, 73, 175, 215
  in obese patients, 327–328
  for parenteral nutrition, 41–42
  refeeding syndrome and, 113, 114
Glutamine
  in burn trauma, 251
  gastrointestinal tract and, 280, 283
  in immune enhancing formulas, 231
  in neutraceuticals, 359–360
  in parenteral nutrition, 40–41, 241
  in processed foods, 368
  in protein metabolism, 349–350
Glutathione, 368–369
Gramlich, Lean, 347–356
Grapefruit, 161, 166, 167
Growth hormones, 241, 252, 351–354
Gut
  gut-associated lymphoid tissue, 126, 127, 357
  gut integrity, 271–273
  gut permeability, 125–126
  immunity and, 347, 385–386
  lactic acid bacteria in, 390
  mucosal immunity in, 127–128

H

Hakmiller, Karl, 219–228
Harris-Benedict Energy Equation, 33, 112, 177, 191, 225
Hassoun, Paul, 1–10
Head injuries
  Glasgow Coma Score, 259
  intracranial pressure, 259, 260
  mortality rate in, 259, 260
  nutritional support, 122, 262–264
  in pediatric patients, 264–265
  prevention of, 260
  severe brain injuries in, 260–262
  statistics, 259
Heart disease. *See* Cardiac disease
Hemodialysis, 75, 106, 239
Hepatic failure, 199–208
  acid/base issues, 206
  causes of, 199
  with diabetes, 204–206
  fluid restricted patients, 204
  hypophosphatemia in, 204, 205
  liver transplants, 200, 202–203
  malnutrition in, 200, 201
  metabolic issues, 204–205
  nutritional support, 199–200, 201
  nutrition requirements for, 202–204
  patient evaluation, 200–201
  specialty formulas for, 200
Hepatic proteins, 3
Hepatic steatosis, 112
Hermann, Virginia, 51–60
HIV/AIDS patients
  nutritional support, 339
  predicting mortality in, 6
  probiotics for, 394
  weight loss in, 3, 6
  zinc and, 54
Howdieshell, Thomas, 287–296
Hydrochloric acid, 108–109
Hyperalimentation, 39, 111
Hypercalcemia, 95–96
Hypercaloric feeding. *See* Overfeeding
Hypercatabolism, 245–246
Hyperemesis gravidarum, 292, 293
Hyperglycemia
  in brain injury, 261
  in burn trauma, 246, 247
  causes of, 111, 112, 124–125, 176, 180
  in children, 312
  chromium supplementation and, 73
  in diabetes, 176, 178, 179, 180
  during hypermetabolic stress, 15
  enteral vs. parenteral feeding and, 124–125
  in trauma patients, 240
Hyperinsulinemia, 183
Hyperkalemia, 92–93, 94, 223, 299
Hypermagnesemia, 99
Hypermetabolism
  body water retention from, 17
  in brain injury, 26
  lipid metabolism and, 16
  nutrient alterations during, 14–15
  in respiratory failure, 192
  in stress responses, 2, 14–15, 189
Hypernatremia, 88–89
Hyperparathyroidism, 95
Hyperphosphatemia, 98, 171
Hypertriglyceridemia, 112
Hyperventilation, 105
Hypervolemia, 46–47, 85
Hypoalbuminemia, 176, 177
Hypocalcemia, 94–95, 99, 224, 299
Hypocaloric feeding. *See also* Starvation
  body energy stores used during, 14
  of children, 312
  drug administration and, 168
  energy expenditure and, 14, 35
  in enteral feeding, 329
  fat oxidation and, 328–329
  fed state vs., 168, 272
  in healthy vs. critically ill persons, 2
  infections decreased with, 241
  in nutritional support, 7, 28
  protein sparing and, 329
Hypoglycemia, 179–180, 202–203, 300
Hypokalemia, 90–92, 113, 223
Hypomagnesemia, 99, 113, 223–224
Hyponatremia, 87–88, 300
Hypophosphatemia
  causes of, 96–97, 113, 114, 224
  in hepatic failure, 204, 205
  refeeding syndrome and, 96–97, 113
  in respiratory failure, 5, 188
  treatment, 97–98

I

Immune enhancing diets. *See* Immunonutrition
Immunity. *See also* Immunonutrition
  fatty acids for, 191, 247–248
  feeding formulas for, 231–233, 234, 248, 358, 386, 404
  feeding the gut and, 347
  gastrointestinal tract and, 271, 357, 366, 385–386
  immunosuppression drugs, 341–342
  impaired, 112–113, 194–195, 372
  lifestyle effects on, 385
  measuring competence of, 26
  mucosal immunity, 127–128
  parenteral nutrition and, 194–195

in preoperative starvation, 372
Immunocompromised diseases, 335–340
cancer, 338
HIV/AIDS, 3, 6, 54, 339
nutrition algorithm for, 335–337
sepsis, 337–338
Immunoglobulin production, 387
Immunonutrition. *See also* Neutraceuticals
in burn trauma, 248
clinical evidence, 361–363
controversy over, 386
cost of, 361–362
enteral nutrition formulas, 358
feeding formulas, 231–233, 234, 248, 358, 386, 404
initiating, 362
for trauma patients, 231–233, 234, 361
Immunosuppression drugs, 341–342
Indirect calorimetry
in burn trauma, 246
in children, 314
circulatory indirect calorimetry, 331
energy expenditure measured with, 32–33
respiratory indirect calorimetry, 191–192, 330, 331
Infants. *See also* Neonatal issues
birth weight, 289, 300
breast feeding, 305–306
of diabetic mothers, 299
energy requirements, 300–301, 313
enteral feeding formulas, 319
neural tube defects in, 291
protein needs, 302
sepsis in, 303
Infection. *See also* Sepsis
antibiotics and, 135, 366
cather-related, 134–135, 240, 298
gastrointestinal secretions and, 375
hypocaloric feeding and, 241
iron and, 75
multiple organ failure from, 229
nutrition and, 264, 357, 361, 362
in postoperative patients, 384
probiotics for, 389
Inflammatory bowel disease, 123, 283
Inflammatory response. *See* Acute phase response; Stress response
Injury Severity Score, 120
Insoluble fibers, 382
Insulin
as anabolic agent, 351
for diabetes, 179, 180, 181–183, 204–206, 238
drip therapy guidelines, 182
insulin resistance, 178
protocol for diabetes, 238
Intestinal diseases, 279–285. *See also* Gastrointestinal tract
enterocutaneous fistula, 279, 280, 282
gut specific substrates, 280–281
inflammatory bowel disease, 123, 283
low blood flow states, 284
macronutrients for, 280–281
nonocclusive bowel necrosis, 240–241
nutritional support, 126–127, 279, 280, 282, 284
short bowel syndrome, 279, 281–282
small bowel access, 144, 233, 411–412
therapy principles, 279–280
Intracellular fluid, 79, 80
Intragastric feeding, 140, 263
Intravenous therapy, 131–137
central venous access, 131–132, 249
complications in, 134–136
intravenous lipid emulsions, 42–43, 44, 387
used in burn trauma, 246
venous cannulation techniques, 133–134
Iodine, 74, 292
Ireton-Jones, Carol, 31–37
Ireton-Jones Equations, 33–34, 191, 330
Iron
anemia, 23, 72–73, 305
in burn trauma, 251
in critical illness, 52–54
deficiency, 69
in erythropoietin therapy, 74
needs during pregnancy, 290, 291
toxicity, 69
vitamin C interaction with, 55
Isoniazid, 169

J

Janeway gastric tube technique, 147
Jejunal feeding, 144–146
nasojejunal tubes, 140, 201, 233
in pancreatitis, 270–271, 274, 275
percutaneous gastrojejunostomy, 144–145, 337
in perioperative enteral nutrition, 372–373
in trauma patients, 240
tube placement, 146, 147–148
Jensen, Gordon, 111–118
Joint Commission on Accreditation of Healthcare Organizations (JCAHO), 153, 408

K

Kayexalate, 93, 94
Kidney disease, 343, 344
Kidney stones, 55
Koutkia, Polyxeni, 175–185
Kozar, Rosemary, 229–244
Kudsk, Kenneth, 119–130
Kutsogiannis, Demetrios, 347–356

L

Lactic acid bacteria, 387–393
apoptosis stimulated by, 387
for colitis, 391
combinations of, 395
in cytokine release, 388–389
for diarrhea, 390–391
in immunoglobulin production, 387
for intensive care patients, 391–392
in lymphocyte functions, 388
in macrophage function, 387
mucin production increased by, 389
in mucosal growth, 390
for multiple organ failure, 392–394
toxins and mutagens eliminated by, 389–390
Western lifestyle and, 384
Lactic acidosis, 105, 106
Lactobacillus bacteria. *See* Lactic acid bacteria
Laparoscopic surgery, 333
Lean body mass
body weight and, 24
increased with anabolic steroids, 351
loss of, 348, 349, 357
in obese patients, 330
Lee, Mark, 259–267
Levodopa, 169
Linoleic acid, 360
Lipids. *See also* Fatty acids
acute myocardial infarction and, 220
in burn trauma, 247
in hepatic failure, 203–204
intravenous lipid emulsions, 42–43, 44, 387
lipid-based medication, 17, 73, 260
metabolism of, 16–17, 350
monitoring, 28, 29
for obese patients, 328
in parenteral nutrition, 42–43
requirement for, 177–178
in respiratory failure, 193
Liver disease. *See also* Hepatic failure
comorbid disease assessment and, 237
nutrient problems in, 343
nutrition needs in, 344
risk of sepsis in, 121
Loop diuretics, 94, 95, 169–170
Lowell, Jeffrey, 341–346
Lukan, James, 269–277
Lymphocyte functions, 388

M

Macronutrients. *See also* Carbohydrates; Fat; Lipids; Protein
for burn trauma, 247–248
determining requirements for, 45–47
micronutrients and, 52, 61
overfeeding hazards and, 111–113
for parenteral nutrition, 40–43, 45–57
for respiratory failure, 192–193
Macrophage functions, 387
Magnesium, 98–99, 113, 223–224
Malnutrition. *See also* Nutrition assessment
in AIDS patients, 6, 339
in cancer patients, 338
cost of, 401, 402–403
defined, 1, 2, 407
during hospitalization, 401, 404, 407
during pregnancy, 289–290, 292
enteral vs. parenteral feeding and, 119–120
in hepatic failure, 199
identifying, 1–4, 21, 25, 177, 225
in nutritional support, 6–7
in obesity, 6
in postoperative patients, 6
protein energy malnutrition, 1, 4, 229
refeeding syndrome and, 113–114, 115
in renal failure, 6, 212
in respiratory failure, 4–5, 187, 188, 189, 190, 191
Malnutrition Cost Survey, 402–403
Manganese, 54, 69
Martindale, Robert, 11–19, 287–296, 357–364
Mason, Joel, 61–77
McCarthy, Mary, 153–173, 187–197
McClave, Stephen, 269–277
McNally, Therese, 407–416
McQuiggan, Margaret, 229–244
Medications. *See* Drugs
Melatonin, 253
Metabolic acidosis, 102, 103, 104, 105–108, 206
Metabolic alkalosis, 103, 104, 107, 108–109, 188
Metabolic response to stress. *See* Stress response
Methotrexate, 169
Metoclopramide, 140
Micronutrients, 51–60. *See also* Drug-nutrient interactions; Electrolytes; Minerals; Trace elements; Vitamins
in acute phase response, 51–52
combinations of, 53
in critical illness, 51, 52–58
in feeding formulas, 71–72
interactions, 52, 54, 55
laboratory measurements, 57
macronutrients vs., 61
for organ transplant patients, 345
requirements for, 52, 61, 62, 72, 291
for respiratory failure, 193–194
single micronutrient supplementation, 53, 58
special considerations, 75–76
supraphysiologic supplementation, 72–74
in trauma patients, 58
Minerals. *See also* Electrolytes; *specific minerals*
deficiencies, 22, 23, 24
for infants and children, 315, 317
recommended requirements, 17, 294
for respiratory failure, 193
Mithramycin, 95
Mogensen, Kris, 1–10, 401–406
Molybdenum, 253
Monoamine oxidase inhibitors, 162, 166
Moore, Frederick, 229–244
Mucosal alterations, 125–126
Mucosal-associated lymphoid tissue, 127, 272
Mucosal immune system, 126–128, 272, 390
Multiple organ dysfunction syndrome, 126
Multiple organ failure, 229, 230, 279, 392–394
Muscle function tests, 3–4
Muscle groups, 22
Myocardial infarction, 181–182

N

Nasoduodenal tubes, 140
Nasoenteric nutritional access, 139–143
alternate feeding tube technology, 143
contraindications, 139
in immunocompromised patients, 336–337
intraoperative tube placement, 142
post-operative feeding, 140, 141
timing of, 140
tube placement, 139–141, 142, 263
Nasogastric tubes, 140, 280, 293, 305, 336
Nasojejunal tubes, 140, 201, 233
Nasraway, Stanley, 401–406
National Research Council, 312
Naylor, Michael, 11–19, 325–334
Necrotizing enterocolitis, 304
Neonatal issues, 297–309. *See also* Pregnancy
anemia, 305
breast feeding, 305–306
enteral nutrition, 303–305
intravenous fluid and electrolytes, 298–299
nutritional goals, 300–301
nutrition and developmental outcome, 306
parenteral nutrition, 297–298, 301–303
Neostigmine, 252
Neutraceuticals, 357–364
about, 357–358
arginine, 358–359, 385
clinical evidence on, 361–363
defined, 357
glutamine, 359–360
nucleotides, 360
omega-3 fatty acids, 360–361
Neutrophil, 126–127
Nishikawa, Reid, 11–19
Nitric oxide, 280, 358, 373, 375–376
Nitrogen, 2, 26, 43, 261
Nitrogen balance, 2, 26, 27, 371
Nonocclusive bowel necrosis, 240–241
Nucleotides, 360
Nutrient formulas. *See* Neutraceuticals
Nutritional support. *See also* Enteral nutrition; Nutrition support team; Parenteral nutrition
comorbid disease assessment in, 237–238
determining energy requirements and, 31, 35–36
goals, 17–18, 27, 35, 111
high carbohydrate intake, 5
inadequate delivery, 6–7, 41
monitoring, 5, 28–29, 56
for organ transplant patients, 345–346
protein catabolism and, 15
Nutrition assessment, 21–30
biochemical measurements, 26–27
body composition measurements, 24–26
in cardiac disease, 225
case study, 29
clinical assessment, 21–22
energy and protein requirements, 27–28
fluid requirements, 24, 28
identifying malnutrition, 21
monitoring nutritional support, 5, 28–29, 56
nutrition screening criteria, 22
physical examination for, 22–24
of pre-transplant patients, 342–343
weight loss and, 177
Nutrition support team, 407–416
about, 407–408
certification, 408
dietitian's role, 408–410
efficacy of, 407–408, 413–415
nurse's role, 411

nutrition research by, 413
pharmacist's role, 410–411
physician's role, 408
postpyloric feeding tube placement by, 411–412
responsibilities, 170, 408, 412–413

O

Obese patients, 325–334. *See also* Overfeeding
comorbidities, 326–327
defined, 3, 325–326
with diabetes, 177
energy expenditure in, 34–35
estimating caloric requirements, 329–331
with hepatic failure, 202
hypocaloric feeding for, 35, 241, 328–330, 331
malnutrition in, 6
nutrition access issues, 331–333
nutritional support hazards, 327–328
prevalence of, 326
protein requirements, 202
as trauma patients, 237–238
Olson, Diane, 311–323
Omega-3 fatty acids, 191, 194, 247–248, 360–361
Omega-6 fatty acids, 358, 360, 361
Onithine supplementation, 251–252
Oral naloxone, 252
Organs
multiple organ dysfunction syndrome, 126
multiple organ failure, 229, 230, 279, 392–394
sepsis in, 121
Organ transplants, 341–346. *See also* Surgery
complications, 384
enteral vs. parenteral feeding in, 124, 345, 376
immunosuppression drugs for, 341–342
indications/contraindications, 341
monitoring and follow-up, 345–346
nutritional support, 124, 345, 346
post-transplant phase, 343, 345
pre-transplant phase, 342–343
rejection rate, 376
waiting lists, 341
Orlistat, 162
Overfeeding, 111–118
case presentation, 115–117
in children, 312
diabetes and, 177
hyperglycemia caused by, 111, 112, 124–125
of macronutrients, 111–113, 371
in parenteral nutrition, 39, 45
prevention of, 111, 114
refeeding syndrome and, 96–97, 113–114, 115
in respiratory failure, 104, 112, 189
risks, 45, 371
Overnutrition. *See* Overfeeding
Oxandrolone, 241, 252, 351

P

Pancreatitis. *See* Acute Pancreatitis
Parathyroid hormone, 93
Parenteral nutrition, 39–49. *See also* Parenteral vs. enteral nutrition; Total parenteral nutrition
ASPEN guidelines for, 47
in burn trauma, 248, 249
in cancer patients, 338
complications, 194–195, 303
drug-nutrient interactions and, 154–156
enteral nutrition vs., 139, 230–231, 263, 365–366
feeding formulas, 47, 71, 72
indications for using, 409
intravenous access, 131–136, 249
macronutrients for, 40–43, 45–47
malnutrition and, 119–120
micronutrients for, 52, 53, 56, 62, 71
for nontrauma patients, 122–124
overfeeding in, 39, 45
sepsis in, 124–128
supraphysiologic supplementation, 72–74
for trauma patients, 120–122
undernutrition in, 43–44
Parenteral vs. enteral nutrition, 119–130
impact on clinical outcome, 119–120
in nontrauma patients, 122–124
septic complications in, 124–128, 366
for surgery patients, 365–366, 371–372
in trauma patients, 120–122
Parish, Anjali, 297–309
Pectin, 382
Pediatric patients, 311–323
basal metabolic rate, 312–314
case study, 321–322
energy requirements, 312–314
head injuries in, 264–265
height and weight measurements, 312
hyperglycemia in, 312
neurologic impairment in, 321
nutritional assessment, 311–312
nutritional support, 124, 315, 318–321
nutrition requirements, 71, 312–315
preoperative starvation, 372
Percutaneous endoscopic gastrostomy, 143–146, 263–264, 280, 293, 337
Percutaneous gastrojejunostomy, 144–145, 337
Perioperative enteral nutrition, 365–380
acute phase response in, 369, 370
antioxidants in, 368–369
calorie needs, 371
cytokine response in, 370–371
early feeding for, 366–367
gastrointestinal secretions in, 373–375
immune control in, 371–372
immunonutrition, 367–368, 377
jejunal feeding, 372–373
nitric oxide in, 375–376
nitrogen balance and, 371
organ rejection and, 376–377
starvation in, 367, 372
therapeutic window for, 366, 369–370
pH. *See also* Acidosis; Alkalosis
acid-base abnormalities and, 101, 102, 103
assessing, 102, 103
defined, 101
of gastrointestinal secretions, 375
of the stomach, 382
of urine, 169, 170
Pharmaceuticals. *See* Drugs
Pharmacokinetics, 246
Phenytoin, 162, 169
Phosphorus, 98, 171. *See also* Hypophosphatemia
Physical examinations, for nutrition assessment, 22–24
Physiologic functions, 13, 14
Physiologic State Classification system, 13
Pipkin, Walter, 279–285
Polyunsaturated fatty acids, 360
Pomposelli, James, 199–208
Postoperative patients, 6, 21, 22, 140, 384
Postpyloric feeding tube placement, 411–412
Potassium, 89–93, 94, 113, 223, 299
Potassium chloride, 108
Prebiotics, 381, 382–383
Pregnancy, 287–296. *See also* Neonatal issues
anatomic and physiologic changes, 287–288
hormonal changes, 288
maternal weight gain, 288–289
metabolic changes, 288
nutrient requirements, 290–292
nutritional assessment, 290, 293
nutritional support during, 292–294
placental transfer of nutrients, 289–290

Probiotics. *See also* Lactic acid bacteria; Prebiotics
- about, 383–384
- antibiotics and, 281, 383, 386
- effects of, 390
- for intestinal disease, 281, 283
- in pancreatitis, 384
- postoperative morbidity and, 384
- superinflamation and, 384–385
- synbiotics and, 381, 382
- for transplant patients, 376

Progesterone, 288
Prognostic Nutritional Index, 201
Prokinetic therapy, 264
Propofol, 17, 73, 260
Propranolol, 95
Prospective randomized controlled trials, 230–233
Protein
- assessing requirements for, 27–28, 202
- for burn trauma patients, 247, 248
- for cardiac patients, 225
- deficiency, 23, 24
- in diabetes, 177
- drug-nutrient interactions, 169
- excessive intake, 45, 349
- guidelines, 28
- for hepatic failure, 202
- high protein diet, 169, 234, 248
- loss during critical illness, 14, 15, 348, 349
- metabolism, 349–350
- in parenteral nutrition, 40–41
- for post-transplant patients, 344, 345
- for pregnancy, 291
- protein energy malnutrition, 1, 4, 229
- protein sparing, 328, 329
- for renal failure, 213
- requirements, 25, 28–29, 202
- for respiratory, 192
- serum protein, 26–27, 28, 176–177, 212, 262
- storage, 14, 22
- underfeeding and, 35

Proton pump inhibitors, 162
Pulmonary cachexia syndrome, 4
Pulmonary ventilation changes, 101

R

Radiographic techniques, 132, 134, 135
Reactive oxygen species, 51, 52
Recommended Dietary Allowance (RDA)
- for folate, 291
- for healthy persons, 61, 202
- for micronutrients, 52, 56, 72, 291
- for pregnancy, 294
- for protein, 202
- for vitamins, 350

Refeeding syndrome
- body weight and, 113, 114
- in cardiac disease, 225–226
- hypophosphatemia and, 96–97, 113
- malnutrition and, 113–114, 115
- overfeeding and, 96–97, 113–114, 115
- in trauma patients, 240

Renal failure. *See* Acute renal failure
Resistant starch, 383
Respiratory acidosis, 103, 104–105
Respiratory alkalosis, 103, 105
Respiratory failure, 187–197
- acute respiratory distress syndrome, 190–191
- acute respiratory failure, 188–189
- case study, 195–196
- chronic obstructive pulmonary disease, 4–5, 189–190, 191
- energy expenditure in, 191–192
- malnutrition and, 4–5, 187, 188, 189, 190, 191
- nutritional support, 187–188, 189, 190–191, 192–195
- overfeeding and, 104, 112, 189
- ventilation requirements, 189

Respiratory quotient, 32, 112
Resting energy expenditure, 2, 112, 191, 312–313
Reticuloendothial system, 112–113

S

Saliva, 373–374
Saltzmann, Edward, 1–10
Schmidt, Hank, 357–364
Schwaitzberg, Steven, 139–151
Schwenk, W. Frederick, 311–323
Seashore formula, 314
Selenium, 52, 224, 250–251
Sepsis
- catheter related, 240, 298
- described, 337–338
- in infants, 303
- neutraceuticals and, 362
- nutrition assessment and, 21–22, 337
- in parenteral vs. enteral nutrition, 124–128, 366
- reducing, 124–128, 231, 338
- risks for, 120, 121

Serosal adhesions, 384, 385
Serum anion gap, 105, 106
Serum osmolality, 80, 86, 87
Serum protein, 26–27, 28, 176–177, 212, 262
Shikora, Scott, 11–19, 325–334
Short bowel syndrome, 279, 281–282
Siepler, John, 11–19
Small bowel, 126–127, 144, 233, 411–412
Sodium, 86–89, 94, 106–108
Soluble fibers, 382–383
Somatostatin, 95
Sorbitol, 162, 163, 164–165
Starvation, 14, 113–114, 126, 367, 372. *See also* Hypocaloric feeding
Steroids, 260
Stress response, 11–19. *See also* Acute phase response; Hypermetabolism
- anabolic agents, 347–348
- carbohydrate metabolism in, 15–16
- described, 11–13, 176
- fluid and electrolytes in, 17
- hypercatabolism in, 245–246
- lipid metabolism in, 16–17
- mediators, 13–14
- nutrient alterations during, 14–15, 262
- protein metabolism in, 15
- vitamins and minerals in, 17

Stroke, 182
Subjective global assessment, 6, 26, 342–343
Supplemental oxygen, 104, 105
Supraphysiologic supplementation, 72–74
Surgery. *See also* Organ transplants; Perioperative enteral nutrition; Postoperative patients
- enteral feeding after, 365
- nutritional support in, 122–123, 365–366, 371
- postoperative morbidity, 384
- surgically placed enteral access, 146–149
- surgical tube placement in obese patients, 332–333

Sweat, 81
Synbiotics, 381, 382
Systemic inflammatory response syndrome. *See* Acute phase response
Szeszycki, Elaina, 407–416

T

Tea, 407–408
Testosterone, 252–253, 351
Theophylline, 169
Thiamine, 114, 224
Tolerated upper intake, 63–67, 68–70
Torso trauma. *See* Abdominal trauma
Total parenteral nutrition. *See also* Parenteral nutrition
- antibiotics and, 154
- ASPEN guidelines for, 47
- cost of, 402–404, 405
- in diabetes, 178, 180
- drug-nutrient interactions, 154–156
- for ex vivo biopharmaceutical inactivations, 154–156
- in hepatic failure, 200, 201
- insulin for diabetics, 205–206
- iodide supplementation and, 74

pros and cons, 194–195
trace elements in, 62, 71
Trace elements. *See also* Minerals; *specific minerals*
assessing status of, 68–70, 71
biochemistry and physiology, 68–70
deficiencies, 62, 68–70, 71
for infants and children, 317
for pregnancy, 291–292, 294
for respiratory failure, 193–194
toxicity, 68–70
Transplant patients. *See* Organ transplants
Trauma patients, 229–244. *See also* Burn trauma
abdominal trauma, 120–122, 140
case study, 241–242
comorbid disease assessment, 237–238
complications, 240–241, 384
controversies, 241
head injuries, 122
immune enhancing diets for, 231–233, 234, 361
multiple organ failure, 229, 230, 279, 392–394
nutritional assessment, 21, 22
nutritional support, 120–122, 230–231, 233–237, 238–240
renal failure in, 239–240
Trendelenburg positioning, 132
Tube feeding. *See also* Jejunal feeding; Nasoenteric nutritional access
alternate feeding technology, 143
complications, 148–149, 201
contraindications for, 139
drug absorption and, 161
dual lumen single tube, 252
G-tube placement, 146, 147
interruptions in, 72
irrigation, 157
nasoduodenal, 140
nasoenteric, 139–141, 263, 336–337
nasogastric, 140, 280, 293, 305, 336
obstructions in, 157, 160, 161
percutaneous endoscopic gastrostomy, 143–144, 263–264, 280, 293, 337
postpyloric feeding tube placement, 411–412
push & pull techniques, 144
Tumor-necrosis factor, 13, 14, 222
Tunneled catheters, 132, 134

U

Ultrasound, 132, 134, 141
Underfeeding. *See* Hypocaloric feeding
United Network of Organ Sharing (UNOS), 341
U.S. National Academy of Sciences, 61
U.S. Public Health Service, 291
U.S. Summit on Immune-Enhancing Enteral Therapy, 362
Urine
drugs eliminated through, 169
fluid losses and, 81
nitrogen excretion and, 261
output, 83–84, 113
pH of, 169, 170

V

Valproic Acid, 168–169
Vanek, Vincent, 79–100, 101–109
Vegetables, 368–369, 383, 384
Vender, John, 259–267
Venous cannulation techniques, 133–134
Venous thrombosis, 384, 385
Ventilator support, 104, 189, 190–191, 192
Veterans Affairs Cooperative Study, 403
Vitamin A
in burn trauma, 250
in critical illness, 54
deficiency, 23, 63
in renal insufficiency, 75
for respiratory failure, 193
toxicity, 63, 75
Vitamin C
in burn trauma, 250
in critical illness, 55
deficiency, 23–24, 66
for respiratory failure, 193
toxicity, 66
Vitamin cocktails, 55–56
Vitamin D, 63
Vitamin E
in burn trauma, 250
in critical illness, 55
deficiency, 64
drug-nutrient interactions, 168
for respiratory failure, 193
toxicity, 64
Vitamin K
in critical illness, 55
deficiency, 23, 64
drug-nutrient interactions, 168
toxicity, 64
in warfarin therapy, 75–76
Vitamins, 61–77. *See also* Drug-nutrient interactions; Micronutrients; *specific vitamins*
deficiencies, 22, 23–24, 64–67
fat-soluble, 55, 62, 63–64
for infants and children, 315, 316
for pregnancy, 291
recommended requirements, 17, 294, 350–351
for renal failure, 213
for respiratory failure, 193
water-soluble, 62, 64–67

W

Warfarin, 75–76, 168
Water-soluble vitamins, 62, 64–67
Weight. *See* Body weight
Weight loss. *See also* Starvation
assessing, 25
in cancer patients, 338
cardiac cachexia and, 222
in HIV patients, 6
in malnutrition, 3
in nutritional assessment, 177
refeeding syndrome and, 113, 114
respiratory disease and, 4
Wernicke's encephalopathy, 114
Witzel jejunostomy, 148
World Health Organization, 357

X, Y, Z

Ziegler, Thomas, 407–416
Zinc
in burn trauma, 250, 251
deficiency, 23, 24, 70, 73, 74
in head injuries, 262
needs in pregnancy, 291–292
toxicity, 54, 70

Appendix

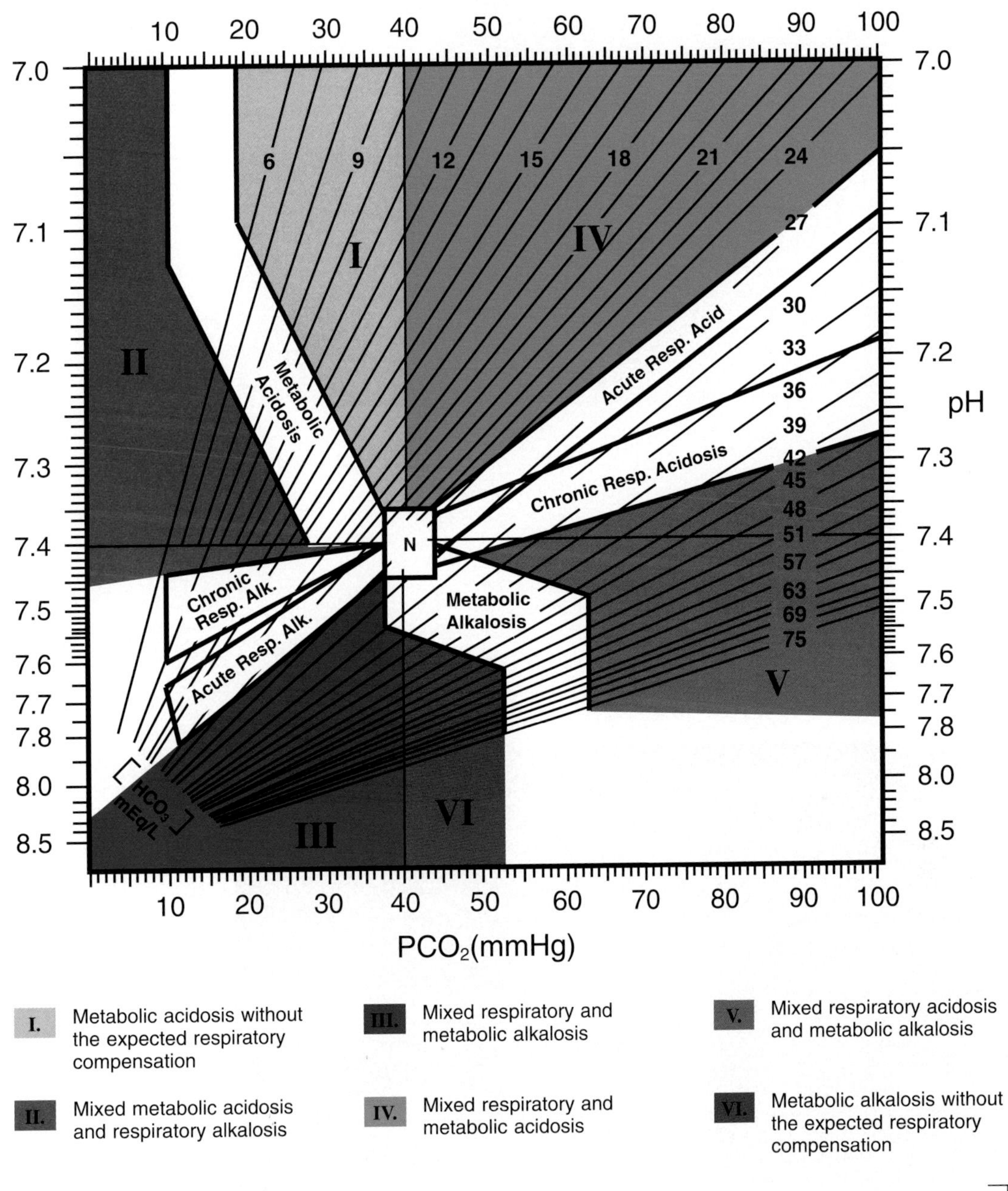

+Mixed disturbance

Figure 9.2

A nomogram, such as the Acid-Base Card shown here, can be used to determine which type of acid-base abnormality is present. It comes with a transparency with horizontal and vertical crosshairs. The vertical cross hair is lined up on the patient's pCO2 and the horizontal crosshair is lined up on the patient's pH. The section of the nomogram where the two cross hairs intersect represents the acird-base abnormality in that patient. These Acid-Base Cards can be purchased by writing to Acid-Base Cards, Pulmonary & Critical Care Medicine, Box 26901 WP 1310, University of Oklahoma Health Sciences Center, Oklahoma City, OK, 73190. Acid-Base Card was copied with permission from the Pulmonary & Critical Care Medicine Department.

Map adapted from M.S. Goldberg, et al. JAMA 223:269, 1973. Acid-base card prepared by B.E. Pennock, Ph.D. © 1978.

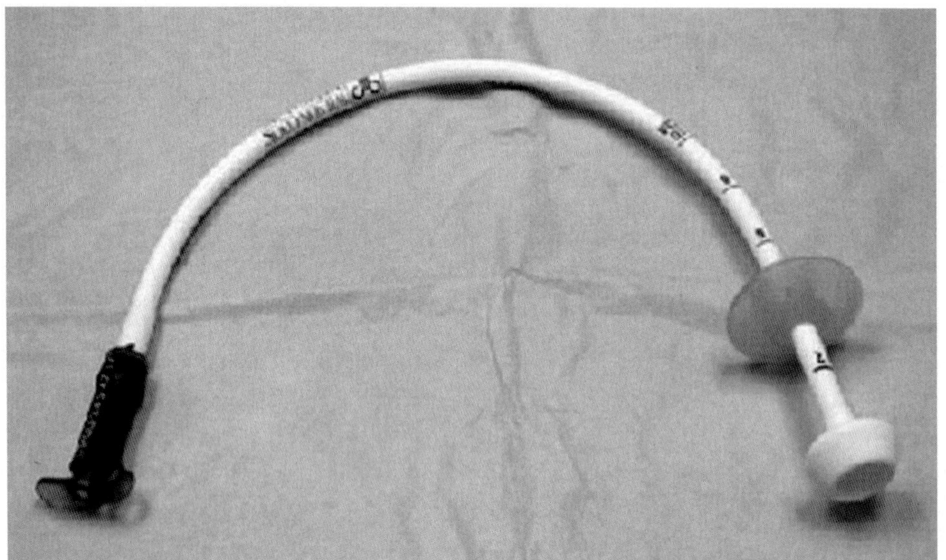

Figure 13.1a

PEG with Attached Bolus Adaptor

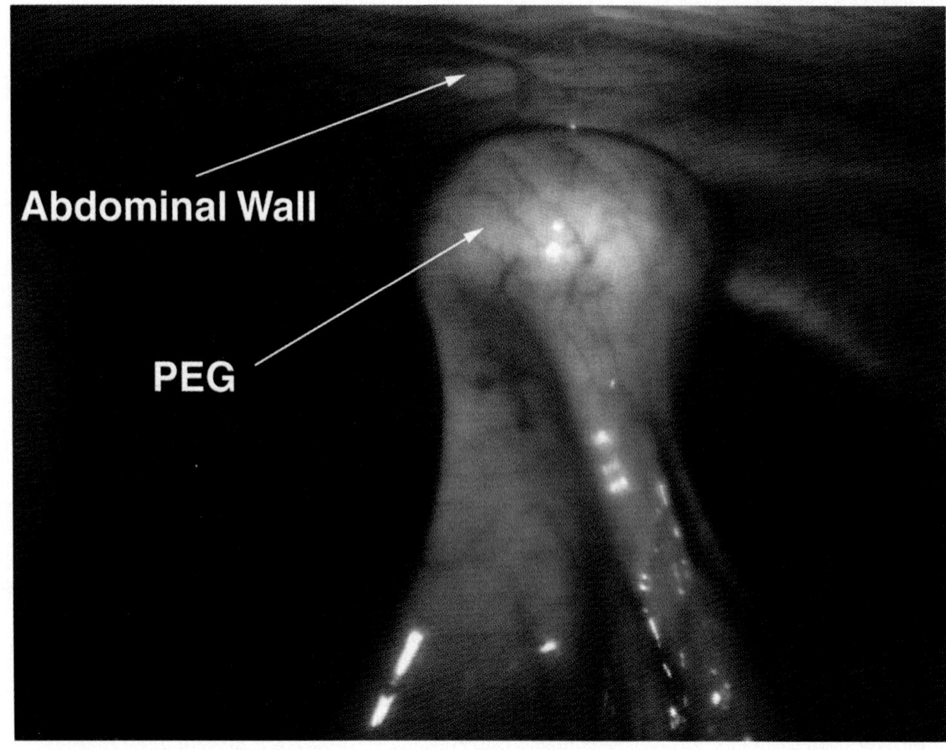

Figure 13.1b

PEG Placement Intra Abdominal View

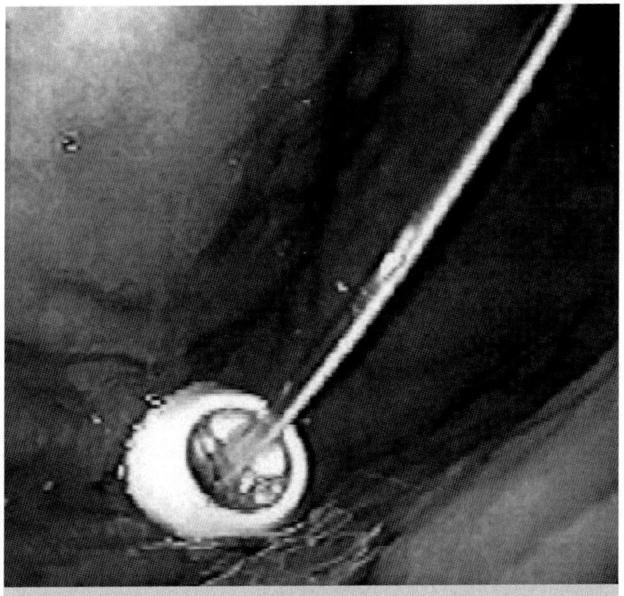

Figure 13.2

Jejunal tube with no looping exiting PEG on the way to the outside of patient

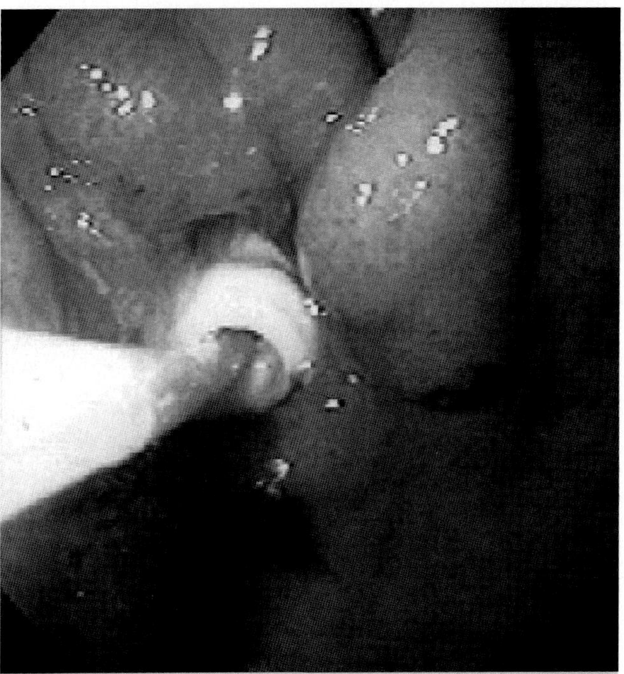

Figure 13.3

Alligator Forceps Being Passed Up through PEG to the Outside of Patient

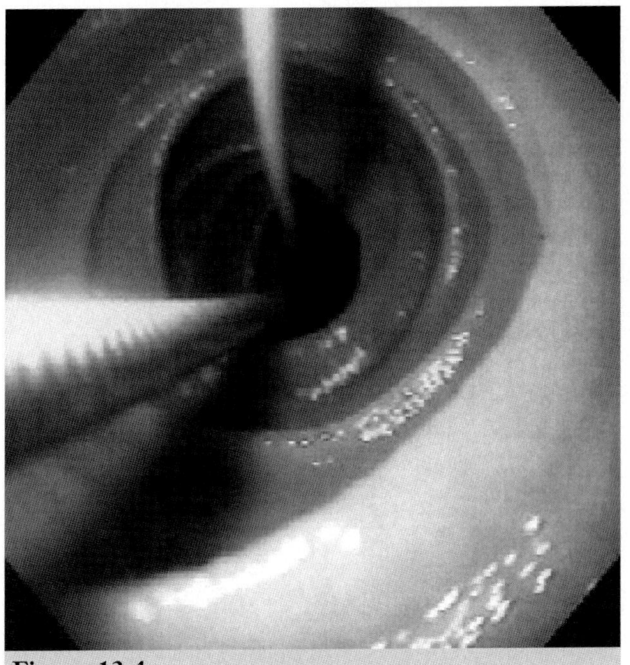

Figure 13.4

Guide Wire Being Dragged Down into Small Intestine

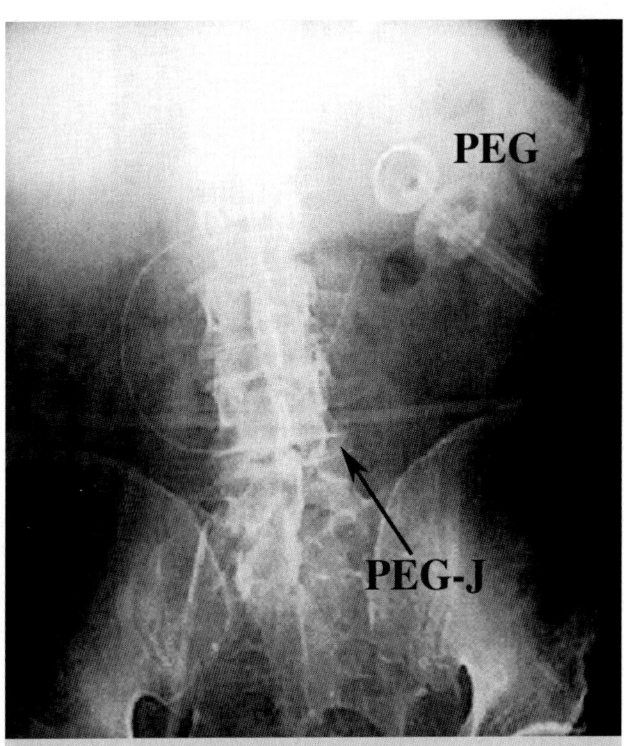

Figure 13.5

Radiograph of a Properly Placed PEG/J

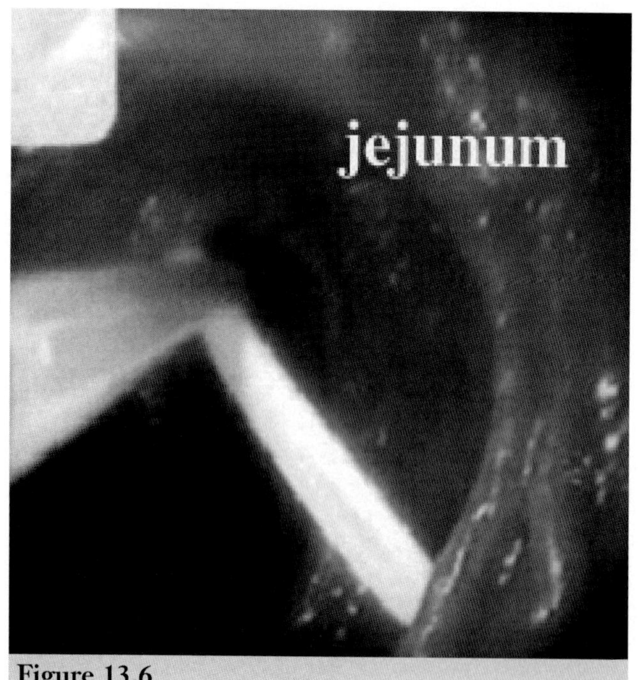

Figure 13.6

Needle Catheter Device Entering the Small Bowel Lumen

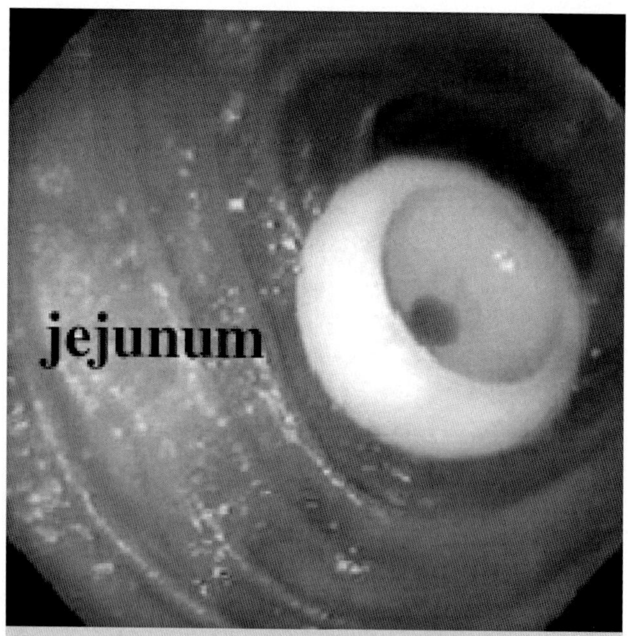

Figure 13.7

PEG Tube Internal Bolster in the Small Lumen after Successful Placement

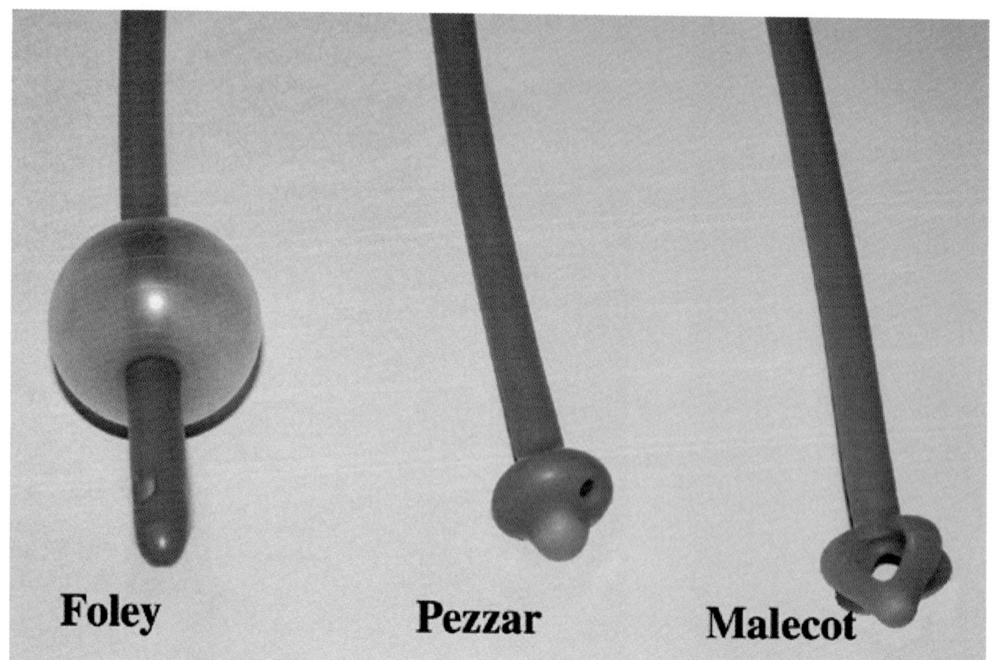

Figure 13.8

Feeding Tubes Used to Create Surgical Gastrostomy

Figure 13.9

Creation of Laparoscopically Placed G-tube

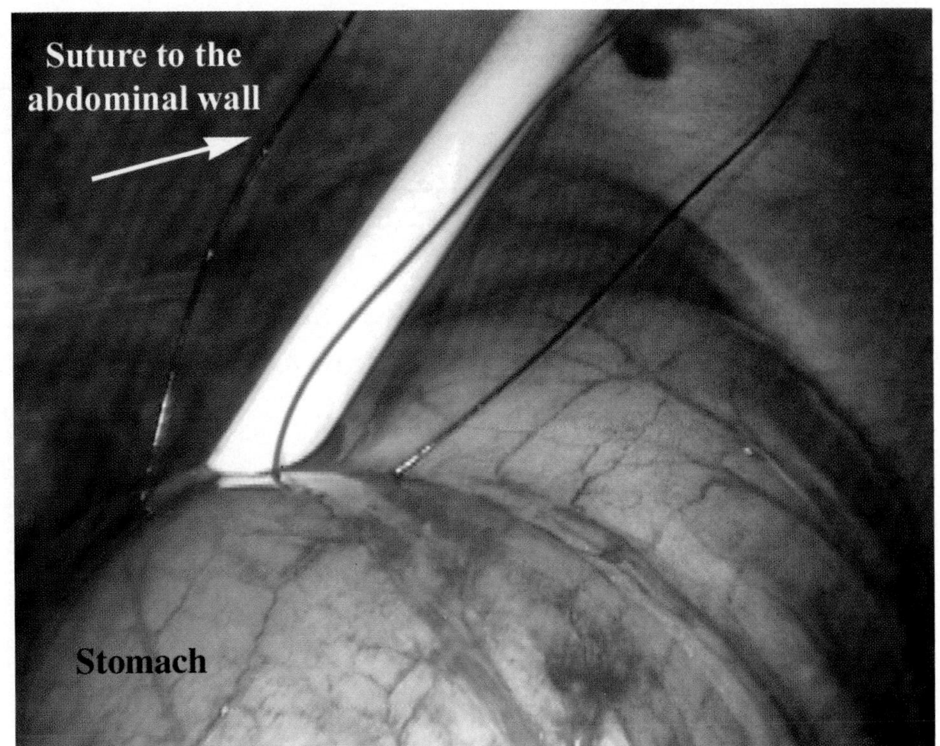

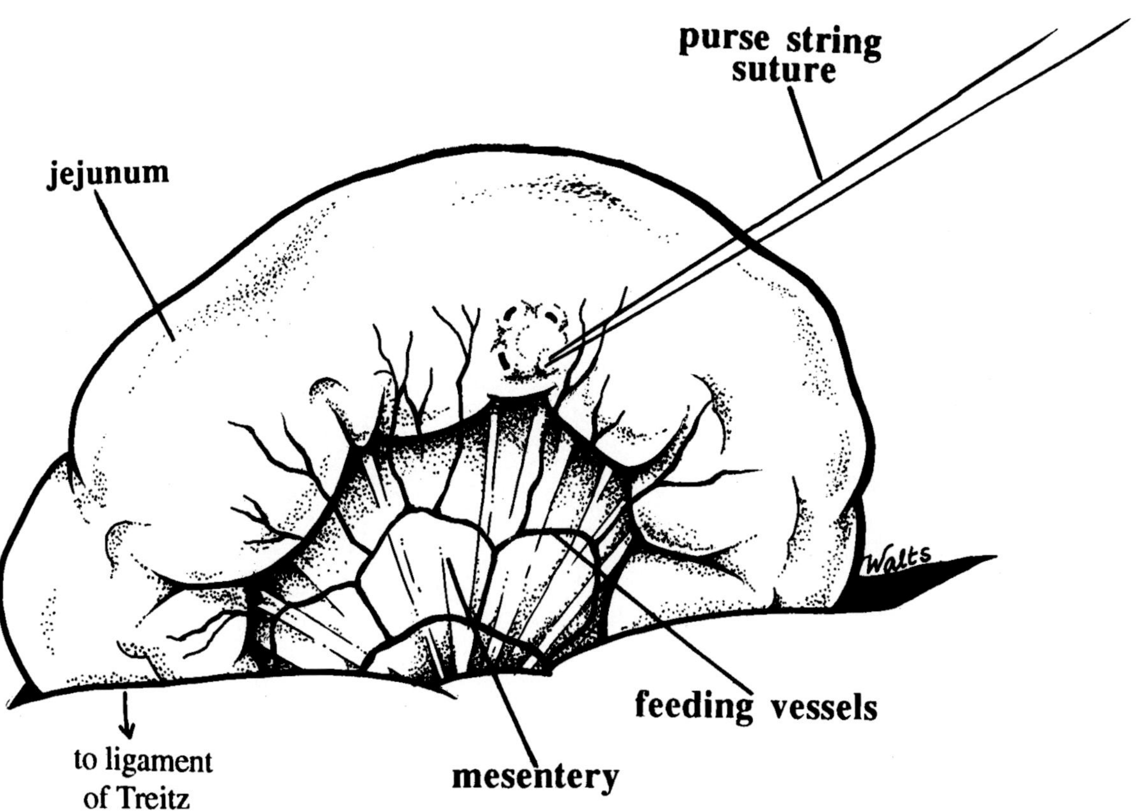

Figure 13.10a

Creation of Transverse Witzel Feeding Jejunostomy

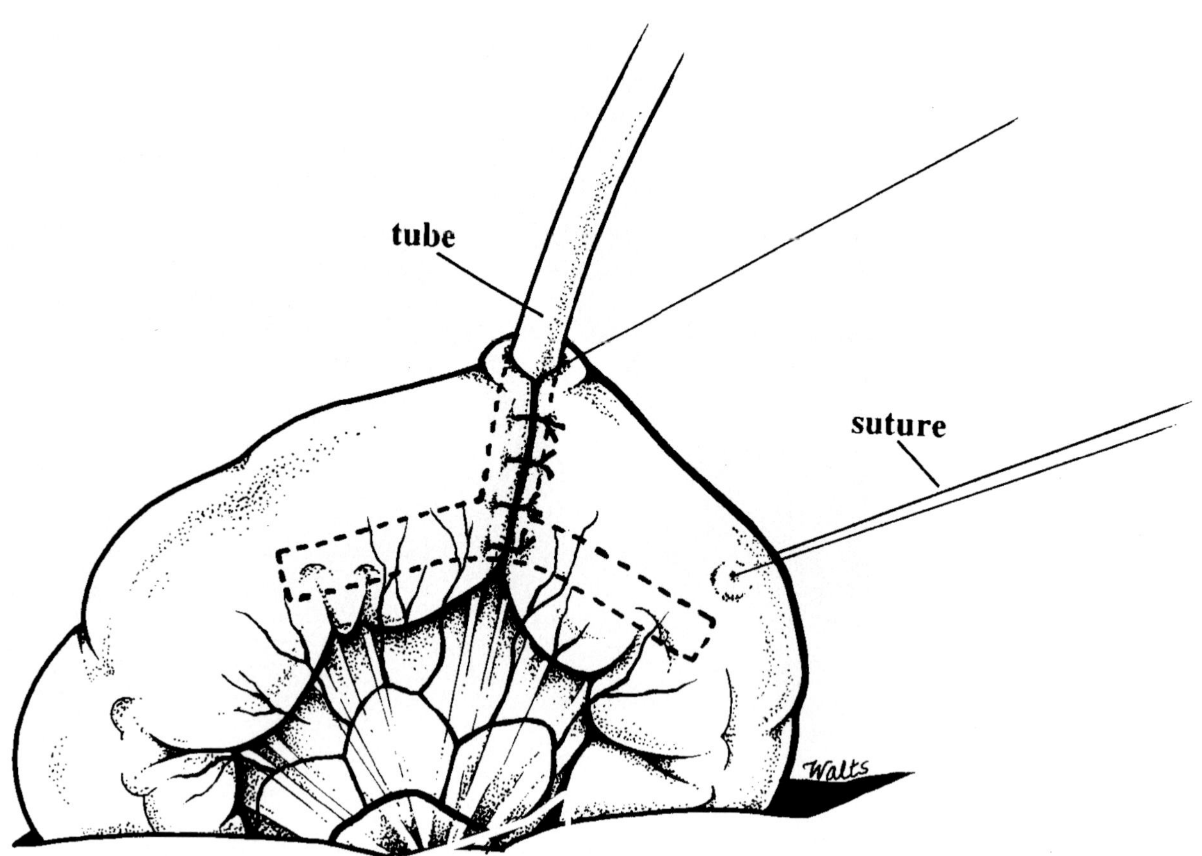

Figure 13.10b

Creation of Transverse Witzel Feeding Jejunostomy

Recommended Requirements for CD-ROM Use

Macintosh

200 MHz PowerPC or faster recommended
Mac OS 8.1 or later
64 MB of RAM
Monitor capable of displaying thousands of colors
6X or faster CD-ROM drive

Windows

Windows 95 or above
200 MHz Pentium or faster recommended
64 MB of RAM
Monitor capable of displaying thousands of colors
6X or faster CD-ROM drive